The Immunology of Horses and Donkeys

The Immunology of Horses and Donkeys

Ian R. Tizard

Distinguished Professor Emeritus, Texas A & M University, College Station, TX, United States

ELSEVIER

ACADEMIC PRESS

An imprint of Elsevier

Academic Press is an imprint of Elsevier
125 London Wall, London EC2Y 5AS, United Kingdom
50 Hampshire Street, 5th Floor, Cambridge, MA 02139, United States

ISBN: 978-0-443-44863-8

For information on all Academic Press publications visit our website at https://www.elsevier.com/books-and-journals

Publisher: Andre Wolff
Acquisitions Editor: Wendi Baker
Editorial Project Manager: Soumya Yadav
Production Project Manager: Omer Mukthar
Cover Designer: Mark Rogers

Typeset by TNQ Tech

To Fiona

Contents

Preface

The role of this book is to integrate the foundational research on the immune system of the equids, specifically horses (*Equus caballus*) and donkeys (*Equus asinus*). These are two closely related species that have contributed immeasurably to the development of human society over millennia. They have generally been lumped together when their infectious diseases and immunity have been investigated. Nevertheless, the fossil and molecular records indicate that the two ancestral equids separated about two million years ago. Two million years make a difference, and it must not be assumed that their immune systems are identical. Donkeys are not simply ponies with long ears and shaggy coats. As the reader will find, there are numerous subtle differences between the two. Unfortunately, relative to the horse, immunologists have been derelict in their duties concerning donkeys. There are about the same number of donkeys in the world as horses. They are a critically important means of transport in much of the world. Nevertheless, the resources available for horse research vastly exceed those for donkeys. The amount of basic data available on their immunology for these two species matches this allocation of resources. I hope that this book will encourage immunologists to take a closer look at the donkey.

This text is focused on the biology of the immune system in these two equids. It is not a clinical text, and it generally avoids extensive discussions on disease diagnosis and treatment. There are other excellent texts available for that purpose. The goal of this text is to provide an integration and synthesis of the basic biology of the subject for these specific species. This integration is not possible to the same extent with review articles or individual papers. In fact, I have been struck by the nature of much of the immunological research conducted on horses. Reflecting the sources of research support, while applied and clinical research studies are plentiful, there are many frustrating gaps in our knowledge of the basic features of the equine immune system. For example, how much IgD do they have? Is it expressed? Horses are not, obviously, the easiest or cheapest research animals to work with, especially when compared to laboratory rodents. As a result, the research studies performed reflect, not unreasonably, the interests of their sponsors.

Two areas in which equine immunological studies have excelled are cancer therapy and the effects of exercise. The emphasis on the former reflects the intrinsic value of horses, the fact that many live to a ripe old age, and the importance of treating individual beloved animals. The latter reflects the current role of horses in Western societies, namely, competition and recreation. This has been studied in depth and revealed many fascinating connections between physical stress, training, extreme exercise, and immune system functionality.

Some of the gaps in our knowledge of basic horse immunology reflect the recent rapid advances in other areas of basic immunology, and the fact that horse studies have lagged somewhat. Fortunately, the equine genome has been mapped. This has proved to be an invaluable resource, especially in confirming that important proteins described in the immune systems of laboratory rodents and humans are also present and functional in horses and donkeys.

A word of caution.

Recent developments in the world of scientific publishing, such as the rise of predatory journals, have resulted in an increase in the production of fraudulent papers. The rise of artificial intelligence has also resulted in the production of fabricated scientific papers. I have not knowingly encountered any such papers while writing this text, but should you, the reader, come across data and statements that you know to be incorrect or fabricated, please do not hesitate to let me know. There are obvious gaps in our knowledge of equine immunology that need to be filled, but not by scientific fraud.

Ian Tizard
College Station, Texas
itizard@cvm.tamu.edu
September 2024

Acknowledgments

As always, a book such as this could not be written without the support of colleagues and family. I am especially grateful to the Department of Veterinary Pathobiology at Texas A&M University for providing me with an office with easy access to the current literature, free coffee, and a photocopier! I would especially like to thank my colleagues, Drs. Brian Porter, Mark Johnson, and Leslie Easterwood, for providing excellent photographs of normal and diseased horses and their tissues.

I would also like to acknowledge the professionalism and assistance provided by the staff of Academic Press. Especially my editor, Ms. Wendi Baker.

Finally, of course, I must thank my wife Claire for her continuing encouragement and support, without which none of this would be possible.

Ian Tizard
College Station, Texas
September 2025

CHAPTER

The evolution and domestication of horses and donkeys

1

Perissodactyls are hindgut fermenting herbivores that constitute one of the two groups of ungulates that walk on their toes. The perissodactyls have an odd number of toes that range from one in horses to three in rhinoceroses. This is distinctly different from the even-toed artiodactyls, such as cattle and pigs that walk on two or four toes. Perissodactyls are completely terrestrial and herbivorous. They gather their food through their mouth since their feet have no grasping ability. This emphasis on limb structure is a result of their adaptation to rapid movement, especially flight from predators. Thus, equids are agile and can run very fast. In the case of the horse, their ability to travel fast while, at the same time, tolerating a human riding on their back was a prime reason for their domestication. Donkeys, however, were domesticated because they could carry other heavy burdens on their backs.

The origins of the Equidae

The Perissodactyls diverged from the other mammalian orders in the great radiation that followed the K–P event and the extinction of the dinosaurs around 65 million years ago (mya). The first equids appeared about 10 million years later during the lower Paleocene in Laurasia (modern North America and Asia). The rich fossil record and their wide distribution have resulted in the Equids being classic exemplars of macroevolution. The earliest recognized ancestor of the domestic horse, Eohippus, appeared in the early Eocene, around 52 mya. It is well represented among North American fossils. Eohippus was dog-sized and probably a browser. It had three toes on each foot. As the equine ancestors evolved, however, the fossil record shows increasing reliance on the single central digit and the development of enlarged hoofs. They also became grazers. While initially small and slow, as the equids evolved, they grew progressively larger and faster. The perissodactyls appear to have been the dominant herbivores across what is now Eurasia and North America, and the fossil record shows an incredible variety of extinct forms. They thrived during the Eocene about 38 million years ago, when climate change resulted in the massive expansion of grasslands. At that time, they were probably the most abundant herbivores in Laurasia. However, while they prospered for a time, they were eventually outcompeted by the more efficient ruminants. In the late Eocene and early Oligocene, about 35–30 mya, many failed to adapt to climate change that involved

The Immunology of Horses and Donkeys. https://doi.org/10.1016/B978-0-443-44863-8.00015-6

the world becoming the cooler and drier. Some subsequently migrated to Africa during the Miocene, eventually giving rise to modern rhinos and zebras (the Ceratomorpha and Equidae).

The equids continued to flourish during the Miocene, between 23 and 5 million years ago. They appear to have been most successful in North America. During the early Miocene, they underwent massive radiation and explosive diversification. By the end of the Miocene and the beginning of the Pleistocene, about 5 mya, they were highly diverse.

Over the past 65 million years however, the Earth's climate has repeatedly changed. One reason for this has been (until recently) a progressive decline in atmospheric CO_2 levels. This has resulted in "CO_2 starvation," which affected many plant populations. There are two major photosynthesis pathways, termed C_3 and C_4. Plants that use the C_4 photosynthetic pathway are more efficient users of CO_2 and were thus better able to adapt to this change than plants that use the C_3 pathway.

During the late Miocene epoch, 11.6–5.3 mya, there was a progressive change in the world's climate. Instead of the previous hot, moist conditions, there was a trend toward decreased rainfall. This was a result of global cooling and the decreased ability of cold air to hold moisture. As a result, a "tipping point" was reached about 8–5 million years ago. At that time, C_3 plants declined and C_4 plants gained such an advantage that, within a relatively short time, they came to dominate many terrestrial ecosystems. Sixty percent of C_4 species are grasses (Edwards et al., 2010). As a result, forests fragmented and retreated; subtropical grasses and sedges came to dominate, and savannah grasslands and open woodlands expanded massively at the expense of forest ecosystems. Consequently, between 8 and 5 mya, there was a major expansion of these grasslands, and the equids evolved with them. The grasses that thrived could withstand drought and assimilate CO_2 more efficiently than their predecessors. (CO_2 also levels dropped during the late Miocene.) Grasses that preferentially use a C_4 photosynthesis pathway rather than the previous C_3 pathway could thrive in a climate with lower levels of CO_2 and higher levels of sunlight (Edwards et al., 2010). This expansion of grasslands was associated with the coevolution and expansion of some grazing herbivores. Not all grazers could eat and digest the newly abundant, tough, silica-rich grasses, and many large herbivores went extinct. However, horses prospered, as did ruminants (Cerling et al., 1998). The ancestral carnivores also adapted to these changes and followed the herbivores onto the grasslands. Some herbivores, in response, evolved defensive horns and antlers, whereas others acquired the ability to escape by running at a very high speed (Edwards et al., 2010).

The structure of grass leaves helps them reduce water loss and survive in dry environments. However, grass leaves are much tougher and richer in silica than leaves from bushes and shrubs. As a result, they are harder to break off, chew, and digest. These changes meant that browsing mammals were also obliged to adapt in order to effectively exploit these new resources. Among those that exploited it most successfully were the evolving ruminants and horses (Cerling et al., 1998). Ruminants used their foregut to develop fermentation chambers such as the rumen. Horses, in contrast, became hindgut fermenters with a very large cecum and colon. Grass is a challenging diet. It is very tough and difficult to chew into small fragments. Eating tough herbage requires tough teeth, such as molars and premolars (Hypsodont teeth) that can withstand constant grinding; it requires the presence of an intestinal microbiota that produces cellulases that can break down the plant fibers. Mammals are unable to break the beta [1–4] glycoside bonds in cellulose since they lack the enzyme cellulase. The gastrointestinal bacteria can however, hydrolyze cellulose, hemicellulose, pectins, starch, and plant proteins. They generate fatty acids in addition to carbon dioxide and methane. This requires the development of large fermentation chambers such as the rumen or cecum, where microbial fermentation can take place and the cellulose broken down. These bacteria can effectively consume about 10% of the carbon, 80% of the nitrogen, and 60% of the dietary phosphorus. The remainder is available for the animal's own use.

Foregut fermentation in the rumen that allows the food bolus to be repeatedly chewed and exposed to the microbiota is very efficient at extracting plant energy, especially when compared with hindgut fermenters such as horses and related perissodactyls. As a result, wild horses spend up to 70% of their time feeding by nibbling on grasses and consuming small pieces of forage.

The products of this fermentation, the volatile fatty acids, provide much of the animal's caloric needs. In addition, the bacterial proteins provide much of their protein needs. Rumens are much more effective at this process than caeca since they release these nutrients before their passage through the small intestine. As a result of this increased efficiency, ruminants have been more successful than hindgut fermenters such as the perissodactyls. This is reflected in the relatively small number of modern perissodactyl species when compared with the ruminants.

The modern Equidae are a relatively small family consisting of horses, asses, and zebras. Based upon an analysis of the genome of a horse found in the permafrost at Thistle Creek in the Yukon, it has been estimated that the most recent common ancestor of the equids, both non-caballine (zebras and asses) and caballine equids (domestic and wild horses), emerged between 4.0 and 4.5 mya (Jonsson et al., 2014). The Thistle Creek horse has been dated at 700,000 years before the present. Its DNA also provides evidence for continuous selection of the immune system and olfaction throughout equine evolution (Orlando et al., 2013).

The Old World was likely colonized several times by equids from North America. The first wave occurred about ~2.6 mya. However, about 900,000 years ago, there was a second wave. A massive migration consisting of the true horses and ancestral equids spread from North America across the Bering land bridge into Eurasia. They thrived there. However, by the late Pleistocene and the early Holocene, during the last Glacial maximum, there was another cycle of rapid extinction, especially in the Americas. As a result, many large mammals, including the perissodactyl populations of North America, such as the rhinoceroses and three-toed horses, eventually died out. Their extinction was largely a result of climate change. The grasses in the tundra were replaced by unpalatable shrubs. In addition, their first interactions with the newly arrived humans almost certainly involved horses being hunted for food. Butchered horse bones have been identified at Paleolithic-era sites. For example, bones from a horse species, *E. occidentalis*, have been found in large numbers in the La Brea tar pits in California. This horse was short and stocky and somewhat resembled modern zebras. Their final extinction in North America occurred about 11,700 years ago and has been attributed to rapid climate change in addition to hunting and overkill by the newly arrived humans from Asia. The remaining equid species persisted over a much-reduced range in Asia and Africa. The tapirs remained a jungle species, and some migrated to South America, where three species survive. The remaining wild perissodactyls are all endangered as a result of hunting and habitat destruction.

The extant equids

Perissodactyls are exclusively herbivores. Unlike the ruminants, they retained their single stomachs but became hindgut fermenters in order to exploit the nutritional properties of the carbohydrates in the grasses. In effect, therefore, food that has already passed through the intestine is stored and further digested in the cecum. Thus, ideally, it extracts every possible calorie before the residue is excreted.

Herbivores such as the horse are naturally prey to large carnivores such as wolves, large cats, and bears. Lacking horns, the horse relies on flight as its primary defensive mechanism. It must be capable of outrunning predators. If flight is not possible, it must resort to kicking and biting. Horses also need to be perceptive. If they are to evade predators, they must be able to detect them at a distance and respond promptly. Horses are easily "spooked." This must be accompanied by a rapid response time. Their young foals are also precocious, so that they too can escape predators as soon as possible after birth.

Equid diversity

The extant members of the Equidae consist of seven species belonging to the genus *Equus* (Fig. 1.1).

Thus, there are relatively few living equid species, and their modern distribution and range are fragmented. They occupy only a very small fraction of their prehistorical ranges (Librado & Orlando, 2021). The order Perissodactyla currently consists of two suborders. The suborders are the Hippomorpha (horses, donkeys, and zebras), and the Ceratomorpha (rhinoceroses and the tapirs). The most successful of these suborders is the Hippomorpha. Collectively, they include 17 species classified into three families: the Equidae, including horses, asses, and zebras; the Rhinocerotidae (rhinoceroses); and the Tapiridae (tapirs) (Kefena et al., 2012). The donkey and zebra clades emerged about 2 million years ago (mya) and subsequently diversified into multiple species (Musilova et al., 2013). The Equidae currently consists of a single genus, *Equus*, and this consists of three species of zebra, three species of wild ass, and the true horses (the Cabellines). The wild horse currently consists of two

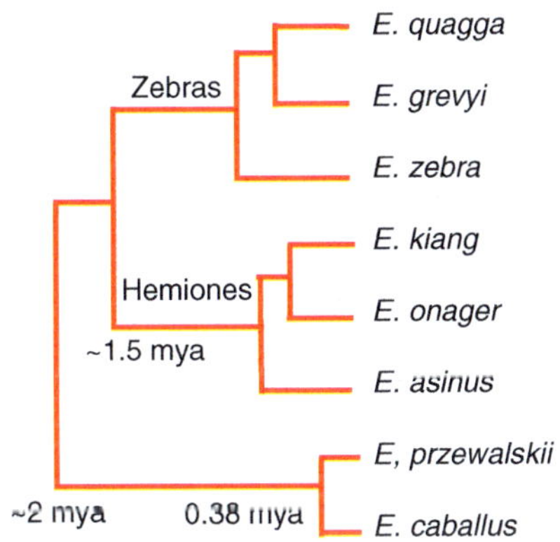

FIGURE 1.1 The phylogeny of the modern Equidae.

Note that the ancestral horse clade diverged about 2 million years ago and the donkey and zebra clades diverged about one and a half million years ago.

living subspecies: Przewalski's horse and the domestic horse. A third wild horse species, the Tarpan (*Equus ferus lenensis*), survived until 1909 but is now considered extinct.

Horse domestication

As pointed out above, the initial interactions between early humans and horses almost certainly involved hunting horses for their meat. Neanderthals are known to have hunted horses for food more than 500,000 years ago during the late Pleistocene period (Hutson et al., 2025; Taylor, 2025). While some horse populations died out, especially in North America, in other locations, they thrived. They did so, especially on the steppes of central Eurasia.

Horses are believed to have been domesticated at several different locations within the western Eurasian steppes around the end of the third millennium BCE. This was several thousand years after the domestication of cattle, sheep, goats, and pigs. Evidence also indicates that donkeys were domesticated significantly earlier in North Africa and the Middle East (Frantz, 2025). Genetic evidence and mitochondrial DNA analysis have indicated that domestic horses were derived from several different wild horse populations on multiple occasions over an extended time period. They appear to fall into six distinct clades. Thus, the taming and utilization of wild horse foals occurred repeatedly across this region.

Around 5500 years ago, the first domesticated horses were primarily used as a source of meat and milk. This was probably rapidly followed by the taming and subsequent riding of young horses (Frantz, 2025). Wild horses live in bands where they are dominated by some of their peers. Thus, a dominant hierarchy is readily established. Humans could also learn to establish their dominance over captive horses.

Once horseback riding was mastered, the advantages of the technique would have been obvious to everyone. It revolutionized transport and warfare. The subsequent development of reins, the saddle, and the stirrups would have greatly facilitated the process. The knowledge of horse domestication methods would have spread among the tribes, who would also have domesticated some of their local horses. This would have greatly facilitated livestock herding and permitted the diffusion of goods and ideas. It would also have dramatically altered people's sense of distance.

Domestic horses are very diverse concerning phenotypic differences such as size, color, and shape. However, they are all classified as a single species. *E. caballus*. Wild horses have been classically considered a single species, *E. ferus*, divided into two distinct subspecies. Of these, the Tarpan (*E. ferus lenensis* survived until the beginning of the 19th century in Ukraine. Przewalski's horse, *E. ferus przewalskii* survives in managed populations to the present day and originated in Mongolia. Genetic analysis has demonstrated that Przewalski's horses have made no contribution to the domestic horse gene pool (Kefena et al., 2012).

The earliest evidence for horse domestication comes from archeological studies on the Botai culture located in North–central Kazakhstan. Modern domestic horses are not the descendants of this earliest domestic horse lineage. This lineage (classified as DOM1) is associated with archeological evidence of human management in the form of corrals, bridling, and milking, dating to around 3000–3500 BCE. Evidence from the skulls and teeth of these animals suggests that they had worn some sort of bit. Sequencing of these DOM1 genomes has, however, shown that they cluster with Przewalski's horse and show very little affinity with modern horse breeds. These first domesticated horses did not persist and likely became feral. The earliest visual evidence of horseback riding dates to 2000–1500 BCE (Fig. 1.2).

Similarly, the ancient domestic horse remains from the Iberian Peninsula dated to 2000–3000 BCE have been sequenced and also shown to be members of a different lineage than modern horses (IBE). They appear to have made only a minimal contribution to the genome of DOM2 horses (Orlando, 2020).

However, it has proved possible to map other horse lineages accompanying domestication in ancient horse genomes. This points to Western Eurasian steppes as the site of origin of the modern horse. Specifically, the genetic evidence of horse domestication points to a population (classified as DOM2) originating in the Volga-Don region of Western Eurasia north of the Caucasus around 3500 years ago. Horses from this region expanded rapidly across Eurasia and replaced other local domestic populations. Thus, DOM2 horses moved westward and by 2200–2000 BCE could be found in Bohemia, in the Lower Danube region, and in central Anatolia. This spread occurred at the same time as the development of horse-associated material culture, especially the spread of spoke-wheeled chariots. These were often buried with the remains of rulers. The earliest chariot burial has been dated to about 2000 BCE on the Ural steppes. Recently, 2100-year-old graves have been excavated in Bulgaria, where warriors were buried with their horses in addition to valuable grave goods!

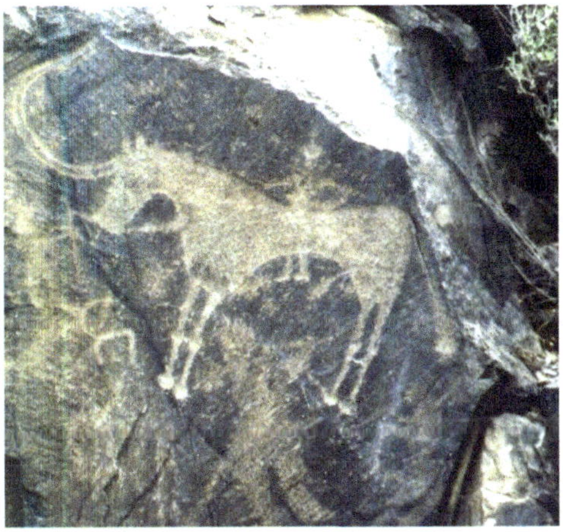

FIGURE 1.2 Stone horse etching.

An etching of a horse and rider on a rock at Tanbaly gorge, Kazakhstan. The figures at this World Heritage site are believed to have been drawn around 2000 BCE. These are some of the earliest images of horse domestication.

Analysis of the genomes of ancient, domesticated horses has also identified many genes that have undergone positive selection. (DNA can be extracted from skeletal remains at tissue sites such as the inner ear and the roots of teeth.) These modified genes largely involve muscular and limb development, joints, and the cardiovascular system. They also include a group of genes associated with social behavior, learning ability, and temperament. Unfortunately, modern horse genomes also contain multiple deleterious mutations as a result of current breeding practices (Schubert et al., 2014).

The development of equestrianism appears to have involved selection for genes such as *GSDMC* and *ZFPM1*. The *GSDMC* gene encodes gasdermin C, which is associated with chronic back pain. and lumbar spinal stenosis. The *ZFPM1* gene is located on chromosome ECA 3 and encodes a zinc finger protein that is associated with serotonergic neurons involved in mood regulation and aggressive behavior. A key variant of the *GSMDC* gene is associated with structural back changes and increased endurance (Liu et al., 2025). Within a few hundred years, the prevalence of this variant in domesticated horses went from 1% frequency to almost 100% as a result of artificial selection. Thus, the early selection of these genes suggests that these humans selected for docile, resilient horses well able to undergo endurance running and weight-bearing (Librado et al., 2021). It is clear, however, that there were multiple subsequent domestication events and even feralization of some breeds (Librado et al., 2021). Nevertheless, DOM2 horses eventually replaced all the other local domestic horse populations.

An alternative method of determining the origins of a species is by analysis of their mitochondrial genomes. Mitochondria are present in the cytoplasm of the ovum, and as a result, their genealogy reflects the maternal origins of the species. Thus, mitochondrial DNA studies in over 650 diverse horses have demonstrated that there were 93 different mitochondrial types grouped into 17 distinct clusters. Several of these clusters correspond to specific breeds or restricted geographical areas. Thus, cluster As2 is specific for Przewalski's horse. Cluster C1 is characteristic of Northern European ponies, while cluster D1 is restricted to Iberian and West African breeds. This analysis has indicated that the founding population of the domestic horse consisted of at least 77 different mares recruited from the wild. Because these 77 mares were genetically diverse, it suggests that they were derived from multiple different wild horse populations (Jansen et al., 2002).

Cultural issues

The domestication of the horse has been a long process. It has had profound and significant effects on the development of human civilizations. No other domestic animal has influenced social development, the spread of people, and the establishment of empires to the extent that horses have. By vastly increasing the speed of human travel, horses revolutionized the spread of human populations around the globe. It also revolutionized the speed of human communications. For example, the Pony Express delivered the results of the US Presidential election of 1860 to California newspapers within 8 days of them being announced on the East Coast. It is important to remember that before the development of railroads, humans could only travel long distances on land, either by walking or riding horses.

Burdens

On average, a horse can carry up to 30% of its own weight. However, as pointed out above, the ability of horses to carry loads and perform other functions depends in large part upon their specific conformation. Horses tasked with carrying heavy burdens have a very different conformation than those used primarily for racing or sport. Thus, a different type of horse was required to carry a man in armor rather than a conventionally dressed individual. Similarly, horses can pull more weight than they can carry, but this, too, depends upon the animal's conformation (and fitness). These large, heavy horses used for draft work are generally calm and docile and are classified as cold-blooded breeds (reflecting temperament rather than temperature). They mainly originated in Northern Europe.

Warfare

The domestication of the horse revolutionized warfare. While riding was the first trait selected for, it was soon followed by the development of chariots. The earliest known chariots have been excavated from burial sites associated with the Sintashta culture in Eurasia and dated to 1900 BCE. They employed light, spoked wheels that enabled them to move fast. Once invented, chariot use spread widely and rapidly. By 1600 BCE, it dominated warfare in Eurasia and the Middle East. By 1250 BCE, the use of chariots for warfare was commonplace and had extended across Eurasia from Greece to China. The great Asian empires of Genghis Khan could never have been achieved without horses. Horses changed the nature of warfare. Raids were more effective. Chariots and cavalry charges could be used to decimate enemies on foot. The trained, aggressive warhorse was one of the most potent weapons employed in Medieval warfare. Consider the "great" warriors such as Alexander the Great and Napoleon. Their conquests would not have been possible without cavalry. One of the most famous horses in antiquity was Bucephalus, the horse of Alexander the Great. When Bucephalus died, Alexander named the city of Bucephala after him! It is relevant to point out here that successful horse warfare required healthy horses. Outbreaks of infectious diseases such as glanders that killed large numbers of horses could make the difference between victory and defeat.

Horses had been extinct in the Americas for thousands of years until they were reintroduced by Columbus and his successors beginning in 1493. Many escaped and were readily integrated into Native American cultures, especially those living on the prairies of North America, so that by the mid-1700s, they had spread across the continent. These were local Iberian horses from southern Spain. They were first used on the West Indian Islands. They reached the Continent when Hernán Cortés, with 16 horses, invaded Mexico in 1519. Their numbers increased greatly as the Spaniards bred them in the Caribbean islands. Spanish soldiers on horseback massacred native American warriors when they fought in pitched battles.

These early introduced horses were relatively small animals, since they had to be transported by ship. Crossbreeding began in the early 19th century when larger European draft horses were introduced. Horses provided the only significant means of long-distance human transportation until railroads were built, and were absolutely required for handling cattle as large ranches developed. In effect, the North American beef industry was horse-dependent.

Hunting

Given the enormous increase in speed and range conferred on humans by horseback riding, it is unsurprising that they radically improved hunting successes. As in warfare, it was easier to kill one's prey if they could be effectively pursued and closely approached. An obvious example is the ability North American natives acquired to hunt and kill stampeding bison once they had mastered their newly introduced horses. At the other extreme, English foxhunting was so enjoyable that it was regarded as a sport (except by the fox)!

Sports

While horses were the most important mode of transport for thousands of years, they were inevitably replaced by motor vehicles once the internal combustion engine was invented. Nevertheless, they have been increasingly used for sports and recreation. More than 70% of the 6.9 million horses in the United States at present are involved in showing or recreation, including showjumping and racing. It has been estimated that 7.1 million Americans participate in the horse industry (Bailey & Binns, 1998).

Religion

The critical importance of horses to many early human societies is reflected in the fact that they were respected and often worshiped. They were recognized as playing a key role in warfare and were, in effect, considered indispensable. This, in turn, developed into an ideology so that the horse not only became a symbol of prestige but also a means of influencing sacred powers. They could be sacrificial animals or components of religious beliefs. Thus, as early as the Bronze Age, the horse was seen as divine. Horse figurines have been found in graves dating back to 4000 BCE in Central Asia. The spectacular Uffington White Horse in England dates from around 500 BCE. The Gods also needed horses! Gods such as Poseidon and Apollo were carried on chariots pulled by horses. (Alternatively, Poseidon's chariot could be pulled by horse-headed fish-like beasts called hippocampuses). It was useful if they also possessed wings, such as Pegasus. In the Hindu religion, Hayagriva, one of the avatars of the god Vishnu, has a human body and the head of a white horse. He is worshiped for his strength, knowledge, and wisdom.

It is also of interest to note that medieval Christianity condemned the eating of horsemeat (hippophagy), although the prohibition does not appear to have been rigidly enforced. Some societies enforced the ban, whereas others totally ignored it (Bartosiewicz & Gal, 2025). Even today, European societies differ in their taste for horse meat. There is no religious or moral prohibition, but horses are generally considered "pets" in much of Western society (Haspel, 2025).

Feral horses

When domestic horses are permitted to roam freely in the wild, they are considered feral. While originating as domesticated animals, their behavior reverts to that found in truly wild horses.

Feral horses are social animals that live in small herds or bands. These bands consist of one or more stallions, a group of mares, and their foals. The herd itself is generally led by a dominant, older, experienced mare. However, the stallion considers himself to be in overall control and serves as the herd's guardian. He considers the mares in the herd to be his harem. There is a steady turnover of stallions as they are constantly replaced by younger and fitter males. Colts may leave the natal herd to meet with others and form bachelor herds.

Important feral horse populations include those in Western North America. These populations are healthy and can double every 4 or 5 years. As a result, the US Bureau of Land Management is obliged to keep about 60,000 horses in holding facilities. While contraceptive vaccines are available (Chapter 15), it is often difficult to round-up widely dispersed herds (Haspel, 2025). Isolated, smaller pony populations occur on islands along the Atlantic coast, such as the Sable Island horse and the Chincoteague pony from Virginia and Maryland. Populations of small wild ponies also present in the British Isles including the Welsh pony, the Exmoor pony, the Fell pony from Cumbria and the Connemara pony from the West of Ireland. Many of these are not truly feral but are owned by their landowners.

Modern horse breeds

As described above, the genetics of the domestic horse have been significantly modified by human breeding practices. Many societies have, over the centuries, bred their horses from a limited number of selected stallions. As a result, diverse horse breeds have been developed for specific applications. Thus, very large, heavy draft horses such as the Clydesdale, Percheron, and Belgian horses were developed to move heavy loads (hence the term horsepower). As a result, they are relatively docile. Conversely, smaller, lighter breeds have been developed for riding and entertainment purposes. This requires speed and agility, and they are classified as hot-blooded breeds. Many originated in the Middle East and North Africa. Examples include Thoroughbred racehorses and Arabians. Breeds suitable for children's use, such as Exmoor and Shetland ponies, have been developed. Even smaller miniature horses around 40 inches in height or less have also been developed multiple times through aggressive selection of small ponies, especially the Shetland breed. Some miniature horse lines may be significantly inbred (Fig. 1.3).

This selective breeding can have significant adverse consequences for the species. For example, there has been a sharp decline in equine genetic diversity, especially over the past 2000 years (Orlando, 2020). The original DOM2 lineage has experienced severe diversity losses, especially in the Y chromosome. This loss of diversity reflects the use of a limited number of stallions. This started about 2000 years ago when the diversity was halved. It has continued to drop since then. In addition, overall genetic diversity has dropped significantly over the past 250 years. This decrease has also been accompanied by an increase in mutational load (Orlando, 2020).

The overall loss of equine genetic diversity, especially over the past 250 years, is exemplified by the Thoroughbred breed. The breed was developed in England when local mares were crossbred with three imported stallions - The Byerley Turk in the 1680s, the Darley Arabian in the 1700s, and the Godolphin Arabian around 1730. Other stallions also contributed to the development of the breed, but about 50% was derived from the Arabian bloodlines. The thoroughbred population is essentially closed. Analysis of microsatellite and pedigree information has demonstrated that the breed has a very narrow genetic base. Seventy-eight percent of alleles in the current population are derived from 30 founder animals. Of these, 27 were male! 10 founder females account for 72% of maternal lineages, while 28 maternal lineages account for 89% of the modern population. In addition, a single founder stallion, the

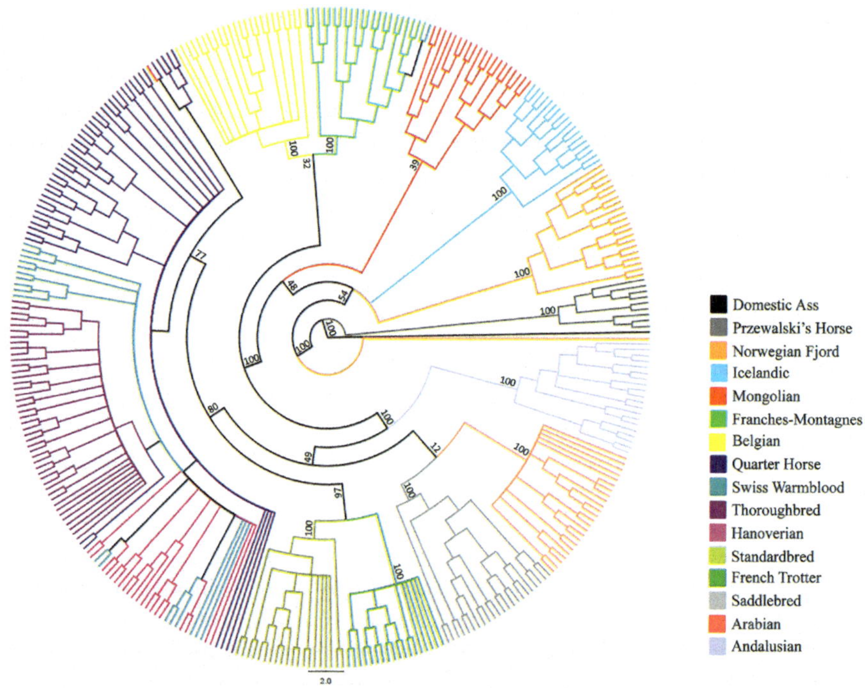

FIGURE 1.3 Phylogeny of domestic horse breeds.

Phylogenetic tree of domestic horse breeds and Przewalski's horse. Parsimony analysis across 46,244 autosomal loci in the Domestic and Przewalski's horse. The tree is rooted in the Domestic donkey.

- OPEN ACCESS SOURCE: Adapted from McCue ME, Bannasch DL, Petersen JL, Gurr J et al. A high density SNP array for the domestic horse and extant Perissodactyla: Utility for association mapping, genetic diversity, and phylogeny studies. PLOS Genetics, *8(1): e1002451. https://doi.org/10.1371/journal.pgen.1002451*

Darley Arabian, is responsible for 95% of paternal lineages (Cunningham et al., 2001). The breed is estimated to have 13% inbreeding. This has failed to improve racing performance in addition to significantly increasing foal mortality (Lawson et al., 2024). Similar recent inbreeding, depending upon the use of a single ancestral stallion, has also been detected in Clydesdales (Todd et al., 2023).

An even more extreme example of restricted equine genetic diversity has resulted from the growth of the horse cloning industry. This is accomplished by somatic cell nuclear transfer into a mare's oocytes and has been relatively successful. It has been employed to preserve and duplicate high-performing horses such as those engaged in polo. Some individual horses have been cloned multiple times. This is regarded as cheating by many, and the authorities have prohibited the use of gene-edited and cloned horses in the sport. Presumably, these horses have identical immune systems and equal susceptibility to infectious diseases (Kavanagh, 2025).

Donkeys

The last common ancestor of modern horses and donkeys lived about 2 million years ago when they diverged from their ancestral donkeys. The donkeys and zebras subsequently diverged around 1 mya (Jonsson et al., 2014). Like the horse, the domestication of the donkey radically transformed ancient societies. Donkeys have been traditionally used as beasts of burden. They can carry heavy loads over high-altitude, rough, and mountainous terrain and are sure-footed. However, with the mechanization of agriculture, their use has declined, especially in developed countries. Their number has been falling over the past 30 years as they are replaced by motor vehicles. They are primarily found in less developed societies, where they are used as draft animals. Their formal scientific name is *Equus africanus asinus*.

While the use of donkeys as pack animals has declined, in countries such as China, they have become an increasingly important source of meat (Wang et al., 2022). The global donkey population is estimated to be about 44 million, while there are estimated to be about 11 million mules (Barrandeguy & Carossino, 2018). It is estimated that there are 12 million donkeys in China alone. In addition to China, large populations of donkeys are found in Ethiopia (8 million), as well as in other regions of sub-Saharan Africa, the tropical Andes in South America, and Northern India.

Donkeys are primarily working animals used for transportation. However, their meat is considered very delicious, with large amounts of intramuscular fat deposits. There is also a high demand for ejaio, a traditional Chinese medicine and beauty product made from donkey skin gelatin. (The gelatin is mixed with herbs and other ingredients for use as medicines and cosmetics. The ejaio industry requires millions of donkey skins annually to keep up with the demand.) In addition, there is a growing market for donkey milk. It is claimed to be nutrient-rich and an effective substitute for human breast milk. As a result, donkey breeding is increasing in some societies. Donkeys are also an increasingly prized source of leather.

Donkeys, like horses, were first introduced into the Americas by Christopher Columbus when he arrived in Hispaniola in 1495. They were highly valued as pack animals and progressively spread across both North and South America. They were especially valued as sires for breeding to horse mares and so producing mules. Mules were in especially high demand during the gold rushes as well as for working in mines.

Wild donkeys

There are three living species of the wild ass. The African wild ass (*E. africanus*) and two Asian wild asses or hemionids that consist of the Onager (*E. hemiones onager*) and the Tibetan wild ass or Kiang (*E. kiang*) (Figs. 1.4 and 1.5).

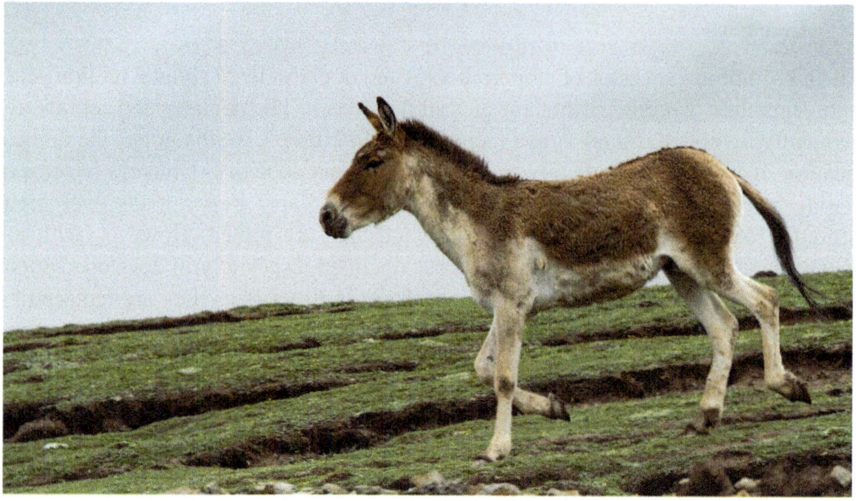

FIGURE 1.4 Tibetan Kiang.

A Tibetan Kiang (*Equus kiang*). Qumarlêb County, Yushu, Qinghai, China.

- Courtesy of Robert Tizard.

Hemiones are morphologically similar to Kiangs but are genetically distinct. There are multiple subspecies of Hemionids and Kiangs. The third groups of modern equids are the well-recognized species of zebras, confined to sub-Saharan Africa (Fig. 1.6).

The African wild ass consists of two subspecies, the Nubian wild asses (*E, africanus africanus)* and the Somali wild ass (*E. africanus somaliensis*). However, recent genetic studies have indicated that the Somali wild ass may, in fact, be

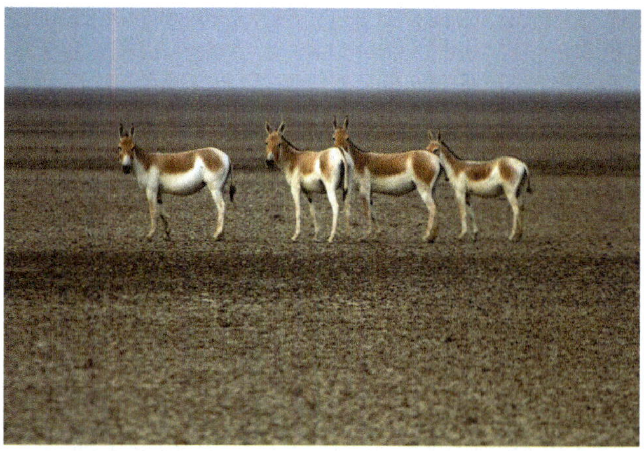

FIGURE 1.5 Asian wild asses.

Asian wild asses in the Rann of Kutch, India (*E.hemiones onager).*

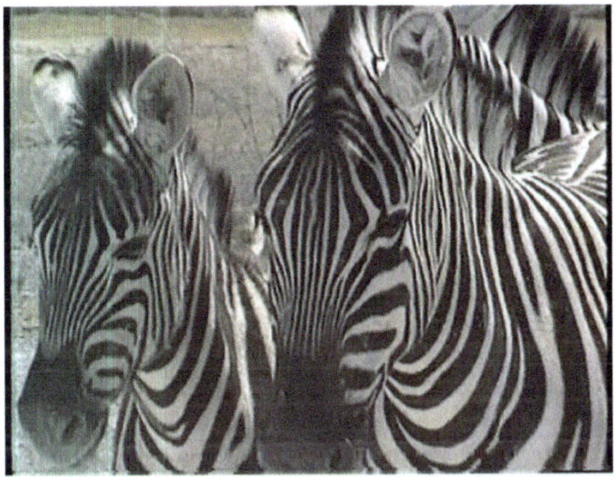

FIGURE 1.6 Plains zebras.

(Equus quagga burchellii), in Etosha National Park, Namibia.

- Courtesy of Fiona Tizard.

more closely related to the zebras than to the other wild asses. It appears to be a stripeless zebra! The complete mitochondrial genome of the donkey has been sequenced and compared with that of the horse (Xu et al., 1996). Both appear to be highly conserved, containing 37 genes, including 13 protein-encoding genes (Du et al., 2025). The donkey genome has also been completely assembled (Renaud et al., 2018).

Donkey domestication

The most recent genetic data suggests that the African Wild Ass was first domesticated and used for carrying heavy loads in the Horn of Africa (modern Eritrea) around 6000–5000 BCE. Phylogenetic analysis indicates that they were also domesticated in what is now Egypt around 5000 BCE, well before the domestication of the horses in Central Eurasia (Rossell et al., 2008). Donkey domestication was probably motivated by the drying of the climate following a humid period and a reduction in water availability across North Africa. Donkeys, however, could carry heavy loads for long distances across the arid landscape (Librado & Orlando, 2021).

Domestic donkeys cluster in two distinct mitochondrial clades, suggesting that there were two independent domestication events (Wang et al., 2022). Both were derived from African wild asses, although the original subspecies is unclear. One clade is clearly derived from the extinct Nubian wild ass that inhabited Northeast Sudan. The source of the second clade is probably the Somali wild ass. There is also evidence of hybridization by a third lineage that emerged in the Eastern Mediterranean area around 200 BCE. This likely contributed to the ancestry of the

Eurasian donkeys (Todd et al., 2022). Nevertheless, the Nubian wild ass appears to be the primary species of origin of Asian donkeys (Ahlawat et al., 2023).

The newly domesticated donkeys were subsequently traded to the West and North, soon reaching what are now Egypt and the Arabian Peninsula (Todd et al., 2022). Donkeys proved so useful that they rapidly expanded out of Africa into Eurasia.

Archaeological remains of 10 small-bodied donkeys have been found in Egypt, dated to 4000–3000 BCE, and have been considered to reflect domestication (Rossel et al., 2008). Thus, skeletal data from ~3400 BCE discovered in Abydos, in middle Egypt, exhibit osteopathologies consistent with confinement and prolonged heavy load bearing. (Compression of the spinal vertebrae, spondylosis, and osteophyte formation in addition to spavin). Thus, the first evidence of equids pulling carts dates from the Nile valley around 3000 BCE (Taylor, 2025). Their size was midway between that of wild asses and modern donkeys, and they presumably pulled light carts. The fact that they were deliberately buried also suggests that these animals were highly valued. Similarly, wall carvings in Abydos depicting walking cattle, sheep, and donkeys have also been interpreted as evidence of domestication. Genetic analysis supports this location insofar as modern donkeys are more closely related to the African wild ass than to the Asian species. Unlike the horse, genomic data indicate very limited introgression from wild asses.

An intact donkey skeleton dated to 4350–3950 years ago has been excavated from a site in Shaanxi Province in Central China. The skeleton also showed evidence of domestication. Nevertheless, analysis of Chinese domestic donkey genomes has indicated that they are also descended from the African wild ass rather than from local wild equids.

Donkeys, like horses, were also selectively bred, and the production of horse-donkey hybrids and mules appears to have occurred since the earliest times. For example, the Romans bred donkeys so that they could produce improved mules that were employed both for economic and military purposes. Roman mules were relatively large and strong (Box 1.1). Mules, like horses, were used to support human

Box 1.1 Horse-donkey hybrids

Horses and donkeys are sufficiently closely related that both domesticated species have been successfully interbred since earliest times. The mule is the offspring of a horse mare with a donkey stallion, while a hinny is the offspring of a donkey mare and a horse stallion. In both cases, the hybrids are normally sterile. This is because horses have 64 chromosomes while donkeys have 62. As a result, mules have 63 chromosomes and therefore one chromosome cannot be paired during meiosis. Since meiosis is a key step in the formation of germ cells, ova and sperm, these cells are not produced by mules and hinnies.

It should also be pointed out, however that mules and hinnies exhibit significant hybrid vigor. As a result, they have greater stamina and cognitive ability than either horses or donkeys (Renaud et al., 2018). From an immunological viewpoint, however, the immune systems of mules and hinnies are intermediate in their properties between horses and donkeys. This is seen in many examples throughout this text.

warfare, primarily as pack animals but occasionally for riding. Mules were especially well-suited to more strenuous tasks, especially carrying heavy loads over difficult terrain. More recently, they have been used to deliver vaccines to remote rural communities in parts of Africa where instability has made road travel hazardous (Box 1.2).

Box 1.2 An early iron-age mule

It has long been assumed that the production of donkey-horse hybrids, - mules, originated in Roman times. This is incorrect! In 1986, the skeleton of a female equid was discovered in an archeological site in North-East Spain near Barcelona. It was dated from the early Iron Age, the 8–6th century BCE. The animal was found, together with the remains of a woman in a pit-silo. Recent DNA and structural analysis of these remains have demonstrated that it was actually an adult female mule. The maxillary and mandibular bones of the animal showed lesions consistent with bit use and riding. Carbon and nitrogen isotope analysis showed that it was fed a diet of cereal grains. These are the earliest genetically confirmed mule remains found in Western Europe. It is speculated that African donkeys may have been imported into the Iberian Peninsula through Phoenician-developed trade networks and were subsequently bred with local Iberian horses. Alternatively, this mule may have been bred elsewhere and subsequently imported (Albizuri et al., 2025).

References

Ahlawat, S., Sharna, U., Arora, R., Sharma, R., et al. (2023). Mitogenomic phylogeny reveals the predominance of the Nubian lineage of African wild ass in Indian donkeys. *Gene, 880*, Article 147627.

Albizuri, S., Nadal, J., Cuervo, M. M., Grandal-D'Anglade, A., et al. (2025). The oldest mule in the Western Mediterranean. The case of the early iron age in Hort d'en Grimau (Penedes, Barcelona, Spain). *Journal of Archaeological Science: Reports*. https://doi.org/10.1016/j.jasrep.2025.105506

Bailey, E., & Binns, M. M. (1998). The horse gene map. *ILAR Journal, 39*(2–3), 171–176.

Barrandeguy, N. E., & Carossino, M. (2018). Infectious diseases in donkeys and mules: An overview and update. *Journal of Equine Veterinary Science, 65*, 98–105.

Bartosiewicz, L., & Gal, E. (2025). Hippophagy in medieval Hungary: A quantitative analysis. *Antiquity*. https://doi.org/10.15184/aqy.2025.10138

Cerling, L. E., Ehleringer, J. R., & Harris, J. M. (1998). Carbon dioxide, starvation, the development of C_4 ecosystems, and mammalian evolution. *Philosophical Transactions of the Royal Society of London - Biological Sciences,, 353*, 159–171.

Cunningham, E. P., Dooley, J. J., Splan, R. K., & Bradley, D. G. (2001). Microsatellite diversity, pedigree relatedness and the contributions of founder lineages to thoroughbred horses. *Animal Genetics, 32*, 360–364.

Du, W., Sun, O., Hu, S., Yu, P., et al. (2025). *Equus* mitochondrial pangenome reveals independent domestication imprints in donkeys and horses. *Scientific Reports*. https://doi.org/10.1038/s41598-025-91564-1

Edwards, E. J., Osborne, C. P., Strömberg, C. A. E., Smith, S. A., et al. (2010). The origins of C_4 grasslands: Integrating evolutionary and ecosystem science. *Science, 328*, 587–591.

Frantz, L. (2025). The rise of rideable horses. *Science, 389*(6763), 874–876.

Haspel, T. (2025). *The case for eating wild horses out West.* https://www.washingtonpoast.com.food/2025/08/01/wild-horses-overpopulation-food-eating/.

Hutson, J. M., Bittmann, F., Fischer, P., Garcia-Moreno, A., et al. (2025). Revised age for Schöningen hunting spears indicates intensification of Neanderthal cooperative behavior around 200,000 years ago. *Science Advances.* https://doi.org/10.1126/sciadv0752

Jansen, T., Forster, P., Levine, M. A., Oelke, H., et al. (2002). Mitochondrial DNA and the origins of the domestic horse. *Proceedings of the National Academy of Sciences.* https://doi.org/10.1073/pnas.152330099

Jonsson, H., Schubert, M., Seguin-Orlando, A., Ginolhac, A., et al. (2014). Speciation with gene flow in equids despite extensive chromosomal plasticity. *Proceedings of the National Academy of Sciences, 111*(52), 18655–18660.

Kavanagh, K. (2025). First CRISPR horses spark controversy: What's next for gene-edited animals? *Nature.* https://doi.org/10.1038/d41586-025-02800-7. Science News.

Kefena, E., Mekasha, Y., Han, J. L., Rosenbom, et al. (2012). Discordance between morphological systematics and molecular taxonomy in the stem line of equids. A review of the case of taxonomy of genus *Equus. Livestock Science, 143*, 105–115.

Lawson, J. M., Shilton, C. A., Lindsay-McGee, V., Psifidi, A., et al. (2024). Does inbreeding contribute to pregnancy loss in thoroughbred horses? *Equine Veterinary Journal, 56*(4), 711–718. https://doi.org/10.1111/evj.14057

Librado, P., Khan, N., Fages, A., Kusliy, M. A., et al. (2021). The origins and spread of domestic horses from the Western Eurasian steppes. *Nature, 598*, 634–639.

Librado, P., & Orlando, L. (2021). Genomics and the evolutionary history of equids. *Annual Review of Animal Biosciences,, 9*, 81–101.

Liu, X., Jia, Y., Pan, J., Zhang, Y., et al. (2025). Selection of the GSDMC locus in horses and its implications for human mobility. *Science, 389*(6763), 925–930.

Musilova, P., Kubickova, S., Vahala, J., & Rubes, J. (2013). Subchromosomal karyotype evolution in Equidae. *Chromosome Research, 21*, 175–187.

Orlando, L. (2020). Ancient genomes reveal unexpected horse domestication and management dynamics. *BioEssays, 42*, Article 1900164.

Orlando, L., Ginolhac, A., Zhang, G., Froese, et al. (2013). Recalibrating Equus evolution using the genome sequence of an early middle Pleistocene horse. *Nature, 499*, 74–78.

Renaud, G., Petersen, B., Seguin-Orlando, A., Berteksen, M. F., et al. (2018). Improved de novo genomic assembly for the domestic donkey. *Science Advances.* https://doi.org/10.1126/sciadv.aaq0392

Rossell, S., Marshall, F., Peters, J., Pilgram, T., et al. (2008). Domestication of the donkey: Timing, processes, and indicators. *Proceedings of the National Academy of Sciences, 105*(10), 3715–3720.

Schubert, M., Jonsson, H., Chang, D., Sarkissian, C. D., et al. (2014). Prehistoric genomes reveal the genetic foundation and cost of horse domestication. *Proceedings of the National Academy of Sciences.* https://doi.org/10.1073/pnas.1416991111

Taylor, W. T. T. (2025). Understanding horse domestication and horse health care in the ancient world. *Journal of Equine Veterinary Science, 148.* https://doi.org/10.1016/j.jevs.2025.105419

Todd, E. T., Fromentier, A., Sutcliffe, R., Collin, Y. R. H., et al. (2023). Imputed genomes of historical horses provide insights into modern breeding. *Science, 26*, Article 107104.

Todd, E. T., Tonasso-Calvière, L., Chauvey, L., Schiavinato, S., et al. (2022). The genomic history and global expansion of domestic donkeys. *Science, 377*, 1172–1180.

Wang, Y., Hua, X., Shi, X., & Wang, C. (2022). Origin, evolution, and research development of donkeys. *Genes*. https://doi.org/10.3390/genes13111945

Xu, X., Gullberg, A., & Arnason, U. (1996). The complete mitochondrial DNA (mtDNA) of the donkey and mtDNA comparisons among four closely related mammalian species-pairs. *Journal of Molecular Evolution, 43*, 438–446.

CHAPTER

Equine immune ontogeny, reproduction, and lactation

2

The gestation period of the mare is a relatively long 340 days. Horse foals are precocious at birth. They have to be able to avoid predators and run with the herd as soon as possible after birth. That is why the equine gestation period is so long. However, throughout this pregnancy, the mare's immune system must also learn to tolerate the presence of a semi-allogeneic fetus within her uterus. The immune system and the reproductive system must cooperate if a successful pregnancy is to be achieved.

Mating-induced endometritis

Natural and artificial breeding procedures introduce cell debris and bacteria in addition to spermatozoa and seminal plasma into the uterine lumen. This results in the development of a transient bacterial endometritis, which is considered to be a normal physiological response. Healthy mares can clear this foreign material within about 24–48 hours. This is critical since a sterile uterine environment is essential for the survival of the conceptus when it arrives in the uterus about 5–6 days later. Unfortunately, a subset of mares may be unable to remove this contamination, and as a result, their endometritis may be persistent. This persistent endometritis is a significant cause of equine subfertility (Woodward & Troedssen, 2013).

The reasons for microbial persistence within the uterus are complex. Thus, it may simply be a result of its conformation. A uterus that droops anteriorly cannot drain. Studies on endometrial lymphatics suggest that in susceptible mares, lymphatic drainage is slower than in resistant mares (LeBlanc et al., 1995). Susceptibility is affected by the mare's age as well. However, it is believed to mainly reflect defects in the endometrial innate immune defenses of susceptible mares. Studies have demonstrated that susceptible mares express higher levels of the genes encoding the chemokine CCL2, phospholipase A2, lipocalin 2, lactoferrin, equine beta-defensin 1, lysozyme, and secretory leukoprotease inhibitor (Marth et al., 2018). Collectively, these changes may interfere with the normal uterine innate defenses and microbial clearance mechanisms.

The Immunology of Horses and Donkeys. https://doi.org/10.1016/B978-0-443-44863-8.00017-X

Equine pregnancy

The fertilized equine ovum develops into a blastocyst between days 6 and 22 post-conception. It is covered by an elastic glycoprotein layer. The developing fetus within this blastocyst then moves progressively down the uterine lumen propelled by smooth muscle contractions. Uterine "milk," secreted by endometrial glands, provides nutrition and lubrication during this stage. The developing embryo also releases chemical signals that inform the endometrium that the mare is pregnant. This blastocyst migration ends on day 17 once the embryo has reached the base of one of the uterine horns (Allen & Stewart, 2001). Around day 22 postconception, the blastocyst disintegrates as a result of the actions of trophoblast proteases. The allantois then begins to expand. and fuses with the chorion to form the chorioallantois. Subsequently, the trophoblast begins to differentiate into invasive and non-invasive regions and thus forms a diffuse epitheliochorial placenta. The majority of the placental surface area formed in this way is non-invasive. Thus, the trophoblast simply binds very tightly to the endometrial epithelium. There is, however, a relatively small region, the chorionic girdle, that is invasive. This division of the placenta into invasive and noninvasive regions is unique to equids.

Placentation

Beginning around day 40 post-conception and thus well after trophoblast invasion occurs, the non-invasive region of the trophoblast begins to bind to the endometrial epithelium. It develops large numbers of microvilli that penetrate and thus come into stable contact with the endometrial epithelium (Pozor, 2016). These microvilli then progressively develop into complex, multi-branched structures that interdigitate with the endometrium and form unique microcotyledons that cover the entire surface of the diffuse placenta (Fig. 2.1).

These microcotyledons maximize the contact area between the endometrium and trophoblast and are, as a result, the primary route by which oxygen and nutrients reach the developing foal. Each microcotyledon is supplied with a maternal artery and a placental vein. These surfaces must remain in close contact throughout the pregnancy in order to support the developing fetus. Any loss of chorioallantois or endometrial contact can reduce fetal nutrition and put the pregnancy in jeopardy (Enders & Carter, 2004).

Once pregnancy is established, six tissue layers (two vascular endothelia, two connrective tissue layers as well as the trophoblast and endometrial epithelia) separate the maternal and fetal circulations. As a result, in order to provide sufficient oxygen and nutrition for the fetal foal, the entire surface of the placenta must be functional and tightly attached to the maternal endometrium. Consequently, only one foal fetus is usually supported at a time. As another consequence, no large proteins such as immunoglobulins can cross the placenta, and foals are therefore born agammaglobulinemic. In addition to its basic structure, the equine placenta also

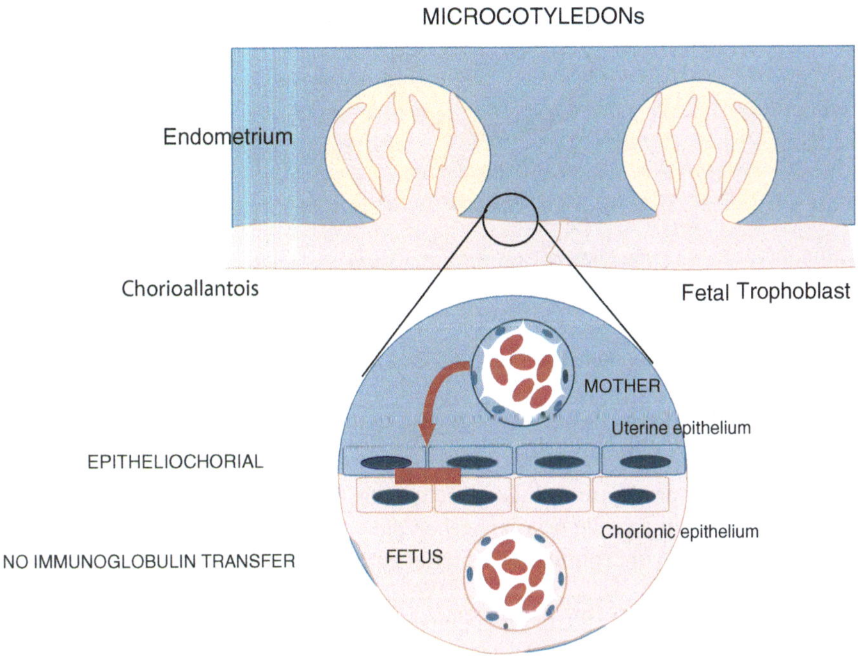

FIGURE 2.1 Trophoblast-derived microcotyledons form within the endometrium but do not penetrate the epithelial barrier. They effectively increase the area of contact between the placenta and the endometrium.

This is therefore an epitheliochorial placenta and its microcotyledons. As a result of the number of layers between foal and mare there is no immunoglobulin transport across it. Nor is it attacked by the cells of the mare's immune system.

contains allantoic pouches and vesicles, hippomanes (thick elastic aggregates of allantoic fluid), amniotic plaques, and remnants of the foal's yolk sac.

Endometrial cups

The invasive regions of the trophoblast, in contrast, are generated by specialized cells that develop at the margin of the yolk sac and chorioallantois and so form the chorionic girdle. The chorionic girdle begins to develop on the outer surface of the chorion around 30 days post-conception. It develops as a ring or horseshoe-shaped structure on the surface of the blastoderm, where it exhibits alternating ridges and pits (Fig. 2.2).

The trophoblast cells in the girdle invade the endometrial tissues, remodel the nearby extracellular matrix, and complete the process of differentiating into endometrial cups by day 38.

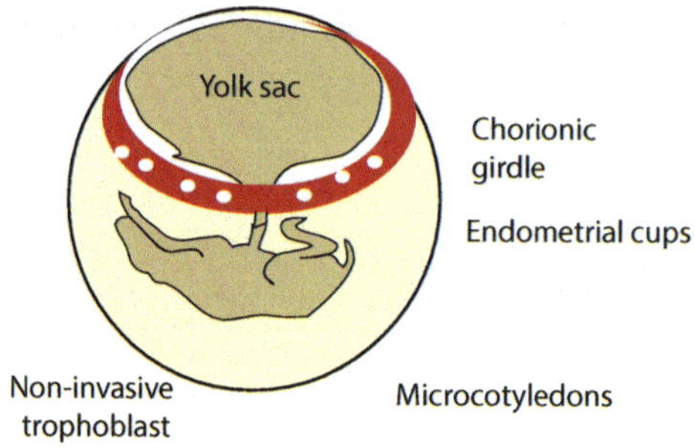

FIGURE 2.2

The location of equine endometrial cups and the chorionic girdle on the surface of the equine blastocyst.

Structure

Endometrial cups are dense cellular structures that can be recognized as pale raised plaques arranged in a circle or a horseshoe pattern. The cups reach maximum size around day 70 post-conception. Endometrial cups are structures unique to the equids (Fig. 2.3).

Between days 40 and 100, these endometrial cups are responsible for the production of the hormone equine chorionic gonadotrophin (eCG) that is required to maintain pregnancy. eCG synergizes with follicle-stimulating hormone from the pituitary to induce secondary development and persistence of the corpus luteum as well as progesterone secretion by the mare's ovaries.

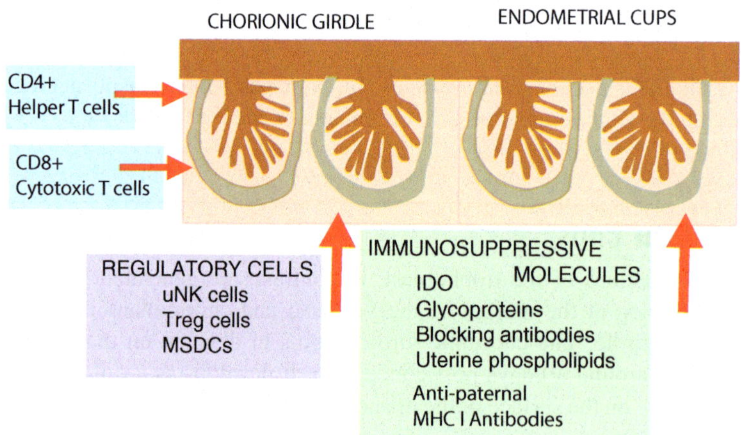

FIGURE 2.3 Endometrial cups bud off the chorionic girdle.

They consist of clusters of MHC -positive fetal cells and as a result trigger an immune response by the mare. This response is subsequently suppressed by multiple immunoregulatory mechanisms as shown here.

Immune attack

Since the endometrial cup cells are derived from the invasive trophoblast of the fetus, they express cell surface major histocompatibility (MHC) molecules inherited by the fetus from both its parents. The MHC antigens from the sire, therefore, stimulate both humoral and cell-mediated immune responses by the mare. As a result, an immune response is directed against the semi-allogeneic fetal cells in the cups (Allen & Stewart, 2001).

The cells forming the surface of the equine conceptus do not express MHC antigens until approximately 30 days post-conception. Thereafter, they are only expressed by the chorionic girdle cells. The invasive chorionic girdle trophoblast cells express high levels of MHC class I molecules. They express them at levels 10-fold higher than on resting somatic cells and are comparable to the levels expressed on lymphoid cells. Their MHC expression level remains high until the cup cells differentiate into trophoblast cells and subsequently drops to low levels by day 45 (Noronha & Antczak, 2010). Significantly, noninvasive trophoblast cells do not express MHC class I molecules.

Antibodies

Following the events described above, mares develop high titers of antibodies to the paternal stallion's MHC antigens by 10–14 days following the initial trophoblast invasion of the endometrium. Antibodies thus appear in the mare's serum by day 60 in primiparous mares. Antibodies are detectable in multiparous mares around day 40. These antibodies persist throughout pregnancy, and if a mare is repeatedly bred by the same stallion, they are stimulated to produce even higher titers of these antibodies. Acting in conjunction with complement, these antibodies are highly cytotoxic. These antibodies, however, are not known to influence equine pregnancy in a negative fashion (Antczak, 2020).

Cell-mediated responses

In addition to making antibodies against paternal MHC antigens, maternal cytotoxic $CD4^+$ and $CD8^+$ T cells also accumulate around the endometrial cups. The numbers of these cytotoxic T cells increase significantly by 60–70 days. There is also an increase in IFN-γ-producing T cell numbers (de Amorim et al., 2023). Other infiltrating cell populations include macrophages, plasma cells, and eosinophils. These cells accumulate to form a thick layer and subsequently invade the cups and attack the fetal cup cells, eventually resulting in the total destruction of the cups between days 100 and 120 (Lunn et al., 1997). The uterine epithelium then regrows over the cups. At the same time, mononuclear leukocytes accumulate around the degenerating cups. Cup destruction is mediated in part by the T cell-derived cytokine, IL-22, between days 32 and 35 (Brosnahan et al., 2012). Mares also mount a T cell-mediated response to the foreign girdle cells; however, this is not intense (Noronha & Antczak, 2010). The equine placenta is usually expelled intact within 1–2 hours of the delivery of the foal (Pozor, 2016).

Maternal immune tolerance

For any successful pregnancy to occur, mammalian mothers must be prevented from mounting a lethal immune response against the paternal antigens expressed by their fetus and its placenta. Suppression of this rejection process must be achieved if the benefits of the closest possible proximation of the fetal and maternal blood systems are to be obtained. Suppression of the maternal graft rejection process occurs within the decidua, that part of the uterine wall that is in contact with, the endometrial cups. Among the uterine genes with enhanced expression in the preimplantation uterus are those that regulate the development of immune and inflammatory responses. Activation of these genes results in functional changes in immune regulation.

Immune regulation

Neither antibody- nor cell-mediated immune responses nor the destruction of the endometrial cups appears to compromise equine pregnancy (Baker et al., 1999). This is the consequence of the development of multiple immune tolerance mechanisms. The infiltrating cells mount suppressive Th2 and Treg responses dominated by TGF-β production that do not threaten the pregnancy, rather than cytotoxic Th1 and inflammatory Th17 responses that would otherwise cause fetal allograft rejection.

As part of this regulatory process, the equine placenta produces multiple immunosuppressive factors. For example, extracts from 90-day equine placentas decrease lymphocyte proliferation and cytokine production. One of the conceptus-derived immunosuppressive factors is a protein derived from 20-day embryo culture supernatants. Equine trophoblast cells secrete pregnancy-specific glycoproteins (PSGs). In other mammals, these are known to modulate immune, angiogenic, and platelet responses during pregnancy. They are found at high levels in species with a hemochorial invasive placenta (Aleksic et al., 2016). Analysis has shown that horses possess seven genes encoding Carcinoembryonic Antigen Cell Adhesion Molecules (CEACAMs). Four of these are expressed in purified chorionic girdle cells and endometrial cup cells. One of these glycoproteins is CEACAM49. CEACAM49 binds to a latency-associated peptide and, as a result, activates the suppressive cytokine, transforming growth factor-β1. TGF-β1, in turn, contributes to the generation of regulatory T cells and helps maintain immune tolerance (Kammerer et al., 2020). The endometrium also produces immunosuppressive prostaglandins.

Transforming growth factor-beta

Among the immunosuppressive cytokines produved in the placenta and endometrium during equine pregnancy are members of the transforming growth factor beta (TGF-β) family. This family consists of three related glycoproteins (TGF-β1, TGF-β2, and TGF-β3). They are secreted as inactive precursors that are activated on the cell surface by proteases after binding to integrins. TGFs are produced by platelets, activated macrophages, neutrophils, B cells, and T cells and act on T and B cells, dendritic cells, macrophages, neutrophils, and fibroblasts. It is relevant to note, therefore, that endometrial cups are surrounded by an environment rich in transforming growth factor beta 1 (TGF-β1). TGF-β1 induces Treg activity by inducing the production of $FoxP3^+$ Treg cells.

TGF-β1 mRNA. begins to accumulate in the luminal and glandular cells of the equine endometrium beginning on day 33 at the time of implantation. Its concentration remains high for the duration of the pregnancy. It is expressed at high levels in the mononuclear cells that accumulate around the endometrial cups. In addition to being immuosuppressive, it probably also plays a role in regulating trophoblast growth (Lennard et al., 1995).

TGF-β1 also regulates macrophage activities. It may be either inhibitory or stimulatory, depending on the presence of other cytokines. Thus, it can enhance integrin expression as well as phagocytosis by blood monocytes. On the other hand, it suppresses the respiratory burst and nitric oxide production and blocks monocyte differentiation and the cytotoxic effects of activated macrophages. TGF-β1 is also required for optimal dendritic cell development and regulates the interaction between follicular dendritic cells and B cells. Apoptotic T cells release more TGF-β1, contributing to the suppressive environment. TGF-β1 also influences the differentiation of helper T cell subsets. It tends to promote Th1 responses and the production of IL-2 in naïve T cells, but it also antagonizes the effects of IFN-γ and IL-12 on memory cells. It also controls the development and differentiation of B cells, inhibiting their proliferation, inducing apoptosis, and regulating IgA production.

Interleukin-10

In other mammals suh as humans, ile regulatory cytokine, interleukin 10 plays an important role in the maintenance of pregnancy. Regulatory T cells (Treg cells) produce two major suppressive cytokines, interleukin-10 and transforming growth factor-β. Equine IL-10 has been cloned and sequenced (Singha et al., 2015). IL-10 inhibits both innate and adaptive immune responses and, as a result, is a potent anti-inflammatory cytokine. It is produced in especially large amounts by Treg cells in response to TGF-β. Blood IL-10 levels have been measured in pregnant mares. Its concentration rises to reach peak levels in the 6th month of pregnancy. (These are double those in non-pregnant mare serum) These levels subsequently declined significantly as parturition approached (Figarska et al., 2023).

Another immunosuppressive cytokine is interleukin-1 receptor antagonist (IL-1RA). As its name implies, it binds and blocks the receptors for the proinflammatory cytokine, IL-1. In pregnant mares, blood levels of IL-1RA are elevated in the early stages of pregnancy but decline as parturition approaches. It is known that IL-10 regulates the production of IL-1RA (Figarska et al., 2023).

Indoleamine 2,3-dioxygenase-1

Indoleamine 2,3-dioxygenase-1 (IDO) is an enzyme that has immunosuppressive properties. It degrades the amino acid tryptophan, resulting in a local tissue deficiency. Effector T cells require tryptophan to function. In its absence, effector T cell functions are inhibited. In other domestic species, such as cattle, IDO is produced by placental cells. This serves an immunosuppressive function and inhibits the local maternal anti-fetal immune response (Durr & Kindler, 2013; Munn et al., 1998). This has yet to be demonstrated in the mare. However, IDO is present in the normal healthy equine endometrium, especially in the glandular epithelium. Presumably, it plays an immunomodulatory role in this location (Schoniger et al., 2018).

Natural killer cells

Among the most important of the regulatory processes that support maternal tolerance are those mediated by uterine natural killer (uNK) cells. uNK cells have distinctly different properties from the NK cells found in the circulation and the rest of the body. The circulating NK cells are primarily cytotoxic, while the uterine NK cells produce both cytokines and chemokines and are poorly cytotoxic. These uNK cells mediate the vascular adaptations in the uterus needed for a successful equine pregnancy (Croy et al., 2006).

Uterine NK cells are the predominant population of immune cells present in the endometrium during the establishment of the placenta (Colucci et al., 2011). The placental decidua contains huge populations of uNK cells and macrophages, as well as the key effector cells of the adaptive immune system, namely dendritic cells, and T cells (especially Treg cells). In the first trimester of human pregnancy, about 70% of these immune cells are uNK cells, and about 20%–25% are macrophages (Ander et al., 2019). T cells constitute about 3%–10% of this cell population, while dendritic cells (DCs), B cells, and mast cells are only present in low numbers. Presumably, these leukocytes are attracted to the decidua by chemokine gradients generated by stromal and trophoblast cells. The population of uNK cells undergoes a major expansion during early pregnancy when they invade the embryonic implantation site (Matson & Caron, 2014). They occupy the decidual basalis and form the mesometrial lymphoid aggregate of pregnancy. These uNK cells proliferate until mid-gestation. They subsequently decline and are gradually replaced by T cells that predominate at term.

Uterine natural killer cells are present in large numbers among the dense lymphocyte infiltration that surrounds equine endometrial cups (Noronha et al., 2012). Through the use of real-time PCR, it has been demonstrated that there is extensive NKP46 and CD16 gene expression in the CD3-negative lymphocytes around the cups. This is characteristic of equine NK cells (Fig. 2.4).

In the case of equine pregnancy, the composition of the infiltrating lymphoid cell populations is slightly different from that in humans. Analysis of the endometrial lymphoid cell populations from biopsies taken beginning at 33 and 42 days of gestation in mares shows that the main immune cell populations include natural killer cells (46%), $CD3^+$ lymphocytes (T cells) 36%, monocytes (14.5%), innate lymphoid cells (ILCs) 3% and B cells (1.3%). Novel subpopulations that are also present

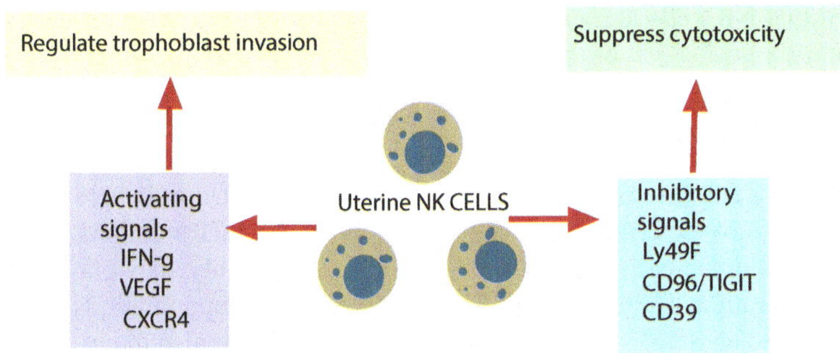

FIGURE 2.4 The functions of uterine NK cells.

Some of the functions of uNK cells that contribute to the success of equine pregnancy.

include resident innate lymphoid cells and mucosal-associated invariant T cells. There are also natural killer T (NKT) cells present that express CD161 (Noronha et al., 2012).

Four major subpopulations of equine uterine NK (uNK) cells have been identified based upon their expression of cell surface receptors. This suggests that they may be activated at different levels. All four are CD56-negative. Subpopulation 1 is $CD39^+$ $Ly49F^+$; subpopulation 3 is $CD39^+$, $Ly49F^-$. The other two uNK subpopulations are $Ly49F^+$ and $CD39^{low}$ respectively. Subendometrial NK cells are the most abundant lymphocyte population found at the time of implantation. These NK cells not only express surface receptors such as Ly49F that can interact with equine MHC class I antigens, but they also express immunoregulatory receptors such as CD96/TIGIT. Upregulation of the chemokine receptor CXCR4 has been detected in several of these immune cell populations. Thus, mares utilize many of the same immunoregulatory mechanisms mediated by uNK cells in other mammals.

uNK cells produce a diverse mixture of growth factors, angiogenic factors, and cytokines. As described above, subpopulations of uNK cells have been identified in the equine decidua based on their surface antigen expression and gene expression profiles. However, they also have many other receptors and ligands that are unique in their extreme diversity. Different combinations may have different effects on trophoblast invasion and the development of a successful pregnancy (Colucci et al., 2011). There is, in effect, a balance between MHC class I expression on the trophoblast and uNK cells in the uterine wall that together regulate trophoblast growth and immune invasion.

The binding of MHC ligands to their receptors on uNK cells suppresses their cytotoxicity and also triggers epigenetic changes in their DNA, especially during a first pregnancy. This subgroup of uNK cells, called pregnancy-trained uterine NK cells, is present in the decidua after repeated pregnancies. They have a unique transcriptome and epigenetic signature (Valencia-Ortega et al., 2020). Their activation leads to increased production of interferon (IFN)-γ and vascular endothelial growth factor (VEGF)-α. In effect, this results in a form of “trained” immunity that plays a role in facilitating subsequent pregnancies (Colucci, 2019). It should be noted that NK cells are also present in the uterus of non-pregnant mares. They constitute about 2%–3% of their endometrial lymphocyte population.

Regulatory T cells

Regulatory T cells (Tregs) are also present in the endometrium, where they constitute 14%–15% of the lymphocyte population. However, their numbers vary greatly between individual mares (Jaworska et al., 2022). Presumably, they play a defensive role in this location. There are four CD3-negative T cell subpopulations in the endometrium. Most are $CD8^+$ (Jaworska et al., 2025). There are also many Tregs. found at the fetal-maternal interface. Thus, there is a threefold increase in $FoxP3^+$ Treg lymphocytes.

$CD4^+$ $FoxP3^+$ Treg cells play a critical role in preventing fetal rejection. Estrogen treatment and pregnancy both induce FoxP3 activation, as does the presence of seminal plasma (Lenicov et al., 2012). These induced Treg cells suppress maternal responses to paternal antigens, probably through IL-10 and TGF-β production, while at the same time suppressing the production of Th1, Th2, and Th17 cells. Treg numbers steadily increase before declining late in gestation. This decline may assist in promoting parturition. These fetal-specific Treg cells can persist beyond parturition. In subsequent pregnancies, their numbers increase rapidly (Ander et al., 2019). Thus, young foals have significantly higher numbers of Treg cells (47%) than their mothers (18%) and yearlings (26%). These cells also have significantly enhanced suppressive activity. This presumably assists in the development of specific tolerance but may also render the foals more susceptible to some neonatal infections, such as those caused by *Rhodococcus equi* (Hamza et al., 2015). Placental T cells also secrete antiviral molecules, including IFN-γ and some microRNAs that restrict viral infections in a paracrine and autocrine manner. This may be accompanied by a degree of thymic involution in the pregnant mare (Laan et al., 2016).

Foal immune ontogeny

As the embryonic foal develops, so too does its immune system (Fig. 2.5).

Lymphocytes appear first in the fetal foal thymus at about 11–12 weeks post-conception. They are found in the mesenteric lymph nodes at 13 weeks, in the intestinal lamina propria at 13–14 weeks, in the bloodstream at about 17 weeks, in regional lymph nodes at 23 weeks, and in the spleen by 25 weeks (Mackenzie, 1975; Perryman et al., 1980). By about 100 days gestation, the fetal liver and bone marrow are active sites of hematopoiesis. $CD8^+$ T cells are detectable in the fetal spleen by 13–17 weeks gestation. Graft-versus-host disease, a T cell-mediated response, has developed in immunodeficient foals transplanted with tissues from a 79-day-old fetus (Perryman et al., 1979). The equine fetus can make IgG1 antibodies against coliphage T2 at 200 days post-conception and against Venezuelan equine encephalitis virus by 230 days. Plasma cells may be present by 240 days Their antigen binding site (V[D]J) sequence diversity

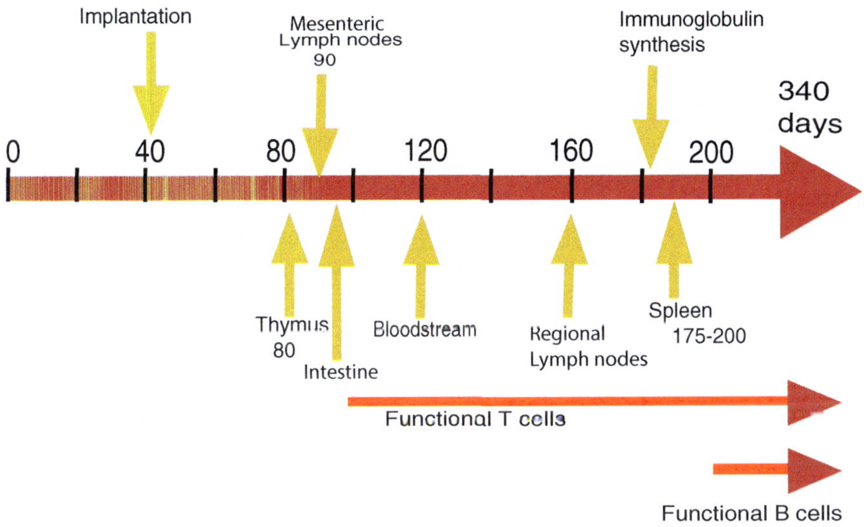

FIGURE 2.5 The ontogeny of the immune system in the fetal foal.

Note that all the components of a functional system appear to be present by around 200 days of gestation. Thereafter, it simply grows with the foal.

increases as the fetus develops and as the foal develops into an adult (Chapter 11). Major B cell markers such as CD20 and CD21 are detectable in the liver, spleen, and bone marrow by 13–17 weeks of gestation. Immunoglobulin isotype switching occurs in these B cells in utero (Tallmadge et al., 2009) and *IGHM* and *IGLC* transcripts are also expressed in the liver, bone marrow, and spleen as they develop (Tallmadge et al., 2013). Thus, gene recombination and immunoglobulin class switching occur during equine fetal life despite the absence of antigenic stimulation (Ander et al., 2019; Roberts et al., 2016). As a result, newborn foals have detectable quantities of IgM and IgG1 in their serum. IgG1 is the only IgG isotype produced by fetal foal B cells.

Neonatal foals have significantly higher levels of Treg cells (47%) than their mothers (18%) and yearlings (26%). These cells also appear to have significantly enhanced suppressive activity. They presumably assist in the establishment of specific tolerance to normal body tissue antigens.

After parturition

Foals are precocial. They can stand, suckle, run, and follow their mother soon after birth. When a foal is born, it emerges from the sterile uterus into an environment where it is immediately exposed to a host of microorganisms. During the foaling process, the foal transitions rapidly from an environment that is largely free of environmental antigens to a whole new world of diverse antigens, and a commensal microbiota in addition to many potential pathogens. Its innate and adaptive immune systems need time to adapt to this new antigenic environment. It cannot change instantly to a fully functional system. This, however, means that for a period of time, the newborn foal is vulnerable to opportunistic pathogens. It requires immune protection that must be provided by its mother, - passive immunity. It needs assistance in defending itself at this time. This temporary help is provided through the mare's colostrum in the form of ingested antibodies, cytokines, and possibly also T cells. The passive transfer of immunity from the mare to her foal is essential for its survival.

Passive immunity

Colostrum

Just before foaling, the mare's mammary gland must develop and produce sufficient colostrum for the first suckling of the foal. Within hours of birth, the foal must be able to stand up, reach the mammary gland, and suckle without assistance. It must nurse repeatedly and consume significant amounts of colostrum.

During late pregnancy, the mammary glands develop under the influence of estrogens and progesterone. Colostrum secretion only begins when progesterone levels drop at birth. Nutritional components are synthesized within the mammary gland itself, whereas the immunological components, such as immunoglobulins, leukocytes, growth factors, and cytokines, are actively transferred from the mare's bloodstream (Tizard, 2001).

Colostrum therefore consists of the accumulated mammary gland secretions obtained over the first 48 hours after birth. It tends to be yellowish and more viscous than milk, reflecting its high protein content. While the foal intestinal tract is fully formed at birth, it is functionally immature and is undergoing colonization by its microbiota. As a result, its digestive functions are initially minimal but increase progressively over time.

Nutrition

Healthy foals can suckle the mare frequently and readily obtain adequate nutrition from her colostrum (Bigler et al., 2022). When foals first suckle immediately after birth, they usually drink, on average, about 2 Liters of colostrum. However, some large foals may drink up to 6 Liters. The most important sources of energy in colostrum are its diverse lipids and carbohydrates. Thus, on average, equine milk contains 6.62% lactose, 1.68% protein, 0.73% fat, and 440 kcal/kg of energy (Barreto et al., 2020). Colostrum, in contrast, contains much more dry matter, 20%–30% as opposed to 10%–12% in mare's milk. It contains 1.53% lactose, 18% protein, and 1.7% fat. It is also a critical water source, as well as providing growth factors and some digestive enzymes. The fluid serves to maintain vascular volume. The nutritional and immunological qualities of colostrum are not correlated.

Immunoglobulins

A large proportion of the proteins found in mare's colostrum consist of immunoglobulins (antibodies). Protease activity in the digestive tract of neonatal foals is low. In addition, colostrum contains multiple trypsin inhibitors. As a result, the colostral immunoglobulins are protected from digestion and, after passing through the esophagus and stomach, can reach the small intestine intact. Once within the intestine, these ingested immunoglobulins are endocytosed by enterocytes that express the neonatal immunoglobulin receptor, FcRn. The FcRn on neonatal enterocytes translocates from the apical to the basal surface of these cells thus allowing the IgG to be captured from the intestinal lumen and then transported across the enterocytes. The immunoglobulins are actively transported across the enterocytes to the lacteals and the intestinal capillaries. These immunoglobulins quickly reach the bloodstream, and, as a result, newborn foals obtain a massive transfusion of maternal antibodies, especially those of the IgG1 subclass (Fig. 2.6).

Before suckling, foals are essentially agammaglobulinemic. Drinking their mother's colostrum provides them with a dose of IgG antibodies that is normally sufficient to protect them against potential pathogens. Ideally, foals should begin to suckle within 2–4 hours after birth. Depending on the time and duration of first suckling, their IgG levels peak between 12 and 24 hours after birth. Once the foal's IgG uptake is completed, the ingested immunoglobulins progressively decline through normal protein catabolism. The persistence of these immunoglobulins in the foal serum and thus the duration of passive protective immunity depend upon the initial quantity of colostral immunoglobulin ingested and absorbed.

Intestinal permeability is highest immediately after birth but declines progressively beginning about 6 hours later. This is because the foal's FcRn-bearing enterocytes are gradually replaced by cells that do not express this receptor. It also results from the maturation of the enterocyte brush border as well as the tight junctions between the epithelial cells. Feeding colostrum tends to hasten intestinal closure, whereas a delay in suckling can result in a delay in closure for several more hours.

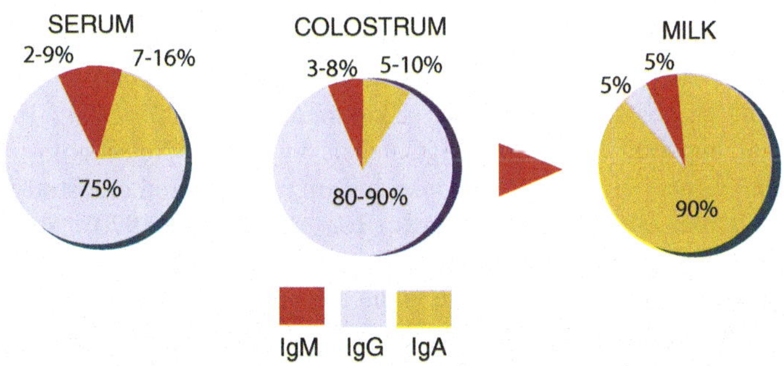

FIGURE 2.6

Relative immunoglobulin class levels in equine serum, colostrum, and milk.

When a foal suckles, the epithelial cells lining its small intestine take up immunoglobulin-rich droplets through pinocytosis and FcRn binding. These immunoglobulin-rich droplets eventually reach the lymphatic system and the foal's bloodstream. The ability to undertake this pinocytosis is limited to the neonatal epithelial cells. As the epithelial cells mature, their expression of FcRn drops so that by 38 hours, immunoglobulin binding and uptake has ceased. The rate of decline is progressive, dropping to less than 1% by about 20 hours.

As in other mammals, the equine IgG receptor, FcRn, is responsible for the maintenance of blood IgG levels in foals. Studies in horses have indicated that the FcRn is also expressed in synovia and respiratory tissues. While gastrointestinal tissues also express significant amounts of this receptor (Guenther et al., 2024). FcRn is an MHC class I-related protein. It is a heterodimer consisting of a 32.3 kDa α chain and a 13 kDa β2M chain (Fig. 2.7).

Immunoglobulins

Serum immunoglobulin levels

In serum collected from Standardbred mares at the time of parturition, their mean concentrations of serum IgG, IgM, and IgA were 1953.3 ± 1635 mg/dL, 33.8 ± 0.4 mg/dL, and 58.4 ± 42.2 mg/dL, respectively. The IgG concentrations in mare serum did not correlate closely with those in colostrum, a reflection of the ativities of the active transport mechanism that moves igG from serum to colostrum (Kohn et al., 1989).

Colostral immunoglobulin levels

Normal equine colostrum contains between 3000 and 12,000 mg/dL of IgG. The average level is about 7000–9000 mg/dL). It also contains about 130 mg/dL (100–350) 1 gM and 1000 mg/dL IgA (500–1500 mg/dL) (Hart & Wong, 2024). For example, in the colostrum of Standardbred mares, the mean concentrations of IgG, IgM, and IgA were 8911.9 ± 628.2 mg/dL, 95.7 ± 108.8 mg/dL and 1223 ± 77.3 mg/dL, respectively (Kohn et al., 1989).

In comparison to the above figures, a study on immunoglobulin levels in the colostrum of Japanese heavy draft horses demonstrated the following levels. From colostral IgG, 10,540 ± 3190 mg/dL; and from foal serum IgG, 1750 ± 919 mg/dL (Aoki et al., 2020). At the other extreme, McGuire et al. reported that IgG levels in Thoroughbred colostrum were only 2354 mg/dL (McGuire et al., 1977) while Kenzig et al. reported the average IgG levels in Quarter horse colostrum to be 3125 mg/dL (Kenzig et al., 2009). Rouse and Ingram reported colostral IgG levels in Shetland ponies averaged 4600 mg/dL (Rouse & Ingram, 1970). An average of about 100 g of IgG is produced per lactation in the mare (Walther et al., 2015).

The ingested colostral immunoglobulins are not only protective, but they also probably exert an imprinting effect on the B cell repertoire of the developing foal. Thus, they delay interactions between these immature B cells and some common environmental antigens until the B cells are able to fully respond (Fink et al.,

2008). Foal serum IgG levels are also correlated with their birthweight and their mare's colostral IgG concentrations. There is no significant correlation between foal IgG concentration and average daily gain (Gallacher et al., 2025). Total IgG levels in the foal serum generally remain in the range of 800–1000 mg/dL for up to 6 months-of-age (Tallmadge et al., 2009).

Immunoglobulins A and M

Most IgA and IgM in colostrum are produced by B cells and plasma cells that have emigrated from the maternal Peyer's patches and reside within her mammary glands,

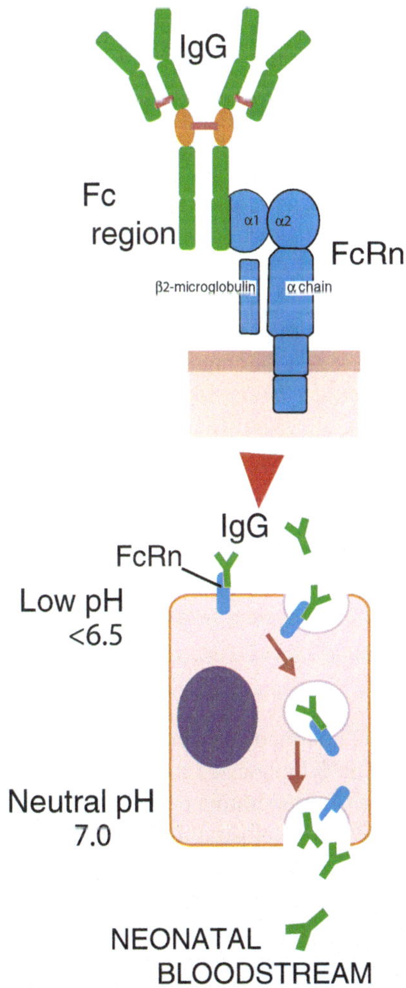

FIGURE 2.7 The mechanism of action of the neonatal FcRn receptor.

This is how colostral immunoglobulins are carried from the foal's gastrointestinal tract across the epithelial cell layer to its bloodstream.

where they produce antibodies directed against intestinal commensals and pathogens (Usami et al., 2021). As a result, IgM and IgA levels remain relatively constant.

Milk immunoglobulin levels

Once the mare's colostrum transitions to milk, its IgG content drops to about 50 mg/dL and IgA to 70 mg/dL (Figs. 2.2–2.5). This IgA eventually becomes the predominant immunoglobulin (90%), with much smaller amounts of IgG and IgM (5% each). As a result of the absence of pancreatic proteases, immunoglobulins in the foal's gut remain intact and functional for many weeks. Thus, the continuing intake of milk protects the intestinal tract from potential pathogens and also helps shape the composition of the developing intestinal microbiota. Other bioactive immune compounds present in colostrum include antimicrobials such as lysozyme and lactoferrin. β-Lactalbumin is a potential antiviral that may be able to prevent pathogen adhesion. α-Lactalbumin is an immunomodulatory protein. Lactoperoxidase is an antimicrobial enzyme that synergizes with immunoglobulins. Colostrum also contains growth factors such as insulin-like growth factor, epidermal growth factor, and nerve growth factor that collectively promote foal development.

Colostral cytokines

Mares' colostrum contains multiple cytokines. These include interleukin-4 (IL-4) - 1141 pg/mL, CXCL8 (IL-8)– ~ 840 mg/mL, IL-13– ~ 333 pg/mL, and IFN-γ - ~ 5050 pg/mL (Mariella et al., 2017). It also contains IL-6 but is lacking IL-10 (Burton et al., 2009). There are significant amounts of IL-4 in mare's colostrum, which may serve to compensate for the very low level of IL-4 production by the young foal (Mariella et al., 2017). IL-13 has not been detected in mare's colostrum, but IFN-γ is present in both colostrum and foal serum at birth. The chemokine CXCL8 (IL-8) is also present in significant amounts (Mariella et al., 2017). Equine colostrum has also been shown to contain TNF-α. These cytokines probably promote the development of the immune system in the young animal (Mariella et al., 2017; Perkins & Wagner, 2015).

Colostral cells

Mare's colostrum also contains many leukocytes, including macrophages, neutrophils, and lymphocytes. The lymphocytes are primarily T cells with few B cells. These T cells may have a similar immune-stimulating function as seen in other mammals (Perkins et al., 2014). Colostral T cells likely serve as a passive source of cell-mediated immunity (Reber et al., 2008a; Reber et al., 2008b). These $CD8^+$ cells are increased relative to their proportion in the serum, suggesting that their migration into the mammary gland is an active process. On exposure to the immunostimulant, phorbol myristate acetate, they produce large amounts of IL-17, normal amounts of IFN-γ, and reduced amounts of IL-4 and IL-10 when compared to peripheral blood T cells. Thus, they appear to have a proinflammatory phenotype (Perkins et al., 2014).

Colostral exosomes

In addition to its obvious contents of proteins, lipids, and cells, equine colostrum and milk are also rich in small vesicles or exosomes (Sedykh et al., 2021). These are nanovesicles composed of a lipid bilayer with a cytosolic content produced by different cell types. Their cargo includes multiple proteins and lipids in addition to nucleic acids such as miRNA. Once within the neonatal intestine, these vesicles can be absorbed intact by intestinal epithelial cells and enter the bloodstream through vascular endothelial cells. Colostral exosomes vary in size between 40 and 100 nm in diameter. Proteomic analysis indicates that they are complex structures containing at least 20 large proteins, such as actin, β-lactoglobulin, lactoferrin, and butyrophilin, as well as numerous small peptides.

Proteinuria

Maximal intestinal absorption of colostral proteins occurs during the first 6 hours after birth. As this intestinal absorption is taking place, simultaneous transient proteinuria also occurs in foals (Jeffcott & Jeffcott, 1974). This presumably reflects the immature state of the foal's kidneys. Protein levels in urine rise progressively to reach a peak at 6–12 hours. They then decline to zero by 24–28 hours. This results from the absorption of very small proteins, such as β-lactoglobulin, that are then excreted in the urine. There are no detectable immunoglobulins in the foal's urine after this period.

Duration of maternal immunity

It has been determined that the average half-life of maternal IgG in the foal is about 23 days (Reilly & Macdougall, 1973). However, this varies between IgG isoforms. For example, IgG4/7 accounts for about 60% of all isotypes and has the longest half-life of 32 days. The half-life of IgG1 is 17.6 days, IgG6 half-life is also 32 days, IgG3/5 is 21 days, and IgA is 3.4 days in foals (Sheoran et al., 2000). The half-life of maternal IgM is 5–16 days (McGuire & Crawford, 1973) (Fig. 2.8). Total IgG levels in foals remain below 1000 mg/dL for up to 6 months (Tallmadge et al., 2009).

Nevertheless, because maternal antibodies exert a negative feedback on B cell immunoglobulin production, it is not usually possible to successfully vaccinate very young foals. If protection is required at this stage, the mare may be vaccinated during the later stages of pregnancy. The vaccinations being timed so that peak antibody levels are achieved at the time of colostrum formation. Once a foal is born, B-cell responses and successful active immunization can occur only after passive immunity has waned. As pointed out above, the foal's immune system develops progressively. For example, at, or just after birth the foal begins to synthesize IgG1, IgG3/5, and IgA. However, the production of other IgG subclasses such as IgG4/7 as well as IgE production, progressively develops over the first year of life (Perkins & Wagner, 2015).

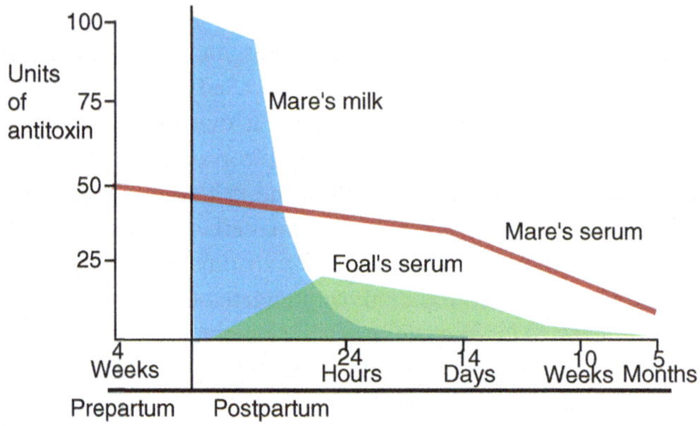

FIGURE 2.8 Passive immunity to tetanus in the neonatal foal.

Clostridium tetani antitoxin levels in serum, colostrum, and milk of six pony mares and in the serum of their foals from birth to 6 months.

- From: Jeffcott, L. B. (1974). Studies on passive immunity in the foal. 1. G-globulin and antibody variations associated with the maternal transfer of immunity and the onset of active immunity. Journal of Comparative Pathology, 84, 93–101.

A similar progressive development occurs with cell-mediated immunity. Thus, IFN-γ production starts soon after birth and increases progressively over the first year of life, whereas IL-4 production only begins about 3 months of age. This delay in Th2 response development is in part responsible for foal susceptibility to opportunistic pathogens such as *R. equi* as well as their poor responses to early vaccination.

Active immunity

In mammals with a long gestation period, such as the horse, the adaptive immune system of the newborn is fully developed at the time of birth but cannot function at adult levels for several months. Thus, it can take up to 12 weeks before a newborn foal can generate an effective, targeted antimicrobial defense. During that period, the foal relies on passively acquired colostral immunity. While neonatal foals have some functional innate immune responses at birth, their development of adaptive responses is uneven. For example, the production of IgG1, starts before birth. IgG3/5 and IgA production start shortly after birth and reach adult levels around 12 weeks. Other antibody responses are much slower to develop. Thus, serum IgG4/7 production is delayed and does not reach adult levels until 1 year of age. Likewise, IgE production begins around 9–11 months of age (Marti et al., 2009; Perkins & Wagner, 2015).

Despite the presence of maternal antibodies, there is a progressive increase in the number of circulating lymphocytes in developing foals. This reflects the animal's ongoing responses to environmental antigens such as those derived from the developing gut microbiota. These include both T and B cells. The majority of the T cells are $CD4^+$ helper cells (Flaminio et al., 2000) (Fig. 2.9).

Cytokine synthesis

Similar delays are also seen in neonatal T cell responses (Perkins & Wagner, 2015). Thus, cytokine responses are generally lower than in adult horses, reflecting T cell immaturity. IFN-γ, IL-4 and IL-10 production are all lower than in adults. However, the balance between the Th1 cytokine, IFN-γ and the Th2 cytokine IL-4 shows a clear Th1 bias (Wagner et al., 2010).

For example, IFN-γ production by $CD4^+$ helper T cells and $CD8^+$ cytotoxic T cells starts slowly shortly after birth and gradually increases over the first year. In contrast, IL-4 is almost undetectable for the first 3 months of life. IL-4 is absent from neonatal foal serum prior to suckling but rises significantly by 24 hours. It is probably absorbed from colostrum (Mariella et al., 2017). These findings, especially

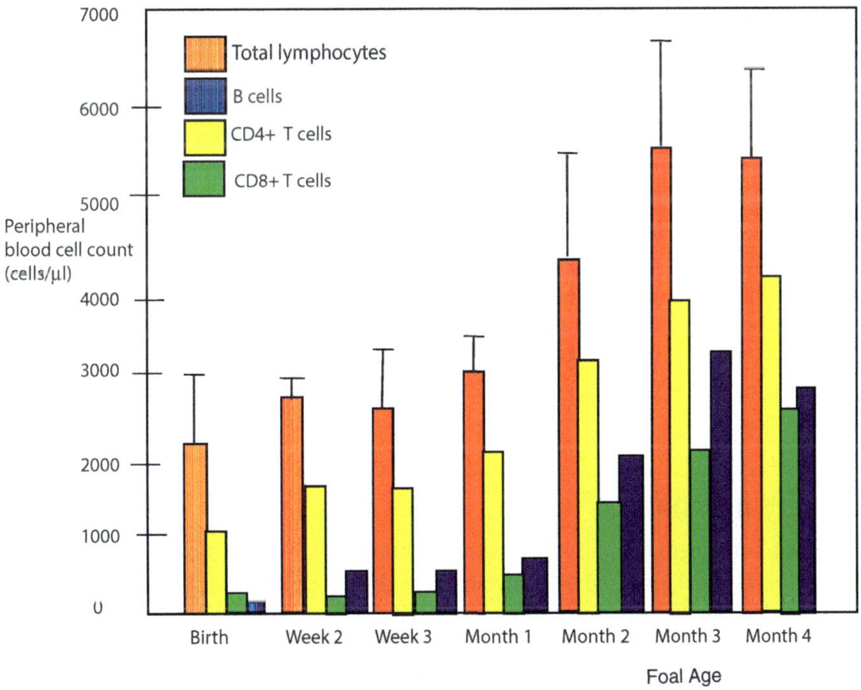

FIGURE 2.9 Peripheral blood total lymphocyte and subpopulation counts in healthy foals from birth to 4 months of age.

Note that the increase involves both T and B cells. The majority of the T cells are $CD4^+$ helper cells. The results represent the mean and standard deviation of 10 foals.

- Selected data derived from a Figure in Flaminio et al. (2000). With permission.

the slow development of type 2 responses, begin to explain how foals are very susceptible to some bacterial infections, such as *R. equi,* during their 1st months of life.

IFN-γ and IL-10 ratios in foals are similar to those in adult horses, suggesting that regulatory T cell function is not impaired in neonatal animals (Wagner et al., 2010).

The production of other cytokines by neonatal foals has also been investigated (Liu et al., 2009). It is clear that the basal production of IFN-γ and IL-6 is relatively low in neonatal foals. Conversely, the basal production of CXCL8, IL-12p35/p40, and IL-23p19/p40 is either comparable to or greater than adult levels. Prior to suckling, neonatal foals had significant quantities of the chemokine CXCL8 in their serum in addition to both IL-13 and IFN-γ.

Mule pregnancy

In a normal horse pregnancy, as described above, the mare mounts an immune response to the paternal MHC antigens expressed on her fetal endometrial cups. The fetal foal is, in effect, a semi-allograft since half its genes come from its sire. When, however, a donkey sire breeds a horse mare to produce mules, the mule fetus is in effect a semi-xenograft since half its genes come from another species. In a normal horse pregnancy, as described above, there are significant decreases in MHC-restricted cytotoxic T cell activity in pregnant mares. Thus, there is, in effect, a shift away from a cellular toward a humoral immune response during horse pregnancy. This pregnancy-associated decline in cytotoxic T cell activity is, however, not observed in mares carrying mule fetuses (Baker et al., 1999). In a normal horse pregnancy, the endometrial cups are progressively destroyed between days 80 and 120. In interspecies mule pregnancies, there is a marked increase in the maternal cytotoxic lymphocyte reaction around the endometrial cups. For example, when horse mares are mated to male donkeys (Jacks) to produce mules, the endometrial cups tend to be destroyed by around day 60 (Antczak & Allen, 1984).

Donkey pregnancy

The gestation length of the Jenny averages about 12 months (It ranges from 11 to 14 months). The donkey placenta is structurally similar to that of the horse in that it is diffuse epitheliochorial and non-invasive. The donkey chorioallantois does, however, have a relatively greater density of microcotyledons. As a result, it is somewhat more efficient than that of the horse, and twin donkey foals are therefore more common.

An analysis of the immune cells infiltrating the endometrium of Jennies found that T cells predominated while large numbers of macrophages were also present. Eosinophils, neutrophils, and B cells were relatively uncommon. Unfortunately, NK cell numbers were not measured in this study (Radar-Chafirovitch et al., 2025).

Donkey colostrum

It is of interest to note that donkey foals are not totally agammaglobulinemic at birth. When born, they have a significant concentration of IgG (897 ± 50 mg/dL) in their serum. In contrast, IgG concentrations in the serum of neonatal horse foals averaged only 300 mg/dL (Turini et al., 2020). As in horses, inadequate intake of colostral immunoglobulins and failure of passive transfer make foals more susceptible to infectious agents. In a study of Ragusana crossbred jennies, it was demonstrated that of 20 foals, 70% demonstrated complete transfer of immunoglobulins (>800 g/dL). whereas the remaining 30% showed evidence of partial failure (400–800 mg/dL), although none of these mules developed clinical disease. This failure was not affected by age, parity, or the season (Nervo et al., 2021).

An analysis of colostrum from nine jennies indicated that at birth, it contained, on average, 195 ± 142 mg/dL of IgG. By 24 hours, this had dropped to 140 ± 97 mg/dL. In this same study, the IgG concentration in donkey foal serum at 24 hours of age, had reached 1491 ± 50 mg/dL (Turini et al., 2020).

References

Aleksic, D., Blaschke, L., Missbach, S., Hanske, J., et al. (2016). Convergent evolution of pregnancy-specific glycoproteins in human and horse. *Reproduction*. https://doi.org/10.1530/REP-16-0236

Allen, W. R., & Stewart, F. (2001). Equine placentation. *Reproduction, Fertility and Development, 13*, 623–634.

Ander, S. E., Diamond, M. S., & Coyne, C. B. (2019). Immune responses at the maternal-fetal interface. *Science Immunology,, 4*, Article eaat6114.

Antczak, D. F. (2020). Immunological memory and tolerance at the maternal-fetal interface: implications for reproductive management of mares. *Theriogenology, 150*, 432–436.

Antczak, D. F., & Allen, W. R. (1984). Invasive trophoblast in the genus Equus. *Annals of Immunology, 135D*, 325.

Aoki, T., Chiba, A., Itoh, M., Nambo, Y., et al. (2020). Colostral and foal serum immunoglobulin G levels and associations with perinatal abnormalities in heavy draft horses in Japan. *Journal of Equine Science, 31*(2), 29–34.

Baker, J. M., Bamford, A. I., & Antczak, D. F. (1999). Modulation of allospecific CTL responses during pregnancy in equids: An immunological barrier to interspecies matings. *Journal of Immunology, 162*, 4496–4501.

Barreto, I. M. L. G., Urbano, S. A., Oliveira, C. A. A., Macedo, C. S., et al. (2020). Chemical composition and lipid profile of mare colostrum and milk of the Quarter horse breed. *PLoS One*. https://doi.org/10.1371/journal.pone.0238921

Bigler, N. A., Bruckmaier, R. M., & Gross, J. J. (2022). Implications of placentation type on species-specific colostrum properties in mammals. *Journal of Animal Science, 100*, 1–9.

Brosnahan, M. M., Miller, D. C., Adams, M., & Antczak, D. F. (2012). IL-22 is expressed by the invasive trophoblast of the equine (*Equus caballus*) chorionic girdle. *Journal of Immunology, 188*, 4181–4187.

Burton, A. B., Wagner, B., Erb, H. N., & Ainsworth, D. M. (2009). Serum interleukin-6 (IL-6) and IL-10 concentrations in normal and septic neonatal foals. *Veterinary Immunology and Immunopathology, 132*, 122–128 (LOOK UP).

Colucci, F. (2019). The immunological code of pregnancy. *Science, 365*, 862–863.

Colucci, F., Boulenouar, S., Kleckbusch, J., & Moffett, A. (2011). How does variability of immune system genes affect placentation? *Placenta, 32*(8), 539–545.

Croy, B. A., van den Heuvel, M. J., Borzychowski, A. M., & Tayade, C. (2006). Uterine natural killer cells: A specialized differentiation regulated by ovarian hormones. *Immunological Reviews, 214*, 161–185.

de Amorim, M. D., Byron, M., Giudici, A. J. L., Chong, L., et al. (2023). Characterization of interferons in the equine conceptus and endometrium. *Journal of Equine Veterinary Science, 25*, Article 104764.

Durr, S., & Kindler, V. (2013). Implication of indoleamine 2,3 dioxygenase in the tolerance towards fetuses, tumors, and allografts. *Journal of Leukocyte Biology, 93*, 681–687.

Enders, A. C., & Carter, A. M. (2004). What can comparative studies of the placenta tell us? - A review. *Placenta, 25*, 1–7.

Figarska, A., Domino, M., Masko, M., & Witkowska-Pitasewicz, O. (2023). Serum cytokine reactions during pregnancy in healthy mares. *Agriculture*. https://doi.org/10.3390/agriculture13020331

Fink, K., Zellweger, R., Weber, J., et al. (2008). Long-term maternal imprinting of the specific B cell repertoire by maternal antibodies. *European Journal of Immunology, 38*, 90–101.

Flaminio, J. B. F., Rush, B. R., Davis, E. G., Hennessey, K., et al. (2000). Characterization of peripheral blood and pulmonary leukocyte function in healthy foals. *Veterinary Immunology and Immunopathology, 73*, 267–285.

Gallacher, K., Champion, L., & Denholm, K. S. (2025). Mare colostrum quality and relationship with foal serum immunoglobulin G concentrations and average daily weight gains. *Equine Veterinary Journal, 57*, 904–914.

Guenther, M. C., Borowicz, P. P., Hirchert, M. R., Semanchil, P. L., et al. (2024). Identifying the immunoglobulin G transporter in equine tissues: A look at the neonatal Fc receptor. *Journal of Equine Veterinary Science, 139*, Article 105131.

Hamza, E., Mirkovitch, J., Steinbach, F., & Marti, E. (2015). Regulatory T cells in early life.: Comparative study of $CD4^+$ $CD25^{high}$ T cells from folks and adult horses. *PLoS One*. https://doi.org/10.1371/journal.pone.0120661

Hart, K. A., & Wong, D. (2024). Humoral Immunity and transfer of maternal Immunity. In D. M. Wong, & P. A. andWilkins (Eds.), *Equine neonatal medicine* (1st ed.). John Wiley and Sons Inc.

Jaworska, J., de Mestre, A. M., Wisniewska, J., Wagner, B., et al. (2022). Populations of NK cells and regulatory T cells in the endometrium of cycling mares. - A preliminary study. *Animals*. https://doi.org/10.3390/ani12233373

Jaworska, J., Tobolski, D., Salem, S. E., Kahler, et al. (2025). Single-cell atlas of the pregnant equine endometrium before and after implantation. *Biology of Reproduction, 112*(3), 458–473.

Jeffcott, L. B., & Jeffcott, T. J. (1974). Studies on passive immunity in the foal. III. The characterization and significance of neonatal proteinuria. *Journal of Comparative Pathology, 84*, 455–465.

Kammerer, R., Ballesteros, A., Bonsor, D., Warren, J., et al. (2020). Equine pregnancy-specific glycoprotein CEACAM49 secreted by endometrial cup cells activates TGFB. *Reproduction*. https://doi.org/10.1530/REP-20-0277

Kenzig, A. R., O'Meara, K. M., Kremer, C. J., Jogan, K. S., et al. (2009). Colostral milk and serum immunoglobulin G concentrations in quarter horse mares and their foals. *Journal of Equine Veterinary Science, 29*, 486–487.

Kohn, C. W., Knight, D., Hueston, W., Jacobs, R., & Reed, S. M. (1989). Colostral and serum IgG, IgA, and IgM concentrations in Standardbred mares and their foals at perurition. *Journal of the American Veterinary Medical Association, 195*(1), 64–68.

Laan, M., Haljasorg, U., Kisand, K., Salumets, A., & Peterson, P. (2016). Pregnancy-induced thymic involution is associated with suppression of chemokines essential for T-lymphocyte progenitor homing. *European Journal of Immunology, 46*, 2008–2017.

LeBlanc, M. M., Johnson, R. D., Calderwood Mays, M. B., & Valderrama, C. (1995). Lymphatic clearance of India ink in reproductively normal mares and mares susceptible to endometritis. *Biology of Reproduction, 1*, 501–506.

Lenicov, F. R., Rodrigues, C. R., Sabatte, J., CabriniM, et al. (2012). Semen promotes the differentiation of tolerogenic dendritic cells. *The Journal of Immunology, 189*, 4777–4786.

Lennard, S. N., Stewart, F., & Allen, W. R. (1985). Transforming growth factor β1 expression in the endometrium of the mare during placentation. *Molecular Reproduction and Development, 42*, 131–140.

Liu, T., Nerren, J., Liu, M., Martens, R., & Cohen, N. (2009). Basal and stimulus-induced cytokine expression is selectively impaired in peripheral blood mononuclear cells of newborn foals. *Vaccine, 27*, 674–683.

Lunn, P., Vagnoni, K. E., & Ginther, O. J. (1997). The equine immune response to endometrial cups. *Journal of Reproductive Immunology, 34*, 203–216.

Mackenzie, C. D. (1975). Histological development of the thymic and intestinal lymphoid tissue of the horse. *Journal of the South African Veterinary Association, 46*(1), 47–55.

Mariella, J., Castagnetti, C., Prosperi, A., Scagliarini, A., & Peli, A. (2017). Cytokine levels in colostrum and in foals' serum pre- and post-suckling. *Veterinary Immunology and Immunopathology*, 34–37.

Marth, C. D., Firestone, S. M., Hanlon, D., Glenton, L. Y., et al. (2018). Innate immune genes in persistent mating-induced endometritis in horses. *Reproduction, Fertility and Development, 30*, 533–545.

Marti, E., Ehrensperger, F., Burger, D., et al. (2009). Maternal transfer of IgE and subsequent development of IgE responses in the horse (*Equus caballus*). *Veterinary Immunology and Immunopathology, 127*, 203–211.

Matson, B. C., & Caron, K. M. (2014). Uterine natural killer cells as modulators of the maternal-fetal vasculature. *International Journal of Developmental Biology, 58*, 199–204.

McGuire, T. C., & Crawford, T. B. (1973). Passive immunity in the foal: Measurement of serum immunoglobulin classes and specific antibody. *American Journal of Veterinary Research, 34*(1), 1299–1303.

McGuire, T. C., Crawford, T. B., Hallowell, A. L., & Macomber, L. E. (1977). Failure of colostral immunoglobulin transfer as an explanation for most infections and deaths in neonatal foals. *Journal of the American Veterinary Medical Association, 17*, 1302–1304.

Munn, D. H., Zhou, M., Attwood, J. T., et al. (1998). Prevention of allogeneic fetal rejection by tryptophan catabolism. *Science, 281*, 1191–1193.

Nervo, T., Bertero, A., Donato, G. G., Suffat, E. P., & Vincenti, L. (2021). Analysis of factors influencing the transfer of passive immunity in the donkey foal. *Italian Journal of Animal Science, 20*(1), 1947–1956.

Noronha, L. E., & Antczak, D. F. (2010). Maternal immune responses to trophoblast: The contribution of the horse to pregnancy immunology. *American Journal of Reproductive Immunology, 64*, 231–244.

Noronha, L. E., Huggler, K. E., de Mestre, A. M., Miller, D. C., & Antczak, D. F. (2012). Molecular evidence for natural killer-like cells in equine endometrial cups. *Placenta, 33*, 379–386.

Perkins, G. A., Goodman, L. B., Wimer, C., Freer, H., et al. (2014). Maternal T-lymphocytes in equine colostrum express a primarily inflammatory phenotype. *Veterinary Immunology and Immunopathology, 161*, 141–150.

Perkins, G. A., & Wagner, B. (2015). The development of equine immunity: Current knowledge on immunology in the young horse. *Equine Veterinary Journal*. https://doi.org/10.1111/evj.12387

Perryman, L. R., Buening, G. M., McGuire, T. C., Torbeck, R. L., et al. (1979). Fetal tissue transplantation for immunotherapy of combined immunodeficiency in horses. *Clinical Immunology and Immunopathology, 12*(2), 238–251.

Perryman, L. E., McGuire, T. C., & Torbeck, R. L. (1980). Ontogeny of lymphocyte function in the equine fetus. *American Journal of Veterinary Research, 41*(8), 1197–1200.

Pozor, M. (2016). Equine placenta - A clinician's perspective. Part 1: Normal placenta -physiology and evaluation. *Equine Veterinary Education, 28*(6), 327–334.

Radar-Chafirovitch, A., Quaresma, M., Yanez-Ortiz, I., Leiva, B., et al. (2025). Donkey endometrium. Characterization of resident immune cells. *Research in Veterinary Science, 184*, Article 105516.

Reber, A. J., Donovan, D. C., Gabbard, J., et al. (2008a). Transfer of maternal colostral lymphocytes promotes development of the neonatal immune system I. Effects on monocyte lineage cells. *Veterinary Immunology and Immunopathology, 123*, 186–196.

Reber, A. J., Donovan, D. C., Gabbard, J., et al. (2008b). Transfer of maternal colostral lymphocytes promotes development of the neonatal immune system II. Effects on neonatal lymphocytes. *Veterinary Immunology and Immunopathology, 123*, 305–313.

Reilly, W. J., & Macdougall, D. F. (1973). The metabolism of IgG in the newborn foal. *Research in Veterinary Science, 14*, 136–137.

Roberts, R. M., Green, J. A., & Schultz, L. C. (2016). The evolution of the placenta. *Reproduction, 152*(5), R179–R189.

Rouse, B. T., & Ingram, D. G. (1970). The total protein and immunoglobulin profile of equine colostrum and milk. *Immunology, 19*, 901–907.

Schoniger, S., Grafe, H., Richter, F., & SchoonH-A. (2018). Expression of indoleamine 2,3-dioxygenase 1 as a transcript and protein in the healthy and diseased equine endometrium. *Research in Veterinary Science, 118*, 278–287.

Sedykh, S. E., Purvinish, L. V., Burkova, E. E., Dmitrenok, P. S., et al. (2021). Analysis of peptides and small proteins in preparations of horse milk exosomes, purified on anti-CD81-Sepharose. *International Dairy Journal*. https://doi.org/10.1016/j.idairyj.2021.104994

Sheoran, A. S., Timoney, J. F., Holmes, M. A., Karzenski, S. S., & Crisman, M. V. (2000). Immunoglobulin isotypes in sera and nasal mucosal secretions and their neonatal transfer and distribution in horses. *American Journal of Veterinary Research, 61*(9), 1099–1110.

Singha, H., Goyal, S. K., & Malik, P. (2015). Cloning and sequence analysis of interleukin (IL)-2, IL-4, IL-10, and IL-18 in the Marwari horse. *The Indian Journal of Animal Sciences, 85*(6), 621–627.

Tallmadge, R. L., McLaughlin, K., Secor, E., Ruano, D., et al. (2009). Expression of essential B cell genes and immunoglobulin isotypes suggests active development and gene recombination during equine gestation. *Developmental & Comparative Immunology, 33*, 1027–1038.

Tallmadge, R. L., Tseng, C. T., King, R. A., & Felippe, M. J. B. (2013). Developmental progression of equine immunoglobulin heavy chain variable region diversity. *Developmental & Comparative Immunology, 41*(1), 33–43.

Tizard, I. R. (2001). The protective properties of milk and colostrum in non-human species. In B. Woodward, & H. H. Draper (Eds.), Adv Nutr Res*: Immunological properties of milk* (Vol 10, pp. 139–166). New York: Kluwer/Plenum Publishers.

Turini, L., Bonelli, F., Nocera, I., Battaglia, F., et al. (2020). Evaluation of Jennie's colostrum: IgG concentrations and absorption in the donkey foals. A preliminary study. *Heliyon, 6*, Article e04598.

Usami, K., Niimi, K., Matsuo, A., Suyama, Y., et al. (2021). The gut microbiota induces Peyer's -patch-dependent secrertion of maternal IgA into milk. *Cell Reports*. https://doi.org/10.1016/j.celrep.2021.109655

Valencia-Ortega, J., Saucedo, R., Pena-Cano, M. I., Hernandez-Valencia, M., & Cruz-Duran, G. (2020). Immune tolerance at the maternal-placental interface in healthy pregnancy and pre-eclampsia. *Journal of Obstetrics and Gynaecology Research, 46*, 1067–1076.

Wagner, B., Burton, A., & Ainsworth, D. (2010). Interferon-gamma, interleukin-4 and interleukin-10 production by T helper cells reveals intact Th1 and regulatory Tp1 cell activation and the delay of the Th2 cell response in equine neonates and foals. *Veterinary Research, 41*(4). https://doi.org/10.1051/vetres.2010019

Walther, S., Rusitzka, T. V., Diesterbeck, U. S., & Czarny, C.-P. (2015). Equine immunoglobulins and organization of immunoglobulin genes. *Developmental & Comparative Immunology, 53*, 303–319.

Woodward, E. M., & Troedssen, M. H. (2013). Equine breeding-induced endometritis: A review. *Journal of Equine Veterinary Science, 33*, 673–682.

CHAPTER

Innate immunity in the horse

3

The first steps in the defense of the body against microbial invaders involve the triggering of an innate immune response. If innate immunity is to be effective, it must rely upon rapid cellular and humoral defensive responses to microbial invasion. These responses may be constitutive and active in a normal healthy animal. Additionally, they can be induced by microbial invasion and any consequential tissue or cell damage. Thus, horses employ sentinel cells that can detect the presence of molecules associated with invading bacteria and viruses. These cells can respond to microbial invaders and damaged or dying cells. Once invaders are detected, the sentinel cells emit signals in the form of cytokines that trigger inflammation and attract white blood cells to the invasion site. In addition, these cells make many different antimicrobial proteins, such as complement components, defensins, and cathelicidins, that can either kill invading bacteria, fungi, and viruses directly or promote their destruction by phagocytic cells. Some of these antimicrobial molecules are present in normal tissues, while others are produced in response to tissue damage.

The equine innate immune system lacks specific memory, and as a result, each episode of infection tends to be treated identically. The intensity and duration of innate responses, such as inflammation, therefore, usually remain unchanged no matter how often a specific invader is encountered (However, see Trained Immunity, Chapter 10). These innate responses also come at a price - the pain of inflammation plus the fever, fatigue, and malaise of sickness. More importantly, however, the innate immune responses are among the triggers that stimulate antigen-presenting cells to initiate adaptive immune responses and eventually result in strong, long-term immunity.

Sentinel cells include macrophages, dendritic cells, and mast cells. These are located throughout the body at sites where they can readily detect and capture bacteria or fungi invading by many different routes. Thus, they are especially prominent within epithelial surfaces such as the skin, respiratory tract, and gastrointestinal tract. Their consistent feature is that they express pattern-recognition receptors.

Pattern recognition receptors

The innate immune system is activated when sentinel cells sense that the body is under attack. Alarm signals are generated either by the presence of invading

The Immunology of Horses and Donkeys. https://doi.org/10.1016/B978-0-443-44863-8.00005-3

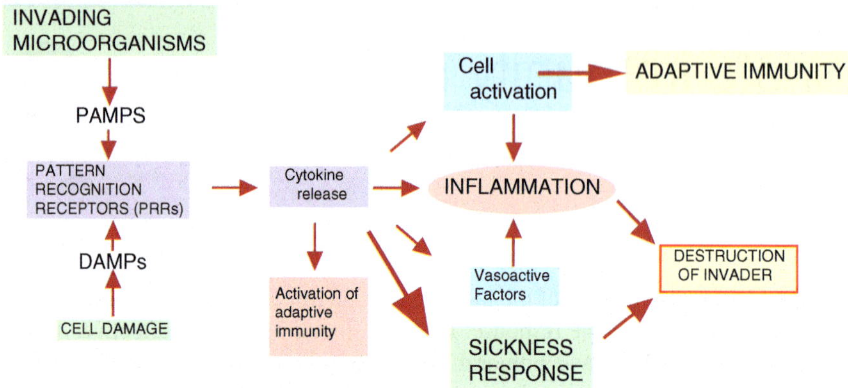

FIGURE 3.1 The basic features of the innate immune response.

It is triggered by microbial invaders and tissue damage. The released cytokines trigger inflammation and sickness that solves both problems.

microorganisms or by dead, damaged, and dying cells. Together, the released pathogen-associated molecular patterns (PAMPs) and damage-associated molecular patterns (DAMPs) bind to pattern-recognition molecules (PRMs) expressed on or in sentinel cells located throughout the body. This binding triggers a cascade of reactions that culminate in local inflammation and the systemic response that we call sickness (Fig. 3.1).

Microbes not only grow very fast but also are highly diverse and can alter their surface structures very rapidly. For this reason, the PRMs of the innate immune system do not try to recognize all possible microbial molecules. Rather, PRMs recognize abundant, essential microbial components. Because they are essential, these components are structurally conserved and are shared by entire classes of pathogens. They form, in effect, conserved molecular patterns. For example, the walls of Gram-positive bacteria are largely composed of peptidoglycans and lipoteichoic acids. Likewise, the walls of Gram-negative bacteria consist of peptidoglycans covered by a layer of lipopolysaccharide (LPS). Acid-fast bacteria are covered in glycolipids. Yeasts have a mannan- or β-glucan-rich cell wall. Viruses contain unique nucleic acid sequences. Horses use many diverse PRMs to ensure the detection of as many of these PAMPs as possible. Most PRMs are cell-associated receptors located on outer cell membranes, within the cytosol, and in cytoplasmic vesicles (endosomes). However, other PRMs, such as the pentraxins, collectins, and ficolins, are soluble PRMs that circulate in the bloodstream.

Toll-like receptors

The most important family of PRMs are the Toll-like receptors (TLRs). In the case of the horse, 12 functional TLR receptors have been identified. TLRs 1, 2, and 4–6 are located on external cell surfaces, where they can bind PAMPs from microbial cell walls. The other TLRs 3 and 7–12 are expressed on endosomal membranes inside cells, where they bind PAMPs from intracellular invaders such as viruses. When triggered, they activate the pathways involved in producing proinflammatory molecules. Thus, they trigger a response immediately they sense the presence of invaders or tissue damage (Akira, 2003; Jungi et al., 2011).

TLRs are mainly expressed on the cell types most likely to encounter invaders (Fig. 3.2).

These sentinel cells include neutrophils, monocytes, macrophages, keratinocytes, and dendritic cells. However, dendritic cells and macrophages consist of multiple subpopulations, and their TLR expression may differ between these subpopulations as well as depending upon their degree of activation. TLRs are also expressed on T and B cells, in addition to some non-immune cells such as the epithelial cells that line the respiratory and intestinal tracts. TLRs are also expressed on bone marrow stem cells, the source of blood leukocytes. Bacterial lipopolysaccharides binding to TLR4 on these stem cells stimulate them to divide, resulting in increased leukocyte production. An increase in leukocyte numbers in the blood (the white cell count) is therefore a consistent feature of equine infectious diseases (Baldridge et al., 2011).

Equine skin keratinocytes are located in an excellent position to encounter and respond to invading pathogens. They express both TLR4 and TLR5. As a result, when exposed to the TLR4 ligand LPS, the keratinocytes increase their production of the three inflammatory cytokines, IL-1β, IL-6, and CXCL8 mRNA. When exposed to the TLR5 ligand flagellin, they produce IL-6 and CXCL8. Keratinocytes do not respond to the ligands of TLR2, TLR9, or NOD (Leise et al., 2010).

TLR4 is expressed in large amounts on the pulmonary intravascular macrophages in equine lungs (Singh Suri et al., 2006). TLR4 and TLR5 recognize bacterial

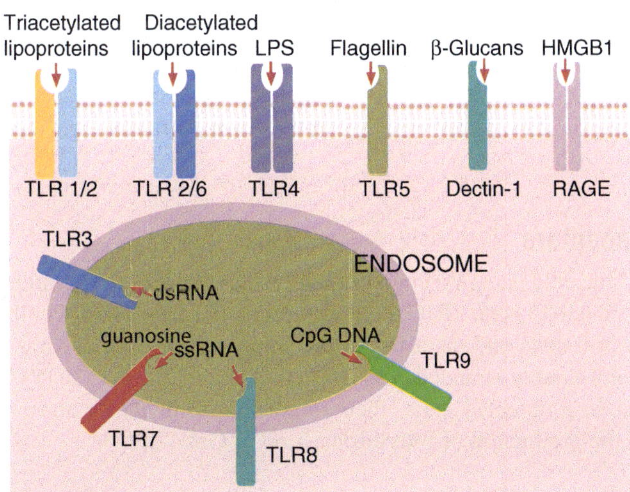

FIGURE 3.2 Equine TLRs.

The equine Toll-like receptors and their sites of expression.

lipopolysaccharide and flagellin, respectively. On exposure to these bacterial PAMPs, neutrophils, peritoneal macrophages, and mononuclear phagocytes produce reactive oxygen species that can kill bacteria and they express the mRNA for proinflammatory cytokines such as TNF-α (Barton et al., 1996). Thus, they all express TLR4. However, on exposure to flagellin from *Salmonella enterica* Typhimurium, only the neutrophils respond! Thus, they express TLR5. Conversely, unlike other domestic mammals, equine mononuclear phagocytes do not appear to express TLR5 (although they contain its mRNA). As a result, they are unresponsive to bacterial flagellin (Kwon et al., 2011). It is also of interest to note that stimulation of equine neutrophils by bacterial lipopolysaccharides through TLR4 prolongs their lifespan by inhibiting their apoptosis. This phenomenon of enhanced neutrophil survival may play a role in the development of a systemic inflammatory response syndrome (Chapter 5) (Anderson et al., 2018).

TLR9 recognizes microbial DNA. There are, however, species differences in its ligand-binding sites. For example, the TLR9 gene sequences in horses and donkeys differ by 1%. Three amino acid substitutions within the binding site account for these differences and they may have a significant influence on its binding specificity. The horse TLR9 also differs significantly in its sequence from other mammals. Thus, it shows 14% divergence from TLR9 in humans (Manuja et al., 2019).

The TLR family in the Perissodactyls is divided into six sub-families based on their gene sequences. For example, TLR4 and TLR5 are clustered together, as are TLR1, TLR6, and TLR10. Among the Equidae, the average evolutionary divergence is only 0.3%, indicating a high degree of conservation. In each of these TLR genes, there are haplotypes shared between equid breeds and species. Twenty-five SNPs have been identified in the TLR6-1-10 cluster alone. Of these, seven are synonymous while 18 are not.

There are 13 single-nucleotide polymorphisms (SNPs) in the coding regions. of the equine TLR3, TLR7, and TLR8 genes. The SNP frequencies vary greatly between different horse breeds (Astakhova et al., 2009). Each horse breed has a predominant major haplotype (Stejskalova et al., 2025). TLR3 and TLR9 show the greatest haplotype variation. There is evidence that genetic selection differs between the TLRs that primarily detect viruses and those with different ligands (Stejskalova et al., 2024).

RIG-like receptors

TLRs are not the only pattern recognition molecules expressed by sentinel cells. Retinoic acid inducible gene (RIG)-like receptors (RLRs) are a family of PRMs expressed within cells and, as a result, are important sensors of viral RNA. They can detect viral double-stranded (ds) RNA molecules. Because dsRNA molecules do not occur in uninfected cells, their interaction with RLRs activates caspases and triggers the production of interferons (Loo & Gale, 2011).

NOD-like receptors

Nucleotide-binding oligomerization domain (NOD), leucine-rich repeat receptors (NLRs) are PRMs that can also detect intracellular PAMPs. Although NLRs differ in their location and function, they react to microbial PAMPs and trigger innate responses to invaders. NOD1 and -2 have been most extensively studied. NOD1 binds bacterial peptidoglycans, whereas NOD2 binds muramyl dipeptides and serves as a general sensor of intracellular bacteria. Ligand binding to the NLRs activates the NF-κB pathway and triggers the production of proinflammatory cytokines. NOD2 binding also triggers the production of antibacterial defensins. NOD3 binds diverse ligands, including many viral nucleic acids as well as inorganic particles such as silica, asbestos, and alum (Elinav et al., 2011).

AIM2 receptors

Absent in melanoma 2 (AIM2) is a pattern recognition receptor expressed within the cytosol of hematopoietic cells that recognizes foreign double-stranded DNA through a 200 amino acid hemopoietic, interferon inducible, nuclear (HIN) domain, and activates interferon responses. It plays an important role in host defense against intracellular bacteria and viruses. The number of AIM2 genes varies between species. For example, in humans, there are four members of the AIM2 family, whereas it is absent from dogs and cats. Horses appear to possess four related genes with a unique HIN–B domain and an intact AIM2 gene (Cridland et al., 2012).

Cyclic GMP-AMP synthase

Another important DNA binding pattern recognition molecule is cyclic GMP AMP synthase (cGAS). dsDNA activates cGAS that then binds and activates an adaptor molecule, known as stimulator of interferon genes (STING). STING then activates the IRF3 and NF-κB pathways. The activation of these pathway by bacterial and viral double-stranded DNA leads to the induction of large quantities of interferons, especially IFN-β as well as the NF-κB-mediated expression of inflammatory cytokines (Motwani et al., 2019). Equine cGAS has been characterized. It contains 510 amino acids and is 57 kDa in size. It is encoded by a gene located on chromosome ECA10.

Equine macrophages, mast cells, and dendritic cells express many other PRMs that can recognize microbial molecules and trigger innate responses. These include C-type lectin receptors (CLRs) that bind carbohydrates, a molecule called CD36 that binds lipoproteins, and CD1 that binds glycolipids. CD1 is an important ligand-binding molecule that is also used for the presentation of selected lipid antigens to T cells and so triggers adaptive immune responses (Chapter 10).

Soluble pattern-recognition molecules

While the TLRs, NLRs, and RLRs are expressed on cell surfaces, soluble PRMs in tissue fluids also bind PAMPs. They promote the destruction of any organisms they encounter by acting as opsonins and so causing them to undergo phagocytosis. In general, soluble PRMs do not induce the expression of inflammatory cytokines. That task is accomplished by the cell-surface receptor PRMs (Werling & Coffey, 2007). It appears, however, that soluble PRMs may have a special role to play on equine body surfaces, such as the epithelial mucosa of the airways. Epithelial cells at these sites produce large quantities of these molecules that contribute to the defenses of the respiratory tract (Smole et al., 2020) (Fig. 3.3).

Since many bacterial PAMPs are glycoproteins and polysaccharides, circulating carbohydrate-binding lectins play important roles in innate immunity. Three extracellular lectin families, the S-, C-, and P-type lectins, are involved in this process. Collagenous (C-type lectins (CTL) lectins are a family of soluble pattern recognition receptors that play an important role in the defense against infections. The best recognized of these collagenous lectins are the pulmonary surfactant proteins SP-A and SP-D, mannose-binding lectins (MBL) 1 and 2, and the ficolins, as well as diverse collectins. Three collagenous lectins have been characterized in the horse: MBL-C, SP-A, and SP-D. All require calcium to bind to their carbohydrate ligands. Each end of a CTL peptide chain has a distinct function; the C-terminal domain binds to carbohydrates, whereas the N-terminal domain interacts with cell receptors or complement components, thereby exerting its biological effect. CTLs may be both soluble and membrane-bound.

Horses possess 11 collagenous lectin genes. These proteins are highly polymorphic, and as a result, 92 variants have been identified in their gene coding regions. Twelve of these may significantly affect the protein structure (Fraser et al., 2018). These mutations have been associated with altered resistance to infectious diseases such as Streptococcal infections, enteritis, septicemia, and herpesvirus infections.

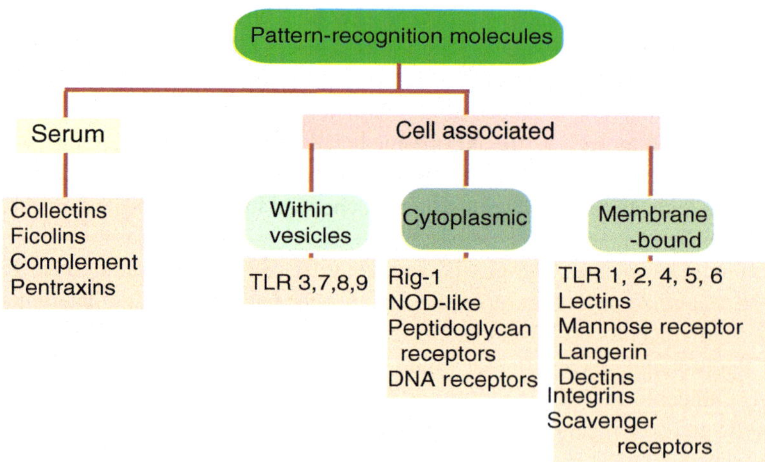

FIGURE 3.3 The diversity of pattern-recognition molecules.

Some circulate in the bloodstream, whereas others are present in different cellular compartments.

The most important of the soluble CTLs are the mannose-binding lectins (MBL). MBLs are synthesized in the liver and are found in large amounts in the bloodstream. They have multiple sites that bind oligosaccharides, such as *N*-acetylglucosamine, mannose, glucose, galactose, and *N*-acetylgalactosamine. MBL thus binds strongly to bacteria such as *S. enterica* and *Listeria monocytogenes*. Bacteria coated by MBL are readily ingested by phagocytic cells. MBLs also play an important role in activating the complement system through the lectin pathway.

CTLs such as the surfactant proteins SP-A and SP-D are produced in the lungs of horses by cells such as pulmonary intravascular macrophages located in the alveolar septa (Bocking et al., 2021) (Chapter 7).

Some CTLs are expressed on cell surfaces where they can bind bacteria, fungi, and some viruses. The most important are the dectins. The dectins bind β-glucans on fungal cell walls and play an important role in antifungal defense by promoting their phagocytosis and intracellular destruction (Chapter 16).

Selectins are CTLs expressed on vascular endothelial cells and play a key role in the emigration of leukocytes from the bloodstream into the tissues during inflammation. Galectins are extracellular S-type lectins. Their name derives from their binding specificity for galactosides. They play a role in inflammation by binding leukocytes to the extracellular matrix. Other soluble collectins include the ficolins (H-, L-, and M-ficolins) produced by the liver and some lung cells. These, too, can bind bacterial carbohydrates and activate the complement system. There are also many cell-associated lectins. DC-SIGN, for example, is a lectin expressed on macrophages and dendritic cells. Not only does DC-SIGN recognize bacterial carbohydrates, but it also interacts with T cells and so is used by dendritic cells to interact with T cells. The collectins are especially important in the defense of foals whose immature adaptive immune system is not yet capable of mounting an effective protective response (Thompsen et al., 2011).

Inflammasomes

The first steps in inflammation occur when PAMPs and DAMPs bind to pattern recognition receptors on sentinel cells and initiate the assembly of the large multiprotein complexes called inflammasomes. Inflammasomes are molecular machines that initiate and then regulate inflammatory responses. Inflammasome-mediated responses are critical in controlling microbial infections as well as in regulating some metabolic processes.

The initial steps following receptor binding involve activation of an adaptor protein called MyD88. This, in turn, activates the nuclear factor-kappa B (NF-κB) pathway (Fig. 3.4).

NF-κB is a transcription factor that, once activated, turns on many different defensive genes, especially those involved in cytokine production (Fig. 3.5).

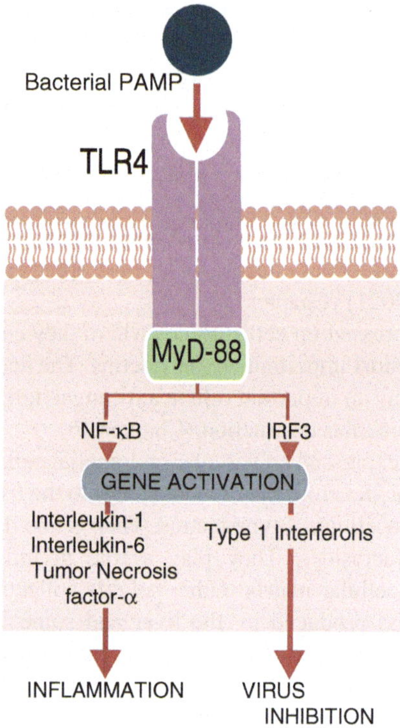

FIGURE 3.4 The role of MyD88.

The first step in TLR signaling is activation of the transcription factor MyD88. This initiates either an inflammatory response mediated by NF-κB or an antiviral response triggered by interferon regulatory factor (IRF).

Structure

Inflammasomes consist of multiple peptide chains arranged in a star-like fashion (Fig. 3.6). Each inflammasome chain consists of three domains. These are a pathogen sensor domain (PRR) that recognizes the PAMPs and DAMPs; an adaptor domain that signals to the cell; and an effector domain such as a pro-caspase that activates the cytokines. Once the inflammasome complex is assembled, binding of its ligand to the sensor domain ensures that caspase-1 is activated and cytokines such as TNF-α, IL-1β, and IL-18 are produced, activated, and released (Fig. 3.6).

Many different inflammasomes have been characterized in mammals, each generated by different PAMPs and DAMPs, and each consists of slightly different components and thus generates different cytokines and proinflammatory molecules (Lamkanfi & Dixit, 2014). For example, one type senses pathogens by using ALRs (AIM2-like receptors) as sensors. AIM2 peptides detect cytoplasmic DNA. Another type of inflammasome uses NLR peptides such as NLRP1, NLRP3, or NLRC4 as

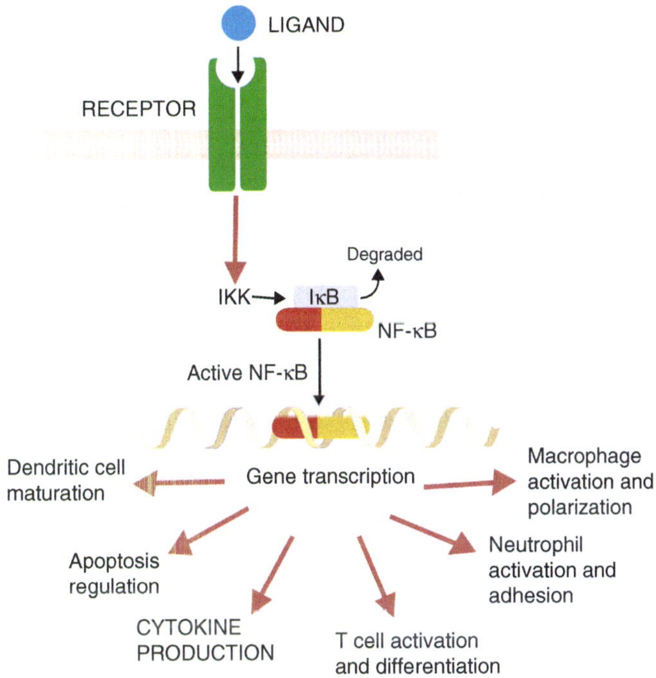

FIGURE 3.5 The role of NF-κB.

The second step in triggering an inflammatory response involves releasing NF-κB to function as a transcription factor by removing its inhibitors.

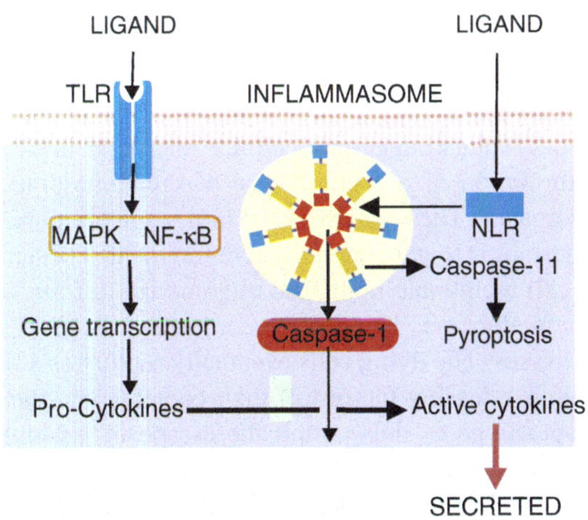

FIGURE 3.6 Inflammasome structure and function.

The role of inflammasomes in equine inflammatory responses.

sensors. These also contain an adaptor ASC (apoptosis-associated speck-like) peptide and an effector protein, caspase-1.

Functions

When a PAMP binds to its corresponding TLR, signals are passed to the sentinel cell. As a result, inflammasomes assemble, signal transduction cascades are initiated, and pro-inflammatory cytokines are produced by the cell. Each step in the process involves multiple biochemical reactions involving different inflammasomes. Additionally, the cell surface TLRs use different signaling pathways than do the intracellular TLRs. All extracellular TLRs except TLR3 use the MyD88 adaptor protein to activate the transcription factors, nuclear factor kappa-B (NF-κB), and IRF3. NF-κB activates the genes for three inflammatory cytokines, interleukin-1 (IL-1), interleukin-6 (IL-6), and tumor necrosis factor-alpha (TNF-α). IRF3 activates the gene for interferon-β (IFN-β) (Kawasaki & Kawai, 2014). Although some inflammasomes require TLR-mediated activation and downstream NF-κB mediated transcription of pro-IL-1 and IL-18, others do not require this transcriptional activation step (Vrentas et al., 2018). Once activated, caspase 1 acts on pro-IL-1 and pro-IL-18 to generate the active forms of these cytokines (Bryant & Fitzgerald, 2009).

In the case of the horse, NLRP3 inflammasomes in peripheral blood mononuclear cells can be activated by exposure to proinflammatory stimuli such as ATP, nigericin, alum crystals and urate crystals. Equine NLRC4 and AIM2 inflammasomes can be activated by cytosolic flagellin and double-stranded DNA. Their activation induces IL-1β secretion. In the presence of potassium efflux blockers, IL-1β production is partially but not completely attenuated (Ahn et al., 2020).

Pyroptosis

Pyroptosis is a form of programmed cell death characterized by the formation of pores in the cell membrane and the escape of IL-1β and IL-18 through these pores. Unlike apoptosis, pyroptosis triggers inflammation. This is normally a defensive process that prevents replication of intracellular microbial invaders. Pyroptosis is triggered by the formation of a specific type of inflammasome, which activates several different caspases. These caspases, in turn, cleave a pore-forming effector protein called gasdermin D to generate an active fragment. The activated gasdermin fragments bind to cell membrane lipids and oligomerize to form large, ring-shaped pores in the plasma membrane. These pores permit the escape of cell contents and cytokines into the tissues. The dying cells eventually rupture as a result of increased osmotic pressure, thus releasing the rest of their contents into the tissues (Evavold et al., 2018). Pyroptosis pores thus permit the escape of inflammatory mediators such as IL-1β, HMGB-1, and ATP that act as "alarmins" and so activate local immune cells. They also release both nuclear and mitochondrial DNA. Mitochondrial DNA is a potent proinflammatory DAMP since its nucleotide composition reflects its microbial origins (Yu et al., 2021).

Necroptosis

Necroptosis is a form of programmed necrosis triggered by death receptors such as TNFR, nucleic acid sensors, or by TLR-signaling. They activate threonine kinases and form molecular complexes called necrosomes. Together with proteases and kinases, necrosomes generate a pore-forming protein that inserts itself into the cell wall and allows the escape of cellular contents. Necroptosis is characterized by cell and organelle swelling, eventually resulting in rupture of the cell membrane. This alerts the immune system by the release of danger signals (DAMPs). It is, in effect, a backup cell death program that is used when apoptosis fails. Like pyroptosis, necroptosis causes inflammation because of the escape of intracellular DAMPs such as HMGB-1 and interleukin 33 (IL-33) into the surrounding tissues (Dondelinger et al., 2016).

Antimicrobial peptides

A key component of constitutive immunity in the horse is the production of multiple antimicrobial peptides. The horse appears to have more than the average number and diversity of these peptides. The reasons for this are unclear, but it may be a consequence of being a hindgut fermenter with a large cecum full of bacteria that need to be monitored and controlled. Horse bactericidal peptides include at least one lysozyme, five cathelicidins, nine defensins, one psoriasin, one hepcidin, and five equinins (Bruhn et al., 2009, 2011). As in other mammals, neutrophils are the major source of these antibacterial peptides. In the horse, these also include lysozyme and the neutrophil antibacterial peptides NAP-1 and -2. Mesenchymal stem cells also release antimicrobial peptides that can kill many bacteria involved in wound infections (Harman et al., 2017).

Lysozyme

Equine lysozyme is a protein of 16.7 kDa encoded by a gene located on chromosome ECA 6. It is a hydrolytic enzyme that attacks bacterial cell walls. It cleaves the beta (1-4) bond between *N*-acetyl muramic acid and *N*-acetyl glucosamine and thus destroys cell wall peptidoglycans in Gram-positive bacteria. This may not necessarily be immediately lethal to invading bacteria, but it can result in the exposure of the vulnerable bacterial cell membrane to other antibacterial pathways, such as complement or the defensins. Equine lysozyme can can oligomerize and form filaments and multimeric complexes with oleic acid. The enzyme contains calcium, which is essential for its proper functioning. Lysozyme can be found in horse serum, synovia, endometrium, colostrum, and milk. It is produced by equine granulocytes as well as by intestinal Paneth cells (Cui et al., 2023). Horse lysozyme can kill Gram-positive bacteria such as *Streptococcus equi* and *Staphylococci*. It also attacks Gram-negative bacteria such as *E. coli*, *Klebsiella pneumoniae*, and *Bordetella bronchiseptica*.

Lysozyme is also a potent opsonin, binding to bacterial surfaces and facilitating phagocytosis in the absence of specific antibodies and under conditions in which its enzyme activity is ineffective (Linde et al., 2008).

Equine lysozyme readily unfolds and then aggregates to form stable "molten globules." These can then assemble into ring-shaped and linear amyloid fibrils (Morozova-Roche, 2007). While important experimentally, this form of amyloid does not appear to cause clinical disease in horses (Chapter 5).

It is interesting to note that in Arabian mares, the activity of lysozyme appears to be seasonal. Thus it tends to be higher in the months of June, July, and August and lower in December, January, and February (Gill et al., 1985). Serum lysozyme levels also tend to decline with increasing age (Sotirov, 2004).

NK-lysin

As described in Chapter 10, natural killer (NK) cells can kill target cells and bacteria using their cytotoxic molecules: perforin, granulysin, and NK-lysin (Chapter 10). Equine NK lysin has been characterized. It is a protein containing 83 amino acids with 67% sequence identity to its pig homolog. It shows 41% identity with neutrophil granulysin. It appears to be expressed by most populations of equine lymphocytes (Davis et al., 2005).

Equinins

Equinins are a group of five closely related proteinase inhibitors found in the granules of equine neutrophils as well as in their tracheobronchial secretions. Like the related chemokine, neutrophil-activating peptide (NAP-2), they inhibit microbial proteinase K and subtilisin, and as a result, have antibacterial and antiviral functions. For example, they can kill *Streptococcus zooepidemicus*, *Escherichia coli*, and *Pseudomonas aeruginosa*. They are also active against equine herpesvirus 2 (Pellegrini et al., 1998).

Psoriasin

Psoriasin is a member of the S100 protein family. It was first isolated from psoriasis lesions in human skin. Equine psoriasin-1 is encoded by a gene on chromosome ECA5. It can be detected in equine skin, trachea, esophagus, intestine, and vulva. It has activity against *E. coli* (Bruhn et al., 2011).

Cathelicidins

Cathelicidins, - otherwise called myeloid antimicrobial peptides, are a heterogeneous family of peptides stored in the secretory granules of neutrophils and macrophages and released when these cells are activated (Zhu & Gao, 2017). The mRNA from three horse cathelicidins has been characterized, eCATH-1, eCATH-2, and

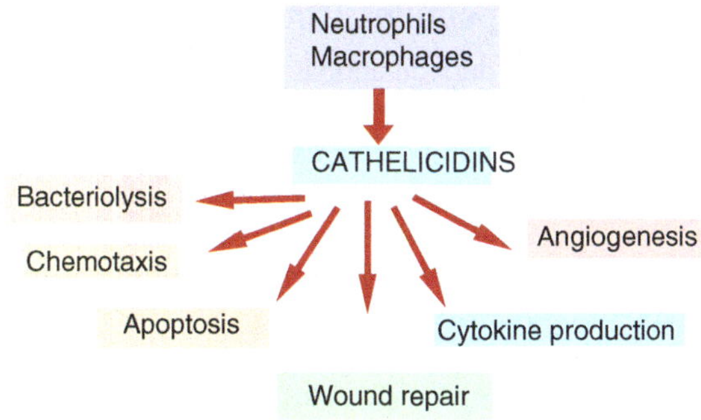

FIGURE 3.7 Functions of cathelicidins.

The diverse functions of the Equine cathelicidins.

eCATH-3. They each have a 99% conserved constant domain but a diverse antigen-binding region. They are 12–100 amino acids in size, with a characteristic "cathelin" domain at their C-terminus. As many as 50% of horses carry a null allele of eCATH-1, while it also appears to be unable to encode a functional protein within myeloid cells. On the other hand, the genes encoding eCATH-2 and eCATH-3 are functional. All horses appear to express eCATH-2 and -3 (Scocchi et al., 1999) (Fig. 3.7).

Cathelicidins are stored as inactive precursors and are activated by proteolytic cleavage when released from leukocytes. In addition to their antibacterial activity, they are also immunomodulatory (van Harten et al., 2018).. They all have broad-spectrum antibacterial activity. eCATH-2 has antifungal activity as well. They are active against both Gram-positive and Gram-negative bacteria as well as fungi, enveloped viruses, and parasites. As with other antimicrobial peptides, they interact with the negatively charged lipid membranes of microorganisms. However, because of their high cationic charge, they can also interfere with their protein synthesis and DNA replication since cathelicidins efficiently bind bacterial nucleic acids. They can then deliver these nucleic acids to dendritic cells and, as a result, trigger a very strong interferon response. Cathelicidins have a variety of immunomodulatory functions, including the control of inflammation by influencing wound repair, angiogenesis, and chemotaxis (Araujo et al., 2022). Cathelicidins are present in the bronchial secretions of horses with chronic obstructive pulmonary disease (Chapter 20).

Donkey cathelicidins

Donkeys produce two unique cathelicidins termed EA-CATH1 and EA-CATH2. They contain 25 and 26 amino acids, respectively, and are thus similar in size to eCATH-2 and eCATH-3. They do not appear to have significant sequence homology to cathelicidins in other species. EA-CATH1 can bind and cause rapid disruption of the surface membrane of *Staphylococcus aureus*, resulting in bacterial lysis. It also possesses hemagglutinating and hemolytic activity.EA-CATH2 does not appear to have antibacterial activity (Lu et al., 2010).

Neutrophil antimicrobial peptides (NAP)

Horses possess two neutrophil-derived antibacterial peptides, eNAP-1 and eNAP-2. These two peptides are structurally unrelated and belong to different peptide families. eNAP-1 is related to granulins, whereas eNAP-2 is related to the equinins. NAP-1 accounts for only about 1% of a typical level in other species. It has antibacterial activity against *Strep equi, E. coli*, and *P. aeruginosa*. Compared to typical defensins, it is a weak antimicrobial agent (Bruhn et al., 2011). eNAP-2 has similar antibacterial properties to eNAP-1 but is present in horse neutrophils at much higher concentrations. It is a peptide of 46 amino acids (4.7 kDa). It appears to act by selectively inhibiting bacterial serine proteases (Bruhn et al., 2011).

Defensins

Defensins are small cysteine-rich proteins 18–45 amino acids in length. They act by binding and disrupting bacterial membranes. Defensins are arranged in a β-sheet crosslinked by three or four disulfide bonds. They are classified into α- and β-defensins based on their origin and on the number and position of these disulfide bonds (Bagnicka et al., 2010). Defensins may be produced at a constant rate (constitutively) or in response to microbial infection. Some defensins attract monocytes, immature dendritic cells, and T cells. Their production is stimulated by the inflammatory cytokines, IL-1β and TNF-α. All defensins identified so far can kill or inactivate bacteria, fungi, or enveloped viruses. Some defensins can also neutralize microbial toxins such as those from *Bacillus anthracis, Corynebacterium diphtheriae,* and *Staphylococcus aureus*. Although present in normal tissues, defensin concentrations increase in response to infections (Machado & Ottolini, 2015). Neutrophils of horses lack defensins, which makes them very different from other mammals (Fig. 3.8).

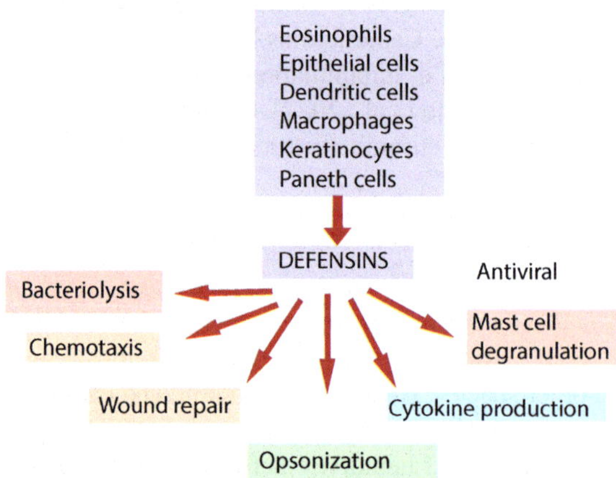

FIGURE 3.8 Equine defensins.

Their origins and multiple functions.

Alpha defensins

The horse appears to rely to a much greater extent than other mammals on intestinal α-defensins. (They are absent from cattle, pigs, and dogs.) Thirty-eight alpha defensin gene transcripts have been detected in equine intestinal tissues, and at least 20 of these are functional antibacterial peptides. These genes are located in a single cluster on chromosome ECA27 (Bruhn et al., 2011).

The α-defensins are found in the granules of Paneth cells in the small intestine (Chapter 13). When released into the intestine, their antibacterial effects influence the composition of the intestinal microbiota (Sahi et al., 2005). The equine defensin DEFA1 is an enteric defensin exclusively produced in Paneth cells. It has potent activity against the major horse pathogens, especially *Rhodococcus equi* and *Streptococcus equi* (Bruhn, Cauchard, et al., 2009; Leonard et al., 2012). However, no other active peptides have been detected, yet. If these transcripts are expressed, the horse would be the first eutherian outside the primates, lagomorphs, and rodents known to possess multiple alpha-defensins (Bruhn, Cauchard, et al., 2009).

Beta defensins

Beta-defensins are constitutively expressed in the epithelial cells that line the airways, skin, salivary gland, reproductive, and urinary systems (Leonard et al., 2012; Patil et al., 2004). Horses possess six beta-defensins that are ~60% identical to those in other mammals (Bagnicka et al., 2010). For example, equine beta-defensin-1 (DEFB1) is 69.5% identical to porcine BD-1. They are expressed in many different tissues, including the heart, liver, lungs, pancreas, and especially the Paneth cells of the gastrointestinal tract. A β-defensin gene cluster is located on chromosome ECA27q17. Analysis has identified nine functional equine β-defensin genes, as well as 10 β-defensin-related pseudogenes (Looft et al., 2006). Six are very similar in sequence to human defensin BD-4.

Hepcidin

As its name suggests, hepcidin is an antibacterial peptide produced by the equine liver. It is a cysteine-rich protein of 25 amino acids (9.1 kDa). It is encoded by a gene on chromosome ECA10 (Filho et al., 2010). It is produced in response to stimulation by IL-6. Hepcidin is an innate antibacterial peptide. It also sequesters iron within cells and as a result, causes a hypoferremia and therefore inhibits bacterial growth (Barton & Acton., 2019). Donkey hepcidin shows 98% sequence homology to that of the horse (Oliveira-Filho et al., 2012).

The equine complement system

Protection from infection requires that the body respond to microbial invaders as rapidly and effectively as possible in order to minimize damage. A critical component of this early constituent response is the complement system. This system can detect and kill invaders long before other defenses have had a chance to respond. The complement system consists of a network of interacting pattern-recognition proteins, enzymes, receptors, and regulatory proteins that once activated, kill invaders fast. The major complement proteins bind covalently (and hence irreversibly) to the surface of invading microbes and this leads to the production of membrane attack complexes. These complexes punch holes in the invaders and so result in microbial killing. The complement system is activated by the presence of microbial surface molecules or by antigen-bound antibodies (Fig. 3.9).

Complement forms an essential innate defense system. Although its main function is to kill pathogens immediately they enter the body, the complement system also alerts the other defensive systems to the presence of invaders, regulates inflammation, removes damaged or altered cells, and regulates adaptive immune responses. It is also involved in the removal of antigen-antibody complexes, blood vessel formation, mobilization of stem cells, tissue regeneration, and lipid metabolism. The first step, complement activation, is triggered through three different pathways, referred to as the alternative, the lectin, and the classical pathways. The alternative and lectin pathways are activated by contact between specific complement proteins in serum, and microbial surface carbohydrates. The classical pathway, in contrast, is activated when antibodies bind to microbial surface antigens and thus works in association with adaptive immune responses (Cagliani et al., 2016).

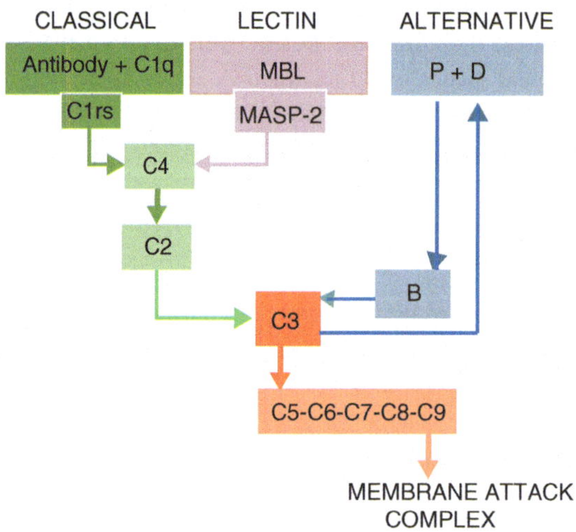

FIGURE 3.9 The three complement pathways act through different routes to activate the most important component, C3.

C3 in turn activates the terminal complement pathway and generates membrane attack complexes that punch holes in invading microorganisms, thus killing them.

Complement proteins

By convention, complement proteins are either labeled numerically with the prefix C (e.g., C1, C2, C3) or designated as "factors" by letters of the alphabet (FB, FD, FP, and so forth). Some of these proteins are found free in serum, whereas others are cell-surface receptors. Collectively, complement components account for up to 10% of the proteins in blood serum - a reflection of the critical importance of this system. Their size varies from 22.5 kDa for factor D (FD) to about 460 kDa for C1q. Complement proteins are synthesized at multiple sites throughout the body. Thus, C3, C6, C8, and FB are made in the liver, whereas C2, C3, C4, C5, FB, FD, FP, and FI are made by macrophages. C1q is also produced by mast cells. Neutrophil granules may store large quantities of C6 and C7. As a result, these proteins are readily available for defense at sites where neutrophils accumulate. Complement components, like other proteins, have multiple allelic variations and collectively these variants form a horses "complotype" (Harris et al., 2012). These variations may influence an animal's relative susceptibility to infectious and inflammatory diseases.

The equine complement system appears to be similar to that in other mammals. It consists of multiple proteins, many of which are pro-enzymes. When activated by bacterial surfaces, bacterial carbohydrates, or antigen-bound immunoglobulins, these pro-enzymes are activated in a cascade fashion. The system plays a critical role in the elimination of invading microorganisms. The three activating pathways are all focused on activating the third component of complement, C3. C3 is central to the protective effects of the system. Equine C3 has been characterized. It is a heterodimeric protein with an alpha chain of 118 kDa and a beta chain of 68 kDa linked by a disulfide bond. It is very similar in structure to human C3 (Boschwitz & Timoney, 1993). It is synthesized by liver cells and macrophages and is the most abundant complement component in horse serum. Equine C3 exists in at least four different allelic forms (Bowling & Dileanis, 1990).

Complement pathways

The alternative pathway

The equine alternative complement pathway has been characterized, and its major components identified. It accounts for 80%–90% of all complement activation. It is activated when microbial cell walls encounter complement proteins. In healthy normal animals, C3 spontaneously breaks down into two fragments called C3a and C3b. This breakdown of C3 exposes binding sites for a protein called factor H (FH). When FH binds to these sites, it permits a protease called factor I (FI) to cleave the C3b, and the C3b is promptly destroyed. In a healthy animal, therefore, there is a continuous low-level activation of C3, but FH and FI destroy the C3b as fast as it is generated.

In contrast, when C3b binds to an invading bacterium, FH cannot bind to the C3b. As a result, FI is inactivated, and the C3b remains attached to the microbial surface. The bound C3b exposes a binding site for another complement protein called factor B (FB) and as a result, an alternative C3 convertase forms. This alternative C3 convertase, C3bBb, cleaves bound C3 to generate more C3b. C3bBb is, however, very unstable, with a half-life of only 5 minutes. If another protein called factor P (FP or properdin) binds to the complex, it forms a stable C3bBbP complex with a half-life of 30 minutes. Since C3b generates more C3bBbP, the net effect of all this is that a positive feedback loop is established where increasing amounts of C3b are produced and irreversibly bound to the surface of the invading organism, leading eventually to its destruction through the teminal complement pathway. (Equine properdin is a protein of 51 kDa whose gene is located on the X chromosome).

Quantitative studies of the alternative complement system in horses, donkeys, and mules have been conducted (Sotirov, 2004). There appear to be significant breed differences, and its activity tends to decline as the animals age. The pathway appears to differ from that in other mammals in that it requires the presence of Ca^{++} to function (Leid et al., 1985).

The lectin pathway

As described above, mannose-binding lectin is a member of the collectin family. It acts as a pattern recognition molecule that binds to mannose residues on microbial surfaces. This binding triggers the lectin pathway by activating MBL-associated serine protease-2 (MASP). The activated MBL-MASP complex first cleaves C4 into C4a and C4b. Another complement component, C2, then binds to the C4b to form a complex, C4b2. The bound C2 is then cleaved by MASP-2 to generate C4b2b. Cell-bound C4b2b is another C3 convertase that acts on C3 to generate C3a and C3b and expose the thioester group on the C3b. The complement terminal pathway is then activated, membrane attack complexes are generated and the invader is killed. Interestingly, in sick horses (intestinal disease, pneumonia, or vasculitis), MBL-MASP activity drops significantly (Podolsky et al., 2006).

The classical pathway

The classical complement pathway differs from the others since it is triggered when the complement component C1q encounters antibody bound to an invading microorganism. Unlike the alternate and lectin pathways, the classical pathway cannot therefore be activated until antibodies are made and this may take 7–10 days after onset of infection.

When antibody molecules bind to an invader, active sites on their Fc regions are exposed. The first component of the classical pathway is a protein complex called C1. C1 consists of three subunits (C1q, C1r, C1s) bound together by calcium. C1q is activated when it binds to activating sites on clustered antibody molecules.

This binding triggers a conformational change and C1s is converted into an active protease. Active C1s then cleaves C4 into C4a and C4b. C2 then binds to C4b to form the complex C4b2. Activated C1s then splits the bound C2, generating a small peptide fragment C2a and the C4b2b complex. The newly formed C4b2b complex is a potent C3 convertase as described above.

Activation of C3 by these convertases results in its cleavage into two fragments, C3a (7 kDa) and C3b (110 kDa). Equine C3b has a reactive thioester side-chain that binds to microbes and marks them for destruction by immune cells. Activation of this thioester side-chain must be carefully regulated to ensure that C3b does not bind and kill normal cells. To prevent such accidents, the thioester group in inactive C3 is normally hidden within the folded molecule (Fig. 3.10). The other breakdown product, C3a is chemotactic for neutrophils and is therefore pro-inflammatory (Fig. 3.10).

The activation of C3b by C4b2b is a major step, because each C4b2b complex can generate as many as 200 C3b molecules. Since these reactions are confined to the microenvironment close to microbial surfaces, the newly formed C3b bind to nearby microbes.

Horse Imm

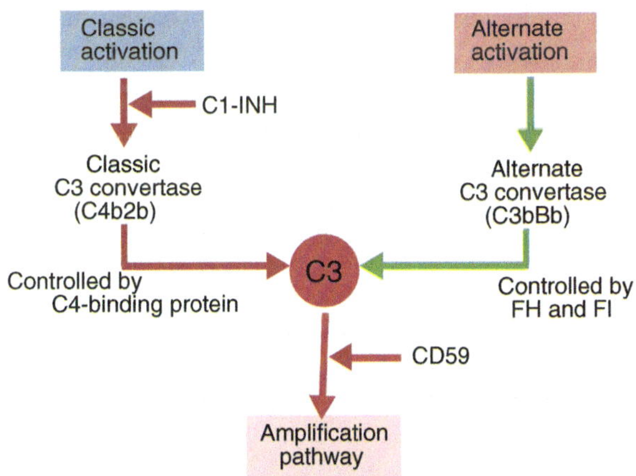

FIGURE 3.10 The classical pathway of complement is triggered by antibodies, especially IgM binding to a bacterial cell surface.

The alternative pathway (which is probably much more important) acts simply by binding to an activating surface such as a bacterial cell wall. Its activities are carefully regulated to prevent excessive activation (C1-INH, C1 inhibitor).

The terminal pathway

The three activating complement pathways, alternate, lectin and classical all converge by generating C3 convertases bound to the microbial surface. Activated C3b is also a convertase, a C5 convertase! The C3b convertase binds and breaks C5 (195 kDa) into a small fragment called C5a, leaving a large fragment C5b attached to the C3b. This exposes a site on C5b that can bind two new proteins, C6 and C7, to form C5b67. The C5b67 complex then inserts itself into the microbial cell wall. The complex first binds a molecule of C8 to form C5b678. Twelve to 18 C9 molecules then polymerize with the C5b678 complex to form tubular structures called membrane attack complexes (MAC). These MACs insert into microbial cell membranes and punch holes in its surface. As a result, the invaders are killed by osmotic lysis.

Just as important as the direct complement-mediated lysis of invaders are the potent inflammatory effects of the small peptide C5a. C5a can degranulate mast cells and stimulate platelets to release histamine and serotonin.C5a is a powerful attractant for neutrophils and macrophages. It increases vascular permeability, causes lysosomal enzyme release from neutrophils and thromboxane release from macrophages and regulates some T cell responses. C5a is not bactericidal although the other small complement peptides, C3a and C4a can kill bacteria such as *E. coli*, *Pseudomonas aeruginosa*, *Enterococcus faecalis*, and *Streptococcus pyogenes*. C3a acts like other antimicrobial peptides, acts by disrupting bacterial membranes.

Equine C5a is rapidly converted to C5a des arg through the removal of its C-terminal arginine. Large quantities of C5a des arg can be found in horse serum when the complement system is activated. C5a des arg acts on blood neutrophils to promote their adhesiveness and cause their aggregation. This permits the neutrophils to swarm and attack invading organisms even more effectively (Slauson et al., 1987).

It is relevant to note here that complement can exacerbate some equine diseases. For example, complement causes erythrocyte lysis in animals suffering from equine infectious anemia (EIA). Thus, the EIA virus binds to the red cell surface. The infected horse makes antibodies that bind to the viral antigens so activating the classical complement pathway and leading to red cell lysis by generating membrane attack complexes (Sentsui & Kono, 1987).

References

Ahn, H., Kim, J., Lee, H., Lee, E., & Lee, G.-S. (2020). Characterization of equine inflammasomes and their regulation. *Veterinary Research Communications, 44*, 51–59.

Akira, S. (2003). Mammalian toll-like receptors. *Current Opinion in Immunology, 15*, 5–11.

Anderson, S. L., Townsend, H. G. G., & Singh, B. (2018). Role of toll-like receptor-4 and caspase -3. -8 and -9 in lipopolysaccharide-induced delay of apoptosis in equine neutrophils. *American Journal of Veterinary Research, 79*(4), 424–432.

Araujo, J. B., Sastre de Souza, G., & Lorenzon, E. B. (2022). Indolicidin revisited: Biological activity, potential applications and perspectives of an antimicrobial peptide not yet fully explored. *World Journal of Microbiology & Biotechnology*. https://doi.org/10.1007/s11274-022-03227-2

Astakhova, N. M., Perelygin, A. A., Zharkikh, A. A., Lear, T. L., et al. (2009). Characterization of equine and other vertebrate TLR3, TLR7, and TLR8 genes. *Immunogenetics, 61*, 529–539.

Bagnicka, E., Strazlkowska, N., Jóźwik, A., Krzyzewsli, J., et al. (2010). Expression and polymorphism of defensins in farm animals. *Acta Biochimica Polonica, 57*(4), 487–497.

Baldridge, M. T., King, K. Y., & Goodell, M. A. (2011). Inflammatory signals regulate hematopoietic stem cells. *Trends in Immunology, 32*, 57–65.

Barton, J. C., & Acton, R. T. (2019). Hepcidin, iron, and bacterial infection. *Vitamins and Hormones, 110*, 223–242.

Barton, M. H., Collatos, C., & Moore, J. N. (1996). Endotoxin induced expression of tumor necrosis factor, tissue factor, and plasminogen activator inhibitor activity by peritoneal macrophages. *Equine Veterinary Journal, 28*(3), 382–389.

Bocking, L., Johnson, L., Singh, A., Desai, A., et al. (2021). Expression of surfactant protein A and D, and CD9 in lungs of 1 and 30-day-old foals. *BMC Veterinary Research*. https://doi.org/10.1186/s12917-021-02943-5

Boschwitz, J. S., & Timoney, J. F. (1993). Purification and characterization of equine complement factor C3. *Veterinary Immunology and Immunopathology, 38*, 139–153.

Bowling, A. T., & Dileanis. (1990). Population data and a fourth allele for equine complement component 3 (C3). *Animal Genetics, 21*, 83–86.

Bruhn, O., Cauchard, J., Schlisselhuber, M., et al. (2009). Antimicrobial properties of the equine a-defensin DEFA1 against bacterial horse pathogens. *Veterinary Immunology and Immunopathology, 130*, 102–106.

Bruhn, O., Grotzinger, J., Cascorbi, I., & Jung, S. (2011). Antimicrobial peptides and proteins of the horse – Insights into a well-armed organism. *BMC Veterinary Research*. https://doi.org/10.1186/1297-9716-42-98

Bruhn, O., Paul, S., Tetens, J., & Thaller, G. (2009). The repertoire of equine intestinal a-defensins. *BMC Genomics*. https://doi.org/10.1186/1471-2164-10-631

Bryant, C., & Fitzgerald, K. A. (2009). Molecular mechanisms involved in inflammasome activation. *Trends in Cell Biology, 19*, 455–464.

Cagliani, R., Forni, D., Filippi, G., Mozzi, A., et al. (2016). The mammalian complement system as an epitome of host pathogen conflicts. *Molecular Ecology, 25*, 1324–1339.

Cridland, J. A., Curley, E. Z., Wykes, M. N., Schroder, K., et al. (2012). The mammalian PYNIN gene family: Phylogeny, evolution, and expression. *BMC Evolutionary Biology, 12*, 140.

Cui, C., Li, L., & Peng, J. (2023). Paneth cells in farm animals: Current status and future direction. *Journal of Animal Science and Biotechnology*. https://doi.org/10.1186/s40104-023-00905-5

Davis, E. G., Sang, Y., Rush, B., Zhang, G., & Blecha, F. (2005). Molecular cloning and characterization of equine NK-lysin. *Veterinary Immunology and Immunopathology, 105*, 163–169.

Dondelinger, Y., Huipiau, P., Saeys, Y., Bertrand, J. M., & Vandenabeele, P. (2016). An evolutionary perspective on the necroptotic pathway. *Trends in Cell Biology, 26*(10). https://doi.org/10.1016/j.tcb.2016.004

Elinav, E., Strowig, T., Henao-Mejia, J., & Flavell, R. A. (2011). Regulation of the antimicrobial response by NLR proteins. *Immunity, 34*(5), 665–679.

Evavold, C. L., Ruan, J., Tan, Y., Xia, S., et al. (2018). The pore forming protein gasdermin D regulates interleukin-1 secretion from living macrophages. *Immunity, 48*(1), 35–44.

Filho, J. P. O., Badial, P. R., Cunha, P. H. J., Cruz, T. F., et al. (2010). Cloning, sequencing, and expression analysis of the equine hepcidin gene by real-time PCR. *Veterinary Immunology and Immunopathology, 135*, 34–42.

Fraser, R. S., Arroyo, L. G., Meyer, A., & Lillie, B. N. (2018). Identification of genetic variation in equine collagenous lectins using targeted resequencing. *Veterinary Immunology and Immunopathology, 202*, 153–163.

Gill, J., Kompanowska-Jeziereska, E., Jakubow, K., Kott, A., & Szumska, D. (1985). Seasonal changes in the white blood cell system, lysozyme activity, and cortisol level in Arabian brood mares and their foals. *Comparative Biochemistry & Physiology, 81A*(3), 511–523.

Harman, R. M., Yang, S., He, M. K., & Van der Walle, G. R. (2017). Antimicrobial peptides secreted by equine mesenchymal stromal cells inhibit th growth of bacteria commonly found in skin wounds. *Stem Cell Research & Therapy*. https://doi.org/10.1186/s13287-017-0610-6

Harris, C. L., Heurich, M., Rodriguez De Cordoba, S., & Morgan, B. P. (2012). The complotype: Dictating risk for inflammation and infection. *Trends in Immunology, 33*, 513–521.

Jungi, T. W., Farhat, K., Burgener, I. A., & Werling, D. (2011). Toll-like receptors in domestic animals. *Cell and Tissue Research, 343*, 107–120.

Kawasaki, T., & Kawai, T. (2014). Toll-like receptor signaling pathways. *Frontiers in Immunology*. https://doi.org/10.3389/fimmu.2014.00461

Kwon, S., Gewirtz, A. T., Hurley, D. J., Robertson, T. P., et al. (2011). Disparities in TLR5 expression and responsiveness to flagellin in equine neutrophils and mononuclear phagocytes. *Journal of Immunology, 186*, 6263–6270.

Lamkanfi, M., & Dixit, V. M. (2014). Mechanisms and functions of inflammasomes. *Cell, 157*, 1013–1022.

Leid, R. W., Coley, S. C., Blanchard, D. P., & Perryman, L. E. (1985). Equine alternative pathway activation by unsensitized rabbit red blood cells. *Veterinary Immunology and Immunopathology, 9*, 71–85.

Leise, B. S., Yin, C., Pettigrew, A., & Belknap, J. K. (2010). Proinflammatory cytokine response of cultured equine keratinocytes to bacterial-pathogen-associated molecular pattern motifs. *Equine Veterinary Journal, 42*(4), 294–303.

Leonard, B. C., Affolter, V. K., & Bevins, C. L. (2012). Antimicrobial peptides: Agents of border protection for companion animals. *Veterinary Dermatology, 23*(3). 177-e36.

Linde, A., Ross, C. R., Davis, E. G., Dib, L., et al. (2008). Innate Immunity and host defense peptides in veterinary medicine. *Journal of Veterinary Internal Medicine, 22*, 247–265.

Loo, Y. M., & Gale, M. J. R. (2011). Immune signaling by RIG-I-like receptors. *Immunity, 34*, 680–692.

Looft, C., Paul, S., Regenhard, P., Kuiper, H., et al. (2006). Sequence analysis of a 212 kb defensin gene cluster on ECA 27q17. *Gene, 376*, 192–198.

Lu, Z., Wang, Y., Zhail, L., Che, Q., Wang, H., et al. (2012). Novel cathelicidin-derived antimicrobial peptides from *Equus asinus*. *The FEBS Journal, 277*, 2329–2339.

Machado, L. R., & Ottolini, B. (2015). An evolutionary history of defensins: A role for copy number variation in maximizing host innate and adaptive immune responses. *Frontiers in Immunology*. https://doi.org/10.3389/fimmu.2015.00115

Manuja, A., Manuja, B. K., & Singha, H. (2019). Sequence and functional variability of toll-like receptor 9 gene in equines. *Molecular Immunology, 105*, 276–282.

Morozova-Roche, L. A. (2007). Equine lysozyme: The molecular basis of folding, self-assembly and innate amyloid toxicity. *FEBS Letters, 581*(14), 2587–2592.

Motwani, M., Pesiridis, S., & Fitzgerald, K. A. (2019). DNA sensing by the cGAS-STING pathway in health and disease. *Nature Reviews Genetics*. https://doi.org/10.1038/s41576-0151-1

Oliveira-Filho, J. P., Marques, J. A., Cunha, P. H. J., Medeiros, G. X., et al. (2012). Sequencing and expression analysis of hepcidin mRNA in donkey (*Equus asinus*) liver. *Pesquisa Veterinaria Brasileira*. https://doi.org/10.1590/s100-736x2012001000019

Patil, A., Hughes, A. L., & Zhang, G. (2004). Rapid evolution and diversification of mammalian a-defensins as revealed by comparative analysis of rodent and primate genes. *Physiological Genomics, 20*, 1–11.

Pellegrini, A., Kalkinc, M., Hermann, M., Grünig, B., et al. (1998). Equinins in equine neutrophils: Quantification in tracheobronchial secretions as an aid to the diagnosis of chronic pulmonary disease. *The Veterinary Journal, 155*, 257–262.

Podolsky, M. J., Lasker, A., Flaminio, M. J. B. F., Gowda, L. D., et al. (2006). Characterization of an equine mannose-binding lectin and its roles in disease. *Biochemical and Biophysical Research Communications, 343*, 928–936.

Sahi, H.-G., Pag, U., Bonness, S., et al. (2005). Mammalian defensins: Structures and mechanism of antibiotic activity. *Journal of Leukocyte Biology, 77*, 466–475.

Scocchi, M., Bontempo, D., Boscolo, S., Tomasinsig, L., et al. (1999). Novel cathelicidins in horse leukocytes. *FEBS Letters, 457*, 459–464.

Sentsui, B., & Kono, Y. (1987). Complement-mediated hemolysis of horse erythrocytes treated with equine infectious anemia virus. *Archives of Virology, 95*, 53–66.

Singh Suri, S., Janardhan, K. S., Parbhakar, O., Caldwell, s, et al. (2006). Expression of toll-like receptor 4 and 2 in horse lungs. *Veterinary Research, 37*, 541–551.

Slauson, D. O., Skrabalak, D. S., Neilsen, N. R., & Zwahlen, R. D. (1987). Complement induced equine neutrophil adhesiveness and aggregation. *Veterinary Pathology Online, 24*, 239–249.

Smole, U., Kratzer, B., & Pickl, W. F. (2020). Soluble pattern recognition molecules: Guardians and regulators of homeostasis at airway mucosal surfaces. *European Journal of Immunology, 50*(5), 624–642. https://doi.org/10.1002/eji.201847811

Sotirov, L. (2004). Lysozyme and complement concentrations in horses, donkeys, and mules. *Revue de Médecine Vétérinaire, 155*(4), 221–225.

Stejskalova, K., Janova, E., Splichalova, P., Futas, J., et al. (2024). Twelve toll-like receptor (TLR) genes in the family Equidae - Comparative genomics, selection and evolution. *Veterinary Research Communications, 48*, 725–741.

Stejskalova, K., Vychodilova, L., Janova, E., Oppelt, J., & Horin, P. (2025). Innate immunity toll-like triad TLR6-1-10 and its diversity in distinct horse breeds. *Veterinary Medical Science*. https://doi.org/10.1002/vms3.70230

Thomsen, T., Schlosser, A., Holmskov, U., & Sorensen, G. L. (2011). Ficolins and FIBCD1: Soluble and membrane bound pattern recognition molecules with acetyl group selectivity. *Molecular Immunology, 48*, 369–381.

Van Harten, R. M., van Woudenbergh, E., & Haagsman, H. P. (2018). *Cathelicidins: Immunomodulatory antimicrobials*. Vaccines. https://doi.org/10.3390/vaccines6030063

Vrentas, C. E., Schaut, R. G., Boggiatto, P. M., Olsen, S. C., et al. (2018). Inflammasomes in livestock and wildlife: Insights into the intersection of pathogens and natural host species. *Veterinary Immunology and Immunopathology, 201*, 49–56.

Werling, D., & Coffey, T. J. (2007). Pattern recognition receptors in companion and farm animals: The key to unlocking the door to animal disease? *The Veterinary Journal, 174*, 240–251.

Yu, P., Zhang, X., Liu, N., Tang, L., et al. (2021). Pyroptosis: Mechanisms and diseases. *Signal Transduction and Targeted Therapy.* https://doi.org/10.1038/s41392-021-00507-5

Zhu, S., & Gao, B. (2017). Positive selection in cathelicidin host defense peptides: Adaptation to exogenous pathogens or endogenous receptors. *Heredity, 118*, 453–465.

CHAPTER

The hematology of horses and donkeys

4

The leukocytes of the equids play a central role in both their innate and adaptive immune systems. If leukocyte numbers decline, then adverse consequences may result. If their numbers increase, this may be diagnostically important. Changes in the hemogram of horses and donkeys are common and are not necessarily associated with diseases or infections. For example, as horses age, their erythrocyte count drops steadily. Likewise, their total leukocyte counts drop as a result of a decline in lymphocyte numbers (Allen, 1989). Breed differences also affect blood neutrophil counts. Thus, hot-blood horse breeds tend to have higher leukocyte counts than cold-blood breeds. Likewise, Thoroughbreds and Arabians have approximately equal numbers of neutrophils and lymphocytes, whereas cold-blood horses and miniature horses have neutrophil: lymphocyte ratios of 1.7 and 0.67, respectively (Freeman et al., 2022). Other physiological factors affect leukocyte counts, including training, exercise, and reproductive status (Satue et al., 2014) (Fig. 4.1) (Tables 4.1 and 4.2).

Equine leukocytes

The structural features of the leukocytes of the Equidae are generally unremarkable and very similar to those of the other domestic mammals. The only exceptions are equine eosinophils, which contain many, relatively large granules (Table 21.1) (Burden et al., 2016).

Neutrophils

Neutrophils are produced by stem cells in the bone marrow. After they have completed their development, neutrophils are released into the bloodstream. Here, they divide into two populations (or pools). A circulating pool that flows freely through the bloodstream with other blood cells and a marginal pool of neutrophils attached to vascular endothelial cells in organs such as the lungs and intestines. The marginal pool, in effect, acts as a reservoir of cells that can be mobilized on demand. The two pools are of roughly equal size (Carakostas et al., 1981). The mean total blood granulocyte pool has been estimated to be about $5.65 \pm 1.514 \times 10^8$ granulocytes/kg body weight of which about 2.1×10^8 granulocytes/kg are

The Immunology of Horses and Donkeys. https://doi.org/10.1016/B978-0-443-44863-8.00030-2

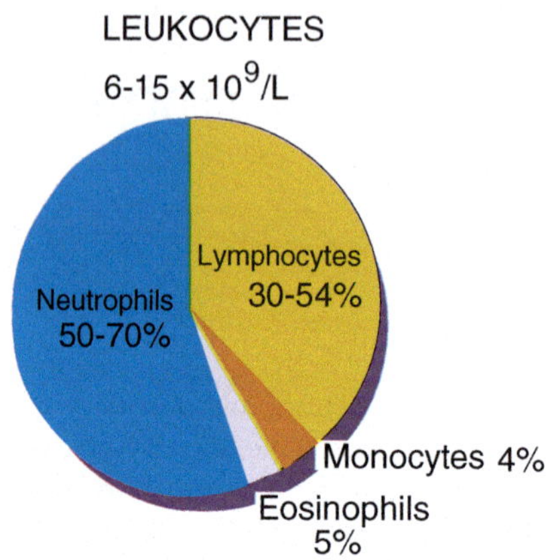

FIGURE 4.1 The composition of leukocyte populations in equine blood.

Note that these numbers are highly variable. They vary with breed, age, and seasonality.

Table 4.1 The leukocytes of the horse.

Cell	Total count	Percentage
WBCs	6–15 × 10^9/L	
Neutrophils	3.7–6.0	58 ± 12
Lymphocytes	0.9–5.9	29 ± 11
Monocytes	0.1–0.6	5 ± 2.5
Eosinophils	0.1–3.0	7 ± 3.5
Basophils	0	-

WBCs, *white blood cells.*

Data from Allen, B. V. (1989). Age differences in the haemogram of the National Hunt trained racehorse. Equine Veterinary Journal, 21*(4), 309–310.*

Table 4.2 The leukocytes of the donkey.

Cell	Total count	Percentage
WBCs	6–15 × 10^9/L	
Neutrophils	3.7 (2.3–5.9)	38 (23–59)
Lymphocytes	5.7 (2.2–9.6)	54 (34–69)
Monocytes	0.3 (0–0.75)	3.0 (0–7.5)
Eosinophils	0.4 (0.1–0.9)	4.0 (0.94–9.1)
Basophils	0.005 (0–0.66)	0.05 (0–0.5)

WBCs, *white blood cells.*

*Data from Burden, F. A., Hazell-Smith, E., Mulugeta, G., & Patrick, V., et al. (2016). Reference intervals for biochemical and haematological parameters in mature domestic donkeys (*Equus asinus*) in the UK.* Equine Veterinary Education, 28*(3), 134–139.*

circulating, and 2.94×10^8 granulocytes/kg are in the marginal pool. All these numbers increase in horses suffering from infections (Carakostas et al., 1981). Neutrophils are the most abundant leukocytes in equine blood, accounting for 50%–70% of the total number of blood leukocytes. They average about $5 \pm 2.5 \times 10^9$ cells/L, although this can vary greatly between individual animals. Mature neutrophils in the horse are about 10–15 μm in diameter. They have a clear gray or pale blue cytoplasm with pinkish cytoplasmic granules (Fig. 4.2).

Neutrophil populations respond strongly to inflammatory stimuli and, as a result, are considered to be the primary indicators of inflammation. Many diseases appear to be driven by the presence and activities of large numbers of neutrophils. These include sepsis, systemic inflammatory response syndrome, some inflammatory airway diseases, and endotoxemia caused by Gram-negative bacterial infections. Circulating equine neutrophils have a mean half-life of 10.5 hours and are thus renewed about 1.5 times daily (Freeman et al., 2022). Once they migrate into the tissues, they do not return to the bloodstream. They survive in tissues for 1–2 days before undergoing apoptosis. Unlike human neutrophils, equine neutrophils are

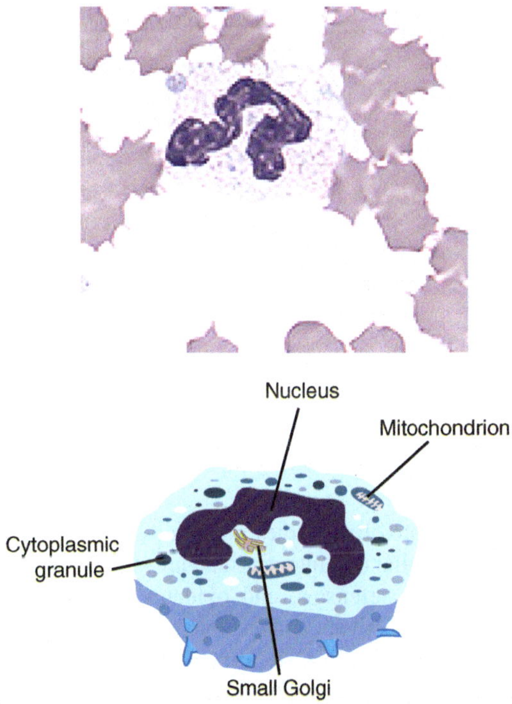

FIGURE 4.2

An equine neutrophil and its structure.

- Courtesy of Dr Mark Johnson.

not attracted by formylated peptides such as *N*-formyl-methionyl-leucyl-phenylalanine (Anderson & Singh, 2018).

When newly produced in response to severe inflammatory stimuli, neutrophils may develop so-called "toxic" changes, including basophilic staining in the cytoplasm, vacuole formation in the cytoplasm, and toxic granulation. They usually have highly segmented nuclei. and there tend to be fewer band forms found in the horse when compared to other domestic mammals (0–0.3 $\times$ 10^9 cells/L). These band forms are immature neutrophils recently produced by the bone marrow. It appears that horses do not generate a major "left shift" in response to inflammatory stimuli (Blais & Penedo, 2022). In fact, in cases of systemic inflammation, horses may undergo a temporary neutropenia. Their numbers rebound however, so that this is followed by a neutrophilia. Increased numbers of immature band forms in the bloodstream result from bone marrow stem cell activation and are indicative of an ongoing innate immune response. This increase is often accompanied by increased monocyte and eosinophil numbers. Elevated neutrophil counts over 15 $\times$ 10^9/L are also indicative of infection. Other "toxic" changes in neutrophils include alterations in cell size, the presence of Döhle bodies, and changes in nuclear morphology. These changes are especially associated with severe inflammation and infections. (Döhle bodies are blue or grayish-blue cytoplasmic inclusions that consist of free ribosomes or fragments of rough endoplasmic reticulum.)

Neutrophil granules contain large amounts of myeloperoxidase. It is released when the cells are activated and plays a key role in generating the neutrophil oxidative burst. This occurs just as the cell is generating a phagolysosome and thus acts as a powerful and lethal source of oxidants. Neutrophil granules also contain elastase, a serine protease that plays a key role in digesting ingested microorganisms within the phagolysosome. Equine neutrophils appear to have less potent elastases than do human neutrophils, but this likely depends upon the nature of the activating stimulus and the presence of cytoplasmic inhibitors (Anderson & Singh, 2018).

Equine neutrophil granules also contain lysosomal acid hydrolase as well as peroxidase. Acid phosphatase is also present in these granules, as well as lysozyme. Secondary granules can release metalloproteases, lactoferrin, cathelicidin, and lipocalin 2 (Coignoul et al., 1984).

Activation

Neutrophils must be activated before they attack and destroy invaders. Thus, when neutrophils bind to endothelial cell integrins and are stimulated by CXCL8 (IL-8) or C5a, they secrete elastase, defensins, and oxidants. The elastase promotes their adhesiveness. The oxidants activate tissue proteases, which in turn release TNF-α from macrophages. The TNF-α, in turn, attracts more neutrophils, thus providing feedback amplification. Platelet-activating factor also activates neutrophils, confirming the close functional linkage between neutrophils and blood platelets.

Equine neutrophils depend upon the presence of arachidonic acid to synthesize eicosanoids. This is different from human neutrophils. It appears that this results from the equine phospholipase A2 being less phosphorylated and hence less efficient (Anderson & Singh, 2018). There are also age-related differences in neutrophil functionality since neutrophils from foals less than 1 week of age have less intense chemotactic responses to complement-activated serum. Their ability to phagocytose *Staphylococcus aureus* is also reduced in comparison to neutrophils from adults. In fact, the neutrophil killing ability in foals declines for the first 100 days after birth before rising to adult levels. Foals appear to be born with higher neutrophil numbers that may compensate for these functional deficiencies. However, this early age unresponsiveness does not apply to other stimuli or neutrophil functions. For example, foal neutrophils are sensitive to formylated methionine stimulation at birth. They can generate an oxidative burst and transcribe significant quantities of mRNA encoding IFN-γ, CXCL8, and IL-23p35 while, at the same time, reducing TNF-α mRNA. Additionally, foal neutrophils stimulated by *Rhodococcus equi* increase their mRNA production of IL-6. CXCL8, IL-23p19, and TNF-α (Liu et al., 2009) (Fig. 4.3).

Equine neutrophil functionality also appears to increase significantly in response to intense exercise such as racing. Thus, they show increased reactive oxygen species production and increased phagocytic activity. They may also develop a transient neutropenia within 72 hours after a race (Donovan et al., 2007) (Chapter 24).

Equine neutrophils express a complete panel of cell surface toll-like receptors (TLRs 1, 2, and 4–6.) On exposure to TLR ligands, such as bacterial

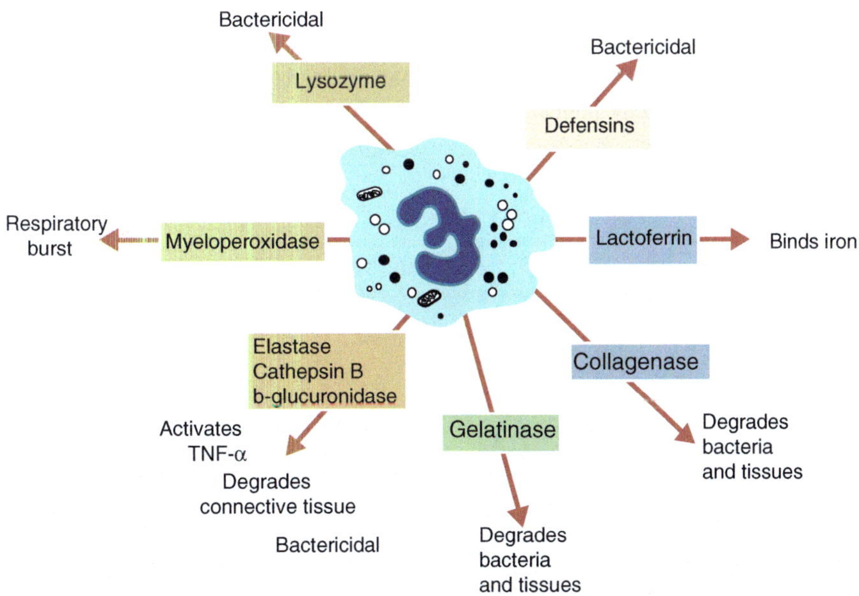

FIGURE 4.3

Some of the bioactive molecules produced by activated neutrophils.

lipopolysaccharides, these cells are activated. In addition to secreting newly synthesized cytokines, these activated neutrophils are larger, with decreased granularity as well as increased expression of certain cell surface adhesive molecules such as CD11 and CD18.

Activated neutrophils are a feature of inflammatory diseases, including inflammatory bowel disease (Weiss & Evanson, 2003). The presence of band cells and toxic neutrophils is a feature of horses suffering from severe systemic inflammatory response syndrome (Lambert et al., 2016) (Chapter 5).

Extracellular traps

In addition to their phagocytic functions, neutrophils can trap and kill extracellular bacteria. This happens when the neutrophils undergo a form of cell death termed NETosis as an alternative to apoptosis or necroptosis (Papayannopoulos & Zychlinsky, 2009). After activation by the chemokine CXCL8, bacterial lipopolysaccharides, or phorbol esters, equine neutrophils release the contents of their azurophil granules (Rebordao et al., 2014). These enzymes rupture the nuclear and plasma membranes, and as a result, the cell releases long strands of sticky nuclear chromatin and its associated proteins into the extracellular environment. These neutrophils die within 3–8 hours, but the released chromatin strands accumulate to form an extensive network of decondensed DNA called neutrophil extracellular traps (NETs) (Tan et al., 2021). On occasion, neutrophils may also release their NETs in a rapid, oxidant-independent process that is not suicidal (Fig. 4.4).

The NETs are densely coated with antimicrobial proteins, including citrullinated histones and bactericidal granule components such as elastase, myeloperoxidase, cathepsin G, calreticulin, lactoferrin, and gelatinase. NETs can also activate the alternative complement pathway. As a result, the NETs not only trap nearby

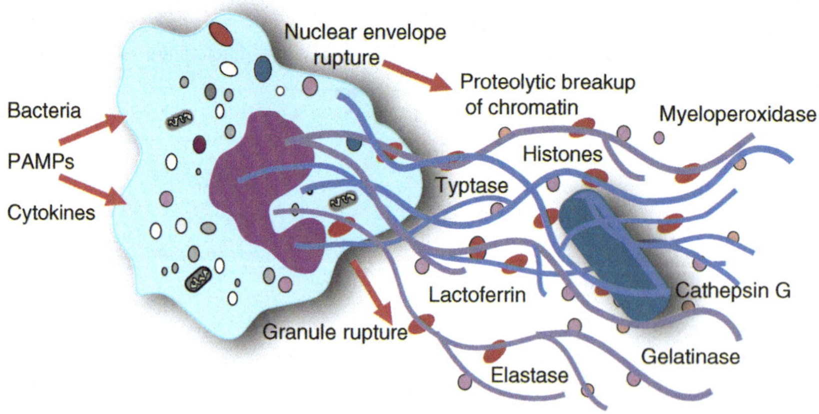

FIGURE 4.4

The structure and composition of neutrophil extracellular traps.

bacteria, but they can also kill them. It is also possible that neutrophils can sense the size of their microbial targets and resort to NETosis when their targets are "too large to eat."

NET formation has been investigated in horse neutrophils responding to diverse stimuli (Quiroga et al., 2024). As in other mammals, equine NETs are web-like structures composed of DNA with its associated histones. They also contain antimicrobial granule contents such as myeloperoxidase and elastase. These NETS can trap pathogens. However, they may also cause tissue damage and so contribute to disease pathology.

Neutrophils are activated by PAMPs and DAMPs acting through PRMs. Experimentally, it has been shown that equine neutrophils release NETs in response to exposure to PMA (phorbol myristate acetate) and platelet-activating factor. Interestingly, LPS and cytokines such as CXCL8, TNF-α, and GM-CSF did not do so. It also appears that peptidyl-arginine deaminases are necessary for NET release in the horse, NETs play a very important role in containing microbial invaders by acting as physical barriers and preventing their spread from their initial invasion sites. However, under some circumstances, excessive neutrophil trap formation may itself cause tissue damage. They can be deposited on vessel walls and so cause a vasculitis and immunothrombosis. They can also be deposited in the kidneys, where they may cause glomerulonephritis. Normally, however, once their task is completed, the NETs are degraded by DNAse, and normal blood flow is restored.

Pelger–Huët anomaly

Pelger–Huët anomaly is an inherited disorder characterized by a failure of granulocyte nuclei to segment into lobes. The neutrophils, therefore, appear on first sight to be very immature (a left shift). The anomaly is usually detected when an animal is observed to have a persistent left shift that cannot be reconciled with its good health. Although Pelger–Huët neutrophils closely resemble band forms, their nuclear chromatin is condensed, reflecting their maturity. In humans, the anomaly is due to a mutation in the gene coding for lamin B, a nuclear membrane receptor that interacts with chromatin to determine the shape of the nucleus. Pelger–Huët anomaly has been reported to occur in Arabian horses (Gill et al., 2006; Grondin et al., 2007). In the affected animals, hyposegmented neutrophils constituted $1–8 \times 10^3$/mL compared to $0.0–0.2 \times 10^3$/mL in healthy control animals. This nuclear hyposegmentation also affected the nuclei of their eosinophils and basophils. The anomaly is inherited as an autosomal dominant trait. It appears to have a minimal effect on the health of affected horses.

Lymphocytes

Lymphocytes are the second most common leukocyte found in equine blood. The neutrophil: lymphocyte ratio is normally around 1.5:1. Most of these appear to be typical "small" lymphocytes, 7–9 μm in diameter, with a dark-staining round nucleus and a thin rim of basophilic cytoplasm. Of these, between 38% and 66% are T cells, while 17%–38% are B cells, and about 5% are NK cells. Antigen-stimulated, reactive lymphocytes are slightly larger with a greater amount of cytoplasm. Some lymphocytes may contain purple granules within their cytoplasm. These may be T cells or NK cells (Fig. 4.5).

Absolute lymphocyte counts decline in aged horses over 20 years of age when compared to young animals under 12 years. This drop involves both $CD4^+$ and $CD8^+$ T cells as well as B cells (McFarlane et al., 2001). This decline in $CD8^+$ T cells is associated with an increase in the CD4:CD8 ratio in the aged population. Thus, it averages about 4.07 ± 1.54 in aged horses but only 3.30 ± 1.31 in young animals (Fig. 4.6).

The half-life of equine blood lymphocytes varies greatly between subpopulations, and ranges from 20 to 200 days. However, they circulate constantly and emigrate from the bloodstream into lymphoid tissues. As a result, large numbers are found in the efferent lymph. These return to the bloodstream through the thoracic duct and other large lymphatic vessels in the thorax and abdomen.

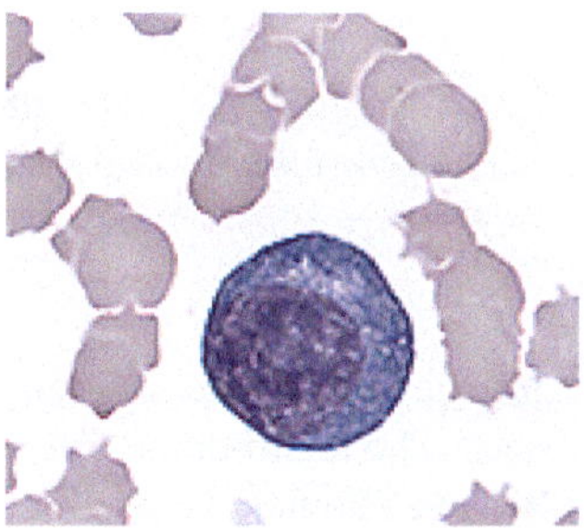

FIGURE 4.5

A typical equine small lymphocyte.

- Courtesy of Dr Mark Johnson.

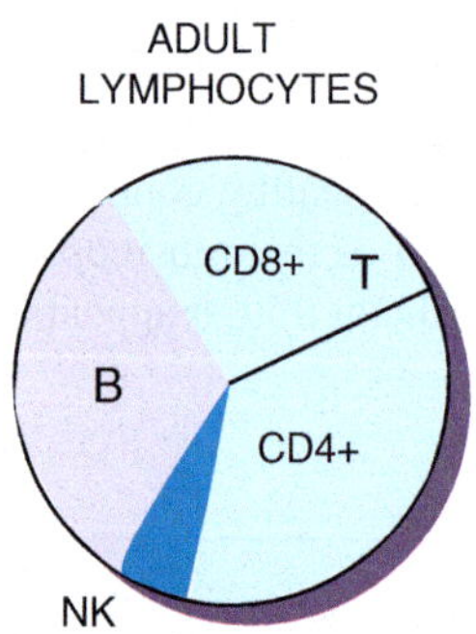

FIGURE 4.6 The composition of the lymphocyte populations found in normal equine blood.

As with other leukocyte counts, these can differ greatly between individual animals.

In a small proportion of these lymphocytes, there may be small pink-purple granules present in their cytoplasm. Reactive lymphocytes are rare in the blood of healthy horses. Epinephrine produced by stressed or excited horses can cause a temporary lymphocytosis.

Monocytes

Monocytes are the largest of the circulating blood leukocytes and are the precursors of tissue macrophages and some dendritic cells (Chapter 7). They are the third most common leukocyte and account for less than 10% of the total count in adult horses. Like the other leukocyte populations, they originate in the bone marrow. They range from 15 to 20 μm in diameter and are thus generally larger than neutrophils. Their nuclear shape is very variable, ranging from round to band-shaped, to trilobed or S-shaped. Unlike neutrophils, their nuclear chromatin is much less condensed. Their cytoplasmic staining depends on the amount of rough endoplasmic reticulum and the presence of ribosomes. Their cytoplasm may contain a few clear cytoplasmic vesicles as well as some blue-staining small granules clustered on one side. A monocytosis is associated with inflammation. Most blood monocytes are found in the marginal pool. Their half-life in the bloodstream is 8.5 hours (Freeman et al., 2022).

Equine blood monocytes attach to glass surfaces and thus can be readily cultivated in vitro. They progressively develop a series of morphological changes as they mature into macrophages. Thus, they develop an increased number of granules and vesicles. Their dense granules are rich in acid phosphatase. The number and size of their mitochondria also increase. These cultured cells are effectively phagocytic (Bennett & Cohn, 1965). Equine infectious anemia virus selectively infects cells of the monocyte-macrophage lineage, so these cultured monocytes are an important tool in studying this disease (Raabe et al., 1998). A marked monocytosis is associated with the onset of equine herpesvirus-1 infection and is thus a useful diagnostic tool (Mason et al., 1989).

Eosinophils

Eosinophils are present in low numbers in the bloodstream of healthy adult horses. They tend to be slightly larger than neutrophils. They have a bilobed nucleus with a cytoplasm packed with large, prominent reddish-orange granules that vary in size. In horses, their numbers range from 100 to 1200 eosinophils/mL. Unlike basophils, eosinophils are phagocytic. They readily take up foreign particles such as yeast cells. They discharge the contents of their granules into the phagocytic vacuoles in a manner similar to neutrophils (Archer & Hirsch, 1963) (Fig. 4.7).

Their pink/orange granules are so large and plentiful that they may obscure the bilobed nucleus. Eosinophil granules are about 450 nm in diameter in most mammals, but in horses, these can aggregate to form much larger structures. Thus,

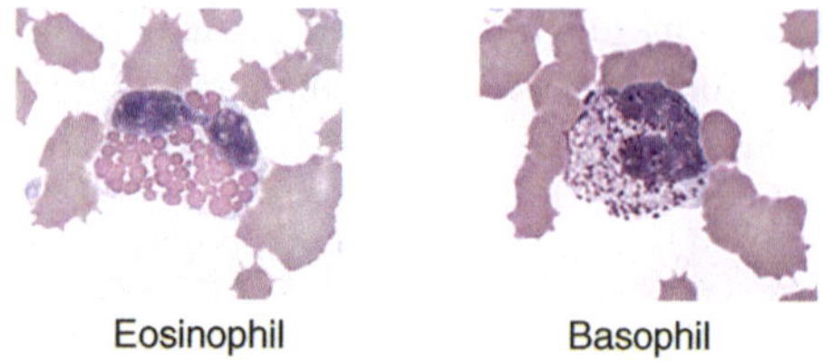

FIGURE 4.7

Photomicrographs of an equine eosinophil and basophil. Note the very large eosinophil granules.

- Courtesy of Dr Karen Russell.

they range from 0.3 to 2.35 μm and average about 1 μm (Sonoda, 1972). Horse eosinophil granules have a dense core that varies in position within each granule and does not appear to be crystalline in nature. This is surrounded by a dense matrix and an outer membrane. Some of the granules appear to have internal structures such as vacuoles. These granules contain large amounts of peroxidase, ribonuclease, cathepsin, acid phosphatase, arylsulfatase, β-glucuronidase, and α- and β-mannosidases. Collectively, these have potent antibacterial and antiparasitic properties. The granules are released by the cells on the surface of invaders such as parasitic worms. Horse eosinophils express the receptor CCR3 on their surface. Its ligand is the chemokine, eotaxin (Brosnahan, 2018).

Eosinophils have been identified in fetal lymphoid organs, especially the fetal thymus (Fig. 8.2). Despite this, they are absent from the blood of newborn foals. They first appear in the bloodstream at about 1 week of age. Their numbers increase progressively during the first year of life.

Circulating eosinophil numbers do, however, differ between breeds (Brosnahan, 2020). Diurnal alterations in eosinophil counts have been reported to occur in Arabian horses, with peak numbers occurring during daylight hours. Their numbers in stallions (2.6%) are higher than in mares (1.2%). As in other species, these numbers fluctuate, reflecting changes in parasite load. There are also seasonal variations in these counts, with lower numbers present in January through March. In Thoroughbreds, eosinophil counts do not follow a normal distribution, and there are very many outliers. This is probably a consequence of different parasite burdens. In addition, the majority of eosinophils migrate into tissues, especially on body surfaces such as the gastrointestinal tract. The half-life of circulating eosinophils in the horse is 2–12 hours (Freeman et al., 2022).

Eosinophilia is uncommon in horses, and if it occurs tends to be relatively mild. It is associated with the presence of parasitic or fungal infestations or ongoing allergic responses. Eosinopenia is difficult to confirm since normal eosinophil numbers are relatively low. Decreased numbers of eosinophils are found in endurance horses undergoing strenuous training. Three-year-old Thoroughbreds racing over 12–16 furlongs had higher eosinophil counts than horses racing over 5–6 furlongs (Allen, 1986).

Basophils

Basophils are major effector cells in equine allergic responses (Chapter 19). Basophils are rare in equine blood (0%–1%). They, too, are slightly larger than neutrophils and similar in size to eosinophils (10–15 μm in diameter) (Fig. 4.7). They tend to have a long, bilobed or convoluted nucleus. Their cytoplasm contains multiple round purple granules that vary in size, shape, and number, which may partially hide their nucleus. Their nucleus tends to have only a few lobules. Basophilia is rare but may be associated with an eosinophilia and hypersensitivity responses. For example, a chronic basophilic enterocolitis has been reported in a horse. This may simply be a variant of an eosinophilic enterocolitis (Pass et al., 1984).

Platelets

Blood platelets play a key role in hemostasis and thrombosis as well as managing vascular injury. However, it has also become increasingly apparent that platelets play important roles in the defense of the body against microbial pathogens. They are abundant in equine blood at 100–250 × 10^9/L. On stained smears, they are small, variably sized, round or oval cell fragments. Activated platelets can release antiviral proteins such as kinocidins and thrombocidins (Aquino -Dominguez et al., 2021). They can phagocytose viral pathogens and produce lethal reactive oxygen. They play important roles in autoimmune and inflammatory diseases such as immunothrombosis and vasculitis, as well as in sepsis (Li et al., 2011). One way they do this is by producing a complex mixture of cytokines. For example, equine platelet lysate contains IL-1β, IL-4, IL-6, IL-10, IFN γ, and TNF-α (Moellerberndt et al., 2023). Interestingly, Lipopolysaccharide-stimulated equine monocytes cultured in the presence of platelet lysate show a significant reduction in their production of these cytokines (Naskou et al., 2018).

White cell counts and cytopenias

Mature and immature neutrophils are released from the bone marrow, as well as from the marginating pool in response to cytokines generated by infection and inflammation. Inflammatory cytokines stimulate neutrophil production. These are mainly growth factors together with interleukins-1, IL-3, and IL-6. As a result, the normal neutrophil development time of 7–9 days is accelerated to as few as 3–4 days. In cases of severe inflammation and endotoxemia, there may be an initial neutropenia as the storage pool is depleted, affecting segmented neutrophils and eosinophils, as well a cortisol and lysozyme levels. Thus, in a study of Arabian mares and their foals, it was found that the mean leukocyte count was highest in young foals compared to mares. It was especially low in pregnant mares during August, October, and November in the Northern hemisphere (Gill et al., 1985).

Exercise or excitement in a horse can trigger a leukocytosis (<20 × 10^9/L). This is physiological. The trigger activates the sympathetic adrenal axis, resulting in the release of epinephrine. The epinephrine can cause splenic contraction, causing the release of sequestered neutrophils, and resulting in a temporary leukocytosis, associated with a neutrophilia and lymphocytosis (Satue et al., 2014). Stress associated with the release of endogenous glucocorticoid levels can also cause a moderate leukocytosis, neutrophilia, monocytosis, lymphopenia, and eosinopenia. These changes are transient, generally lasting no more than 30 minutes. The subsequent leukopenia is due to increased margination and lymphocyte emigration from the bloodstream into tissues (Chapter 24).

A neutrophilia is associated with stress, as described above. It can also be pathological and develop in the presence of acute inflammation, often initiated by an infection. It may also be caused by endotoxemia. An endotoxemia may result in neutropenia as the activated neutrophils leave the circulating pool to join the marginating pool. It may reflect a disease affecting the bone marrow. Corticosteroids also affect neutrophil numbers. Thus, both endogenous and exogenous glucocorticoids can cause a neutrophilia and a lymphopenia. There is a shift in neutrophil populations from the marginating pool to the circulating pool. This neutrophilia is generally not associated with a left shift or toxic changes. Horses do not develop a monocytosis in response to glucocorticoids.

Erythrocytes

Equine blood groups

Erythrocytes are covered, like other cells, by a cell membrane consisting of a lipid bilayer containing numerous embedded glycoproteins. These glycoproteins differ chemically between individual horses. As a result, they are antigenic if transfused into another horse. The antigenic molecules expressed on the surface of red blood cells are called blood group antigens or erythrocyte antigens (EAs). Under some conditions, they can trigger pathologic immune responses. Blood group antigens vary in their antigenicity, some being more potent and therefore of greater importance than others. The expression of blood group antigenic proteins is inherited in a conventional fashion. For each blood group antigen gene, there are a variable number of alleles - molecular variants that also differ in their antigenicity. Although most blood group antigens are integral cell membrane components, some are also found free in serum, saliva, and other body fluids and passively adsorbed onto red cell surfaces.

Blood group glycoproteins are not restricted to erythrocyte surfaces. They are expressed and can be detected and isolated from many other tissues and cell types. In the case of horses, they have been isolated in large amounts from the gastric mucosa. Thus, group A molecules are highly glycosylated proteins found in mucosal tissues (Newman & Kabat, 1976).

Horses possess eight independent blood group systems - A, C, D, K, P, Q, U, and T (Stormont & Suzuki, 1964). All except group T are recognized by the International Society for Animal Blood Group Research. Each of these blood group loci consists of two or more alleles. The alleles within each system are denoted by lowercase letters. Some, such as C, K, and U, and T are simple, one-gene, two-allele, two-phenotype systems. For example, the C system consists of C^a and C^-. However, the blood group A system contains 7 alleles (Aa-Ag), group O and group P contain 4 (a-d), and group Q also has 7 (Qa-Qg). On the other extreme, the D system is very complex, with about 27 alleles identified to date. In addition, these alleles can occur in combinations such as Dadl, and Qbc. These combinations are termed phenogroups. As a result, horse blood groups are very diverse, and it is estimated that there may be as many as 400,000 potentially different equine blood types. It is very unusual, therefore, for two horses to share the same blood type. As a result of this enormous blood group diversity, there are no "universal donor" horses (Blais & Penedo, 2022).

Blood group A

Blood group A is the most potently antigenic of the equine blood groups. It stimulates a strong antibody response. As a result, it is the factor most commonly involved in neonatal isoerythrolysis (Sandberg & Cothran, 2000). The distribution of blood groups varies across horse breeds in addition to geographical variations. For example, 95% of thoroughbreds, 82% of Arabians, and 57% of Standardbreds are Aa positive. However, only 53% of Shetland ponies are Aa positive (Stormont & Suzuki, 1964).

Blood group D

As described above, equine blood group D is by far the most complex, with about 27 different alleles identified to date. It consists of at least 10 subloci grouped into six blocks The entire spectrum of these antigens has probably resulted from repeated mutations. Six of these alleles appear to be due to point mutations. Two appear to have involved neighboring subloci, while four resulted from at least two consecutive mutations. Analysis has shown that these can be classified into 12 "mutant" alleles and 15 "recombinant" alleles based on their origins (Knyazev & Nikitin, 2007).

Alloantibodies

Horses may make antibodies against foreign blood groups. These "alloantibodies" may form naturally or be induced by human procedures. About 10% of normal horses have naturally occurring alloantibodies against foreign equine blood groups, especially against Aa, Qa, and Ca. These antibodies are present at birth and develop without obvious prior sensitization. For example, foals that do not express the Aa antigen frequently possess anti-Aa antibodies. Likewise, foals that do not express Ca make anti-Ca antibodies. Anti-Ca antibodies have minimal clinical significance. Alloantibodies to Aa, on the other hand, are high titered and thus primarily responsible for blood transfusion reactions in the horse. Anti-Qa antibodies also mediate these reactions.

Antibodies against foreign blood groups may also be readily induced by incompatible blood transfusions or, on occasion, by incompatible pregnancies. Anti-Aa and -Qa antibody production, is often associated with severe transfusion reactions and neonatal isoerythrolysis.

Neonatal isoerythrolysis

Neonatal isoerythrolysis (NI), otherwise called, hemolytic disease of the newborn, occurs in foals born to mares that have been sensitized to their paternal blood groups by previous blood transfusions or by administration of vaccines containing equine tissues. Most commonly, however, mares are sensitized by exposure to fetal red cells as a result of repeated pregnancies. The mechanism of this sensitization is unclear, but fetal red cells are assumed to gain access to the maternal circulation as a result of transplacental hemorrhage. Mares have been shown to mount an antibody response to their fetal red cells as early as day 56 after conception. The greatest leakage probably occurs during the last month of pregnancy and during foaling, as a result of the breakdown of placental blood vessels (Becht, 1983).

The alloantibodies produced by these mares during pregnancy are subsequently ingested by the foal through her colostrum, reach the bloodstream, and may result in the development of a hemolytic anemia or a thrombocytopenia (Magdesian, 2024). These antibodies can also cause severe reactions following incompatible transfusions. Their major significance lies in the fact that neonatal isoerythrolysis in newborn foals is relatively common.

In mules, in which the antigenic differences between dam and sire are much greater, about 8%–10% of foals may be affected by NI (McClure et al., 1994). In Thoroughbreds and Standardbreds, the prevalence of NI) is considerably less, ranging from 0.05% to 2% of foals. This is despite the fact that in up to 14% of pregnancies, the mare and the stallion have incompatible red cells (Bailey, 1982) (Fig. 4.8).

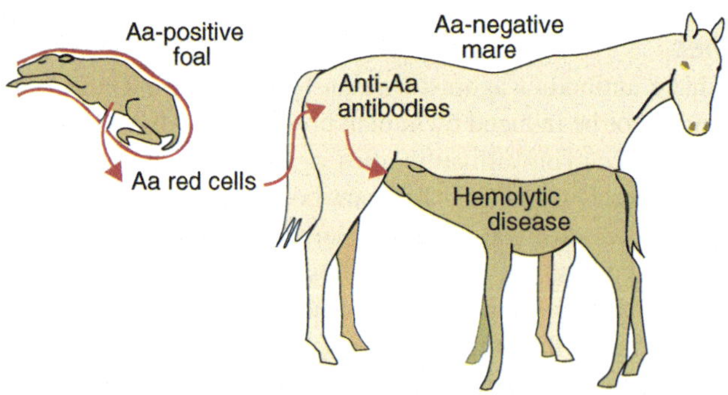

FIGURE 4.8 The pathogenesis of equine neonatal isoerythrolysis.

The mare is commonly sensitized by foal erythrocytes leaking into her circulation at the time of foaling. It may take several pregnancies involving the same sire to generate a pathogenic level of isoantibodies in her colostrum.

Maternal sensitization to foreign red cells is usually minimal following a first pregnancy. However, if the mare is repeatedly mated to the same sire, her antibody responses will be boosted until the antibodies eventually reach harmful levels. NI is therefore usually only a problem in mares that have had multiple foals. The most severe form of the disease results from the production of antibodies directed against the Aa antigen. Natural antibodies to Qa do not occur, so sensitization against this blood group requires prior exposure to Qa + red cells. Anti-Qa produces a less severe disease of slower onset. In practice, 90% of clinical cases are attributable to anti-Aa and anti -Qa alloantibodies as well as to "donkey antigen." Other less antigenic blood groups, such as Pa, Ab, Ac, and Ka. Pa, Qc, Qrs, R, S, Ua, Da, Db, Dc, and Dg have been implicated in some NI cases (Magdesian, 2018). Mares that lack Aa and Qa are therefore most likely to produce affected foals. Pregnant mares often produce antibodies to Ca, but these are rarely associated with clinical disease. Indeed, preexisting antibodies to Ca may reduce sensitization by Aa (Magdesian, 2018). This is because presence of this anti-Ca in a mare rapidly eliminates any fetal red cells that enter her bloodstream and so prevents further sensitization. There are also breed differences in the prevalence of NI. A case of NI caused by a non-specific hemolytic alloantibody has been recorded in a foal from a Fresian filly. The antibody involved caused hemolysis of the red cells in all tested horses except for the mare herself. These horses represented a complete spectrum of equine blood groups. Thus, the antibody was not directed at a specific blood group antigen (De Graff-Roelfsema et al., 2007) (Fig. 4.8).

NI affected foals are therefore born healthy but sicken several hours after suckling. Some may not sicken for 2–3 days, depending upon the volume of colostrum consumed and its antibody titer. The severity of the disease is determined by the amount of antibody absorbed and by the sensitizing blood group. The earliest clinical signs are weakness and depression. The mucous membranes of affected foals may be pale and may eventually show a distinct icterus. Some foals sicken by 6–8 hours and die from shock so rapidly that they may not have time to develop icterus. More commonly, the disease presents as lethargy and weakness between 12 and 48 hours of age. Icterus of the mucous membranes and sclera is consistent in foals that survive for at least 48 hours. Hemoglobinuria, although uncommon, is diagnostic in a newborn foal. As a result of anoxia, some foals in the terminal stages of the disease may convulse or become comatose. The most common causes of death in these foals are liver failure, brain damage, and bacterial sepsis (Whiting & David, 2000).

NI is readily diagnosed by clinical signs alone. Hematological examination is of little diagnostic use but hematocrits may be of assistance in measuring disease severity. Definitive diagnosis requires that immunoglobulin be demonstrated on the surface of the red cells of the foal. In the case of anti-Aa or anti-Qa, the addition of a source of complement (fresh normal rabbit serum) causes rapid hemolysis. If hemolytic disease is anticipated, the serum of a pregnant mare may be tested for antibodies by an indirect antiglobulin test. By using red cells from horses with a major sensitizing blood group, it is possible to show that the mare's antibody titer increases significantly in the month before parturition.

A test that may be useful for detecting the presence of anti-erythrocyte antibodies in colostrum is the jaundiced foal agglutination test. This involves making serial dilutions of colostrum in saline. A drop of anticoagulated foal blood is then added to each tube, and the tubes are centrifuged so that the red cells form a pellet at the bottom. In the presence of antibodies, the cells clump tightly, and the pellet remain intact when the tubes are emptied. Non-agglutinated red cells, in contrast, flow down the side of the tube. Concentrated colostrum is viscous and tends to induce rouleaux formation that mimics agglutination. However, if the mare's blood is used as a negative control, this can be accounted for. The foal's blood should also be tested to ensure that the foal has not already absorbed antibodies and that false-positive results are not obtained.

Mildly affected foals, with a packed cell volume (PCV) of 15%–25% and a red cell count greater than 4×10^6 /μL, will continue to nurse. Those with a PCV of less than 10% will stop nursing and become recumbent.

The prognosis of uncomplicated NI is good, provided the condition is diagnosed sufficiently early and the appropriate treatment is instituted rapidly. Management of HDN includes prevention of further antibody absorption, adequate nutrition, oxygen therapy, fluid and electrolyte therapy, and maintenance of the acid-base balance. Warmth, adequate hydration, and antimicrobial therapy are also critically important. In acute cases, blood transfusion is necessary. A red cell count of less than 3×10^6/mL or a PCV of less than 15% warrants a blood transfusion. Transfused equine red cells have a half-life of only 2–4 days, so transfusion is only a temporary life-saving measure. Compatible blood may be difficult to find because of the high prevalence of Aa and Qa in the normal equine population. A donor should not only be Aa or Qa negative but should also lack antibodies to these antigens. Exchange transfusion, although efficient, requires a donor capable of providing at least 5 L of blood as well as a double intravenous catheter and an anesthetized foal. A much simpler procedure that avoids many difficulties is the transfusion of washed red cells from the mare. About 3–4 L of blood is collected in sodium citrate and centrifuged, after which the plasma is discarded. The red cells are washed once in saline and transfused slowly into the foal. The blood is usually given in divided doses about 6 hours apart. Milder cases of hemolytic disease may require only careful nursing.

If NI is anticipated as a result of either a rising antibody titer or the previous birth of a hemolytic foal, stripping off the mare's colostrum and giving the foal colostrum from another mare will prevent its occurrence. The foal should not be allowed to suckle its own mare for 24–36 hours. Once suckling is permitted, the foal should only be allowed to take small quantities at first and should be observed carefully for adverse side effects.

Horse blood groups may be identified by tube agglutination, hemolytic, and antiglobulin tests. Gel-based agglutination tests and immunochromatographic techniques have produced encouraging results (Luethy et al., 2016). Each blood group system has a preferred test system.

Neonatal thrombocytopenia

Immune-mediated neonatal thrombocytopenia has been recorded in foals. In these cases, maternal colostral antibodies are directed against glycoproteins expressed on the foal's platelets. As a result, affected foals develop thrombocytopenia and a decline in platelet function. Affected foals develop mucosal hemorrhages, especially in the oral and vulvar mucus membranes, as well as obvious skin bruising. Hematomas may develop at sites of venipuncture. As with NI, the severity of the disease is highly variable, reflecting variations in alloantibody levels in the mare. It is believed that mares may be sensitized as a result of previous pregnancies, placental damage, or prior blood transfusions. Mule foals are at significantly increased risk since donkey platelets are highly antigenic in horses. Breeds such as American Quarter horses and Paint horses may also be more susceptible (Magdesian, 2024). Diagnosis is based on finding IgG and IgM bound to the foal's platelets. Immunoglobulins can be detected on the foal's platelets, and antibodies to these platelets can be found in the mare's serum (Buechner-Maxwell et al., 1997).

Neonatal neutropenia

A neonatal neutropenia has been reported in a 12-hour-old Arabian colt that was otherwise healthy. Its neutrophils were shown to be coated with IgG. Other cases have been reported to occur in Thoroughbred foals. For example, a 3-day-old Thoroughbred colt had been described that developed neonatal isoerythrolysis and a persistent neutropenia in the absence of any infection. The mare's serum agglutinated the foal's granulocytes. It was not until day 20 that the foal's neutrophil count stabilized. This syndrome is similar to the neonatal agranulocytosis that affects other species, such as calves (Magdesian, 2024; Wong et al., 2012).

Neonatal dermatitis

A syndrome that occurs in foals less than 4 days of age is associated with the development of a transient ulcerative dermatitis accompanied by a mild neutropenia and severe thrombocytopenia. These foals come from multiparous mares, and the disease can be prevented by withholding colostrum. It is believed to be caused by a passive alloimmune response. Affected foals develop an ulcerative, crusting dermatitis around the eyes, muzzle, and perineum, oral vesicles, mucosal hemorrhages, epistaxis, and hematomas. Histology shows subepidermal vesicular changes, dermal edema, and hemorrhage. IgG has been detected in the epidermis and basement membrane of affected foals and the dermatitis is therefore believed to be antibody-mediated (Perkins et al., 2008).

Donkeys and mules

Leukocytes

The morphology of mule leukocytes has been studied in detail (Mrigesh et al., 2016). Thus, mule neutrophils are round cells averaging about 12.25 μm in diameter, slightly larger than those of donkeys (11.75 μm diameter). They possess 2–5 lobes. Monocytes are 13.4 μm in diameter and are similar in size to those of donkeys. Eosinophils are 13.4 μm in diameter and basophils 13.8 μm diameter. In general, they resemble those of horses. The leukocytes of donkeys are similar to those of horses when stained and viewed by light microscopy. They do, however, differ to a limited extent in their chemical composition (Rocha et al., 1978). As in horses, blood parameters in donkeys are influenced by age, sex, environmental factors, and physical exhaustion (Zakari et al., 2016). Donkeys subjected to extensive packing expeditions have increased numbers of blood eosinophils (Olaifa et al., 2015) (Figs. 4.9–4.13).

Blood groups

A high percentage of horses possess anti-donkey antibodies. These are directed at a red blood cell antigen found only in donkeys and mules, and absent in horses. These antibodies develop to high titers when mares are bred by donkey sires to produce mules. The "Donkey antigen" is distinctly different from all known horse blood groups. As a result, it can be classified as a horse xenoantigen. All donkeys and mules tested share this antigen. As a result, all mule pregnancies are at risk of NI (McClure et al., 1994). Donkeys also possess three characterized blood group antigens, B, M, and N. They are also present in mules (Podliachouk, 1964). The genetic differences between the blood group antigens of the horse and donkey are reflected

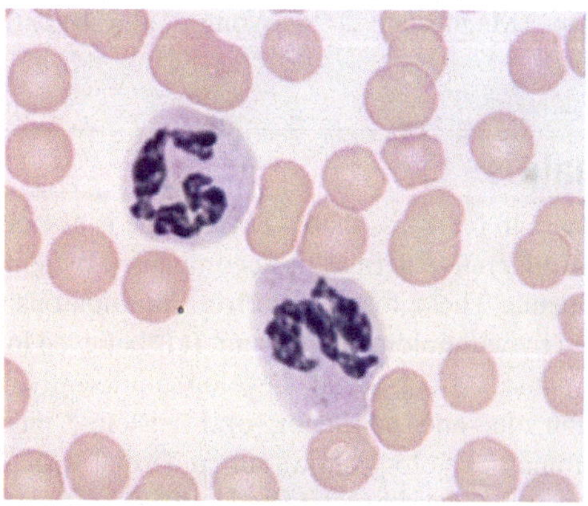

FIGURE 4.9 A segmented neutrophil from a Jenny.

Original Mag. x 100.

- Courtesy of Dr Mark Johnson.

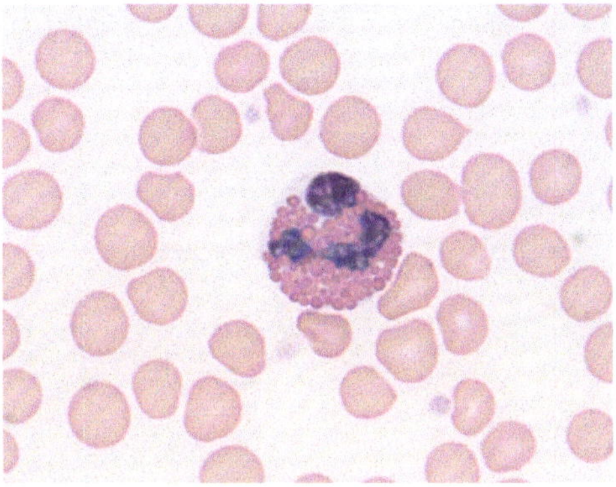

FIGURE 4.10 An eosinophil from a Jenny.

Note the large eosinophilic granules. Original Mag. x 1000.

- Courtesy of Dr Mark Johnson.

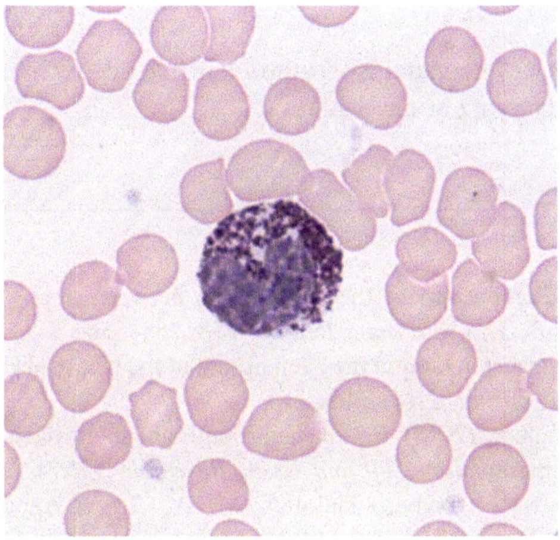

FIGURE 4.11 A dasophil from a Jenny.

Original Mag. x 100.

- Courtesy of Dr Mark Johnson.

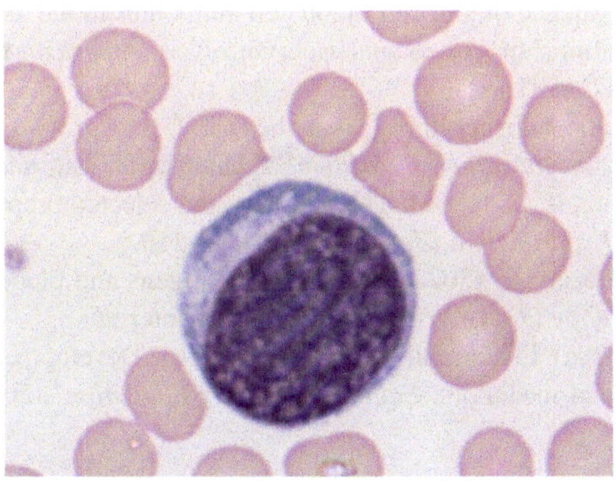

FIGURE 4.12 A donkey lymphocyte.

Original Mag x 100.

- Courtesy of Dr Mark Johnson.

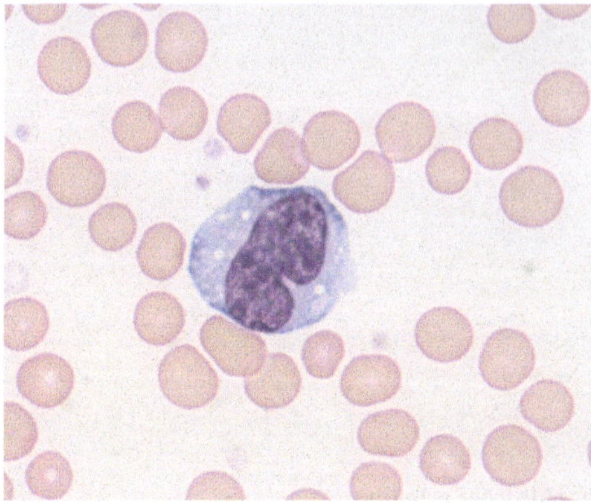

FIGURE 4.13 A donkey monocyte.

From a Jenny. Original magnification × 100

- Courtesy of Dr Mark Johnson.

in the high prevalence of neonatal isoerythrolysis that occurs in mule foals (McClure et al., 1994; Traub-Dargatz et al., 1995).

References

Allen, B. V. (1986). Comparison of the haemogram between three-year-old thoroughbred stayers and sprinters. *The Veterinary Record, 118*, 555–556.

Allen, B. V. (1989). Age differences in the haemogram of the National Hunt trained racehorse. *Equine Veterinary Journal, 21*(4), 309–310.

Anderson, S. L., & Singh, B. (2018). Equine neutrophils and their role in ischemia reperfusion injury and lung inflammation. *Cell and Tissue Research, 371*(3), 639–648.

Aquino-Dominguez, A. S., Romero-Tlalolini, M. A., Torres-Aguillar, H., & Aguilar-Ruiz, S. R. (2021). Recent advances in the discovery and function of antimicrobial molecules in platelets. *International Journal of Molecular Sciences, 22*, Article 10230. https://doi.org/10.3390/ijms221910230

Archer, G. T., & Hirsch, J. G. (1963). Motion picture studies on degranulation of horse eosinophils during phagocytosis. *Journal of Experimental Medicine, 118*, 287–293.

Bailey, E. (1982). Prevalence of anti-red blood cell antibodies in the serum and colostrum of mares and its relationship to neonatal isoerythrolysis. *American Journal of Veterinary Research, 43*, 1917–1921.

Becht, J. L. (1983). Neonatal isoerythrolysis in the foal. I. Background, blood group antigens and pathogenesis. *Compendium: Continuing Education for Veterinarians, 5*, 591–599.

Bennett, W. E., & Cohn, Z. A. (1965). The isolation and selected properties of blood monocytes. *Journal of Experimental Medicine, 123*, 145–159.

Blais, M.-C., & Penedo, M. C. (2022). Erythrocyte antigens and blood groups. In *Schalm's veterinary hematology* (7 ed). Wiley Blackwell (Chapter 96).

Brosnahan, M. M. (2020a). Eosinophils of the horse: Part 1: Development, distribution, structure and biochemical mediators. *Equine Veterinary Education, 32*(10), 545–552.

Brosnahan, M. M. (2020b). Eosinophils of the horse: Part II: Eosinophils in clinical diseases. *Equine Veterinary Education, 32*(11), 590–602.

Buechner-Maxwell, V., Scott, M. A., Godber, L., & Kristensen, A. (1997). Neonatal alloimmune thrombocytopenia in a quarter horse foal. *Journal of Veterinary Internal Medicine, 11*, 304–308.

Burden, F. A., Hazell-Smith, E., Mulugeta, G., Patrick, V., et al. (2016). Reference intervals for biochemical and haematological parameters in mature domestic donkeys (*Equus asinus*) in the UK. *Equine Veterinary Education, 28*(3), 134–139.

Carakostas, M. C., Moore, W., & Smith, J. E. (1981). Intravascular neutrophilic granulocyte kinetics in horses. *American Journal of Veterinary Research, 42*, 623–625.

Coignoul, F. L., Bertram, T. A., Roth, J. A., & Cheville, N. F. (1984). Functional and ultrastructural evaluation of neutrophils from goals and lactating and nonlactating mares. *American Journal of Veterinary Research, 45*(5), 898–902.

De Graff-Roelfsema, E., Boerma, S., van Haeringen, H., & Van der Kolk, J. H. (2007). Nonspecific haemolytic alloantibody causing equine neonatal isoerythrolysis. *The Veterinary Record, 161*, 202–204.

Donovan, D. C., Jackson, C. A., Colahan, P. T., Norton, N. N., et al. (2007). Assessment of exercise-induced alterations in neutrophil functions in horses. *American Journal of Veterinary Research, 68*, 1198–1204 (READ).

Freeman, K. P., Farr, A. J., & Barrelet, A. (2022). Hematology of equids. In *Chapter 10. Schalm's Veterinary Hematology* (7ed). Wiley Blackwell.

Gill, A. F., Gaunt, S., & Sirninger, J. (2006). Congenital Pelger-Huet anomaly in a horse. *Veterinary Clinical Pathology, 35*, 400–462.

Gill, J., Kompanowska-Jezierska, E., Jakubow, K., Kott, A., & Szumska, D. (1985). Seasonal changes in the white blood cell system, lysozyme activity and cortisol level in Arabian brood mares and their foals. *Comparative Biochemistry & Physiology, 81A*(3), 511–523.

Grondin, T. M., DeWitt, S. F., & Keeton, K. S. (2007). Pelger-Huet anomaly in an Arabian horse. *Veterinary Clinical Pathology, 36*(3), 306–319.

Knyazev, S. P., & Nikitin, S. V. (2007). Modeling the structure of supergenes controlling some polyallelic blood group systems in the pig, *Sus scrofa*, and horse *Equus caballus*. *Russian Journal of Genetics, 43*(3), 299–308.

Lambert, J. L., Fernandez, N. J., & Roy, M.-F. (2016). Association of presence of band cells and toxic neutrophils with Systemic Inflammatory Response syndrome and outcome in horses with acute disease. *Journal of Veterinary Internal Medicine, 30*, 1284–1292.

Li, Z., Yang, F., Dunn, S., Gross, A. K., & Smyth, S. S. (2011). Platelets as immune mediators. Their role in host defense responses and sepsis. *Thrombosis Research, 127*(3), 184–188.

Liu, M., Liu, T., Bordin, A., Nerren, J., & Cohen, N. (2009). Activation of foal neutrophils at different ages by CpG deoxynucleotides and *Rhodococcus equi*. *Cytokine, 48*, 280–289.

Luethy, D., Owens, S. D., Stefanovski, D., Nolen-Walston, R., & Giger, U. (2016). Comparison of tube, gel, and immunochromatographic strip methods for evaluation of blood transfusion compatibility in horses. *Journal of Veterinary Internal Medicine, 30*, 1864–1871.

Magdesian, K. G. (2018). Equine blood groups and factors. In N. Pusteria, & J. Higgins (Eds.), Interpretation of equine laboratory diagnostics. *1st*. John Wiley and Sons.

Magdesian, K. G. (2024). Alloimmune conditions in the neonatal foal. *Veterinary Clinics of North America: Equine Practice, 40*, 189–206.

Mason, D. K., Watkins, K. L., & Luk, C. M. (1989). Absolute monocyte counts as an aid to early diagnosis of equine herpesvirus 1 (EHV1) infection in Hong Kong thoroughbred horses. *Journal of Equine Veterinary Science, 9*(3), 133–136.

McClure, J. J., Koch, C., & Traub-Dargatz, J. (1994). Characterization of a red blood cell antigen in donkeys and mules associated with neonatal isoerythrolysis. *Animal Genetics, 25* (22), 119–120.

McFarlane, D., Sellon, D. C., & Gibbs, S. A. (2001). Age-related quantitative alterations in lymphocyte subsets and immunoglobulin isotypes in healthy horses. *American Journal of Veterinary Research, 62*(9), 1413–1417.

Moellerberndt, J., Hagen, A., Niebert, S., Buttner, K., & Burk, J. (2023). Cytokines in equine platelet lysate and related blood products. *Frontiers in Veterinary Science, 2023*. https://doi.org/10.3389/fvets.2023.1117829

Mrigesh, M., Singh, I., Singh, B., Arora, N., & Yadav, G. C. (2016). Morphological study on blood cells of mule. *Indian Journal of Veterinary Anatomy, 28*(2), 17–20.

Naskou, M. C., Norton, N. A., Copland, I. B., Galipeau, J., & Peroni, J. F. (2018). Innate immune responses of equine monocytes cultured in equine platelet lysate. *Veterinary Immunology and Immunopathology, 195*, 65–71.

Newman, W., & Kabat, E. (1976). Immunochemical studies on blood groups: Purification, chemical and immunochemical properties of blood group-active glycoproteins from horse gastric mucosae. *Archives of Biochemistry and Biophysics, 172*, 510–523.

Olaifa, F., Ayo, J. O., Ambali, S. F., & Rekwat, P. L. (2015). Hematobiochemical responses to packing in donkeys administered ascorbic acid during the harmattan season. *Journal of Veterinary Medical Science, 77*, 133–138.

Papayannopoulos, A., & Zychlinsky, A. (2009). NETS: A new strategy for using old weapons. *Trends in Immunology, 30*(11), 513–521.

Pass, D. A., Bolton, J. R., & Mills, J. N. (1984). Basophilic enterocolitis in a horse. *Veterinary Pathology Online, 21*, 362–364.

Perkins, G. A., Miller, W. H., Divers, T. J., Clark, C. K., et al. (2008). Ulcerative dermatitis, thrombocytopenia, and neutropenia in neonatal foals. *Journal of Veterinary Internal Medicine*. https://doi.org/10.1111/j.1939-1676.2005.tb02684.x

Podliachouk, L. (1964). In J. Matousek (Ed.), *Proceedings of the 9th European Animal blood group conference* (pp. 229–235). Springer . com. The blood groups of Equidae.

Quiroga, J., Cortes, B., Sarmiento, J., Moran, G., & Henriquez, C. (2024). Characterization of extracellular trap production and release by equine neutrophils in response to different stimuli. *Developmental & Comparative Immunology, 155*, Article 105151.

Raabe, M. R., Issel, C. J., & Montelaro, R. C. (1998). Equine monocyte-derived macrophage cultures and their applications for infectivity and neutralization studies on equine infectious anemia virus. *Journal of Virological Methods, 71*, 87–104.

Rebordão, M. R., Carniero, C., Alexandre-Pires, G., Brito, P., et al. (2014). Neutrophil extracellular traps formation by bacteria causing endometritis in the mare. *Journal of Reproductive Immunology, 106*, 41–49.

Rocha, M., Cabezas, M., & Cabezas, J. A. (1978). Isolation and chemical composition of the leucocytes from donkey, horse, mule and pig. *Comparative Biochemistry & Physiology, 60B*, 239–244.

Sandberg, K., & Cothran, E. G. (2000). Blood Groups and Biochemical Polymorphisms. Chapter 5. In A. T. Bowling, & A. Ruvinsky (Eds.), *The genetics of the horse* (pp. 85–108). CAB International.

Satue, K., Munoz, A., & Garlon, J. C. (2014). Interpretation of the equine leukogram. *Journal of Hematological Research*. https://doi.org/10.12974/2312-5411.2014.01.01.4

Sonoda, M. (1972). Electron microscopy of eosinophils in the peripheral blood of clinically healthy horses. *Nihon Ketsueki Gakkai Zasshi, 35*, 39–46.

Stormont, C., & Suzuki, Y. (1964). Genetic systems of blood groups in horses. *Genetics, 50*, 915–929.

Tan, C., Aziz, M., & Wang, P. (2021). The vitals of NETs. *Journal of Leukocyte Biology, 110*, 797–802.

Traub-Dargatz, J. L., McClure, J. J., Coch, C., et al. (1995). Neonatal isoerythrolysis in mule foals. *Journal of the American Veterinary Medical Association, 206*(1), 67–70.

Weiss, D. J., & Evanson, O. A. (2003). Evaluation of activated neutrophils in the blood of horses with colic. *American Journal of Veterinary Research, 64*(11), 1364–1368.

Whiting, J. L., & David, J. B. (2000). Neonatal isoerythrolysis. *Compendium on Continuing Education for the Practicing Veterinarian, 22*, 968–976.

Wong, D. M., Alcott, C. J., Clark, S. K., Jones, D. E., et al. (2012). Alloimmune neonatal neutropenia and neonatal isoerythrolysis in a thoroughbred colt. *Journal of Veterinary Diagnostic Investigation, 24*(1), 219–226.

Zakari, F. O., Ayo, J. O., Rekwot, P. I., & Kawu, M. U. (2016). Effect of age, sex, physical activity and meteorological factors on hematological parameters in donkeys (*Equus asinus*). *Comparative Clinical Pathology, 25*, 1265–1272.

CHAPTER

The equine sickness response

5

When horse tissues are invaded by infectious agents such as bacteria or viruses, they trigger an innate response that involves the production of multiple proinflammatory cytokines by sentinel cells. This initial cascade of cytokines not only acts locally, but it also results in a systemic response. The three key inflammatory cytokines TNF α, IL-6, and IL-1β not only cause local inflammation, but they also act on the brain and the liver. As a result, infected horses suffer malaise, lassitude, fatigue, loss of appetite, and muscle and joint pains, as well as developing a fever. In response, their liver produces diverse acute-phase proteins (Fig. 5.1).

Effects on the brain

The major inflammatory cytokines, interleukin-1β (IL-1β), IL-6, and TNF-α, signal to the brain using two pathways. One pathway acts through the sensory neurons that serve damaged tissues. Stimulation of the vagus nerve by IL-1β can signal directly to the brain. (IL-1β will not trigger a fever if the vagus nerve is cut.) Bacterial lipopolysaccharide binding to TLR4 on intestinal cells can also trigger these vagal signals. The signals, in turn, initiate fever, nausea, and other sickness responses in the brain. Alternatively, these cytokines can either diffuse directly into the brain tissue from the bloodstream or be produced within the brain itself. These inflammatory cytokines act on brain cells to modify its behavior and alter an animal's pain perception. Type 1 interferons can also enter the brain and trigger malaise, depression, and sickness behavior.

Fevers

The most obvious systemic response to infection is the development of a fever resulting from an increase in metabolic rate. In the horse, the normal body temperature is considered to range from 37.5 to 38.5°C (99.5–101.3°F). A body temperature greater than 102°F (39.4°C) is considered to be a fever. Many cytokines can trigger this increase. They include IL-1α, IL-1β, IL-6, IFN-α, TNF-α and TNF-β. These cytokines induce cyclooxygenase-2 production in the pre-optic nucleus of the hypothalamus as well as in the limbic system. This results in local prostaglandin-E_2 (PGE_2) production. The PGE_2 acts on heat-sensitive neurons to slow their firing rate and, as a result, alter the body's thermostatic set-point. The

The Immunology of Horses and Donkeys. https://doi.org/10.1016/B978-0-443-44863-8.00006-5

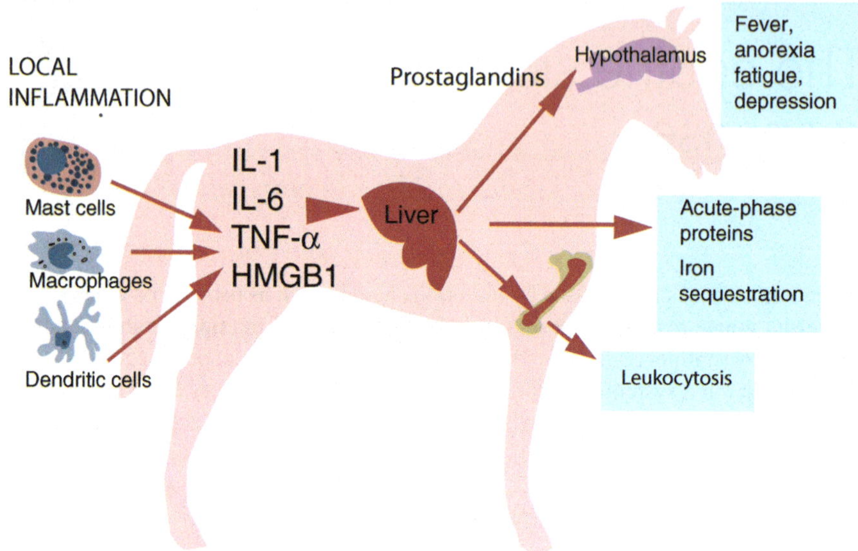

FIGURE 5.1 The equine acute-phase response.

Inflammatory cytokines act on the liver to trigger the production of prostaglandins, acute phase proteins, and cytokines. These in turn trigger a fever, an increase in white cell count, anemia, and sickness behavior.

changes in the set-point result in behavioral changes. For example, febrile animals conserve heat by vasoconstriction and increase their heat production by shivering, thus raising their body temperature until it reaches the new set-point.

Fevers and innate immunity

Combating infection requires a major shift in metabolic priorities. Thus, the development of a fever, 2°C above baseline body temperature, requires a 20% increase in basal metabolism. Given that sickness consistently suppresses food intake, horses must mobilize reserves of protein and energy to support the initial innate response, as well as this increased thermogenesis.

Fever is protective in that it enhances many innate and adaptive immune responses. Fever reduces virus replication and increases the sensitivity of bacteria to complement-mediated lysis. Fever increases blood flow to infected tissues, thus speeding the mobilization of effector cells (Evans et al., 2015). A high body temperature enhances many neutrophil functions. It promotes their release from the bone marrow, their trans-endothelial migration, and their chemotactic responses, thus increasing their accumulation within tissues. Fever-range temperatures stimulate their respiratory burst. Warm body temperatures also enhance multiple macrophage functions such as phagocytosis, release of nitric oxide, and cytokines, as well as the expression of TLR2, TLR4, and MHC antigens. Warmed macrophages upregulate their production of TNF-α through the actions of heat shock protein 70 (HSP70).

Fever upregulates phagocytosis by dendritic cells (DCs) and their expression of TLR2 and TLR4. It enhances DC migration into lymphoid organs. Activated DCs enhance $CD4^{+}$ T cell proliferation and directs them toward Th1 responses (Walter et al., 2016).

Fevers and T cell functions

Higher body temperatures increase the binding affinity of many immune system receptor-ligand pairs. As a result, they enhance lymphocyte, specifically T cell, behavior and effectiveness. Fevers enhance the passage of T cells across high endothelial venule walls, promote immunological synapse formation, and inhibit T cell apoptosis. Fevers act on T cells through a pathway that involves heat shock protein 90 (HSP 90) and α4 integrins. Thus, when mouse T cells are held at 40°C for 12 hours, they develop an increased ability to bind to these integrins. As a result, these heat-treated T cells have an enhanced ability to migrate across membranes. When mice are exposed to elevated temperatures for 6 hours, their T cells show increased adherence to high endothelial venules and trafficking into lymph nodes and Peyer's patches (Fig. 5.2).

Fever-range temperatures also enhance $CD8^{+}$ effector cell differentiation. Febrile temperatures modulate cytokine production by T cells. Thus, when primed

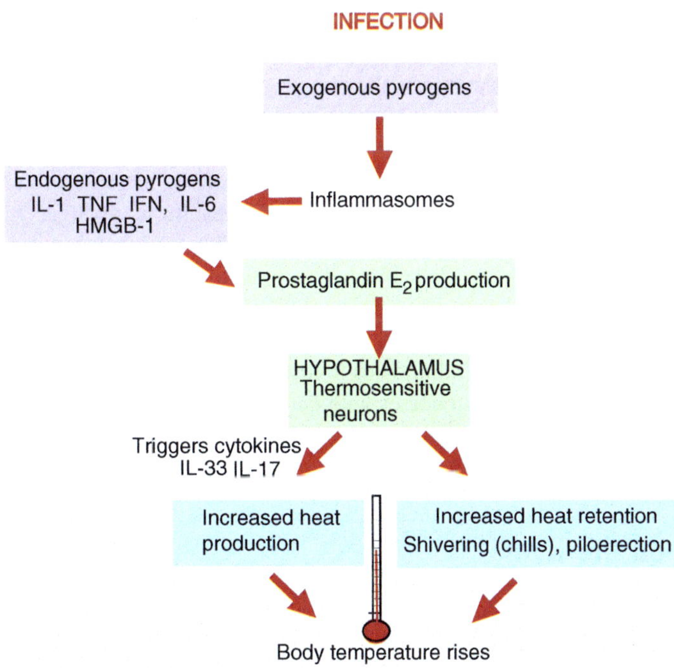

FIGURE 5.2 The mechanisms by which a horse develops a fever.

$CD4^+$ T cells are maintained at a moderate fever temperature (39°C), they tend to function as Th2 cells producing IL-4, IL-5, and IL-13 while suppressing production of the Th1 cytokine IFN-γ. This is also associated with upregulation of the transcription factor, GATA3, and downregulation of another factor, T-bet.

It is also clear that febrile temperatures control the differentiation and plasticity of Th17 cells. As a result, they produce greater quantities of IL-17F and IL-22. These cells and the interleukins they produce play a critical role in stimulating acute inflammation and neutrophil activation. Treatment with antipyretic drugs reduces Th17 cell differentiation in vivo (Wang et al., 2020). Changes in body temperature also influence B cell responses, but this is largely a consequence of alterations in helper T cell functions.

Lethargy

While on balance, the ability to develop a fever is a positive adaptive response, it does result in a temporary inability of an animal to function normally in a social context. Thus, sickness behavior has significant costs. This would have been especially the case in wild horses, especially if it resulted in separation from the rest of the herd and increased vulnerability to predators.

In addition to causing a fever, inflammatory cytokines, especially IL-1β, promote the release of lethargy and fatigue-inducing molecules (Roerink et al., 2017). This response reduces the energy demands on an animal and increases that available for defense and repair. Sick horses move slower (Herz & Kipnis, 2016).

IL-1β, IL-18, and leptin suppress the hunger centers in the hypothalamus and so are responsible for the loss of appetite associated with infections. The benefits of this are unclear.

IL-1β, IL-6, and TNF-α also act on skeletal muscle to increase protein catabolism and release free amino acids. Although this results in myalgia and muscle wastage, the newly available amino acids are available for increased antibody and cytokine synthesis. If horses are subjected to long-term, low-grade inflammation, they will be exposed to chronic, low doses of TNF-α. As a result, they lose weight, become anemic, and protein-depleted. TNF-α inhibits the uptake of lipids by pre-adipocytes and causes mature adipocytes to lose stored lipids. TNF-α is thus responsible for the weight loss seen in horses with cancer or chronic parasitic and bacterial diseases.

Effects on the liver

The acute-phase response

Under the influence of inflammatory cytokines, and especially IL-6, hepatocytes are induced to synthesize many new proteins (Eckersall & Bell, 2010). Because this increase is associated with acute infections and inflammation, these newly produced

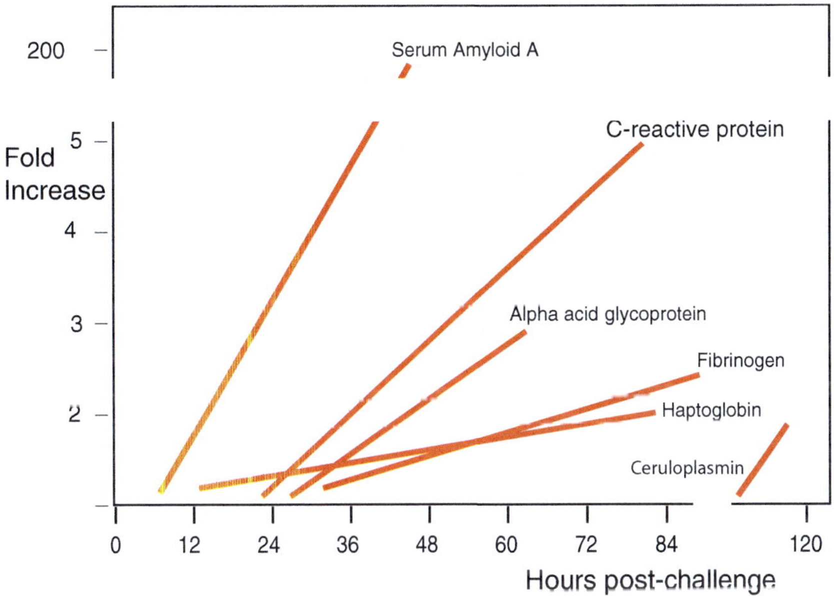

FIGURE 5.3 The acute-phase protein responses of the horse.

Note the time of onset of the rise, the time when peak levels are reached, and the magnitude of the increase.

- Data from: Jacobsen, S., & Andersen, P. H. (2007). The acute-phase protein serum amyloid A (SAA) as a marker of inflammation in horses. Equine Veterinary Education. 19(1), 38–46.

proteins are called acute-phase proteins (APPs). APPs are also synthesized in lymph nodes, tonsils, and the spleen, as well as by blood leukocytes. Mantovani & Garlanda, 2023) The increase in APP levels begins within hours after injury or the onset of systemic inflammation. They subsequently drop between 48 and 100 hours later. APP responses may also occur as a result of prolonged stress, such as confinement or transportation. The acute phase proteins of the horse include soluble PRMs, complement components, clotting molecules, protease inhibitors, and iron-binding proteins. Based upon the level of change in their concentrations, they are classified as major, moderate, or minor APPs (Fig. 5.3).

Major APPs

Serum amyloid A

Serum amyloid A (SAA) is the only major APP produced by horses. Its concentration in the bloodstream increases dramatically as a result of inflammation, infections, or trauma. It is mainly produced in the liver under the influence of inflammatory cytokines. However, it is also produced by mammary epithelial cells, synovial chondrocytes, and endometrial cells (Witowska-Pilaszewicz et al., 2019).

In the healthy horse, SAA concentrations in serum are normally lower than 12 mg/L. These concentrations change with age but not with gender. SAA is a major acute-phase protein, and its levels climb rapidly in cases of systemic inflammation. They can, under some circumstances, climb as high as 4000 mg/L. However, the average high value is about 1600 mg/L. They usually begin to increase around 6–12 hours after the onset of inflammation and peak at around 48 hours (Jacobsen, 2007). Once the inflammation resolves, SAA concentrations drop (Long & Nolen-Walston, 2020).

Equine SAA is a lipoprotein of 9–11 kDa (Witowska-Pilaszewicz et al., 2019). It is not a single homogeneous protein, but some molecules have amino acid insertions, confirming the existence of multiple genes (Sletten et al., 1989). There are three isoforms of SAA found in the horse: SAA1, SAA2, and SAA3. SAA1 and SAA2 are produced by hepatocytes and are found in the bloodstream. SAA3, in contrast, is produced locally within inflamed tissues such as within joints (Jacobsen & Andersen, 2007). SAA tends to circulate complexed to other high-density lipoproteins. SAA has a short half-life, so its levels drop rapidly once synthesis ceases.

Serum amyloid A normally plays a role in lipid metabolism since it binds and scavenges cholesterol from dying cells and transports it to hepatocytes, thus preventing its accumulation. SAA also modulates innate immunity since it binds to TLR2 and may also be an endogenous TLR4 agonist (Cheng et al., 2008). This binding results in NF-κB activation and the production of multiple inflammatory cytokines. SAA is a chemoattractant for neutrophils and monocytes, as well as T cells. It acts through their formylated methionine (fMLP) receptors. SAA can recruit lymphocytes to inflammatory sites and activate enzymes that degrade the extracellular matrix. It regulates the intensity of inflammation by inhibiting myeloperoxidase release and inhibiting lymphocyte proliferation. It also upregulates mucin production. SAA is also a pattern recognition molecule. It opsonizes Gram-negative bacteria such as *E. coli. Klebsiella, Vibrio*, and *Pseudomonas* by binding to their outer membrane protein A (Omp A).

Many different inflammatory stimuli can trigger a rise in equine SAA levels. These include relatively innocuous procedures such as routine vaccination against tetanus or influenza, or minor surgical procedures, where the horses show no other evidence of illness (Baumgarten et al., 2024). SAA levels may also rise in horses following serial injections of procaine penicillin (Gordon et al., 2022). More importantly, elevated SAA levels provide evidence of significant disease occurring. For example, they are elevated in the serum and peritoneal fluid of some horses with colic. The levels depended upon the duration of the colic and can be used to assess the severity of the causal inflammation (Pihl et al., 2015). SAA levels are thus useful markers in determining the prognosis of colic and the effects of treatment (Souto et al., 2019). SAA is also elevated in horses with respiratory diseases such as Rhodococcus infection (Long & Nolen-Walston, 2020). SAA levels are also high in synovial fluid from horses with septic arthritis. It appears to be produced by the inflamed synovium (Stack et al., 2019).

SAA (but not haptoglobin or CRP) is also produced by horses subjected to long races or endurance rides or to strenuous training. This may result in as much as a 10-fold increase in serum SAA levels (Witowska-Pilaszewicz et al., 2019). Likewise, in racing Thoroughbreds that suffer from orthopedic injury, SAA levels can remain high and appear to be a better measure of inflammation than leukocyte counts. There is also a correlation between SAA levels and poor performance (Back et al., 2015).

It is of interest to note that one isoform of SAA (SAA3) is present in significant amounts in mare's colostrum and early milk. It is present in higher concentrations than in periparturient maternal serum. As noted above, however, serum SAA levels rise in mares immediately post-partum, confirming that parturition is an inflammatory event for the brood mare. It is unclear what signal stimulates colostral SAA3 production and what role it may play. It is suggested, however, that it may have a protective effect on the intestinal tract of the newborn foal (Duggan et al., 2008).

Moderate APPs

Haptoglobin

Haptoglobin (Hp) is a protein whose function is to bind free hemoglobin from damaged erythrocytes. It thus scavenges free hemoglobin from the bloodstream. In horses, Hp consists of two peptide chains, alpha and beta. These form a $\alpha_2\beta_2$ tetramer of 85–100 kDa. In plasma, it also exists in polymeric form associated with serum albumin. Because haptoglobin binds any hemoglobin that escapes from erythrocytes, it serves to prevent oxidative tissue damage. Each haptoglobin molecule binds two hemoglobin molecules to form a stable complex. These complexes are phagocytosed by monocytes and macrophages, such as the Kupffer cells of the liver, after binding to the cell surface receptor CD163 (Chapter 10).

Free hemoglobin has a proinflammatory effect, so its removal prevents excessive inflammation. Thus, the binding of Hp-Hb complexes to macrophages upregulates heme-oxygenase-1 and increases IL-10 production. In binding to neutrophils, it inhibits both lipoxygenase and cyclooxygenase and so reduces prostaglandin and leukotriene activity. Hp is also able to effectively bind nitric oxide (NO) and thus limits any damage done by NO when it escapes from phagocytic cells. It has also been reported to inhibit the neutrophil respiratory burst and reduce cathepsin B and lysosomal protease activity. Haptoglobin may also inhibit neutrophil phagocytosis and chemotaxis. It thus tends to minimize the damage caused by neutrophil degranulation. Hp may also modulate T cell function and inhibit Th2 responses. Haptoglobin binds free hemoglobin and, as a result, limits the amount of iron available to growing bacteria such as *E. coli*. There is also evidence to suggest that Hp enhances angiogenesis.

Alpha-1-acid glycoprotein

Alpha-1-acid glycoprotein (AGP) is also a moderate acute-phase protein in horses. It is a glycoprotein containing 219 amino acids and a molecular weight of 20.5 kDa. It is a lipocalin. Lipocalins are a family of proteins that bind and transport hydrophobic molecules such as steroids and prostaglandins. It consists of multiple β-pleated sheets. It binds to receptors on macrophages. Neutrophils exposed to activating agents such as phorbol myristate acetate rapidly release their stores of α_1-acid glycoprotein, resulting in a fivefold increase in serum levels. Increased AGP levels can be detected 24–72 hours after inflammation develops. AGP has four primary functions. It is a major transporter protein that binds inflammatory mediators such as serotonin, histamine, plasminogen-activating factor, and platelet-activating factor. Alpha-1-acid glycoprotein also has immunomodulatory effects. It has an anti-inflammatory function since it inhibits neutrophil chemotaxis and reduces their respiratory burst. It also reduces their degranulation as well as CXCL8 production, and as a result, may reduce the damage caused by excessive inflammation. AGP inhibits complement activities and promotes the release of IL-IRA. It suppresses macrophage oxidant release, as well as granule exocytosis (Ceciliani & Lecci, 2019). It inhibits the chemotaxis of monocytes. AGP is antibacterial for bacteria such as Klebsiella and Mycoplasma. AGP is produced in healthy mammary glands and is present in mare's milk.

Horses also possess a lipocalin that is associated with neutrophil gelatinase. It was originally detected in activated neutrophils; however, it is also present in infected liver and kidneys. Its levels are low in the serum of healthy normal horses but rise significantly in horses with abdominal disease. It is also present in large quantities in peritoneal fluid (Winther et al., 2023).

C-reactive protein

Pentraxins are a family of P-type lectins that act as soluble pattern-recognition molecules (Du Clos, 2013). They come in short and long forms. Two of the most important are short C-reactive protein (also called PTX1) and long pentraxin 3 (PTX3). C-reactive protein (CRP) is a moderate acute-phase protein in horses. It has a discoid pentameric structure (five 23-kDa noncovalently bound subunits arranged in a circle) with two faces and a total molar mass of 118 kDa. One face of the CRP disk binds phosphocholine, a common side chain found in all cell membranes and many bacteria and protozoa. The other face binds to the antibody receptors FcγRI and FcγRIIa on neutrophils. CRP also tends to form stacks. CRP thus acts as an opsonin and promotes the phagocytosis and removal of damaged, dying, or dead cells in addition to invading microorganisms. CRP can bind to bacterial polysaccharides and glycolipids and to necrotic cells, where it activates complement C1q. (Its name derives from its ability to bind and precipitate the C-polysaccharide of *Streptococcus pneumoniae.*) CRP also has an anti-inflammatory role since it inhibits neutrophil superoxide production and degranulation and blocks platelet aggregation.

CRP stimulates fibrosis and may promote healing by reducing damage and enhancing the repair of damaged tissue.

An increase in serum levels of C-reactive protein (CRP) has been reported to occur in horses suffering from inflammatory conditions such as laminitis, enteritis, pneumonia, and arthritis. Its normal concentration is around 7.5 mg/L, but in inflammatory situations it can rise to as high as 35 mg/L. It generally increases within 24 hours of infection and peaks at around 3–5 days. An increased response is seen in old horses compared to young ones (Arfuso et al., 2023). Serum CRP concentrations are low in healthy foals but rise to 14.1 mg/L by 1 year of age. In pregnant mares, serum CRP decreases 2 months prior to foaling, climbs in the days immediately prior to and after parturition, and subsequently increases to relatively high levels by 2 months after (Yamashita et al., 1991). It is also of interest to note that CRP levels in healthy horses are affected by management practices such as diet and exercise, probably reflecting the presence of subclinical inflammation (Hall et al., 2025).

Other pentraxins

Pentraxin 3 is a long pentraxin produced by horses. Short pentraxins, such as CRP and SAP, are produced in the liver. Equine PTX3, in contrast, is produced by inflammatory neutrophils. Horses produce two forms of pentraxin 3 because of alternative splicing. There is a spliced form of 32 kDa and a full-length form of 42 kDa (Ramery et al., 2010). Pentraxin 3 (PTX3) is produced in response to TNF-α, IL-1β, and some microbial components. It can be readily detected in bronchoalveolar monocytes/macrophages, neutrophils, and bronchial epithelial cells in the bronchoalveolar lavage fluid of horses with recurrent airway obstruction. PTX3 levels rise faster than CRP in acute-phase responses since it is stored preformed and rapidly released from neutrophil granules. PTX3 can bind to diverse bacteria, fungi, and viruses and promote their phagocytosis. High PTX3 levels are associated with disease severity and mortality in human patients suffering from a systemic inflammatory response syndrome (Bastrup-Birk et al., 2013). PTX3 can act on alveolar macrophages to enhance their phagocytic abilities. It also appears to be able to bind to pathogens and activate the terminal complement pathway (Townsend et al., 2023).

Equine Serum Amyloid P (SAP) is also a pentraxin (pentraxin-2). It is a protein of 25 kDa encoded by a gene located on chromosome ECA5. It is not an acute-phase protein. Like CRP, it is a pattern recognition molecule, where one face of the disk can bind nuclear constituents such as DNA, chromatin, and histones, as well as cell membrane phospholipids. The other face binds and activates C1q and thus triggers the classical complement pathway. A major function of SAP is to regulate innate immune responses. It interacts with macrophage antibody receptors, reduces binding of neutrophils to the extracellular matrix, reduces the differentiation of macrophages into fibroblasts, so inhibiting fibrosis, and promotes phagocytosis of cell debris.

Fibrinogen

One of the most widely assayed APPs in horses is fibrinogen. Fibrinogen is a β-globulin consisting of a glycoprotein trimer linked by interchain disulfide bonds. It plays a key role in blood clotting. It is a moderate acute-phase protein in the horse. Its normal plasma levels are around 2000–4000 mg/L, and these may rise to 3000–11,000 mg/L beginning around 24–72 hours after disease onset (Borges et al., 2007). Fibrinogen is often increased in cases of systemic inflammatory response syndrome (SIRS). It takes 24–72 hours to reach peak concentrations and is not, therefore, very useful in detecting mild inflammation.

Ceruloplasmin

Ceruloplasmin is a 151 kDa α_2-glycoprotein that contains about eight atoms of copper per molecule. Ceruloplasmin outcompetes invading bacteria for this essential element. It is a moderate APP in the horse. It rises slowly after infections begin around 5 days (120 hours) post-infection. It peaks at 7–10 days and may remain elevated for several weeks (Jacobsen, 2007).

Procalcitonin

Procalcitonin is the 12.5 kDa precursor of the hormone calcitonin. It is produced by the parafollicular cells of the thyroid gland and by neuroendocrine cells in the intestine. Its production is triggered by TNF-α as well as several interleukins. It is thus a useful marker for the diagnosis of intestinal ischemia, such as those with strangulating intestinal lesions (Kilcoyne et al., 2020). It is also elevated in horses with infections such as sepsis, chronic respiratory disease, and inflammatory bowel disease (Barton et al., 2016). Procalcitonin is elevated approximately tenfold in horses suffering from SIRS. As a result, it can be employed as an assay for this syndrome (Bonelli et al., 2015).

Negative APPs

Horses suffering from infections require increased amounts of amino acids for the synthesis of proteins such as immunoglobulins. They acquire these in part by downregulating the synthesis of less essential proteins. Some serum protein levels fall by more than 25% during acute inflammation. These are called "negative" acute-phase proteins. They may drop rapidly over the first 24 hours or decline slowly over several days. Two of the most important are serum albumin and transferrin. The decline may be due to decreased production or increased catabolism. Serum albumin tends to decline gradually and this drop is especially significant in chronic diseases. It serves as a source of amino acids that can be used on demand, such as during infections and inflammation. Transferrin is an iron-transporting molecule and its decline ensures that the iron is unavailable to invading bacteria.

HMGB1

Equine high-mobility group box-1 (HMGB1) is a protein of 24.8 kDa encoded by a gene located on chromosome ECA17. It has several distinct functions. It is a chromatin-associated transcription factor that controls DNA folding. It also acts as a ligand for the receptor for advanced glycation end products (RAGE) and so activates several cell signaling pathways and triggers sickness behavior. Although IL-1β, IL-6, and TNF-α have long been known to cause septic shock and sickness behavior, these three cytokines also induce the slow release of HMGB1 from macrophages (Sha et al., 2008). HMGB1 has been implicated in food aversion and weight loss by its actions on the hypothalamic-pituitary axis. It mediates endotoxin lethality, joint pain, and macrophage activation. The inflammation induced by necrotic cells is caused in part by the escape of HMGB1 from disrupted nuclei and damaged mitochondria (Yang et al., 2005). Serum HMGB1 levels rise rapidly in horses suffering from gastrointestinal disease, increasing about fivefold (Bauquier et al., 2016).

Hepcidin

One of the most important factors that determines the success or failure of bacterial invasion is the availability of iron. Most pathogenic bacteria, such as *Staphylococcus aureus, Escherichia coli, Bacillus anthracis, Pasteurella multocida*, and *Mycobacterium tuberculosis*, require iron for growth. As a result, bacteria and their hosts compete for the same metal. The result of this competition may determine the outcome of an infection (Cassat & Skaar, 2013).

The development of hypoferremia is not uncommon during equine inflammatory diseases. The iron accumulates within macrophages while intestinal absorption is reduced. Almost all of the available iron is bound to iron-binding proteins such as transferrin, lactoferrin, hepcidin, siderocalin, haptoglobin, and ferritin.

Iron is usually absorbed from food by duodenal enterocytes. It binds to the cell surface ferroportin and is transported to the bloodstream, where it is bound by transferrin. This iron is mainly incorporated into hemoglobin in red cells (Filho et al., 2010). Most is derived from recycling aged or damaged red cells. Aged red cells give up their iron when ingested by splenic macrophages. The macrophages phagocytose these cells and catabolize the hemoglobin using heme oxygenase. They release the iron obtained from hemoglobin into the circulation via ferroportin. The exported iron binds to transferrin and is carried to erythroblasts for use in new red cell production (Ganz & Nemeth, 2015).

Horses also respond to microbial invasion by producing the acute-phase protein hepcidin. Equine hepcidin is a 25-amino-acid peptide of 9.1 kDa with a structure similar to that in other domestic mammals. Hepcidin is produced in large quantities by hepatocytes under the influence of IL-1β and IL-6 (Filho et al., 2010). It binds to ferroportin and triggers its internalization and degradation. Hepcidin also suppresses intestinal iron absorption by downregulating ferroportin expression in enterocytes

(Johnson et al., 2010). In healthy individuals, hepcidin production is regulated by systemic iron availability, or by erythropoietic signals and hypoxia. During infections, however, IL-6 and IL-1β stimulate the hepcidin promoter. As a result, hepcidin increases, ferroportin decreases, iron absorption by enterocytes is blocked, and macrophages can no longer export their iron (Drakesmith & Prentice, 2012). Iron availability for red blood cell production drops, and hypoferritinemia develops. Chronically infected horses become anemic —the anemia of inflammation or chronic disease. This is usually a mild normocytic, normochromic, non-regenerative anemia (Nemeth & Ganz, 2014).

The acute phase response in donkeys

Donkeys generally have a high pain tolerance and often express few signs of physical discomfort. As a result their sickness is often missed until too late. However, inflammatory diseases also induce acute-phase responses in donkeys. Measurement of their acute phase response is therefore a useful tool to determine the presence of infection and inflammation. The acute-phase proteins generated in donkeys are very similar to those observed in the horse. Thus, the most significant APP is SAA. Both SAA and α1-acid glycoprotein, are significantly increased in clinically ill juvenile donkeys when compared to young healthy donkeys. In sick adult donkeys, SAA and haptoglobin levels are increased when compared to healthy adult donkeys. There was no difference in CRP levels between sick and healthy donkeys (Li et al., 2021). Normal levels of SAA are higher in Jacks. Donkeys under 5 years of age tend to have higher ceruloplasmin, α1-acid glycoprotein, and procalcitonin levels than older donkeys (Perez-Ecija et al., 2020).

Protein misfolding diseases

Amyloidosis is the name given to the deposition of insoluble proteins in body organs. Amyloidosis is an uncommon disease that develops in older horses. No sex or breed predilection has been reported in this species. Visceral amyloidosis develops secondarily to chronic infections such as tuberculosis, severe Strongylid parasitism, or excessive immune stimulation. When a horse is routinely vaccinated, its serum SAA concentration increases for about 7 days (Baumgarten et al., 2024). When this process is carried out repeatedly, it results in amyloidosis becoming a significant problem in horses used for the commercial production of hyperimmune serum. Cutaneous amyloidosis is not associated with chronic inflammation but possibly with the presence of a malignant histiocytic lymphoma.

Amyloid deposits appear as amorphous, eosinophilic, hyaline protein accumulations in cells and tissues. Amyloid proteins are produced as a result of errors in the folding of newly formed protein chains (Fig. 5.4).

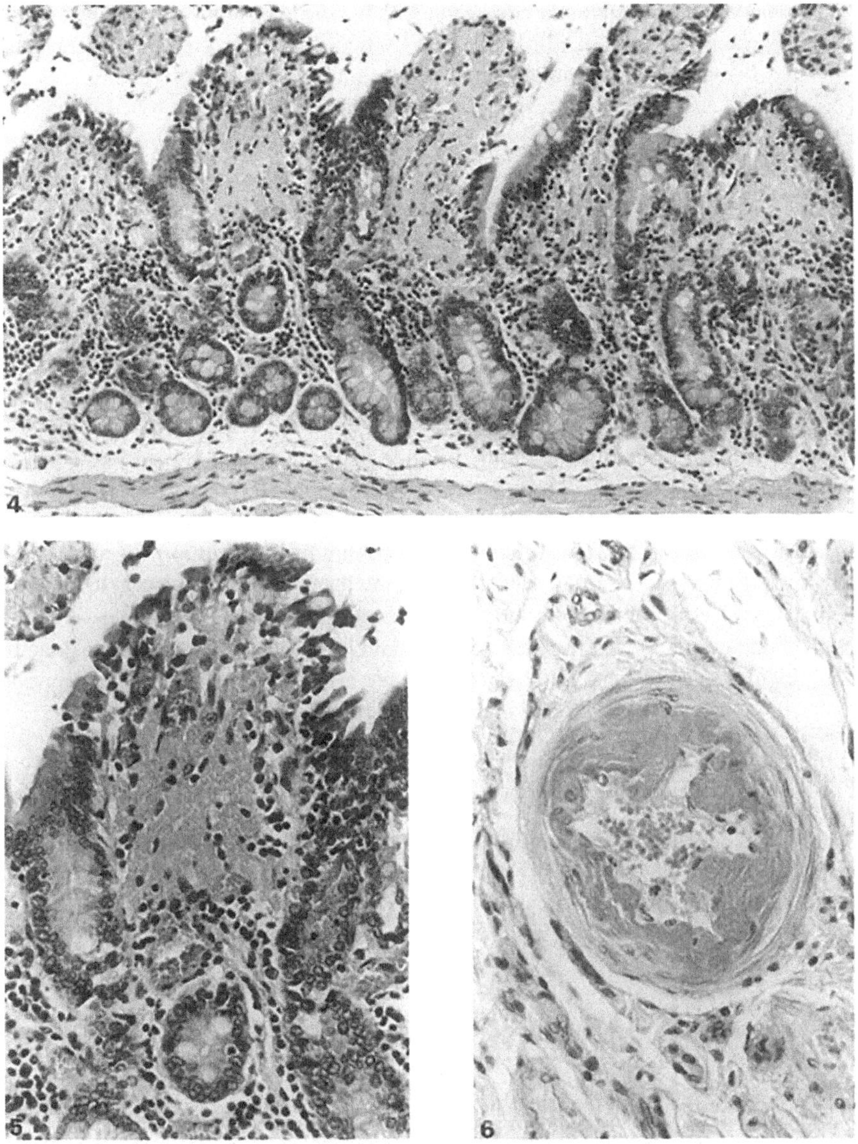

FIGURE 5.4 (A) Amyloid deposits in the jejunum of a horse. Note that it is accompanied by a mononuclear cell infiltration. Congo *red* × 140. (B) A higher magnification of Fig. A showing a villous core filled with amyloid. Congo *red* × 260. (C) Amyloid deposits markedly distort the wall of the submucosal artery in the small colon. Congo *red* × 260.

- From Elsevier paper Hayden, D. W., Johnson, K. H., Wolf. C. B., & Westermark, P. (1988). AA amyloid-associated gastroenteropathy in a horse. Journal of Comparative Pathology. 98, 195–204.

These misfolded chains eventually aggregate. Electron microscopy shows that amyloid proteins consist of fibrils, formed by peptide chains cross-linked to form β-pleated sheets. This molecular conformation makes amyloid proteins extremely insoluble and almost totally resistant to proteases. Consequently, once deposited in cells or tissues, amyloid is very difficult to remove. Amyloid infiltration eventually leads to gradual cell loss, tissue destruction, and death. Amyloidosis may involve multiple organs, or it may be localized, involving only a single organ (Hawthorne et al., 1990; Herczenik & Gebbink, 2008).

AA amyloid.

The most important source of amyloid protein in the horse is the acute-phase protein, SAA. Fragments of SAA tend to accumulate, misfold, form fibrils, and then be deposited extracellularly in organs. This material, the most common form in the horse, is called amyloid AA. This form of reactive amyloidosis is associated with chronic inflammatory diseases such as osteomyelitis, chronic abscesses, and pneumonia. Pentraxin 2, (serum amyloid P) binds and stabilizes SAA amyloid fibrils. Misfolded SAA forms β-pleated sheets. Beta-pleated sheets are insoluble, and when produced excessively, are deposited in organs as AA amyloid (Buxbaum, 2006). Most visceral cases are detected incidentally at necropsy. Amyloidosis may involve the upper respiratory tract, including the nasal cavity, ventral turbinates, the pharynx, larynx, guttural pouch, and associated lymph nodes (van Andel et al., 1988). Cutaneous amyloidosis is associated with the development of tumorlike amyloid nodules, papules, and plaques, and subcutaneous amyloid deposits present on the head, neck, and chest. The disease has a gradual, insidious onset.

Secondary amyloidosis develops gradually in response to chronic inflammation in osteomyelitis, abscesses, or tuberculosis. Horses develop insidious signs of progressive liver and kidney failure, and chronic weight loss leading to emaciation. Protein-losing nephropathy and renal failure secondary to deposition of amyloid within glomeruli may present as nephritic syndrome with proteinuria. Deposition of AA amyloid in glomeruli leads to loss of glomerular function and progressive renal failure. Deposition of AA amyloid in the liver and spleen leads to organ enlargement. Deposition of amyloid in the intestinal tract results in malabsorption and enteric protein loss due to diarrhea (Hayden et al., 1988) (Fig. 5.4). Horses develop insidious signs of progressive liver and kidney failure, and chronic weight loss leading to emaciation. Prognosis and outcome are largely determined by the degree of renal damage. Elimination of the source of inflammation will reduce the rate of disease progression and improve prognosis. Some amyloid deposits are usually present in all elderly horses, but this usually has no detectable effect on renal function.

AL amyloid.

Very rarely, excessive immunoglobulin light chain production by plasma cell tumors (myelomas) or other monoclonal gammopathies may lead to deposition of AL amyloid. AL amyloid is a degradation product of immunoglobulin light chains. AL amyloidosis is common in humans but rare in horses. In equines, it is also associated with excessive light chain production by multiple myelomas (Kim et al., 2005).

Analysis has shown that it is composed of complete λ light chains. Equine AL amyloidosis appears to affect surface structures primarily, such as the nasal and gastrointestinal tracts (Gliatto & Alroy, 1995; Niewold et al., 1996; van Andel et al., 1988). Equine lysozyme is an enzyme that readily unfolds and then aggregates to form stable "molten globules." These globules then assemble into ring-shaped and linear amyloid fibrils (Morozova-Roche, 2007). While important experimentally, this form of amyloid does not appear to cause clinical disease in horses (Chapter 5).

Inflammatory disease syndromes

Tissue damage as a result of trauma or infectious diseases can result in the immediate activation of innate immune responses. These responses serve to limit further damage and initiate healing. However, they can also drive further complications. The innate responses to trauma fall into two phases. In the first phase, additional tissue damage may occur as a result of a systemic inflammatory response. The tissue damage results in the activation of neutrophils and macrophages. Reactive oxygen species (ROS) are generated as a result of their oxidative burst. This may cause additional damage. In the second phase, there is a compensatory anti-inflammatory response syndrome. As a result, the animal may become immunosuppressed. This can result in sepsis and septic shock, leading to organ failure (Hietbrink et al., 2006; Huber-Lang et al., 2018).

Systemic inflammatory response syndrome

Inflammation is an important and necessary defensive process. However, if it is uncontrolled and exaggerated, inflammation can lead to organ damage and death. This uncontrolled inflammation is a greater problem in foals than in adult horses. When foals die from infectious diseases or malignancies, death is not always attributable to a direct effect of the pathogen or its toxins but may be a result of a systemic inflammatory response syndrome (SIRS) (Fig. 5.5).

After massive tissue damage, large quantities of cellular components, including HMGB1, mitochondria, proteases, and oxidants, may escape into the bloodstream and trigger a hyperinflammatory response. These DAMPs activate sentinel cells that, as a result, produce large quantities of inflammatory cytokines and chemokines such as TNF-α, IL-1β, IL-18, IFN-γ, CXCL8, and IL-6 (Lee & Cron, 2023). They also generate large amounts of the complement fragment, C5a. The cytokines and C5a, in turn, trigger the activation of more T cells and the release of yet more cytokines, leading to even greater cell destruction. Combinations of TNF-α plus IL-18, interferon-γ, or IL-1β are especially lethal. Animals develop high fevers, cytopenias, and coagulopathies. This "cytokine storm" may result in multiple organ failure, overwhelming systemic inflammation, and death. The most important of these cytokine storms is generated by massive tissue trauma. However, many viruses, such as

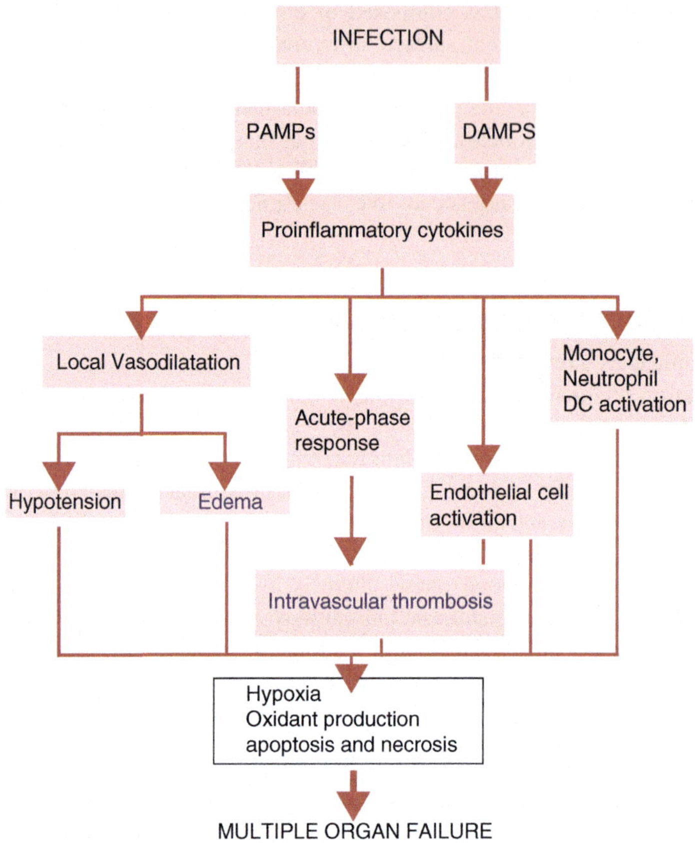

FIGURE 5.5 The pathogenesis of the systemic inflammatory response syndrome.

In effect, the syndrome results from overexpression of multiple cytokines. These cytokines trigger a series of events that result in widespread cell death and multiple organ failure.

influenza and equine viral arteritis, may also trigger excessive cytokine release and death.

It is also of interest to note that stimulation of equine neutrophils by bacterial lipopolysaccharide through TLR4 prolongs their lifespan by inhibiting their apoptosis. This phenomenon may play a role in the development of a systemic inflammatory response syndrome caused by an endotoxemia (Anderson et al., 2018).

Horses that develop SIRS are highly stressed. One characteristic feature of these individuals is an eosinopenia. As a result, eosinopenia has been used as a marker for SIRS in critically ill horses. Horses with the lowest blood eosinophil counts appear to be the least likely to survive (Martin-Cuervo et al., 2022).

Horses possess a histidine-rich glycoprotein in their serum that is involved in the regulation of innate immunity. It appears to play an important role in equine SIRS.

For example, it suppresses neutrophil adherence, reduces neutrophil chemotaxis, inhibits the neutrophil oxidant pathway and the production of reactive oxygen species, but it enhances neutrophil phagocytosis. Its level. is significantly reduced in animals with SIRS, suggesting that this is a major contributing factor to the syndrome (Muko et al., 2021).

Sepsis

Sepsis is the name given to a SIRS accompanied by a bacterial infection, and complicated by reduced blood pressure and unresponsiveness to fluid therapy. It accounts for about 9% of human deaths in the United States and is a correspondingly important cause of equine deaths. It is a common consequence of the failure of passive transfer in foals. Its overall fatality rate is 40%–55% (Taylor, 2015). Both species are relatively sensitive to endotoxin toxicity. It can also result from pleuropneumonia, enterocolitis, meningoencephalitis, metritis, or arthritis. Severe infections may cause excessive triggering of TLRs, leading to a massive and uncontrolled release of HMGB1. Other cytokines that play a major role in equine sepsis are TNF-α and IL-1β, with IFN-γ, IL-6, IL-3, and CXCL8 in a supporting role (Hobbs et al., 2024). These cytokines, in turn, stimulate nitric oxide synthase 2 (NOS2), leading to an increase in serum nitric oxide and COX-2, and resulting in massive prostaglandin and leukotriene synthesis. This excessive mediator release causes severe acidosis, fever, lactate accumulation in tissues, an uncontrollable drop in blood pressure, elevation of plasma catecholamines, and eventually renal, hepatic, and lung failure. Tissue damage, severe systemic inflammation, and the release of damaged cell fragments all act to raise blood levels of "tissue factor," a key initiator of coagulation. Vascular endothelial cell apoptosis may cause their detachment from the basement membrane. The cytokines activate the vascular endothelium so that procoagulant activity is enhanced, leading to blood clotting. The nitric oxide causes vasodilation and a drop in blood pressure. The prostaglandins and leukotrienes cause an increase in vascular permeability. This combination may result in disseminated intravascular coagulation (Lewis et al., 2012).

A defining characteristic of both SIRS and sepsis in horses is an alteration in the numbers of circulating neutrophils. On exposure to bacterial LPS, neutrophil numbers initially fall within hours, and the animal develops neutropenia. Examination of blood smears shows the presence of immature band forms and toxic changes (Lambert et al., 2016). The apoptosis of these neutrophils is delayed. The delayed apoptosis is a result of a decline in caspase 9 activity. These neutrophils also show decreased deformability and, as a result, are unable to pass through some capillary beds. Changes in chemokine levels also affect neutrophil migration patterns. The accumulation of neutrophils within tissues can result in significant organ damage and multiple organ dysfunction. The important target organs in the horse are the kidneys (Aamer et al., 2017). Sepsis causes acute kidney injury. The neutrophil myeloperoxidase, as well as released reactive nitrogen species, also cause epithelial injury as seen in laminitis.

A sepsis staging system has been established for horses. The classification scheme is called PIRO (Predisposition, Insult, Response, and Organ failure) (Sheats, 2019). The predisposition relates to the foal's age and overall health. Insult relates to the nature of the causal bacteria. The response relates to the degree of inflammation triggered in the animal, while the Organ failure is a measure described below.

Multiple organ dysfunction syndrome (MODS)

MODS is defined as altered organ function in an acutely ill animal such that homeostasis cannot be maintained without intervention (Osterbur et al., 2014). It is often a sequel to severe sepsis, septic shock, or acute surgical colic, but can also develop as a result of major trauma or anything else that will induce a systemic inflammatory response syndrome (McConachie et al., 2016). It is characterized by hypotension, insufficient tissue perfusion, uncontrollable bleeding, and organ failure caused by hypoxia, tissue acidosis, mitochondrial dysfunction, cytopathic hypoxia, tissue necrosis, and severe local metabolic disturbances (Fig. 5.6).

The pathogenesis of MODS is unclear, but it appears to result from immune system dysregulation and subsequent mitochondrial dysfunction. The immune system dysregulation may be due to overregulation of the inflammatory response and a compensatory anti-inflammatory response, as well as the excessive release of neutrophil reactive oxygen species, leading to lethal tissue damage. MODS can affect the liver, respiratory system, brain, adrenals, heart, and kidneys. It is often associated with the development of acute laminitis as well as disseminated intravascular coagulation. It permits bacterial translocation from the gastrointestinal tract

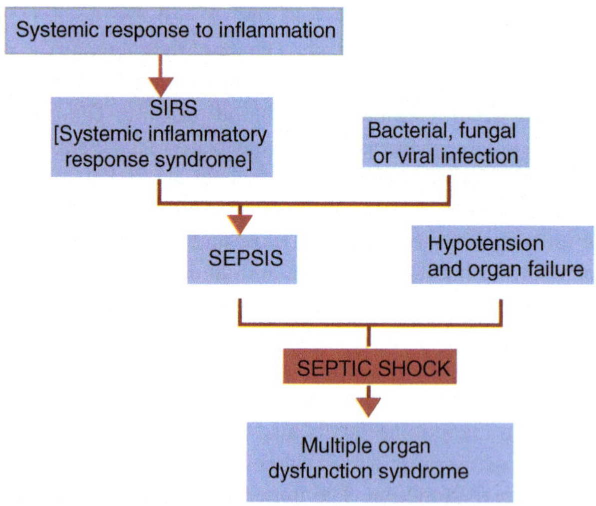

FIGURE 5.6 The progressive development of SIRS, sepsis, septic shock, and multiple organ dysfunction syndrome.

and disseminated intravascular coagulation. Its development is associated with a poor clinical outcome. However, efforts have been made to determine its outcome in horses through the use of a scoring system (McConachie et al., 2016).

Laminitis

Acute laminitis is a common debilitating disease syndrome in horses and ponies as well as donkeys. Animals develop acute inflammation within their hooves that results in failure of the bonds between the hoof wall and the distal phalanx. While traditionally considered a single entity, laminitis is now recognized as a complex inflammatory syndrome resulting from several different trigger factors: These include systemic diseases such as endocrinopathic disease caused by prolonged hyperinsulinemia, disease caused by bacterial endotoxemia or SIRS, local changes in weight bearing, such as support-limb laminitis caused by prolonged weight-bearing on one hoof, and pasture-related laminitis (Patterson-Kane et al., 2018). Experimentally, inflammation sufficient to trigger laminitis can also be triggered by carbohydrate (starch and oligofructose) overload, or by black walnut poisoning (Katz & Bailey, 2012) (Fig. 5.7).

Laminitis caused by sepsis or endotoxemia is associated with infections due to Gram-negative bacteria, metritis, enteritis, and enterocolitis (Steelman et al., 2013).

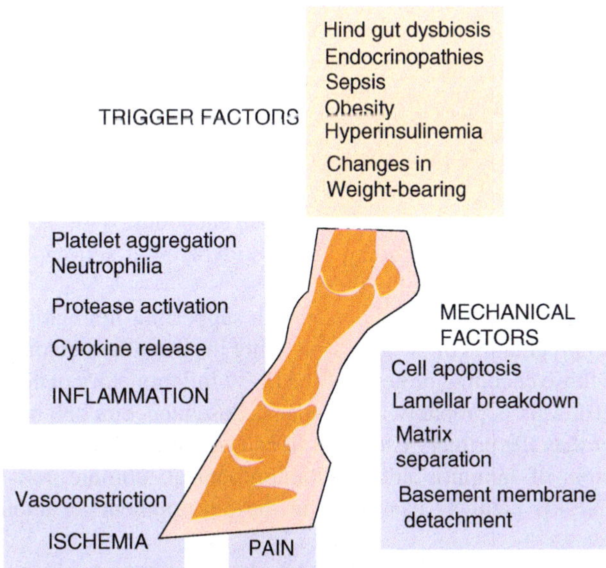

FIGURE 5.7 The pathogenesis of equine laminitis.

Laminitis is, a complex syndrome triggered by diverse inflammatory stimuli that results in tissue breakdown and separation between the hoof wall laminae within the animal's hooves resulting in extreme discomfort and pain.

One common cause is Salmonellosis. In most mammals with sepsis, as described above, internal organs such as the liver or lungs are damaged as a result of a cytokine storm, and this results in organ failure (Woldemeskel, 2012). In the horse, in contrast, the epidermal laminae within the hoof appear to be the most vulnerable organs. (The laminar tissue is formed by the interdigitations between the dermis and epidermis, formed by the basement membrane.) Infections that trigger laminitis may therefore include pleuropneumonia, endometritis, and gastrointestinal injury. In the latter case, this may be due to enterocolitis and severe colic, especially when associated with dysbiosis of the colonic microbiota as a result of carbohydrate overload. Massive overgrowth of Gram-negative bacteria releases large amounts of lipopolysaccharide, resulting in the destruction of the epithelial barrier. Gram-negative sepsis, and endotoxemia. While endotoxin alone cannot induce laminitis, other molecules escaping from the damaged gastrointestinal tract probably play a role. The complex mixture of PAMPs and DAMPs escaping from the colon, presumably acting through PRMs, triggers acute laminar inflammation. Endothelial cells, epidermal cells, and macrophages release cyclooxygenase (COX-2) and ROS, as well as IL-1β, and IL-6, in addition to many different chemokines. There is local production of prostanoids, prostaglandins, prostacyclin, and thromboxanes from arachidonic acid (Marcato & Perillo, 2020). These also trigger neutrophil infiltration and activation. All these reactions collectively result in apoptosis of the basal layer cells and keratinocytes within the lamellar tisue (Faleiros et al., 2004).

In a study examining laminar gene expression in horses with acute laminitis induced by experimental black walnut poisoning it was very clear that an inflammatory response developed in laminar tissues within hours. Thus, as early as 90 minutes after the poison was administered there was significant upregulation of the genes associated with macrophage activation, including, the chemokines CCL7, CCL2, CXCL10, and ICAM-1. At the same time there was downregulation of B cell transcripts encoding IgG3, IgG1 and κ light chains. As the inflammation developed, there was progressive upregulation of the genes encoding SAA, calgranulin C and NF-AT, as well as the genes encoding proteins involved in antioxidant and antimicrobial responses (Noschka et al., 2009).

Studies on lamellar tissue from horses with supporting limb laminitis have also demonstrated upregulation of the genes encoding the proinflammatory cytokine, IL-17, as well as those encoding proteins of the IL-17 inflammatory pathway (Cassimeria et al., 2020). This is probably a secondary consequence of cell stress and tissue damage rather than the primary causation. It can be argued, therefore, that while the initiating factors of laminitis are not immunological, chronic cell stress acting through the NF-κB pathway can result in the development of autoinflammatory processes.

Endotoxin-stimulated peripheral blood leukocytes increase their expression of the inflammatory cytokines, TNF-α, IL-1β, IL-6, and CXCL8. This production is mediated by activation of the mitogen-activated protein kinase (MAPK) pathway (Neuder et al., 2009). The resulting acute inflammation, together with the cytokine-associated tissue damage and loss of integrity within the lamina, upregulates matrix and secreted metalloproteases within the hoof. These, in turn, degrade the proteoglycans in the basement membrane of the lamellae as well as collagen in the intercellular matrix. This leads to basement membrane disruption and the separation of the epidermal and dermal lamellar tissue. The separation may also be due to down-regulation of epithelial cell adherence proteins such as integrins and a loss of hemidesmosomes, oxidative injury, and excessive apoptosis. There is also evidence for the occurrence of a prior subclinical phase that is characterized by gross changes in the hoof capsule with elongation of lamellar cells (van Eps & Burns, 2019).

Studies on horses with chronic laminitis have demonstrated that their leukocytes produce more IFN-γ than leukocytes from normal horses. However, they showed no differences in immunoglobulin levels. Unlike other autoinflammatory diseases, there is no apparent linkage between laminitis susceptibility and the horse's MHC haplotype. Thus, there is no evidence to support the concept that laminitis is autoimmune in nature.

Treatment of laminitis includes prolonged cooling of the foot to reduce blood flow and exudation, pain management, and mechanical support for the damaged hoof. If lamellar damage is not controlled, the disease may become chronic, leading to rotation of the third phalanx, coffin bone remodeling, dropped sole, and development of a lamellar wedge.

Disseminated intravascular coagulation

Disseminated Intravascular Coagulation (DIC) is a severe clinical syndrome characterized by dysregulation of the clotting and fibrinolytic cascades—an imbalance between bleeding and clotting (Berthelsen et al., 2011)! It is a feature of sepsis, pancreatitis, envenomation, immune-mediated hemolytic anemia, protein losing enteropathy and disseminated neoplasia as well as some equine viral diseases. The clotting cascade is initially triggered by injury to vascular endothelial cells caused by ischemia, chemical mediators, or the release of neutrophil NETS. It also results from the excessive production of a transmembrane glycoprotein called "tissue factor" (TF). TF is normally masked and does not trigger blood clotting in healthy tissues. However, TF is released on exposure to cytokines, especially IL-1β and TNF-α. It is also released by massive tissue damage or by exposure to bacteria and bacterial endotoxins in Gram-negative sepsis. For example, tissue factor is expressed in large amounts by horse peritoneal macrophages exposed to bacterial endotoxin. Endotoxin also triggers these cells to produce plasminogen activator inhibitor type 2. It is expressed on macrophages and other cell surfaces and promotes fibrin deposition (Barton et al., 1996) (Fig. 5.8).

The TF transforms prothrombin to thrombin to form fibrin thrombi. Simultaneous down-regulation of anti-coagulant systems results from reduced antithrombin synthesis (it is a "negative" acute-phase protein). In horses suffering from SIRS, activated platelets can also contribute to its pathogenesis and induce complications such as DIC. They can cluster as aggregates or as platelet-

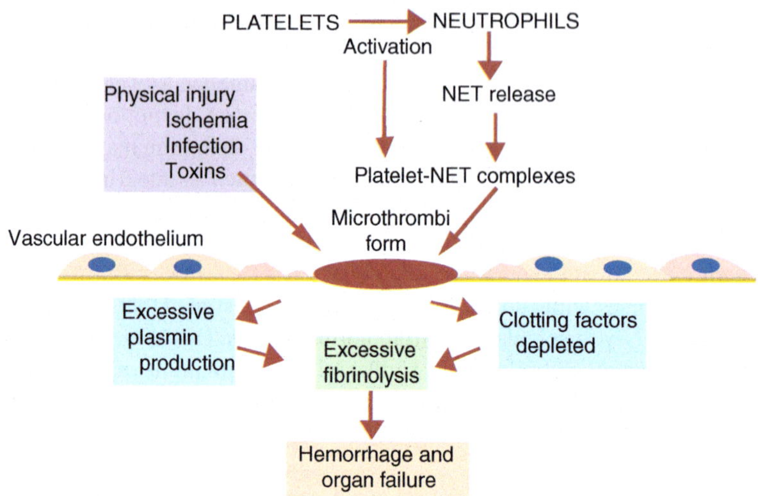

FIGURE 5.8 The pathogenesis of disseminated intravascular coagulation.

leukocyte aggregates (Theuerkauf et al., 2022). Activation of the clotting cascade leads to the formation of fibrin, NETs, and platelet microthrombi in small blood vessels throughout the body. These clots cause intravascular thrombosis and can lead to ischemia, impaired organ perfusion, and widespread damage (Wada, 2004). At the same time, the excessive thrombin released activates plasminogen to generate plasmin, which causes fibrinolysis. When the microthrombi break down, they release fibrin breakdown products such as D-dimer, which promote hemorrhage. In addition, the newly formed thrombi consume clotting factors and platelets. As a result, normal clotting does not occur, and uncontrolled bleeding may result. Plasmin also activates the complement and kinin systems, and these also promote inflammation, hypotension, and increased vascular permeability. The occurrence of DIC carries with it a poor prognosis. An important equine example of DIC is seen in African Horse Sickness. The virus targets vascular endothelial cells, resulting in hemorrhage and edema. It also triggers the coagulation system. Affected horses develop an increase in prothrombin time and D-dimer levels as well as a decrease in many coagulation factors. As a result, DIC is the major cause of death in African Horse Sickness. It is also a significant cause of death in horses with colic resulting from devitalized segments of the intestinal tract (Welch et al., 1992).

References

Aamer, H. G., El-Ashker, Nour, E. M., Wafa, E. W., & Youssef, M. A. (2017). Sepsis-induced acute kidney injury in equine: Current knowledge and future perspectives. *Journal of Equine Veterinary Science, 50*, 84–95.

Anderson, S. L., Townsend, H. G. G., & Singh, B. (2018). Role of toll-like receptor-4 and caspase -3. -8 and -9 in lipopolysaccharide-induced delay of apoptosis in equine neutrophils. *American Journal of Veterinary Research, 79*(4), 424–432.

Arfuso, F., Piccione, G., Guttadauro, A., Monteverde, V., et al. (2023). Serum C-reactive protein and protein electrophoretic pattern correlated with age in horses. *Journal of Equine Veterinary Science, 126*, Article 104561.

Back, H., Penell, J., Pringle, J., Isaksson, M., et al. (2015). A longitudinal study of poor performance and subclinical respiratory viral activity in standardbred trotters. *Veterinary Record Open, 2*, Article e000107.

Barton, M. H., Collatos, C., & Moore, J. N. (1996). Endotoxin induced expression of tumor necrosis factor, tissue factor, and plasminogen activator inhibitor activity by peritoneal macrophages. *Equine Veterinary Journal, 28*(3), 382–389.

Barton, A. K., Pelli, A., Rieger, M., & Gehlen, H. (2016). Procalcitonin as a biomarker in equine chronic pneumopathies. *BMC Veterinary Research, 12*, 281.

Bastrup-Birk, S., Skjoedt, M.-O., Munthe-Fog, L., Strom, J. J., et al. (2013). Pentraxin-3 serum levels are associated with disease severity and mortality in patients with systemic inflammatory response syndrome. *PLoS One*. https://doi.org/10.1371/journal.pone.0073119

Baumgarten, C. M., Delph Miller, C. M., Davis, E. G., Beard, L. A., et al. (2024). Serum Amyloid A increases following routine vaccination of healthy adult horses. *Journal of the American Veterinary Medical Association, 262*(9), 1181–1187.

Bauquier, J. R., Forbes, G., Nath, L., Tudor, E., & Bailey, S. R. (2016). Plasma HMGB-1 and nucleosome concentrations in horses with colic and healthy horses. *Journal of Veterinary Internal Medicine, 30*, 260–268.

Berthelsen, L. O., Kristensen, A. T., & Tranholm, M. (2011). Animal models of DIC and their relevance to human DIC: A systematic review. *Thrombosis Research, 128*(2), 103–116.

Bonelli, F., Meucci, V., Divers, T. J., Jose-Cunilleras, E., et al. (2015). Plasma procalcitonin concentration in healthy horses and horses affected by systemic inflammatory response syndrome. *Journal of Veterinary Internal Medicine, 29*, 1689–1691.

Borges, A. S., Divers, T. J., Stokol, T., & Hussni, M. O. (2007). Serum iron and plasma fibrinogen concentrations as indicators of systemic inflammatory diseases in horses. *Journal of Veterinary Internal Medicine, 21*(3), 489–494.

Buxbaum, J. (2006). The genetics of the amyloidoses: Interactions with immunity and inflammation. *Genes and Immunity, 7*, 439–449.

Cassat, J. E., & Skaar, E. P. (2013). Iron in infection and immunity. *Cell Host and Microbe, 13* (5), 509–519.

Cassimeria, L., Engiles, J. B., & Galantino-Homer, H. (2020). Interleukin 17A pathway target genes are upregulated in *Equus caballus* supporting limb laminitis. *PLoS One*. https://doi.org/10.1371/journal.pone.0232920

Ceciliani, F., & Lecci, C. (2019). The immune functions of α1 acid glycoprotein. *Current Protein and Peptide Science, 20*(6), 505–524.

Cheng, N., He, R., Tian, J., et al. (2008). Cutting edge: TLR2 is a functional receptor for acute-phase serum amyloid A. *The Journal of Immunology, 181*, 22–26.

Drakesmith, H., & Prentice, A. M. (2012). Hepcidin and the iron-infection axis. *Science, 338* (6108), 768–772.

Du Clos, T. W. (2013). Pentraxins: Structure, function, and role in inflammation. *ISRN Inflammation, 2013*, Article 379040.

Duggan, V. E., Holyoak, G. R., MacAllister, C. G., Cooper, S. R., & Confer, A. W. (2008). Amyloid A in equine colostrum and early milk. *Veterinary Immunology and Immunopathology, 121.*

Eckersall, P. D., & Bell, R. (2010). Acute phase proteins: Biomarkers of infection and inflammation in veterinary medicine. *The Veterinary Journal, 185*, 23–27.

Evans, S. S., Repasky, E. A., & Fisher, D. T. (2015). Fever and the thermal regulation of immunity: The immune system feels the heat. *Nature Reviews Immunology, 15*(6), 335–349.

Faleiros, R. R., Stokes, A. M., Eades, S. C., Kim, Y., et al. (2004). Assessment of apoptosis in epidermal laminar cells in clinically normal horses and those with laminitis. *American Journal of Veterinary Research, 65*(5), 578–585.

Filho, J. P. O., Badial, P. R., Cunha, P. H. J., Cruz, T. F., et al. (2010). Cloning, sequencing, and expression analysis of the equine hepcidin gene by real-time PCR. *Veterinary Immunology and Immunopathology, 135*, 34–42.

Ganz, T., & Nemeth, E. (2015). Iron homeostasis in host defense and inflammation. *Nature Reviews Immunology, 15*(8), 500–510.

Gliatto, J. M., & Alroy, J. (1995). Cutaneous amyloidosis in a horse with lymphoma. *The Veterinary Record, 137*, 68–69.

Gordon, D. L., Foreman, J. H., Connolly, S. L., Schnelle, A. N., et al. (2022). Acute phase protein concentrations following serial procaine penicillin G injections in horses. *Equine Veterinary Journal*. https://doi.org/10.1111/evj.13886

Hall, S. M., Friend, M. M., Smarsh, D. N., & Staniar, W. B. (2025). Characterizing the effects of management practices on inflammatory markers in a population of horses in Pennsylvania. *Journal of Equine Veterinary Science*. https://doi.org/10.1016/j.jevs.2025.105465

Hawthorne, T. B., Hawthorne, T. B., Bolon, B., et al. (1990). Systemic amyloidosis in a mare. *Journal of the American Veterinary Medical Association, 196*, 323–325.

Hayden, D. W., Johnson, K. H., Wolf, C. B., & Westermark, P. (1988). AA amyloid-associated gastroenteropathy in a horse. *Journal of Comparative Pathology, 98*, 195–204.

Herczenik, E., & Gebbink, M. F. B. G. (2008). Molecular and cellular aspects of protein misfolding and disease. *The FASEB Journal, 22*, 2115–2133.

Herz, J., & Kipnis, J. (2016). Bugs and brain: How infection makes you feel blue. *Immunity, 44*(4), 718–720.

Hietbrink, F., Koenderman, L., & Leenen, L. P. H. (2006). Trauma: The role of the innate immune system. *World Journal of Emergency Surgery, 1*, 15. https://doi.org/10.1186/1749-7922-1-15

Hobbs, K. J., Bayless, R., & Sheats, M. K. (2024). A comparative review of cytokines and cytokine targeting in sepsis: From humans to horses. *Cells*. https://doi.org/10.3390/cells13171489

Huber-Lang, M., Lambris, J. D., & Ward, P. A. (2018). Innate immune responses to trauma. *Nature Immunology, 19*, 327–341.

Jacobsen, S. (2007). Review of equine acute-phase proteins. *Proceedings of the American Association of Equine Practitioners, 53*, 230–235.

Jacobsen, S., & Andersen, P. H. (2007). The acute-phase protein serum amyloid A (SAA) as a marker of inflammation in horses. *Equine Veterinary Education, 19*(1), 38–46.

Johnson, E. E., Sandgren, A., Cherayil, B. J., et al. (2010). Role of ferroportin in macrophage-mediated immunity. *Infection and Immunity, 78*, 5099–5106.

Katz, L. M., & Bailey, S. R. (2012). A review of recent advances and current hypotheses on the pathogenesis of acute laminitis. *Equine Veterinary Journal, 44*(6), 752–761.

Kilcoyne, I., Nieto, J. E., & Dechant, J. E. (2020). Diagnostic value of plasma and peritoneal fluid procalcitonin concentrations in horses with strangulating intestinal lesions. *Journal of American Veterinary Medical Association, 256*(8), 927–933.

Kim, D. Y., Taylor, H. W., Eades, S. C., et al. (2005). Systemic AL amyloidosis associated with multiple myeloma in a horse. *Veterinary Pathology Online, 42*, 81–84.

Lambert, J. L., Fernandez, N. J., & Roy, M.-F. (2016). Association of presence of band cells and toxic neutrophils with systemic inflammatory response syndrome and outcome in horses with acute disease. *Journal of Veterinary Internal Medicine, 30*, 1284–1292.

Lee, P. Y., & Cron, R. Q. (2023). The multifaceted immunology of cytokine storm syndrome. *The Journal of Immunology, 210*, 1015–1024.

Lewis, D. H., Chan, D. L., Pinheiro, D., Armitage-Chan, E., & Garden, O. A. (2012). The immunopathology of sepsis: Pathogen recognition, systemic inflammation, the compensatory anti-inflammatory response, and regulatory T cells. *Journal of Veterinary Internal Medicine, 26*(3), 457–482.

Li, J., Jiang, G., Zhang, J., Liang, W., et al. (2021). Serum amyloid A as an indicator of infection in donkeys. *Journal of Animal Health and Behaviour Science., 5*, 5–8.

Long, A., & Nolen-Walston, R. (2020). Equine inflammatory markers in the twenty-first century: A focus on serum amyloid A. *Veterinary Clinics of Equine Practice, 36*, 147–160.

Mantovani, A., & Garlanda, C. (2023). Humoral innate Immunity and acute phase proteins. *New England Journal of Medicine, 388*, 439–452.

Marcato, P. S., & Perillo, A. (2020). Equine laminitis: New insights into the pathogenesis, A review. *Large Animal Review, 26*, 353–363.

Martin-Cuervo, M., Gracia-Calvo, L. A., Macias-Garcia, B., Ezquerra, L. J., & Barrera, R. (2022). Evaluation of eosinopenia as a SIRS biomarker in critically ill horses. *Animals*. https://doi.org/10.3390/ani12243547

McConachie, E., Giguere, S., & Barton, M. H. (2016). Scoring system for multiple organ dysfunction in adult horses with acute surgical gastrointestinal disease. *Journal of Veterinary Internal Medicine, 30*, 1276–1283.

Morozova-Roche, L. A. (2007). Equine lysozyme: The molecular basis of folding, self-assembly and innate amyloid toxicity. *FEBS Letters, 581*(14), 2587–2592.

Muko, R., Matsuda, H., Oikawa, M., Shin, T., et al. (2021). Histidine-rich glycoprotein functions as a dual regulator of neutrophil activity in horses. *Journal of Equine Veterinary Science*. https://doi.org/10.1016/j.jevs.2021.103620

Nemeth, E., & Ganz, T. (2014). Anemia of inflammation. *Hematology/Oncology Clinics of North America, 28*(4), 671–681.

Neuder, L. E., Keener, J. M., Eckert, R. E., Trujillo, J. C., & Jones, S. L. (2009). Role of p38 MAPK in LPS induced pro-inflammatory cytokine and chemokine gene expression in equine leukocytes. *Veterinary Immunology and Immunopathology, 129*, 192–199.

Niewold, T. A., Murphy, C., Gruys, E., Weiss, D. T., & Solomon, A. (1996). Equine light-chain-associated amyloidosis. *Experimental and Clinical Investigation, 3*, 183–186.

Noschka, E., Vandenplas, M. L., Hurley, D. J., & Moore, J. N. (2009). Temporal aspects of laminar gene expression during the developmental stages of equine laminitis. *Veterinary Immunology and Immunopathology, 129*, 242–253.

Osterbur, K., Mann, F. A., Kuroki, K., & DeClue, A. (2014). Multiple organ dysfunction syndrome in humans and animals. *Journal of Veterinary Internal Medicine, 28*, 1141–1151.

Patterson-Kane, J. C., Karikoski, N. P., & McGowan, C. M. (2018). Paradigm shifts in understanding equine laminitis. *The Veterinary Journal*, 33–40.

Perez-Ecija, A., Buzon-Cuevas, A., Aguilera-Aguilera, R., Gomzalez-De Cara, C., & Mendoza Garcia, F. J. (2020). Reference intervals of acute phase proteins in healthy Andalusian donkeys and response to experimentally induced endotoxemia. *Journal of Veterinary Internal Medicine*. https://doi.org/10.1111/jvim.16015

Pihl, T. H., Scheepers, E., Sanz, M., Goddard, A., et al. (2015). Influence of disease process and duration on acute phase proteins in serum and peritoneal fluid of horses with colic. *Journal of Veterinary Internal Medicine, 29*, 651–658.

Ramery, E., Fievez, L., Fraipont, A., Bureau, F., & Lekeux, P. (2010). Characterization of pentraxin 3 in the horse and its expression in airways. *Veterinary Research*. https://doi.org/10.1051/vetres/2009066

Roerink, M. E., van der Schaff, E., Dinarello, C. A., Knoop, H., & van der Meer, J. W. (2017). Interleukin-1 as a mediator of fatigue in disease: A narrative review. *Journal of Neuroinflammation*. https://doi.org/10.1186/s12974-017-0796-7

Sha, T., Zmijewski, J., Xu, Z., & Abraham, E. (2008). HMGB1 develops enhanced proinflammatory activity by binding to cytokines. *The Journal of Immunology, 180*, 2531–2537.

Sheats, M. K. (2019). A comparative review of equine SIRS, sepsis, and neutrophils. *Frontiers in Veterinary Science*. https://doi.org/10.3389/fvets.2019.00069

Sletten, K., Husebekk, A., & Husby, G. (1989). The primary structure of equine serum amyloid A (SAA) protein. *Scandinavian Journal of Immunology, 30*(1), 117–122.

Souto, P. C., Fonseca, L. A., Orozco, A. M. O., Lopez, C. J. R., et al. (2019). Acute-phase proteins in healthy horses and horses naturally affected by colic syndrome. *Journal of Equine Veterinary Science, 80*, 1–4.

Stack, J. D., Cousty, M., Steele, E., Handel, I., et al. (2019). Comparison of serum amyloid A measurements in equine synovial fluid with routine diagnostic methods to detect synovial infection in a clinical environment. *Frontiers in Veterinary Science*. https://doi.org/10.3389/fvets.2019.00325

Steelman, S. M., Johnson, D., Wagner, B., Stokes, A. M., & Chowdhary, B. P. (2013). Cellular and humoral immunity in chronic equine laminitis. *Veterinary Immunology and Immunopathology, 153*, 217–226.

Taylor, S. (2015). A review of equine sepsis. *Equine Veterinary Education, 27*(2), 99–109.

Theuerkauf, K., Obach-Schrock, C., Staszyk, C., Moritz, S. A., & Roscher, K. A. (2022). Activated platelets and platelet-leukocyte aggregates in the equine systemic inflammatory response syndrome. *Journal of Veterinary Diagnostic Investigation, 34*(3), 448–457.

Townsend, M., Fowler, B., Aulakh, G. K., & Singh, B. (2023). Expression of pentraxin 3 in equine lungs and neutrophils. *Canadian Journal of Veterinary Research, 87*(1), 9–16.

van Andel, A. C., van Andel, A. C., Gruys, E., & Kroneman, J. (1988). Amyloid in the horse: A report of nine cases. *Equine Veterinary Journal, 20*(4), 277–285.

van Eps, A. W., & Burns, T. A. (2019). Are there shared mechanisms in the pathology of different clinical forms of laminitis, and what are the implications for prevention and treatment? *Veterinary Clinics of Equine Practice, 35*, 379–398.

Wada, H. (2004). Disseminated intravascular coagulation. *Clinica Chimica Acta, 344*(1–2), 13–21.

Walter, E. J., Hanna-Jumma, S., Carreretto, M., & Forni, L. (2016). The pathophysiological basis and consequences of fever. *Critical Care*. https://doi.org/10.1186/s13054-016-1375-5

Wang, X., Ni, L., Wan, S., Zhao, X., et al. (2020). Febrile temperature critically controls the differentiation and pathogenicity of T helper 17 cells. *Immunity, 52*, 328–341.

Welch, R. D., Watkins, J. P., Taylor, T. S., Cohen, N. D., & Carter, G. K. (1992). Disseminated intravascular coagulation associated with colic in 23 horses (1984-1989). *Journal of Veterinary Internal Medicine, 6*(1), 29–35.

Winther, M. F., Haugaard, S. L., Pihl, T. H., & Jacobsen, S. (2023). Concentrations of neutrophil gelatinase-associated lipocalin are increased in serum and peritoneal fluid from horses with inflammatory abdominal disease and non-strangulating intestinal infarctions. *Equine Veterinary Journal, 55*, 426–434.

Witowska-Pilaszewicz, O. D., Zmigrodzka, M., Winnicka, A., Miskiewicz, A., et al. (2019). Serum Amyloid A in equine health and disease. *Equine Veterinary Journal*. https://doi.org/10.1111/evj.13062

Woldemeskel, M. (2012). A concise review of amyloidosis in animals. *Veterinary Medicine International*. https://doi.org/10.1155/2012/427296

Yamashita, K., Fujinaga, T., Okumura, M., Takiguchi, M., et al. (1991). Serum C-reactive protein(CRP) in horses. The effect of aging, sex, delivery and inflammation on its concentration. *Journal of Veterinary Medical Science, 53*(6), 1019–1024.

Yang, H., Wang, H., Czura, C., & Tracey, K. J. (2005). The cytokine activity of HMGB-1. *Journal of Leukocyte Biology, 78*, 1–8.

CHAPTER

Equine cytokines

6

Effective immune responses require that many different cell populations communicate and cooperate. These conversations are mediated, not only by direct cell to cell contact but also through the release of diverse soluble signaling molecules – cytokines. As a result, cells of the immune system generate many different cytokines that control their behavior and interactions (Myers & Murtaugh, 1995). Unlike hormones, which usually affect a single target cell type, cytokine signals can target many different cell types. In addition, immune system cells rarely produce a single cytokine at a time, and cells must respond to complex cytokine mixtures. The composition of these cytokine mixtures and the messages delivered also vary over time as the cytokine environment changes. The most obvious and important roles of cytokines are to trigger acute inflammation and sickness behavior in response to microbial invasion. The four major cytokines generated by responding sentinel cells are TNF-α, IL-1β, IL-6, and IL-18. They act in concert to produce the most effective inflammatory response possible. It must also be remembered however that cells of the immune system are not the only source of complex cytokine mixtures. For example, equine platelet lysate contains a complex mixture of them as well (Moellerberndt et al., 2023). Muscle cells are also a source of many cytokines (Chapter 24) as are adipocytes (Chapter 25).

Inflammatory cytokines

Tumor necrosis factor-α

The precursor of equine tumor necrosis factor-α (TNF-α) is a membrane-bound protein of 234 amino acids produced by endothelial cells, macrophages, T cells, B cells, and fibroblasts in response to TLR stimulation. It has 90.8% sequence identity to human TNF α (Soller et al., 2007). TNF-α is encoded by a gene consisting of four exons located on chromosome ECA20 within the ELA class III region (Chapter 9). The active cytokine consists of a 35 amino acid cytoplasmic domain, a 21 amino acid transmembrane domain, and a 177 amino acid extracellular domain. It is assembled intracellularly to form a non-covalently linked homotrimer that is then expressed on the cell surface. The membrane-bound molecule is subsequently cleaved from the cell surface by a protease called TNF-convertase. The active monomers are 17 kDa in size (Su et al., 1991). The bioactive cytokine is a 55 kDa trimer. TNF-α acts through two receptors: TNFR1 is found on diverse cells, where it can

The Immunology of Horses and Donkeys. https://doi.org/10.1016/B978-0-443-44863-8.00012-0

bind both soluble and membrane-bound TNF-α; and TNFR2, which is restricted to the cells of the immune system and responds only to membrane-bound TNF-α (Fig. 6.1). Soluble TNF-α, in turn, triggers the release of chemokines and cytokines from nearby cells and promotes the adherence, migration, attraction, and activation of leukocytes. Subsequently, TNF-α facilitates the transition from innate to adaptive immunity.

TNF-α is an essential mediator of inflammation because, in combination with IL-1β, it triggers changes in small blood vessels. A local increase in TNF-α causes the classic signs of inflammation, including heat, swelling, pain, and redness. Circulating TNF-α can depress cardiac output, induce microvascular thrombosis, and cause capillary leakage. TNF-α acts on neutrophils to enhance their ability to kill microbes. It attracts neutrophils to sites of tissue damage and increases their adherence to vascular endothelium. It stimulates macrophage phagocytosis and oxidant production. TNF-α induces macrophages to increase its own synthesis through a positive feedback loop together with that of IL-1β. It amplifies and prolongs inflammation by promoting macrophage synthesis of enzymes such as nitric oxide synthase 2 (NOS2) and cyclooxygenase-2 (COX-2), and it also activates mast cells. Mast cell-derived TNF is required for neutrophil recruitment to inflamed skin because it activates endothelial cells and triggers chemokine release (Dudeck et al., 2021). As described in the previous chapter, TNF-α plays a key role in the pathogenesis of some forms of equine laminitis (Hobbs et al., 2024).

As its name implies, TNF-α can kill some tumor cells as well as virus-infected cells. In high doses, TNF-α can also mediate the systemic inflammatory response

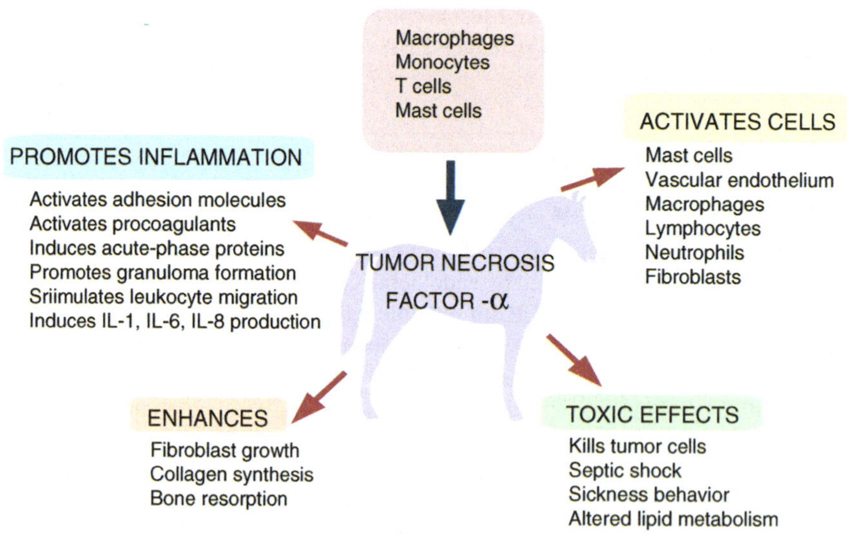

FIGURE 6.1

TNF-α, its sources and its functions in the horse.

syndrome. Other important members of the TNF-α family include TNF-β (or lymphotoxin), CD40L, and FasL (CD95L).

Interleukin-1

When stimulated by microbial products through CD14 and TLR4, sentinel cells synthesize cytokines belonging to the interleukin-1 family (Dinarello et al., 2010). The most important of these are IL-1α and IL-1β. IL-1β is synthesized as a large precursor protein that is cleaved by caspase-1 to form the active 17.5 kDa molecule. The equine IL-1β molecule has 62.8% sequence identity to the human, and it contains 268 amino acids. It has a calculated molecular weight of 30.2 kDa. It is encoded by a gene located on chromosome ECA15. Ten-to 50-fold more IL-1β is produced than IL-1α, and whereas IL-1β is secreted, IL-1α remains attached to the cell surface. As a result, IL 1α acts only on cells that come into direct contact with macrophages. Like TNF-α, IL-1β acts on nearby cells to initiate and amplify inflammation. For example, it acts on vascular endothelial cells to make them adhesive for neutrophils. IL-1β also acts on macrophages to stimulate their synthesis of NOS2 and COX-2 (Dinarello, 2018). Transcription of IL-1β messenger RNA (mRNA) occurs within 15 minutes of ligand binding to TLR4. It reaches a peak 3–4 hours later and levels off for several hours before declining (Sims & Smith, 2010).

Given its function as a proinflammatory cytokine produced by activated neutrophils, it is unsurprising that IL-1β is elevated in inflammatory states such as osteoarthritis, endotoxemia, and septic arthritis (Ehrle et al., 2015). During severe infections, high levels of IL-1β circulate in the bloodstream, where, in association with TNF-α, they are responsible for the horse's sickness behavior. Thus, it acts on the brain to cause fever, lethargy, and malaise. It acts on muscle cells to mobilize amino acids, causing pain and fatigue (and conseuently reduces equine peformance). It also acts on liver cells to induce the production of acute-phase proteins (Dinarello, 2018) (Fig. 6.2).

The most important IL-1β receptors on cells are CD121a and CD121b. CD121a is a signaling receptor, whereas CD121b is not. CD121b thus binds IL-1β, but nothing more happens! If soluble CD121b binds IL-1β, it acts as an antagonist. IL-1β activity is also regulated by IL-1 receptor antagonist (IL-1RA), a protein that binds and thus blocks CD121a. IL-1RA is therefore an important regulator of IL-1β activity and inflammation. It reduces mortality in septic shock and graft-versus-host disease and has anti-inflammatory effects (Heaney & Golde, 1996).

IL-1β is a member of a large family of cytokines that regulate innate immune responses. Other important family members include IL-1RA, IL-18, IL-33, IL-36, IL-37, and IL-38. All these cytokines signal through closely related receptors. Some, like IL-36, have a proinflammatory effect, while others, such as IL-37, have anti-inflammatory effects.

Interleukin-6

Equine IL-6 is a protein of 208 amino acids (23.3 kDa) mainly produced by macrophages. Its production is triggered by bacterial endotoxins, as well as by IL-1β and

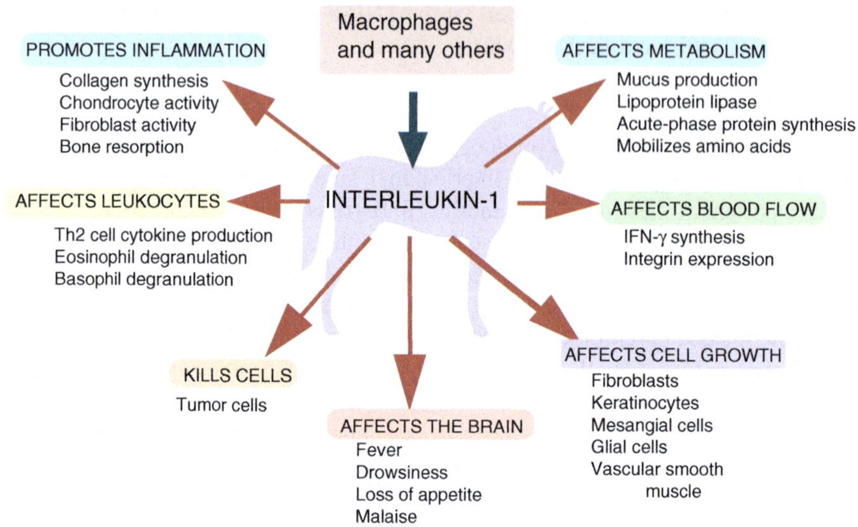

FIGURE 6.2

IL-1, its sources and its functions in the horse.

TNF-α. Like the other inflammatory cytokines, IL-6 is multifunctional (Murakami et al., 2019) (Fig. 6.3).

Thus, IL-6 promotes inflammation, especially in response to tissue damage and severe infections, and it is a major mediator of fever, the acute-phase protein response, and septic shock in the horse. In sepsis and the systemic inflammatory response syndrome (SIRS), the level of IL-6 is correlated with disease severity and its outcome (Hobbs et al., 2024). IL-6 receptors are found on T cells, neutrophils, macrophages, hepatocytes, and neurons. IL-6 also has an anti-inflammatory role in that it inhibits some activities of TNF-α and IL-1β and promotes the production of the suppressive cytokine IL-10. It has been suggested that IL-6 regulates the transition from a neutrophil-dominated process early in inflammation to a macrophage-dominated process later (Kaplanski et al., 2003). IL-6 is released by skeletal muscle cells in response to exercise, where it exerts an anti-inflammatory role (Chapter 24) (Wolf et al., 2014). In the donkey, the IL-6 gene shows an intronic C > T single nucleotide polymorphism (Kumar et al., 2022).

It is of interest to note that IL-6 production undergoes a circadian rhythm in the horse, with peak serum values reaching a maximum at around dawn (0500–0900 hours) and minimal levels occurring around sunset (1700 hours) (Aragona et al., 2025).

IL-6 signals to target cells through a heterodimeric receptor with an antigen-binding chain (IL-6R) and a signal transducing component, (gp130). This can be done in two ways. In its classic signaling pathway the IL-6 can signal directly to target cells such as leukocytes and hepatocytes through the heterodimer. In its trans-signaling pathway, soluble IL-6R can bind and form soluble complexes with

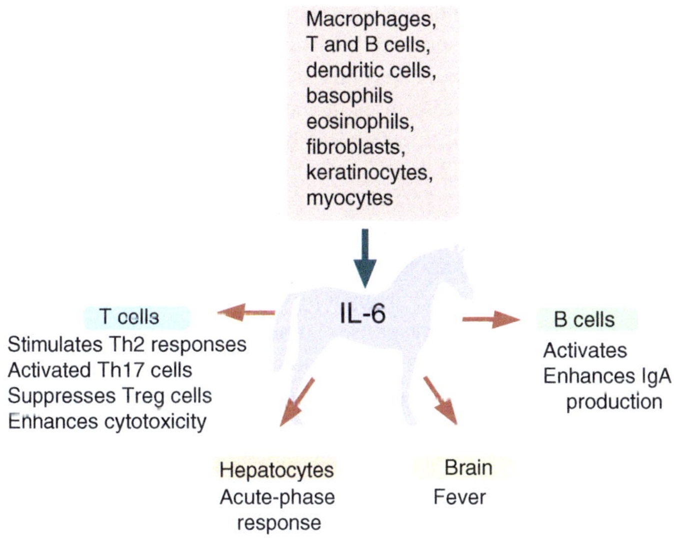

FIGURE 6.3

IL-6, its sources and its functions in the horse.

IL-6. These complexes can then circulate in the bloodstream and act on any target cells that express gp130. (gp130 is ubiquitous, so many different cell types can respond to IL-6). The IL-6 receptor family also includes the receptors for IL-11, IL-27, IL-35, and IL-39 (Murakami et al., 2019).

Interleukin-18

Equine interleukin 18 is an IL-1 family member of about 18 kDa (193 amino acids) encoded by a gene located on chromosome ECA7 (Wu et al., 2004). It is constitutively produced by macrophages and monocytes. It is also produced by keratinocytes and other epithelial cells. Like IL-1β, it is synthesized as an inactive 24 kDa precursor and then activated by caspase 1, yielding the active 18 kDa molecule. Like the other cytokines listed here, IL-18 promotes inflammation by promoting leukocyte nitric oxide and chemokine production. However, it does not induce a fever. IL-18 also activates Th1 and NK cells through the NF-κB pathway to promote the production of IFN-γ, TNF-α, IL-1β, and CD95L, as well as chemokines such as CXCL8, CCL2 (MCP-1), CCL3 (MIP-1α), and CCL4 (MIP-1β). This can lead to positive feedback where the IL-18 and IFN-γ reinforce each other's activities. IL-18 activity is regulated by a naturally occurring, high-affinity IL-18-binding protein (Dinarello et al., 2013; Hayden & Ghosh, 2008).

Regulatory cytokines

When an adaptive immune response is mounted, cytokines derived from antigen-presenting cells such as dendritic cells and macrophages, determine which helper

T cell subsets are activated and hence whether a horse will mount a type 1 or type 2 immune response. (A type 1 response is a cell-mediated immune response regulated by Th1 cells; a type 2 response is antibody-mediated and regulated by Th2 cells.) Cytokines that promote type 1 responses include IL-12 and IFN-γ. These cytokines work by activating the transcription factor T-bet. Cytokines that induce type 2 responses include IL-4, IL-33, and thymic stromal lymphopoietin (TSLP). These activate the transcription factor, GATA3 (Fig. 6.4).

Once presented with an antigen and appropriately co-stimulated with cytokines, helper T cells differentiate into several different families with different roles to play in immunity. Each family produces its own mixture of cytokines that determine the next step in the adaptive immune response. Some helper T cells secrete a mixture of Th1 and Th2 cytokines. These cells may be precursors of Th1 and Th2 or cells that are in transition between the two populations. Some IL-2-secreting T cells may switch to become IL-4-secreting cells after exposure to antigen, implying a change in phenotype from Th1 to Th2. The principal molecules that control this switch are IL-4 and IL-12. When cultured in the presence of IL-4, undifferentiated helper cells become Th2 cells. When cultured in the presence of IL-12, they become Th1 cells. Mixed cell populations are most obvious early after initiation of an immune response, whereas Th1 and Th2 subsets are more obvious in chronic diseases where the antigens are persistent.

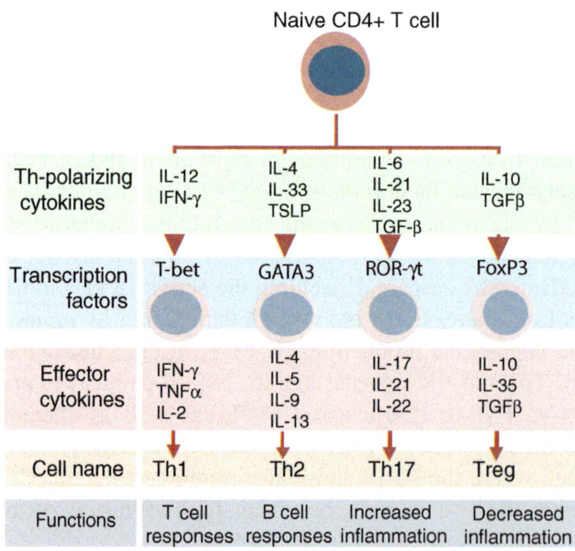

FIGURE 6.4 Antigen processing cells activate selected T cell populations by releasing a complex mixture of cytokines.

Once differentiated, these T cell populations in turn exercise their effects by secreting a specific mixture of other cytokines.

Type 1 immune response inducers

Type 1 helper cells characteristically produce three major cytokines, IL-2, IL-12, and IFN-γ. These act on other T cells to trigger a cell-mediated (type 1) immune response.

Interleukin-2

Equine IL-2 is a protein of 149 amino acids encoded by a gene located on chromosome ECA2 that contains four exons. It has 80% homology to the bovine molecule (Singha et al., 2015). IL-2 is produced by activated $CD4^+$ Th1 cells. Some is also produced by $CD8^+$ cells, NKT cells, dendritic cells, and mast cells (Fig. 6.5). Its targets are T, B, and NK cells as well as macrophages. IL-2 is a potent stimulator of T cell proliferation, IFN production, and antibody production by B cells. It enhances the cytotoxicity of $CD8^+$ T and NK cells. It promotes T cell differentiation into Th1 and Th2 subsets while also inhibiting Th17 differentiation. IL-2 is essential for the survival of regulatory T cells as well as for activation-induced cell death. It may also play a key role in the induction of specific IgG subclass responses in the horse although this has yet to be formally demonstrated (Isakov & Morrow, 1989). Thus, it has a broad range of essential functions (Boyman & Sprent, 2012; Mitra & Leonard, 2018).

The interleukin-2 receptor α-chain is classified as CD25. It is constitutively expressed on the surface of immune cells, especially Treg cells. Thus, equine Treg cells are $CD4^+$, $CD25^+$ $FOXP3^+$. These Treg cells sequester IL-2 and thus make it unavailable to other cells. CD25 may also be transiently expressed on $CD4^+$ and $CD8^+$ T cells (Wagner et al., 2024).

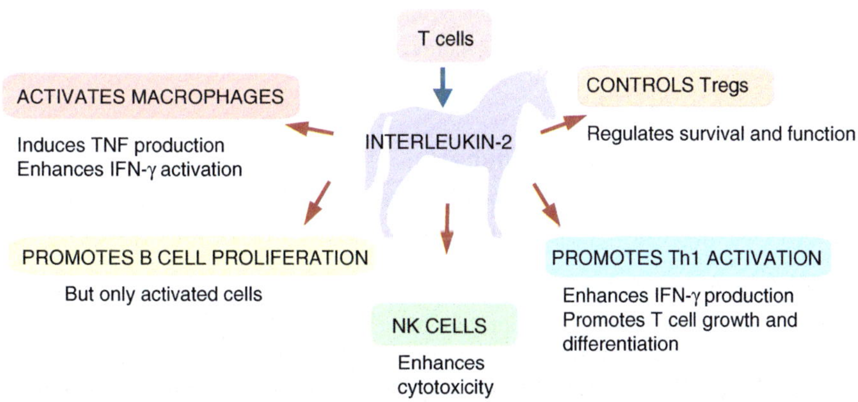

FIGURE 6.5

The origins and functions of equine Interleukin-2.

Interleukin-12

IL-12 is a member of a family of related proteins that also includes IL-23, IL-27, IL-35, and IL-39 (Tait Wojno et al., 2019). These are all heterodimeric proteins. For example, IL-12 is formed by two chains, p35 of 23.6 kDa and p40 of 36.3 kDa. When linked as a heterodimer to p19, it forms IL-23 (Parham et al., 2002). Some of these chains are shared with other family members. All the members of the family regulate T cell function. Thus, IL-12 and IL-27 generate Th1 cells, whereas IL-23 generates Th17 cells (Tait Wojno et al., 2019). The equine IL-12 alpha subunit contains 256 amino acids, and its gene is located on chromosome ECA 19, whereas the beta subunit contains 329 amino acids. It is encoded by a gene on chromosome ECA 14. The equine IL-23 gene contains 579 nucleotides and shares 89% nucleotide homology with the human IL-23 gene (Tompkins et al., 2010).

Interferon-γ

Despite its name, interferon gamma is primarily an immunoregulatory cytokine. Equine IFN-γ has been cloned and sequenced (Grünig et al., 1994). Its major function is the mediation of Th1 cell responses. It is a non-glycosylated homodimer with two chains of 166 amino acids and a molecular weight of 16.9 kDa. It is encoded by a gene located on chromosome ECA6. (In the donkey, *E. asinus*, the IFN-γ gene is located on chromosome EAS 22, and IFN-γ is a 19.3 kDa protein). Each chain is encoded by four exons. IFN-γ is mainly produced by Th1 cells, $CD8^+$ cytotoxic T cells, and natural killer (NK) cells, with lesser amounts from antigen-presenting cells, B cells, and natural killer (NK) T cells. It activates cells through the JAK-STAT receptor pathway (Villarino et al., 2017). It promotes macrophage activation, suppresses Th2 cells, and enhances NK cell activities. IFN-γ plays an important role in regulating equine pregnancy. Together with TNF-α, it regulates the function of the corpus luteum (Galvao et al., 2012). Foals lack IFN-γ at birth (Breathnach et al., 2006). This may explain, in part, their susceptibility to certain bacterial infections, such as those caused by *Rhodococcus equi,* as well as by viruses such as equine herpesvirus 1. However its level increases rapidly in response to antigenic stimulation.

Type 2 immune response inducers

Type 2 immune responses are antibody-mediated. Type 2 helper cells characteristically produce the major cytokines, IL-4, IL-5, IL-9, and IL-13 that activate B cells.

Interleukin-4

Equine IL-4 is a monomeric glycoprotein of 137 amino acids produced by Th2 cells and mast cells. Its targets are T cells, B cells, and macrophages. It is encoded by a gene located on ECA14. Signaling through STAT6, IL-4 activates the Th2-specific transcription factor GATA3. GATA3 is the master regulator of Th2 differentiation. IL-4 promotes IgG and IgE production, inhibits IFN-γ expression, and Th17 cell production. IL-4 is essential for antibody production because it is a key activator of B cells. IL-4 shares overlapping intracellular signaling pathways and biological functions with IL-13. The horse IL-4 gene shows 99.1% homology to that of the donkey (Singha et al., 2015) (Fig. 6.6).

Interleukin-5

Equine Interleukin 5 precursor is a glycoprotein of 134 amino acids (13 kDa) mainly produced by activated Th2 cells, mast cells, NKT cells, and eosinophils. It promotes eosinophil production and basophil differentiation. In the horse, it is an alpha helical glycoprotein that forms a covalently linked heterodimer. It is encoded by a gene located on chromosome ECA14. In the donkey, it is a protein of 15 kDa encoded by a gene on chromosome EAS12.

Interleukin-9

Equine interleukin-9 is a glycoprotein of about 149 amino acids (16 kDa) produced by T cells. It is encoded by a gene located on ECA14. A subset of Th2 cells that can be stimulated to produce large quantities of IL-9 have been called Th9 cells. These Th9 cells are generated by a combination of IL-4 and TGF-β. IL-25 and TSLP treatment of these cells also induces IL-9 release and so enhances allergic responses. Other cells that can produce IL-9 include type 2 innate lymphoid cells (ILC2) and a subset of mucosal mast cells (Pajulas et al., 2023).

IL-9 affects Th2 and ILC2 cells by promoting their differentiation; Th1 cells, where it reduces differentiation; mast cells, where it promotes mediator release; and eosinophils, where it promotes their development and survival. The main

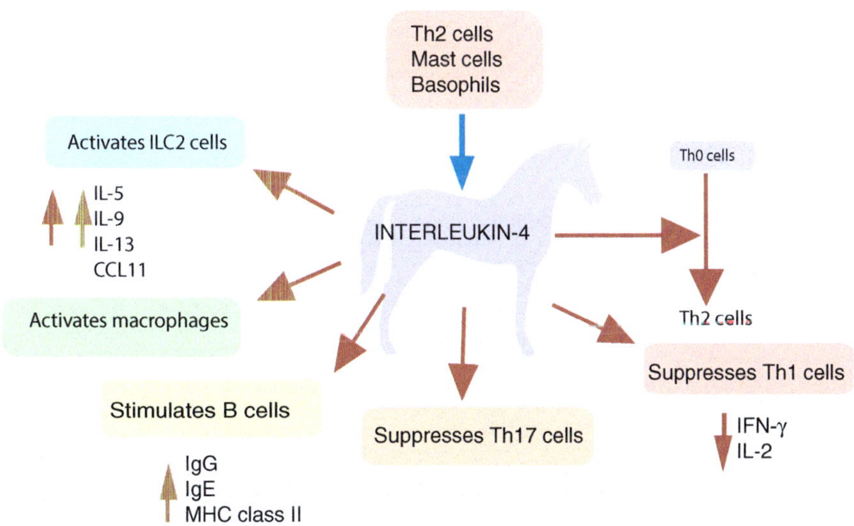

FIGURE 6.6

The sources and properties of equine interleukin 4.

function of these IL-9-producing T cells is probably to defend against parasitic helminths (Chapter 18) (Fig. 6.7).

Interleukin 13

Equine IL-13 is a protein of 133 amino acids encoded by a gene on ECA14. It is produced by activated Th2 cells, cytotoxic T cells, NK cells, mast cells, eosinophils, and dendritic cells. It has biological activities similar to those of IL-4, because it acts through a receptor (CD213) that shares a common α chain with the IL-4R. It regulates IgE synthesis and mucus secretion in the airways and the intestine. IL-13 has anti-inflammatory properties (Fig. 6.8).

Other T cell products

Interleukin -17

A subset of helper T cells generates type 3 immune responses. These are antibacterial inflammatory responses mediated by interleukin-17 (IL-17). Six related cytokines belong to the IL-17 family (IL-17A through IL-17F), but the three most important members are IL-17A, IL-17E, and IL-17F. IL-17A is involved in the development of autoimmunity, inflammation, and some tumors. IL-17F is mainly involved in mucosal defense. IL-17E (also known as IL-25) promotes Th2 responses (Fig. 6.9).

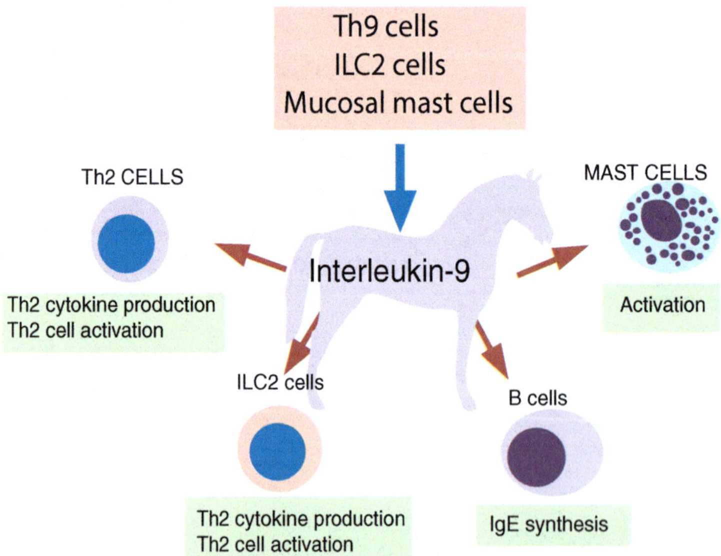

FIGURE 6.7

The sources and properties of equine interleukin-9.

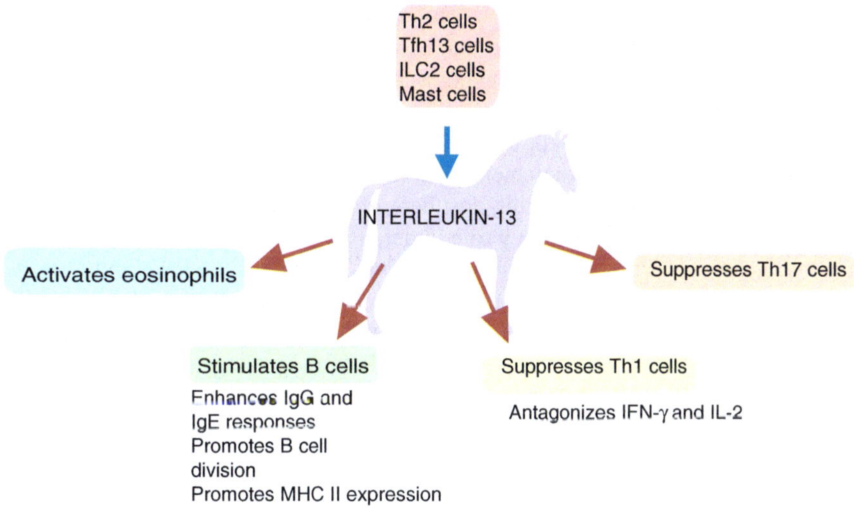

FIGURE 6.8

The sources and properties of equine 1L-13.

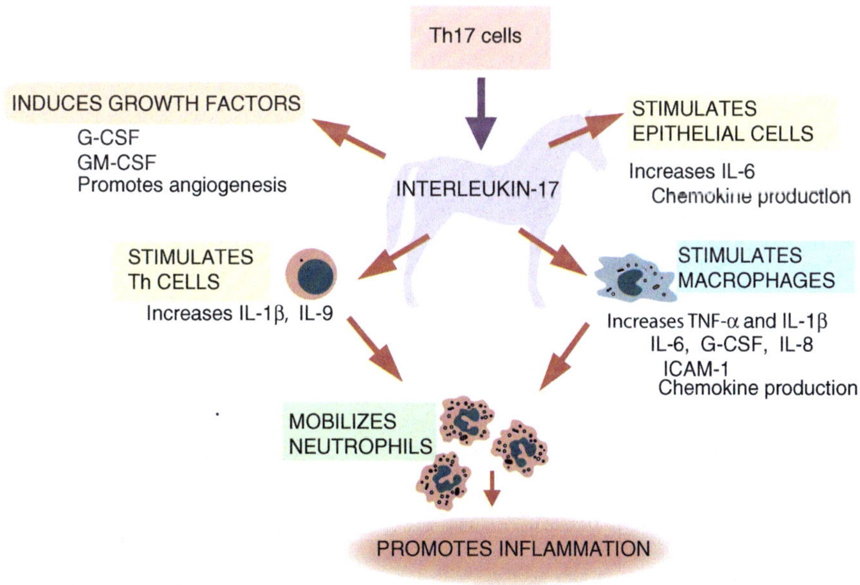

FIGURE 6.9

The sources and functions of equine interleukin-17.

Equine IL-17A is secreted as a disulfide-linked homodimer of 153 amino acids, about 30 kDa, produced by Th17 cells. (The predicted MW of the monomer is 14.8 kDa). Its gene is located on chromosome ECA20. It is also secreted as a 40 kDa heterodimer together with IL-17F. It shares 76% identity with human

IL-17 (Tompkins et al., 2010). IL-17A binds to a family of cell surface receptors (IL-17RA thru RE) that signal through the NF-κB pathway (Hayden & Ghosh, 2008). Endothelial cells and macrophages are the main targets of these cytokines since IL-17 plus TNF-α can stimulate them to produce pro-inflammatory chemokines, G-CSF, GM-CSF, IL-1β, and IL-6, in addition to inflammatory mediators such as acute-phase and complement proteins, and antibacterial defensins.

IL-17 is crucial for coordinating host defenses against many bacteria and fungi. For example, Th17 cells play a key role in defense against pathogens such as *Klebsiella pneumoniae, Salmonella enterica, Mycobacterium tuberculosis,* and *Candida albicans*. They do so by triggering the recruitment of inflammatory cells, leading to rapid pathogen eradication. Engagement of dectin-1 and -2 drives Th17 responses in fungal infections. IL-17 also plays a critical role in the pathogenesis of equine respiratory allergic diseases such as asthma. (Elevated levels of IL-17 can be detected in the bronchoalveolar lavage fluid of affected horses.) (Mensikova et al., 2013) (Chapter 20). Th17 has also been shown to play a key role in the pathogenesis of supporting limb laminitis (Cassimeris et al., 2020). It appears that activation of the IL-17A pathway results from the physical stresses imposed upon the laminitic keratinocytes in the hoof. Th17 cells also play important roles in many autoimmune diseases (Chapter 22) (McGeachy et al., 2019).

Interleukin-10

Regulatory T cells (Treg cells) produce two major suppressive cytokines, IL-10 and TGF-β. Equine IL-10 is a homodimeric protein of 178 amino acids encoded by a gene located on chromosome ECA5. Its calculated molecular weight is 20.4 kDa. It has been cloned and shares 80% sequence homology with bovine IL-10 (Singha et al., 2015) (Fig. 6.10).

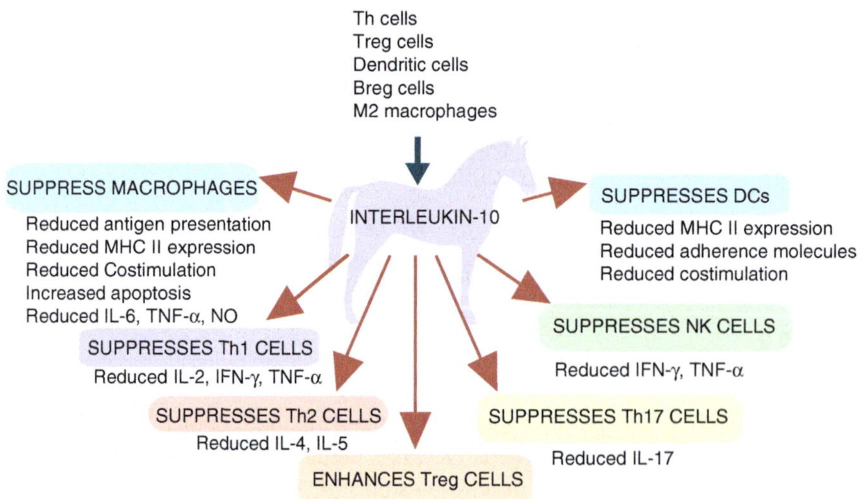

FIGURE 6.10

The sources and properties of the regulatory cytokine, IL-10.

Interleukin-10 inhibits both innate and adaptive immune responses and, as a result, is a potent anti-inflammatory cytokine. It is produced by macrophages (especially M2 macrophages) and classical dendritic cells in response to microbial products (Fickenscher et al., 2002). It is also produced by multiple T cell subsets, including some populations of helper T cells, in response to high antigen doses and IL-12. It is produced in especially large amounts by Treg cells in response to TGF-β. Small amounts of IL-10 may also be produced by B cells, mast cells, neutrophils, and natural killer (NK) cells (Ouyang & O'Garra, 2019).

Interleukin-10 downregulates MHC class II and co-stimulatory molecule expression on dendritic cells and macrophages and hence impairs antigen presentation. IL-10 or IL-10-treated dendritic cells can induce a long-lasting, antigen-specific, anergic state when T cells are activated in their presence. IL-10 inhibits the synthesis of the Th1 cytokines, IL-1β, IFN-γ, and TNF-α, as well as the Th2 cytokines IL-4 and IL-5. Thus, it can suppress both Th1 and Th2 responses. IL-10 also inhibits the production of IL-5, CXCL8, IL-12, granulocyte-macrophage colony-stimulating factor (GM-CSF), and granulocyte colony-stimulating factor (G-CSF). It also downregulates the production of IFN-γ and TNF-α by NK cells (Castillo & Kolls, 2016). It downregulates the expression of the receptors CD40, CD80, CD86, and MHC class II molecules on the surface of antigen-presenting cells (Hobbs et al., 2024). Equine IL-10 also inhibits the development of tissue fibrosis. It does so by inhibiting the profibrotic effects of TGF-β1 and so reducing the production of smooth muscle actin and type 3 collagen (Wise et al., 2020).

Transforming growth factor-β

Transforming growth factor -β (TGF-β) comprises a family of three multifunctional glycoproteins (TGF-β1, TGF-β2, and TGF-β3). They are secreted as inactive precursors and activated on the cell surface by proteases after binding to integrins (Fig. 6.11). TGFs are produced by platelets, activated macrophages, neutrophils, B cells, and T cells and act on T and B cells, dendritic cells, macrophages, neutrophils, and fibroblasts. Equine TGF-β1 is a disulfide-linked homodimer of 47.7 kDa. It contains 414 amino acids. Its gene is located on chromosome ECA30. There are four potential isoforms in the horse (Batille & Massagué, 2019).

As described in Chapter 2, TGF-β plays an important role in the maintenance of equine pregnancy by suppressing the mare's immune responses to her fetal foal. It regulates macrophage activities. It may be either inhibitory or stimulatory, depending on the presence of other cytokines. Thus, it can enhance integrin expression as well as phagocytosis by blood monocytes. On the other hand, it suppresses their respiratory burst and NO production. It blocks monocyte differentiation and the cytotoxic effects of activated macrophages. TGF-β is required for optimal dendritic cell development and regulates the interaction between follicular dendritic cells and B cells. TGF-β inhibits T cell proliferation and stimulates their apoptosis. Apoptotic T cells release TGF-β, contributing to the suppressive environment. TGF-β influences the differentiation of Th subsets. It tends to promote Th1 responses and the

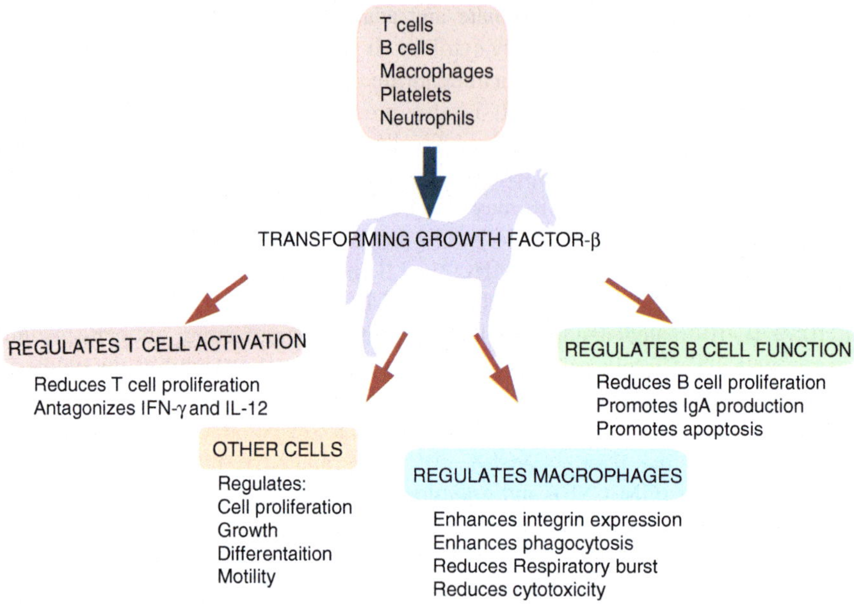

FIGURE 6.11

The origins and functions of equine transforming growth factor-β.

production of IL-2 in naïve T cells, but it also antagonizes the effects of IFN-γ and IL-12 on memory cells. It also controls the development and differentiation of B cells, inhibiting their proliferation, inducing apoptosis, and regulating IgA production. TGF-β1 is found in bronchoalveolar lavage fluid of horses (Desjardins et al., 2004). It is also present in the synovial fluid of young horses and horses with arthritis (Anderson et al., 1997).

Interleukin-22

Interleukin-22 (IL-22) is a member of the IL-10 family of cytokines. In mammals other than the horse, it is known to play an important role in the defense of epithelial surfaces such as the skin. In other mammals, it is also found in both T- and NK cells. It has not yet been well characterized in the horse. However, it is expressed at high levels by cells located within the chorionic girdle of the equine fetus. Its receptor, IL-22R1, is expressed on the maternal endometrium. It is believed that it modulates endometrial immune responses to the developing fetus (Chapter 2) (Brosnahan et al., 2012).

Interleukin-26

The role of interleukin-26 (IL-26) in the horse is uncertain. In other mammals, its production is generally stimulated by exposure to IL-17. As a result, its levels increase in cases of inflammatory diseases. It shares about 25% sequence homology with IL-10. Despite this, it acts through a different cell surface receptor. The IL-26 gene on chromosome ECA6 is located in a cluster bounded by the IFN-γ gene on one side and the IL-22 gene on the other. Studies on the equine IL-26 gene have indicated that it lacks an exon present in other mammals, such as humans. The same deletion is present in the genome of the Przewalski's horse and the donkey. A single-base-pair deletion causes a frame shift in the IL-26 transcript and generates a premature stop codon. Despite this, the IL-26 gene is expressed in the liver and gives rise to five transcript variants. Since IL-26 is a stimulator of T cells and promotes inflammation and autoimmunity in other mammals, this deletion mutation and subsequent inactivation of IL-26 may explain, in part, why some aspects of acute inflammation differ in horses (Shakhsi-Niaei et al., 2013).

Other inflammatory cytokines

Four cytokines play a critical role in triggering and regulating allergic inflammation. These are IL-33, TSLP, IL-25 and IL-31. All four promote Th2 and ILC2 activation as well as cytokine production (Stanbery et al., 2022).

Interleukin-33

Equine inteleukin-33 is a 224 amino acid, 25.1 kDa protein belonging to the IL-1 family. Its gene is located on chromosome ECA23. It is produced by keratinocytes, bronchial epithelial cells, and enterocytes. It is also present in vascular endothelial cells (Haraldsen et al., 2009). IL-33 is not secreted like a conventional cytokine but is stored in the cell nucleus, where it regulates DNA transcription. It is only released by cell death, injury, or stress. It can also be released by living cells following activation of their protease-activated receptors (Enoksson et al., 2011). It promotes allergic diseases while playing a protective role in helminth infections (Liew et al., 2016).

IL-33 functions as an alarm signal (alarmin) when it escapes from damaged or dying cells (Lunderius-Andersson et al., 2012). It is especially potent at activating type 2 innate lymphoid cells (ILC2 cells), but it also activates type 2 dendritic cells (DC2), Th2 cells, and Tfh cells, as well as Tregs and mast cells. The release of IL-33 by epithelial cells, therefore, results in the development of type 2 immunity and allergic inflammation. IL-33 is a key inducer of the type 2 cytokines IL-4, IL-5, and IL-13. (IL-33 together with IL-25 and TSLP all promote Th2 responses, but IL-33 is by far the most potent.) When IL-33 is exposed to neutrophil and mast cell proteases, it is converted into short potent peptides. These peptides also promote type 2 activity by stimulating mast cell and ILC2 cell production of IL-5, IL-6, and IL-13, and thus triggering an eosinophilia. It has been suggested that the production of IL-33 has a significant impact on the severity of equine influenza (Chapter 17) (Rozario et al., 2021).

IL-33 promotes IgE-mediated degranulation of mast cells as well as IgE production, eosinophilia, and goblet cell proliferation. Additionally, it induces mast cell production of leukotrienes and cytokines. IL-33 also binds to sensory neurons, triggering intense pruritus and scratching behavior. IL-33 is thus a key mediator of allergic diseases (Chapter 19).

Thymic stromal lymphopoietin

Equine thymic stromal lymphopoietin (TSLP) is a 233 amino acid, 25.3 kDa member of the IL-2 family that regulates type 2 inflammation at mucosal barriers. It is encoded by a gene on chromosome ECA 14. It is expressed by bronchial and colonic epithelial cells, mast cells, keratinocytes, tuft cells, and lung fibroblasts. Its greatest expression is in bronchial smooth muscle cells and keratinocytes. TSLP production is also upregulated in inflamed skin. TSLP is produced by keratinocytes and mast cells in response to antimicrobial peptides such as β-defensins and cathelicidins. Its release is also stimulated by many allergens (especially those with protease activity), infections, and some chemicals.

TSLP may be considered to be a master regulator that triggers and maintains allergic inflammation on barrier surfaces (Ebina-Shibuya & Leonard, 2023). Its activities overlap significantly with the other two regulatory cytokines, IL-33 and IL-25. Like IL-33, TSLP activates type 2 dendritic (DC2) cells. It stimulates their cytokine production and so promotes IgE production. The activated DC2s also secrete chemokines that attract neutrophils and eosinophils. TSLP also causes DC2 cells to release the chemokines CCL17 and CCL22 that specifically attract Th2 cells. TSLP stimulates basophil production in the bone marrow, and over 70% of activated basophils express TSLP receptors. TSLP receptors are also expressed on the dorsal root ganglia neurons and sensory nerve endings. Thus, when keratinocytes release TSLP, it can act on nearby neurons to cause severe itching (Ziegler et al., 2013).

Interleukin-25

Equine IL-25 is a protein of 168 amino acids and a 19.1 kDa member of the IL-17 family (Its alternative name is IL-17E). Its gene is located on chromosome ECA1. Its major sources are Th2 cells, epithelial cells, tuft cells, and innate lymphoid cells. It is also produced by alveolar macrophages, dendritic cells, mast cells, basophils, eosinophils, keratinocytes, and mucosal epithelial cells. Its release is triggered by exposure to proteases such as tryptase. Mast cells produce IL-25 after cross-linking of their IgE receptor, FcεRI. Basophils also produce it after IgE receptor cross-linking (Borowczyk et al., 2021).

IL-25 induces dendritic cell responses that initiate and sustain type 2 responses. Unlike other members of the IL-17 family that attract neutrophils, IL-25 attracts eosinophils as well as inducing an eosinophilia and promoting IgE production. It is a major activator of ILC2 cells. Eosinophils produce IL-25 after treatment with IL-5 and GM-CSF. Repeated intranasal application of IL-25 results in the production of IL-5 and IL-13 and the induction of airway hypersensitivity. IL-25 also activates Th2 cells and ILC2 cells and induces their IL-9 production. Other targets of IL-25 are fibroblasts and epithelial cells, which it induces to secrete chemokines that can recruit both eosinophils and Th2 cells (Catalan-Dibene et al., 2018).

Interleukin-31

Equine IL-31 is a protein of 153 amino acids17.3 kDa, and a member of the IL-6 family. Its gene is located on chromosome ECA8. It is produced by activated Th2 cells, mast cells, macrophages, basophils, and dendritic cells. Its receptors are expressed on keratinocytes and other epithelial cells, eosinophils, activated macrophages, and especially on dorsal root ganglia neurons and peripheral neurons. When activated, they signal to cells through the Janus kinase pathway. IL-31 is a potent inducer of chronic pruritus and skin inflammation in the horse (Craig et al., 2024). IL-31 is released by Th2 cells, partially in response to histamine acting through H2 receptors.

Growth factors

Growth factors are also known as colony-stimulating factors from their ability to stimulate cultured cells in vitro to grow in clusters and so form colonies. These include granulocyte-macrophage colony-stimulating factor (GM-CSF), macrophage colony-stimulating factor (M-CSF), and granulocyte colony-stimulating factor (G-CSF). GM-CSF not only promotes both granulocyte and macrophage production, but the recombinant protein also appears to stimulate phagocytosis and the respiratory burst (Blecha. 1991). Equine GM-CSF has been cloned and sequenced. It has a single nucleotide deletion at its 3′ end, resulting in an extended reading frame of 24 amino acids. This appears to be unique to the horse. Equine GM-CSH stimulates dendritic cell differentiation from blood monocytes (Mauel et al., 2006) (Chapter 7).

In addition to the colony-stimulating factors, horses also employ a family of cytokines that promote the growth and survival of B cells (Chapter 11). For example, B cell activating factor (BAFF) (CD257) and "a proliferation-inducing ligand" (APRIL) (CD256) are two related cytokines. BAFF is produced by monocytes, dendritic cells, T cells, and neutrophils. APRIL is produced by monocytes, dendritic cells, T cells, and intestinal epithelial cells. They bind to the same or related receptors on B cells. BAFF is expressed on the cell membranes of its producing cells but can be cleaved off as a soluble cytokine. It functions in both situations. APRIL only functions as a soluble cytokine. They both promote B cell division and inhibit their apoptosis. Both BAFF and APRIL are crucial survival factors for B cells and essential for their production and differentiation (Chapter 11).

Chemokines

Chemokines are a large family of relatively small signaling proteins of 8–10 kDa (Baggolini, 1998). They coordinate the migration of leukocytes into inflammatory sites and within lymphoid tissues and hence dictate the course of many inflammatory and immune responses (Luster, 2019). Chemokines are produced by sentinel cells, including macrophages and mast cells. They are classified into four subfamilies based on their amino acid sequences. For example, the alpha (or CXC) chemokines have two cysteine (C) residues separated by a single amino acid (X), whereas the beta (or CC) chemokines have two contiguous cysteine residues. (Chemokine nomenclature is based on this classification, each molecule or receptor receiving a numerical designation. In addition, ligands have the suffix "L" [e.g., CXCL8], whereas receptors have the suffix "R" [e.g., CXCR1].)

Inflammatory chemokines are mainly involved in leukocyte recruitment. Other chemokines promote new blood vessel growth. Some are homeostatic and are found in normal tissues where they regulate cellular migration and homing (Baggolini, 1998).

One of the most important chemokines is CXCL8 (also called interleukin-8). In the horse. It is 8.8 kDa in size (101 amino acids), encoded by a gene on chromosome ECA3. Interestingly, this gene is polymorphic in both horses and donkeys. A G > C mutation causes a nonsynonymous mutation. There are three other synonymous SNPs in the gene as well (Kumar et al., 2022). CXCL8 attracts and activates neutrophils, releasing their granule contents and stimulating their respiratory burst. Another important CXC chemokine is CXCL2 (macrophage inflammatory protein-2, MIP-2), which also attracts neutrophils.

CC chemokines act predominantly on equine macrophages and dendritic cells. Thus, CCL3 and CCL4 (MIP-1α and MIP-1β) are produced by macrophages and mast cells (Schnabel et al., 2018). CCL4 attracts $CD4^+$ T cells, whereas CCL3 attracts B cells, eosinophils, and cytotoxic T cells. CCL2 (monocyte chemotactic protein-1, MCP-1) is produced by macrophages, T cells, fibroblasts, keratinocytes, and endothelial cells. It attracts and activates monocytes, stimulating their respiratory burst and lysosomal enzyme release. CCL5 is a 7.9 kDa protein that attracts monocytes, eosinophils, and some T cells. It activates eosinophils and stimulates histamine release from basophils.

Two chemokines fall outside the CC and CXC families. Equine lymphotactin (XCL1) is a C (only one cysteine residue) chemokine that is chemotactic for lymphocytes. It contains 112 amino acids and is heavily glycosylated, so it has a molar mass of 12.2 kDa. Its gene is located on chromosome ECA5. Its receptor is XCR1. It is specifically chemotactic for T cells. Fractalkine (CX3C ligand 1) is a CXXXC (two cysteines separated by three amino acids) chemokine that triggers adhesion between T cells and monocytes. It is ommonly detected in inflammatory fluids. Its receptor is CX3CR1. It is a disulfide-linked homodimer. It is elevated in inflammatory conditions such as equine recurrent uveitis (Curto et al., 2016). The fractalkine gene is located on chromosome ECA3.

Most chemokines are produced in infected or damaged tissues and attract other cells to sites of inflammation or microbial invasion. It is likely that the chemokine mixture produced by damaged or infected tissues regulates the precise composition of incoming inflammatory cell populations. In this way, the body can adjust the inflammatory response to maximize the destruction of different microbial invaders. For example, eotaxin, CCL2, CCL8, and CCL-13 are all induced by IL-4 in equine dermal fibroblasts and are probably involved in the pathogenesis of allergic skin disease (Benarafa et al., 2000). Many chemokines, such as CXCL4, CCL20, and CCL5, are structurally similar to the antimicrobial defensins and, like them, have antibacterial activity (Gangur et al., 2002) (Box 6.1).

Interferons

Interferons are important antiviral cytokines. Despite its name, interferon-gamma is primarily an immunoregulatory molecule and has been discussed earlier in this Chapter. The remaining interferons are described and discussed in relation to their antiviral properties in Chapter 17.

Cytokine receptors

In general, most cytokines act through receptors that activate tyrosine kinases. However, within this group, some subfamilies share subunits and functions. For example, members of the IL-1/TLR receptor family participate in the responses to injury and infection. The family can be split into the receptors that are IL-1R-like (IL-1R1, IL-18R) and the receptors that are toll-like (TLR). Ligation of these receptors triggers activation of the transcription factor NF-κB and generates inflammasomes (Wietek & O'Neill, 2007).

Another cytokine receptor family shares a common beta (β_c) chain. The β_c family includes among its members the receptors for granulocyte-macrophage

Box 6.1 Chemokines and Lyme borreliosis in horses

Lyme disease is caused by the tick-borne pathogen, *Borrelia burgdorferi*. In both humans and dogs, it is characterized by the development of severe arthritis. The situation in infected horses is less clear, but the development of Lyme arthritis is uncommon. In a study examining the cytokine profile in the synovial fluid of horses infected with *B. burgdorferi*, it was found that there was no statistical difference between inflammatory cytokine levels in the synovia of infected horses and horses with arthritis resulting from trauma or other causes. However, there was a significant negative association between the levels of the chemokine CCL2 and a horse's Lyme disease status. Thus, *B. burgdorferi*-infected horses produce reduced amounts of the inflammatory cytokine, CCL2, in their synovia. As described in the main text, CCL2 is a potent proinflammatory chemokine. In its absence, inflammation is very much reduced (Clark et al., 2025).

colony-stimulating factor (GM-CSF), IL-3, and IL-5 (Pant et al., 2023). These regulate inflammatory responses and hematopoiesis (Dougan et al., 2019). In yet another receptor family, a common gamma chain (γ_c) is shared by the receptors for IL-2, IL-4, IL-7, IL-9, IL-15, and IL-21 (Leonard et al., 2019). These receptor chains dimerize in the presence of the ligand and form complexes with a group of kinases called Janus kinases (JAKs). JAKs, in turn, phosphorylate a cytosolic protein called STAT (signal transducers and activators of transcription). The STAT then dimerizes to form an active transcription factor. Depending on the specific JAKs and STATs used, these may enhance or suppress cytokine signaling. This is called the JAK-STAT pathway.

The members of the group II cytokine receptor family have a very different structure. They bind interferons (α-, β-, γ-, and λ-interferons) as well as members of the IL-10 cytokine family (IL-19, IL-20, IL-22, IL-24, and IL-26). These receptors also form heterodimers in the presence of the ligand and signal through the JAK-STAT pathway (Ouyang & O'Garra, 2019).

References

Anderson, L. D., Raub, R. H., Grieger, D. M., Morris, J., & Weber, J. D. (1997). Transforming growth factor -β1 concentrations in equine synovial fluid. *Journal of Equine Veterinary Science, 18*(2), 109–113.

Aragona, F., Rizzo, M., Arfuso, F., Arrigo, F., et al. (2025). Preliminary insights on the daily rhythm of CRP and IL-6 in athletic horses. *Journal of Equine Veterinary Science*. https://doi.org/10.1016/j.jevs.2025.105702

Baggolini, M. (1998). Chemokines and leukocyte traffic. *Nature, 392*(6676), 655.

Batille, E., & Massagué, J. (2019). Transforming growth factor-β signaling in immunity and cancer. *Immunity, 50*(4), 924–940.

Benarafa, C., Cunningham, F. M., Hamblin, A. S., Horohov, D. W., & Collins, M. E. (2000). Cloning of equine chemokines, eotaxin, and monocyte chemoattractant protein (MCP)-1. MCP2 and MCP-4 mRNA expression in tissues and induction by IL-4 in dermal fibroblasts. *Veterinary Immunology and Immunopathology, 76*, 283–298.

Blecha, F. (1991). Cytokines: Applications in domestic food animals. *Journal of Dairy Science, 74*, 328–339.

Borowczyk, J., Shutova, M., Brembrilla, N. C., & Boehncke, W.-H. (2021). IL-25 (IL-17E) in epithelial immunology and pathophysiology. *The Journal of Allergy and Clinical Immunology, 148*(1), 40–52.

Boyman, O., & Sprent, J. (2012). The role of interleukin-2 during homeostasis and activation of the immune system. *Nature Reviews Immunology,, 12*(3), 180–190.

Breathnach, C. C., Sturgill-Wright, T., Stiltner, J. L., et al. (2006). Foals are interferon gamma-deficient at birth. *Veterinary Immunology and Immunopathology, 112*, 199–209.

Brosnahan, M. M., Miller, D. C., Adams, M., & Antczak, D. F. (2012). IL-22 is expressed by the invasive trophoblast of the equine (*Equus caballus*) chorionic girdle. *The Journal of Immunology, 188*, 4181–4187.

Cassimeris, L., Engiles, J. B., & Galantino-Homer, H. (2020). Interleukin-17A pathway target genes are upregulated in *Equus caballus* supporting limb laminitis. *PLoS One*. https://doi.org/10.1371/journal.pone.0232920

Castillo, P., & Kolls, J. K. (2016). IL-10: A paradigm for counterregulatory cytokines. *The Journal of Immunology, 197*(5), 1529–1530.

Catalan-Dibene, J., McIntyre, L. L., & Zlotnik, A. (2018). Interleukin 30 to interleukin 40. *Journal of Interferon and Cytokine Research, 38*(10), 423–439.

Clark, K. F., Lemcke, R. A., Gasiorowski, J. C., & Wagner, N. (2025). Synovial chemokine and cytokine profiles in horses with and without systemic *Borrelia burgdorferi* infection. *Equine Veterinary Journal*. https://doi.org/10.1111/evj.70123

Craig, N. M., Munguia, N. S., Trujillo, A. J., Chan, A. M., et al. (2024). Interleukin 31 mediates pruritus in horses. *American Journal of Veterinary Research*. https://doi.org/10.2460/ajvr.24.05.0144

Curto, E., Messenger, K. M., Salmon, J. H., & Gilger, B. C. (2016). Cytokine and chemokine profiles of aqueous humor and serum in horses with uveitis measured using multiplex bead immunoassay analysis. *Veterinary Immunology and Immunopathology, 182*, 43–51.

Desjardins, I., Theoret, C., Joubert, P., Wagner, B., & Lavoie, J.-P. (2004). Comparison of TGF-beta 1 concentrations in bronchoalveolar fluid of horses affected with heaves and of normal controls. *Veterinary Immunology and Immunopathology, 101*, 133–141.

Dinarello, C., Arend, W., Sims, J., et al. (2010). IL-1 family nomenclature. *Nature Immunology, 11*, 973.

Dinarello, C. A. (2018). Overview of the IL-1 family in innate inflammation and acquired immunity. *Immunological Reviews, 281*, 8–27.

Dinarello, C. A., Novick, D., Kim, s, & Kaplanski, G. (2013). Interleukin-18 and IL-18 binding protein. *Frontiers in Immunology, 4*, 1–10.

Dougan, M., Dranoff, G., & Dougan, S. K. (2019). GM-CSF, IL-3, and IL-5 family of cytokines: Regulators of inflammation. *Immunity, 50*, 796–811.

Dudeck, J., Kotrba, J., Immler, R., Hoffmann, A., et al. (2021). Directional mast cell degranulation of tumor necrosis factor into blood vessels prims neutrophil extravasation. *Immunity, 54*(3), 468–483.

Ebina-Shibuya, R., & Leonard, W. J. (2023). Role of thymic stromal lymphopoietin in allergy and beyond. *Nature Reviews Immunology, 23*(1), 24–37.

Ehrle, A., Lischer, C. J., Lasarzik, J., Einspanier, R., & Bondzio, A. (2015). Synovial fluid and serum concentrations of Interleulin-1 receptor antagonist and interleukin-1b in naturally occurring equine osteoarthritis and septic arthritis. *Journal of Equine Veterinary Science, 35*, 815–822.

Enoksson, M., Lyberg, K., Moller-Westerberg, C., Fallon, P. C., Nilsson, G., & Lunderius-Andersson, C. (2011). Mast cells as sensors of cell injury through IL-33 recognition. *The Journal of Immunology, 186*, 2523–2528.

Fickenscher, H., Hor, S., Kupers, H., et al. (2002). The interleukin-10 family of cytokines. *Trends in Immunology, 23*, 89–96.

Galvao, A., Skarzynski, D. J., Szostek, A., Silva, E., et al. (2012). Cytokines tumor necrosis factor-α and interferon-γ participate in the modulation of the equine corpus luteum as autocrine and paracrine factors. *Journal of Reproductive Immunology, 93*, 28–37.

Gangur, V., Birmingham, N. P., & Thanesvorakul, S. (2002). Chemokines in health and disease. *Veterinary Immunology and Immunopathology, 86*, 127–136.

Grünig, G., Himmler, A., & Antczak, D. F. (1994). Cloning and sequencing of horse interferon-gamma cDNA. *Immunogenetics, 39*, 448–449.

Haraldsen, G., Balogh, J., Pollheimer, J., Sponheim, J., & Kuchler, A. M. (2009). Interleukin 33 – Cytokine of dual function or novel alarmin? *Trends in Immunology, 30*(5), 227–233.

Hayden, M. S., & Ghosh, S. (2008). Shared principles in NF-κB signaling. *Cell, 132*, 344–362.

Heaney, M. L., & Golde, D. W. (1996). Soluble cytokine receptors. *Blood, 87*, 847–857.

Hobbs, K. J., Bayless, R., & Sheats, M. K. (2024). A comparative review of cytokines and cytokine targeting in sepsis: From humans to horses. *Cells*. https://doi.org/10.3390/cells13171489

Isakov, N., & Morrow, P. R. (1989). Interleukin 2 regulates antigen-specific immunoglobulin response of naive murine B cells. *Cellular Immunology, 120*(2), 366–374.

Kaplanski, G., Marin, V., Montero-Julian, F., Mantovani, A., et al. (2003). IL-6: A regulator of the transition from neutrophil to monocyte recruitment during inflammation. *Trends in Immunology, 24*(1), 25–29.

Kumar, S., Ashraf, M., Pannu, U., & Mehta, S. C. (2022). Single nucleotide polymorphism in interleukin-6 and interleukin-8 genes of equines. *Journal of Equine Veterinary Science, 117*, 104058.

Leonard, W. J., Lin, J.-X., & O'Shea, J. J. (2019). The γ_c family of cytokines, basic biology and therapeutic ramifications. *Immunity, 50*, 832–850.

Liew, F. Y., Girard, J.-P., & Turnquist, H. R. (2016). Interleukin-33 in health and disease. *Nature Reviews Immunology*. https://doi.org/10.1038/nri.2016.95

Lunderius-Andersson, C., Enoksson, M., & Nilsson, G. (2012). Mast cells respond to cell injury through the recognition of IL-33. *Frontiers in Immunology*. https://doi.org/10.3389/fimmu.2012.00082

Luster, A. D. (2019). Introduction: Global positioning by chemokines and other mediators. *Immunological Reviews*. https://doi.org/10.1111/imr.12763

Mauel, S., Steinbach, F., & Ludwig, H. (2006). Monocyte-derived dendritic cells from horses differ from dendritic cells of humans and mice. *Immunology, 117*, 463–473.

McGeachy, M. J., Cua, D. J., & Gaffen, S. L. (2019). The IL-17 family of cytokines in health and disease. *Immunity*. https://doi.org/10.1016/j.immuni.2019.03.021

Mensikova, M., Stepanova, H., & Faldyna, M. (2013). Interleukin-17 in veterinary animal species and its role in various diseases: A review. *Cytokine, 64*, 11–17.

Mitra, S., & Leonard, W. J. (2018). Biology of IL-2 and its therapeutic modulation: Mechanisms and strategies. *Journal of Leukocyte Biology, 103*, 643–655.

Moellerberndt, J., Hagen, A., Niebert, S., Buttner, K., & Burk, J. (2023). Cytokines in equine platelet lysate and related blood products. *Frontiers in Veterinary Science*. https://doi.org/10.3389/fvets.2023.1117829

Murakami, M., Kamimura, D., & Hirano, T. (2019). Pleiotropy and specificity: Insights from the interleukin 6 family of cytokines. *Immunity, 50*, 812–831.

Myers, M. J., & Murtaugh, M. P. (Eds.). (1995). *Cytokines in animal health and disease*. New York: Marcel Dekker.

Ouyang, W., & O'Garra, A. (2019). IL-10 family cytokines, IL-10 and IL-22. From basic science to clinical translation. *Immunity, 50*, 871–891.

Pajulas, A., Zhang, J., & Kaplan, M. H. (2023). The world according to IL-9. *The Journal of Immunology, 211*, 7–14.

Pant, H., Hercus, T. R., Tumes, D. J., Yip, K. H., et al. (2023). Translating the biology of β common receptor-engaging cytokines into clinical medicine. *The Journal of Allergy and Clinical Immunology, 151*, 324–344.

Parham, C., Chirica, M., Timans, J., et al. (2002). A receptor for the heterodimeric cytokine IL-23 is composed of IL-12g1 and a novel cytokine receptor subunit, IL-23R. *The Journal of Immunology, 168*, 5699–5708.

Rozario, C., Martinez-Sibrido, L., McSorley, H. J., & Chauche, C. (2021). Could interleukin 33 (IL-33) govern the outcome of an equine influenza virus infection? Learning from other species. *Viruses*. https://doi.org/10.3390/v13122519

Schnabel, C. L., Wemette, M., Babasyan, S., Freer, H., et al. (2018). C-C motif chemokine ligand (CCL) production in equine peripheral blood mononuclear cells identified by newly generated monoclonal antibodies. *Veterinary Immunology and Immunopathology, 204*, 28–39.

Shakhsi-Niaei, M., Drogemuller, M., Jagannathan, V., Gerber, V., & Leeb, T. (2013). IL26 gene inactivation in equidae. *Animal Genetics, 44*, 770–772.

Sims, J. E., & Smith, D. E. (2010). The IL-1 family: Regulators of immunity. *Nature Reviews Immunology, 10*, 89–102.

Singha, H., Goyal, S. K., & Malik, P. (2015). Cloning and sequence analysis of interleukin (IL)-2, IL-4, IL-10, and IL-18 in the Marwari horse. *Indian Journal of Animal Sciences, 85*(6), 621–627.

Soller, J. T., Murua-Escobar, H., Willenbrock, S., Janssen, M., et al. (2007). Comparison of the human and canine cytokines IL-1(alpha/beta) and TNF-alpha to orthologous other mammalians. *Journal of Heredity, 98*(5), 485–490.

Stanbery, A. G., Smita, S., von Moltke, J., Tait, W. E. D., et al. (2022). TSLP, IL-33, and IL-25: Not just for allergy and helminth infection. *The Journal of Allergy and Clinical Immunology, 150*(6), 1302–1313.

Su, X., Morris, D. D., & McGraw, R. A. (1991). Cloning and characterization of gene *TNF*a encoding equine tumor necrosis factor alpha. *Gene, 107*, 319–321.

Tait Wojno, E. D., Hunter, C. A., & Sturnhofer, J. S. (2019). The immunobiology of the interleukin 12 family: Room for discovery. *Immunity, 50*, 851–870.

Tompkins, D., Hudgens, E., Horohov, D., & Baldwin, C. L. (2010). Expressed gene sequences of the equine cytokines interleukin-17 and interleukin-23. *Veterinary Immunology and Immunopathology, 133*, 309–313.

Villarino, A. V., Kanno, Y., & O'Shea, J. J. (2017). Mechanisms and consequences of JAK-STAT signaling in the immune system. *Nature Immunology, 18*(4), 374–384.

Wagner, B., Babasyan, S., Wilford, S., Robbin, M. G., et al. (2024). Monoclonal antibodies for equine CD25 improve detection of regulatory T cells in horses. *Veterinary Immunology and Immunopathology, 274*, 110790.

Wietek, C., & O'Neill, L. A. J. (2007). Diversity and regulation in the NF-κB system. *Trends in Biochemical Sciences, 32*, 301–309.

Wise, L. M., Stuart, G. S., Sriutaisuk, K., Adams, B. R., et al. (2020). Anti-fibrotic actions of equine interleukin-10 on transforming growth factor beta1-stimulated dermal fibroblasts isolated from limbs of horses. *Frontiers in Veterinary Science*. https://doi.org/10.3389/fvets/2020.577835

Wolf, J., Rose-John, S., & Garbers, C. (2014). Interleukin-6 and its receptors: A highly regulated and dynamic system. *Cytokine, 70*, 11–20.

Wu, D., Murakami, K., Liu, N., Konishi, M., et al. (2004). Expression of equine IL-18 by baculovirus expression system and its biologic activity. *Microbiology and Immunology, 48*(6), 471–476.

Ziegler, S. F., Roan, F., Bell, B. D., Stoklasek, T. A., et al. (2013). The biology of thymic stromal lymphopoietin (TSLP). *Advances in Pharmacology, 66*, 129–155.

CHAPTER

Equine antigen processing cells: Dendritic cells and macrophages

7

In addition to being uncomfortable and damaging, innate immunity, as reflected by inflammation and sickness, is not a foolproof process. If its body is to be defended effectively, a horse must have defenses that detect and eliminate all microbial invaders without the damage and discomfort associated with inflammation and sickness. This is the task of the adaptive immune system.

In order to trigger an adaptive immune response, a sample of the foreign invader must first be captured and processed. Only then can it be presented correctly to the cells that can recognize it. Trapping, processing, and presenting of antigens are the responsibility of dendritic cells, macrophages, and some B cells. These antigen processing cells are attracted by microbial products and tissue damage and are activated by the same stimuli that trigger inflammation. Indeed, dendritic cells and macrophages serve both as sentinel cells and as antigen-processing cells. Once an invader has been eliminated, a horse or donkey can develop adaptive immunity against a second attack by the same organism.

The organisms that trigger adaptive immune responses are of two general types. One type is typified by the bacteria that invade the body from outside and then grow in the tissues and extracellular fluid. These "exogenous" antigens are processed by specialized antigen-processing cells. A second type of invading organism is typified by viruses that invade cells and force them to make viral proteins. These "endogenous" antigens are processed by the cells in which they are produced.

The body employs three cell types: dendritic cells, macrophages, and B cells, to process exogenous antigens. Each of these cell types possesses specialized, antigen-binding receptors. These receptors, encoded by the major histocompatibility complex (MHC), present antigens to T cells. MHC class I molecules present endogenous antigens. MHC class II molecules present exogenous antigens.

Equine dendritic cells

Dendritic cells (DCs) are professional antigen-processing cells that capture and process exogenous antigens and thus initiate adaptive immune responses. They are at least 100 times more effective at this task than are macrophages. As a result, DCs are the only antigen-processing cells that can activate T cells that have never

The Immunology of Horses and Donkeys. https://doi.org/10.1016/B978-0-443-44863-8.00009-0

previously encountered an antigen (naïve T cells). They are therefore essential for initiating primary innate immune responses.

DC populations arise from a common stem cell precursor in the bone marrow. However, they are a heterogeneous cell type. Single-cell RNA sequencing has confirmed that there are two distinct dendritic cell populations present in equine blood. These are, conventional (or classical) DCs (cDCs), and plasmacytoid DCs (pDCs) (Patel et al., 2021). Conventional DCs are responsible for antigen presentation to T and B cells. Plasmacytoid DCs are major sources of IFN-α. The conventional cDCs are further subdivided into cDC1 cells and cDC2 cells. cDC1 cells stimulate T cells to mount cell-mediated (type 1) immune responses. whereas cDC2 cells stimulate B cells to mount antibody (type 2) immune responses.

Location and structure

Equine DCs have typical dendritic cell morphology - irregularly shaped, large cells with multiple, long, cytoplasmic dendrites, a large Golgi, and an extensive endoplasmic reticulum. They express MHC class II, CD1, EqWC1, LFA1, and EqWC2 as would be anticipated from a cell type whose function is to present antigens to T cells. Different subsets have been identified based on their expression of MHC class II and other markers. Thus, dendritic cells from lymph nodes are CD1b positive, but blood DCs are not (Siedek et al., 1997).

Dendritic cells are found in all organs except the brain, parts of the eye, and the testes. They are especially prominent in lymph nodes, skin, and mucosal surfaces - sites where invading microbes are most likely to be encountered. Their long dendrites intertwine so that they collectively form effective antigen-trapping webs.

The two most important subpopulations of equine DCs are derived either from bone marrow stem cells or from blood monocytes. Other important subpopulations are found in the skin (Langerhans cells) and in lymphoid organs (follicular DCs). Each DC subpopulation expresses different surface receptors, and each produces a diverse and complex mixture of cytokines and chemokines (Fig. 7.1).

Most DCs are derived from $CD34^+$ hematopoietic stem cells in the bone marrow. Their production is stimulated by either GM-CSF or by a cytokine called Fms-like tyrosine kinase 3 ligand (flt3L). The developing cells differentiate and emerge as subpopulations optimized to trigger either type 1 or type 2 immune responses. (Summerfield et al., 2015). flt3L is an essential growth factor for the development of both conventional DCs and plasmacytoid DCs.

Monocyte-derived DCs

Blood monocytes are the precursors of tissue macrophages as well as some DCs. Which cell type is produced depends on the cytokines encountered by the monocyte as it differentiates. The main function of these DCs is antigen presentation and induction of T cell responses. Immature monocyte-derived DCs (MoDCs) have typical DC morphology and are characterized by expressing low levels of CD14 as well as a

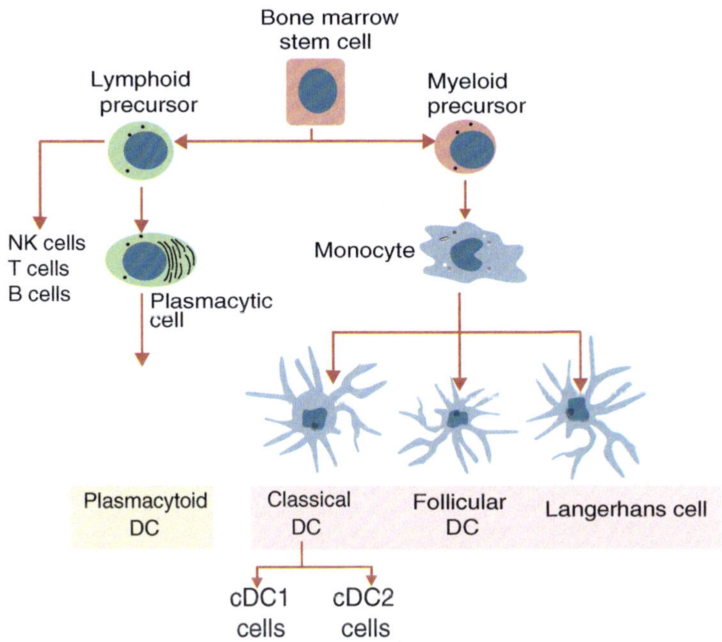

FIGURE 7.1 The origins and diversity of equine dendritic cells.

One population, the plasmacytoid DCs, originates from lymphoid precursors. The second major population arises from myeloid precursors and is closely related to monocytes. These, together with follicular DCs and Langerhans cells, constitute the cDC1 type.

moderate level of expression of MHC class II molecules and CD86. As they mature, they increase their MHC II and CD86 expression while their CD14 expression declines. Compared to humans and mice, in the horse, they take longer to differentiate from monocytes (6–7 days) (Mauel et al., 2006) (Box 7.1).

Equine monocytes are $CD14^+$, $CD86^{low}$, $CD205^-$, and MHC II^+. They upregulate CD206, CD86, and MHC II while downregulating CD14 when induced to differentiate into MoDC. When they mature, this induces CD86, and MHC II expression but downregulates CD206 (in humans but not in horses) (Summerfield et al., 2015).

Two dendritic cell populations can be readily derived from cultures of equine blood monocytes within 3–4 days in vitro. by growing them in the presence of two key cytokines, GM-CSF and interleukin 4 (Mauel et al., 2006). They are both MHC class II and CD14 positive. The two subpopulations differ in size, but it is not known if they are functionally different (Lopez et al., 2020). The size may simply reflect maturity. The small cells express more CD14 and less CD86 than the large cells. The large DCs express more MHC class II and CD86 than do the small cells.

Box 7.1 CD Molecules mentioned in this chapter

CD11. Also called LFA-1, this is an integrin α chain found on leukocytes. Three forms are known, CD11a, CD11b, and CD11c. They bind leukocytes to vascular endothelium.
CD14 This is the receptor for lipopolysaccharide-binding protein and therefore regulates the biological activities of this molecule. It is expressed on macrophages and granulocytes.
CD40 A member of the tumor necrosis factor receptor superfamily. Binding to its ligand CD40L (CD154) on activated helper T cells is essential for a successful antibody response and class switching. It is expressed on all antigen-presenting cells.
CD86 Related to CD80 and also called B7-2, this co-stimulatory receptor is expressed on antigen-presenting macrophages, activated B cells, and dendritic cells. Its ligands are CD28 and CD152 (CTLA-4) on T cells.
CD205. An endocytic cell receptor expressed on dendritic cells that recognizes apoptotic and necrotic dying cells. Its ligands appear to be cell surface keratins.
CD206The mannose-binding receptor found on mature macrophages and immature dendritic cells.
CD209 DC-SIGN found on a subset of dendritic cells. This molecule permits transient binding between T cells and dendritic cells. It is a C-type lectin whose ligand is ICAM-3 (CD50).

Plasmacytoid DCs

Plasmacytoid DCs (pDCs) are long-lived cells found in blood, bone marrow, and lymphoid organs. They account for about 0.5% of the blood mononuclear cell population in humans. Their classification as dendritic cells is disputed since they use different transcription factors than do classical DCs (Summerfield et al., 2015). They lack myeloid antigens but retain some lymphoid characteristics. pDCs serve as an early warning system for viral infections since they are rapidly activated by viral nucleic acids. They respond to viruses by synthesizing massive amounts of the type I interferons (IFN-α and IFN-β). (Ten to a 100-fold more than other cell types). They are also major producers of type III interferons (IFN-λ). pDCs have a unique ability to link innate and adaptive immunity. After producing large amounts of type I interferon, they are still able to differentiate into mature DCs that can stimulate naïve T cells. Because pDCs secrete large amounts of IFN-α, they also activate natural killer (NK) cells (Reizis, 2019). pDC numbers increase dramatically during inflammation and infection.

Equine pDCs have a characteristic cell-surface phenotype. They are $Flt3^{+}$, $CD4^{low}$, $CD13^{-}$, $CD14^{-}$, $CD172a^{-}$, CADM-1^{-}, and MHC class II ^{low}. This low expression of CD4 by equine pDCs contrasts with the situation in other mammals. These pDCs are the only cell subset that is capable of producing large quantities of IFN-α when stimulated by TLR9 agonists. These pDCs also express high levels of the genes *PLAC8, RUNX2*, and *TCF4 t*hat are characteristic of pDCs in other mammals. RUNX2 and TCF4 are transcription factors. The function of the *PLAC8* gene is currentlyunknown (Ziegler et al., 2016).

Langerhans cells

Langerhans cells are specialized, long-lived dendritic cells found in the upper layers of the epidermis of horses. They may also be found within intradermal sweat ducts. They are slightly smaller than macrophages but larger than lymphocytes. While normally diffusely distributed, they sometimes form aggregated foci, especially in lesions caused by insect bite hypersensitivity (Kurotaki et al., 2002) (Chapter 19). Their long dendrites form a network that is ideally situated to capture foreign antigens. Their cytoplasm contains characteristic Birbeck granules in addition to a Golgi apparatus, lysosomes, and multivesicular bodies (Hamada et al., 1992). Langerhans cells influence the development of local inflammatory responses, such as allergic contact dermatitis (Chapter 20). They express multiple pattern-recognition receptors, including the C-type lectins langerin and DC-SIGN that can bind bacteria, fungi, and some viruses. Once antigens are captured, the Langerhans cells migrate to draining lymph nodes, where they present the antigen to T cells. Equine Langerhans cells also express MHC II. Some immunologists regard Langerhans cells simply as specialized macrophages.

Follicular DCs

Specialized DCs called follicular DCs (fDCs) are found in the germinal centers of the spleen, lymph nodes, and Peyer's patches. They are also found around infection sites and chronic inflammatory reactions. In animals that have previously been exposed to an antigen and possess antibodies, follicular DCs take up immune complexes and then shed them in membrane vesicles called exosomes (Hodge et al., 2022). B cells can take up these exosomes and, after processing the antigen, present it to antigen-sensitive T cells (O'Neill & Quah, 2008). Follicular DCs can retain antigens on their surface for more than 3 months. They also integrate signals from toll-like receptors and other sources to support effective germinal center responses.

Pulmonary DCs

The enormous surfaces of the equine lung are highly vulnerable to microbial invasion. As a result, they have evolved many different protective mechanisms. For example, equine lungs contain a large population of specialized dendritic cells whose function is to trap and process inhaled antigens. Their production is stimulated by exposure to GM-CSF and IL-4. These DCs are morphologically similar to blood DCs. They express high levels of MHC class II and CD44, as well as moderate amounts of CD163 and CD204. They are much more avidly phagocytotic when compared to blood DCs. It appears that lung DCs are at an earlier differentiation stage than blood DCs and, as a result, have considerably greater antigen-capturing ability (Lee et al., 2017).

DC products

DCs produce many different cytokines. The precise mixture depends on the stimulus employed. Thus, large amounts of IL-10, IL-12, IL-13, and IFN-α are produced by LPS-stimulated DCs. As in other species, depending upon whether they are Type 1 or Type 2 DCs, they also secrete T cell polarizing cytokines (Siedek et al., 1997).

Dendritic cell maturation

Although there are many DC subpopulations, their most important properties are based on their state of maturity. Thus, immature cDCs are specialized, efficient, antigen-trapping cells. As they mature, DCs undergo cellular reorganization and become specialized, efficient, antigen-presenting cells (Fig. 7.2).

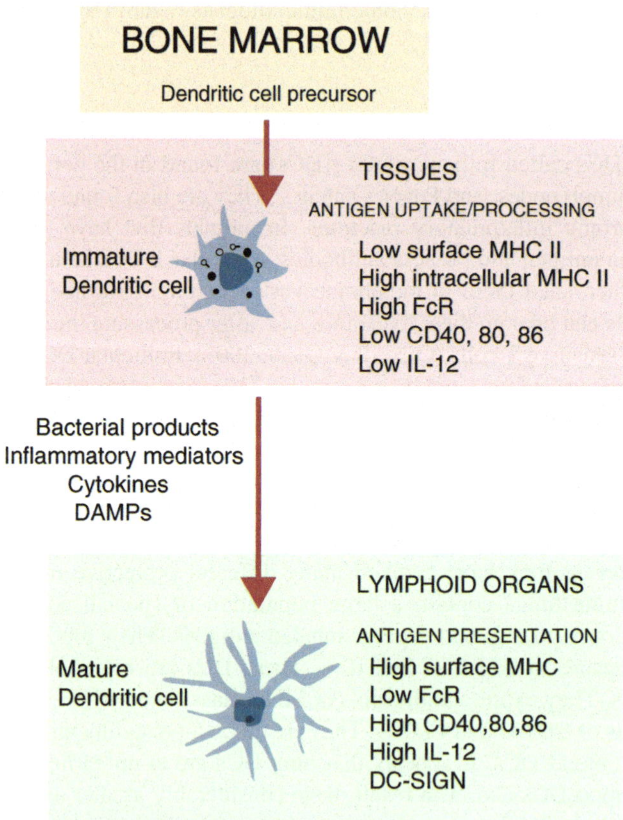

FIGURE 7.2 As DCs mature, they change their function.

Immature DCs are specialized antigen-trapping cells. Mature DCs, on the other hand, are specialized antigen-processing cells.

Immature cDCs

Newly generated cDCs migrate from the bone marrow to lymph nodes and other tissues. Here, they act as disposable antigen-trapping cells. If they do not encounter antigens, they die in a few days. If, however, they encounter antigens and are stimulated by tissue damage or inflammation, they mature rapidly. Immature cDCs have receptors that help them carry out their functions. These include the receptors for interleukin-1β (IL-1R), tumor necrosis factor-α (TNFR), chemokine receptors, C-type lectins, Fc receptors (FcγR and FcεR), mannose receptors (CD206), and heat-shock protein receptors, as well as toll-like receptors.

DCs mature in response to interleukin-1β (IL-1β) and tumor necrosis factor-α as well as to PAMPs and DAMPs. Injured and inflamed tissues release heparan sulfate that binds to TLR4 and also activates these DCs. Breakdown of nucleic acids generates uric acid, another potent dendritic cell activator. Immature DCs are attracted to areas of inflammation by chemokines, defensins, and HMGB1.

DCs capture antigens and cell fragments by phagocytosis, by pinocytosis (cell drinking), and by binding to cell surface receptors. They also capture apoptotic cell bodies. Activation of TLRs by PAMPs ensures that ingested foreign material is processed in such a way that it triggers adaptive immunity. Foreign material that does not activate TLRs is not processed and may not trigger an adaptive response (Chapter 11).

Although the most important functions of DCs are to trap, process, and present antigen to the cells of the immune system, they must also be able to kill any invaders they catch. DCs can kill invaders by producing superoxide and mounting an oxidative burst to generate reactive oxygen species. The pH in the phagosomes of conventional phagocytic cells, such as neutrophils and macrophages, is highly acidic and optimized for proteolytic destruction of foreign material. The pH within dendritic cell phagosomes is, in contrast, relatively alkaline since these phagosomes do not fuse with lysosomes. Proteases are inhibited at these high pH levels, and as a result, the ingested proteins are not completely degraded, but peptides are preserved for presentation to T cells by MHC class II molecules.

Mature cDCs

Dendritic cells are potent T cell stimulators. Once they have captured and processed antigens, immature DCs carry these antigens to sites where they can be recognized by T cells. The activated DCs are attracted to lymphoid organs by chemokines. Infection or tissue damage also promotes the migration of antigen-bearing DCs to lymphoid tissues such as lymph nodes or the spleen. Mature DCs also produce chemokines that attract T cells. The DCs embrace the T cells in a net of dendrites. During this interaction, the T cells examine the DCs for the presence of antigenic peptides. If the T cell receptors can bind the presented peptides, the T cells will be triggered to respond by dividing and producing cytokines.

As DCs mature, their MHC molecules also move to the cell surface. Cell surface expression of their co-stimulatory molecules also increases. As a result, MHC molecules and MHC-peptide complexes are found at levels 100 times higher on the surface of mature DCs than on other cell types such as B cells or macrophages. Their expression of co-stimulatory molecules such as CD86 may also rise 100-fold.

Mature DCs are the only cells that can trigger a primary T cell response. One reason for this is that mature DCs assemble complete T cell activation complexes (antigen-loaded MHC plus co-stimulatory molecules) within the cell before they are carried to the cell surface. Mature DCs also express DC-SIGN (CD209), a C-type lectin that binds a ligand called intercellular adhesion molecule-3 (ICAM-3 or CD50) on naïve T cells. DC-SIGN permits transient binding between DCs and T cells. It allows a single dendritic cell to rapidly screen thousands of T cells to find the few that are expressing a compatible antigen receptor. Because of their potency, only a few DCs are needed to trigger a strong T cell response. Thus, one dendritic cell may activate as many as 3000 T cells. Mature DCs are better at stimulating T cells than are immature DCs. Bone marrow-derived DCs are better at it than monocyte-derived DCs. Mesenchymal stem cells can suppress DC functions. Thus, they can act on monocyte-derived DCs to suppress their response in vitro to LPS (Liu et al., 2013).

In humans, immature and mature DCs can be distinguished by their expression of CD206 and CD83. For example, CD206 expression is a feature of immature DCs, whereas CD83 is only found in the mature cells. Studies on equine monocyte-derived DC populations indicate that this is not the case in the horse. Neither CD83 nor CD206 expression is correlated with dendritic cell differentiation or maturation in this species (Moyo et al., 2013).

cDC1 and cDC2 cells

When classical DCs stimulate helper T cells, they generate three signals. The first signal is delivered when T cell antigen receptors bind antigen fragments attached to MHC class II molecules. The second signal provides the T cells with additional critical co-stimulation through cell surface molecules such as CD40 and CD80/86. The third signal determines the direction in which naïve helper T cells will develop and is provided by secreted cytokines. For example, some microbial antigens trigger cDCs to secrete IL-12. These are called cDC1 cells since their IL-12 activates Th1 cells and triggers type 1, cell-mediated, immune responses. Other microbial antigens induce cDCs to secrete IL-1β and IL-6. These cytokines stimulate Th2 differentiation and are produced by cDC2 cells. They stimulate type 2, antibody-mediated, immune responses.

Equine macrophages

Macrophages and their precursors, the blood monocytes, are the most accessible and best understood of the body's antigen-processing cells. They are very efficient and specialized phagocytic cells that readily ingest and destroy invading microorganisms, especially bacteria. Recent studies have indicated that they also derive significant nourishment from the bacterial amino acids (Lesbats et al., 2025). Once microbial antigens are taken up by macrophages, most are destroyed, but a small portion is processed and presented to sensitized T cells. Macrophages, however, are unable to engage in prolonged interactions with T cells. As a result, they cannot activate naïve T cells. In addition, antigen processing by macrophages is inefficient since much of the ingested antigen is destroyed by lysosomal proteases and oxidants. Indeed, macrophages can be considered cells with other priorities. Their first responsibility is to kill invaders. Macrophages are a heterogeneous family of cells that play key roles as sentinel cells, regulators of inflammation, and as antigen-presenting cells. Thus, the complete population of macrophages throughout the animal body is known as the mononuclear phagocytic system (Fig. 7.3).

Blood monocytes

Equine blood monocytes can be readily isolated and cultured in vitro (Bennett & Cohn, 1965). They consist of three distinct subpopulations in dogs and probably horses as well (Rzepecka et al., 2019). These subpopulations differ in their expression of MHC II and CD4 molecules. One population (Mo1) is MHCII$^+$, CD4$^-$. Another population (Mo2) is MHCII$^+$, CD4$^+$. The third population (Mo3) is MHC II$^-$, CD4$^+$. Mo1 cells are larger than the other two cell types, while Mo3 cells

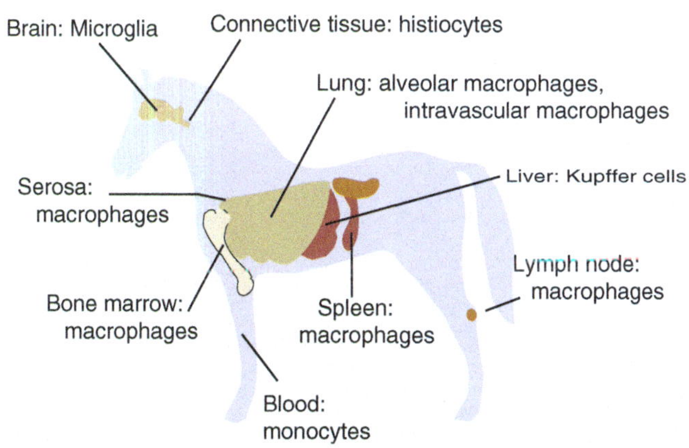

FIGURE 7.3 The mononuclear phagocytic system of the horse.

Large populations of functional macrophages are found in major organs, especially the lungs, liver, and spleen.

are the smallest. It is suggested that these three subpopulations likely have different functions (Karagianni et al., 2020). About 4% of blood monocytes are $CD16^{+}$. These are probably pro-inflammatory cells (Fig. 7.4).

Horse monocytes can bind and grow on glass surfaces where they effectively develop into large, mature macrophages. They produce increased numbers of lysosomes in their cytoplasm, and this is accompanied by an increase in their enzyme contents, - acid phosphatase, and aryl sulfatase. The number and size of their mitochondria also increase. The cultured monocytes develop an increased capacity for phagocytosis of particles such as bacteria or colloidal gold. This phagocytic ability is enhanced by the presence of bacterial lipopolysaccharide (Bennett & Cohn, 1965).

Tissue macrophages

Macrophages are present in almost all equine tissues, where they may account for up to 10% of all the cells. Macrophages are readily cultivated from bone marrow. They characteristically express CD14, CD163 (a hemoglobin-haptoglobin receptor), and MHC class II. MHC II expression but not CD14 is enhanced by exposure to IFN-γ. These cells actively phagocytose IgG-coated erythrocytes, generate superoxide, and secrete TNF-α. However, when cultured equine macrophages phagocytose bacteria such as *Listeria monocytogenes* or *Salmonella enterica* there appears to be no elevation in their nitric oxide production. In addition, there is very weak inducible nitric oxide synthase (iNOS) staining in equine cells exposed to *Salm. enterica* plus IL-1β (Werners et al., 2004).

Although macrophages are competent phagocytes, their phenotype can be modified by different activating pathways. As a result, macrophages can be polarized into two functional subpopulations. Classically activated, or M1 macrophages, are pro-inflammatory effector cells. Alternatively activated, or M2 macrophages, have anti-inflammatory effects and play a role in tolerance induction, resolving inflammation, and tissue repair. This polarization is not necessarily permanent. Macrophages

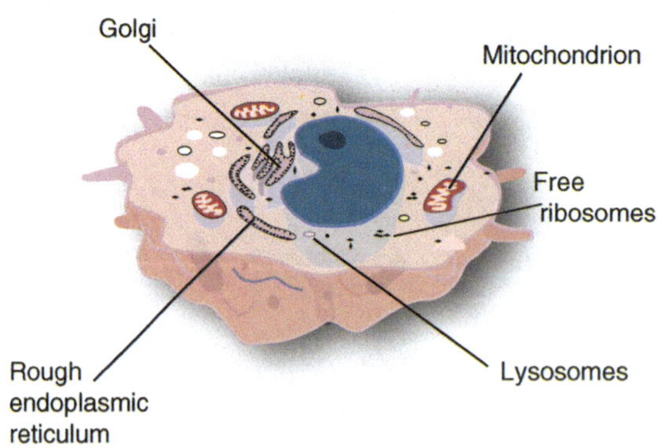

FIGURE 7.4

The structure of a typical macrophage.

can switch their phenotype under the influence of other cytokines and microbial products. M1 and M2 cells should perhaps be considered the extremes of a spectrum of phenotypes rather than distinct subpopulations. M1 cells are produced early in the innate immune process when inflammation is required. M2 cells, on the other hand, tend to appear late in the process when healing is required (Porcheray et al., 2005) (Table 7.1).

Pulmonary intravascular macrophages

The lungs of horses contain a large population of macrophages attached to the lung capillary endothelium (Fig. 7.5).

These pulmonary intravascular macrophages (PIMs) are a distinct subpopulation of cells largely responsible for the clearance of bacteria and other particles from the bloodstream. Thus, in experimental horses, 47%–55% of circulating particles are cleared from the bloodstream at each pass through the lungs during the first hour of infusion. Horses retain the great majority of these bacteria in the lungs rather than in the spleen and liver, as in humans (Longworth et al., 1994).

PIMs are less effective than alveolar macrophages at phagocytosis but are six times more effective in killing virus-infected cells (Chitko-McKown et al., 1991). They develop from blood monocytes that colonize the pulmonary vasculature perinatally. Thus, their relative density in foals doubles between birth and 7 days of age. At birth, they occupy 6% of the capillary volume, but by 30 days, they occupy 25% of the foal's pulmonary vasculature. In addition to being actively phagocytic, they are also responsible for regulating the pulmonary vasculature through their synthesis and release of leukotrienes and prostaglandins. They are relatively small cells (10.2–16.5 μm in diameter). PIMs are irregularly shaped with abundant cytoplasm attached to the capillary endothelium on the thick side of the air-blood barrier (Chitko-McKown & Blecha, 1992). Structurally, they are similar to Kupffer cells.

Table 7.1 Effects of cytokines on macrophage functions.

Cytokine	Major sources	Effect
IL-2	Th1 cell	Activates
IFN-γ	Th1 cell, NK cell	Activates
IFN-α/β	Macrophages, T cells	Activates
TNF-α	Macrophages, Th1 cells	Activates
TNF-β	Th1 cells	Activates
GM-CSF	Many cell types	Activates
IL-4	Th2 cells	Suppresses
IL-10	Th2 cells, macrophages	Suppresses
IL-13	Th2 cells	Suppresses
TGF-β	T Cells	Suppresses

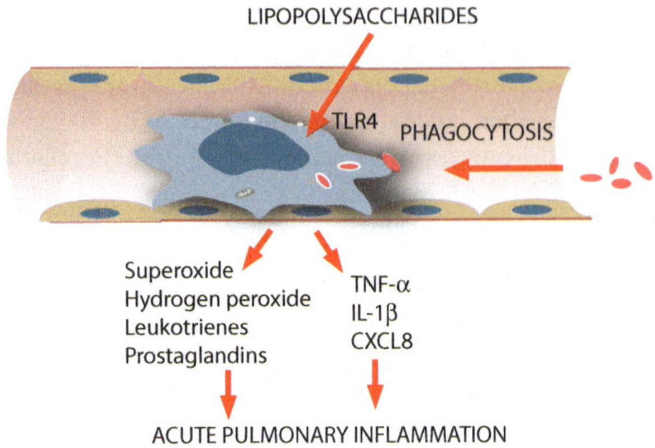

FIGURE 7.5

The location and functions of pulmonary intravascular macrophages.

They are coated with a dense lipoprotein coat (glycocalyx). They form membrane adhesive complexes with the underlying epithelium that resemble intercellular adhesive junctions. They appear to be more active metabolically than alveolar macrophages. They are also more actively phagocytic. When activated, PIMs generate superoxide and hydrogen peroxide and secrete both TNF-α and IL-1β. Mammalian species with these macrophages tend to be acutely sensitive to acute lung inflammation compared to laboratory rodents and humans that lack them. These macrophages secrete inflammatory cytokines such as TNF-α and CXCL8 (Singh et al., 2004).

Endotoxins can activate macrophages in vivo. As a result, they can provoke local inflammation such as laminitis, colic, and neonatal sepsis (Aharonson-Raz & Singh, 2010). Horses appear to be uniquely susceptible to endotoxin-induced cardiopulmonary shock. (The intraperitoneal lethal dose of endotoxin for ponies is 200–400 μg/kg bodyweight, whereas the lethal dose for rabbits and guinea pigs is 3–10 mg/kg) (Berczi et al., 1966; Burrows, 1981). Pulmonary intravascular macrophages therefore significantly increase a horse's sensitivity to inflammation caused by endotoxins (Aharonson-Raz et al., 2012). =In horses exposed to the dust from moldy hay, depletion of these macrophages after gadolinium chloride perfusion significantly reduced the severity of respiratory disease. This depletion also reduced the expression of TLR4 and TLR9 in equine lungs. As a result, it inhibited endotoxin signaling and activation. The complement-derived anaphylatoxins C3qa and C5a may also promote this response.

Alveolar macrophages

Alveolar macrophages play a key role in the defense of the equine lung against inhaled pathogens. They populate the alveoli soon after the birth of the foal and are self-renewing. Alveolar macrophages vary in size from 8.5 to 20 μm in diameter. They possess oval nuclei, a large Golgi, suggesting secretory ability, and numerous cytoplasmic vacuoles. They are adapted to living in this aerobic environment. They have their own unique cell surface phenotype (Karagianni et al., 2013). Horses, especially those confined to dusty stables, inhale significant amounts of soil dusts, fungal spores, and airborne Gram-negative bacteria. For example, following stimulation with bacterial LPS or killed *Salmonella enterica* Typhimurium, alveolar macrophages demonstrate increased production of TNF-α and indole dioxygenase. Horse peritoneal macrophages do not do this. Alveolar macrophages also show high expression levels of CD14, CD163, and TLR4, whereas stimulated peritoneal macrophages express TLR4 only. Alveolar macrophages are much more efficient at phagocytosis than are peritoneal macrophages. One other interesting finding is that, unlike rodent macrophages, equine alveolar macrophages do not produce nitric oxide synthase or reactive nitrogen species on stimulation (Karagianni et al., 2013; Wilson et al., 2020).

Alveolar macrophages express higher levels of CD163 and CD206 than monocyte-derived macrophages. On stimulation with a fungal-lipopolysaccharide mixture, they secrete IL-1β, IL-8, TNF-α, and IFN-γ. Conversely, monocyte-derived macrophages secrete IL-8, IL-10, and TNF-α, suggesting that the alveolar macrophages are more effective in promoting inflammation (Kang et al., 2023).

A comparative analysis of the transcriptome of equine alveolar and peritoneal macrophages has revealed differences in the expression of 451 genes. Alveolar macrophages have a gene expression profile typical of M2 cells, whereas peritoneal macrophages show an M1/M2 hybrid profile. This is reflected in their reduced endotoxin tolerance (Karagianni et al., 2017).

It is essential to remove dead cells and bacteria from the alveoli promptly to avoid local accumulation and inflammation that could result in an inability to exchange oxygen. Alveolar macrophages can migrate between alveoli. By removing the bacteria and keeping the alveoli clean, they prevent harmful inflammation from developing.

Other organs

Macrophages lining the sinusoids of the liver are called Kupffer cells. The red pulp of the spleen also contains extensive periarterial macrophage sheaths that serve as major sites for the clearance of blood particles (Chapter 8). Like other macrophage populations, they can generate the three inflammatory cytokines, TNF-α, IL-6, and IL-1β, on exposure to bacterial lipopolysaccharide. They contain significant quantities of lysozyme as well as nonspecific esterases (Morris et al., 1992).

Macrophage activation

M1 macrophages

When macrophages ingest invading bacteria, they produce enzymes and oxidants that kill the invaders. This response, however, may be insufficient to kill some specialized invaders. For example, bacteria such as *Rhodococcus equi* and *M. tuberculosis* can survive and multiply inside normal macrophages. Antibodies are ineffective against these organisms, so protection against this type of infection requires additional macrophage activation (Fig. 7.6).

These activated macrophages are classified as M1 cells. Thus $CD14^+$ horse macrophages have both inflammatory and regulatory functions. Inflammatory macrophages are activated by LPS plus IFN-γ, whereas the regulatory cells are induced by IL-4 plus IL-10. The activated subset has a rounded granular shape, whereas the regulatory (M2) macrophages tend to be spindle-shaped. Their activation is further stimulated by GM-CSF (Bowlby et al., 2023).

Inflammatory M1 macrophages become fully activated in two stages. The initial activation steps are triggered by exposure to PAMPs and DAMPs from invading bacteria and damaged tissues, as described previously. Molecules that trigger M1 polarization include lipopolysaccharides, CpG DNA, microbial carbohydrates, and heat-shock proteins, as well as many DAMPs. Different levels of M1 activation are recognized, depending on the triggering agent, and some bacteria, such as

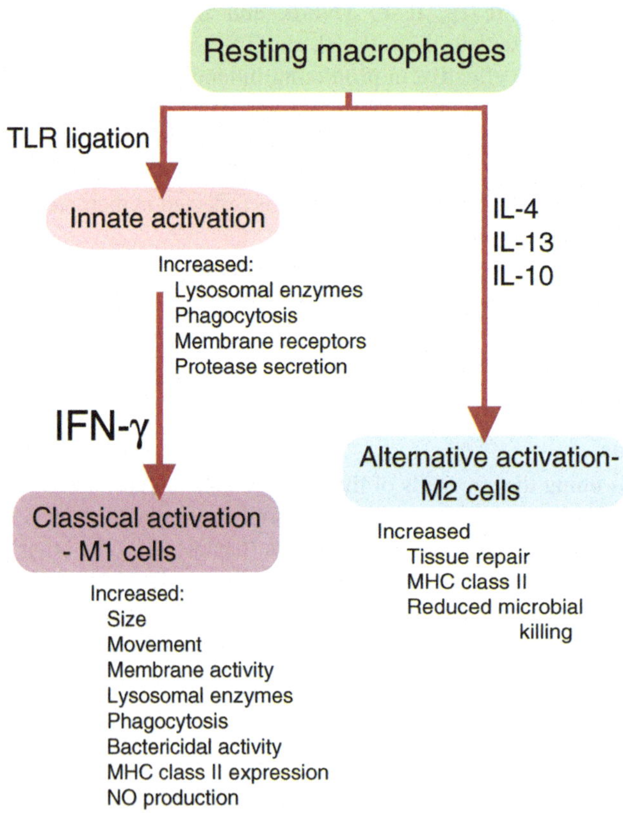

FIGURE 7.6

The activation and differentiation of macrophages into two phenotypically and functionally distinct populations, M1 and M2 cells.

Mycobacterium tuberculosis, are better able to activate macrophages than others. Thus, when monocytes first move into inflamed tissues, they produce increased amounts of lysosomal enzymes, increase phagocytic activity, increase their expression of antibody and complement receptors, and secrete more proteases (Mosser & Edwards, 2008).

The cytokines produced by these activated macrophages, especially TNF-α and IL-12, activate natural killer (NK) cells. NK cells, in turn, secrete IFN-γ, which activates macrophages still further. Some TLR ligands can also activate pathways that result in IFN-β production. This endogenous IFN-β also promotes M1 cell polarization. Stimulation of Th1 cells by IL-12 will also trigger IFN-γ production. These Th1 cells also produce IL-2, which further promotes M1 polarization and complete activation (Fig. 7.7).

Macrophages are activated by IFN-γ through the JAK/STAT pathway. IFN-γ exposure alters the expression of more than 1000 macrophage genes. Activated macrophages secrete proteases that activate complement. They secrete interferons as well as thromboplastin, prostaglandins, fibronectins, plasminogen activator, and the complement components C2 and Factor B. They increase their expression of MHC class II, delay the production of phagosomal proteases, and promote antigen loading onto MHC molecules, so enhancing antigen presentation. M1 macrophages are enlarged and show increased membrane activity (especially ruffling), increased formation of pseudopodia, and increased pinocytosis (uptake of fluid droplets). They move more rapidly in response to chemotactic stimuli, and they are attracted by many different chemokines. They are more avidly phagocytic than resting cells and also take up and employ neutrophil granules with their enzymes (Tan et al., 2006).

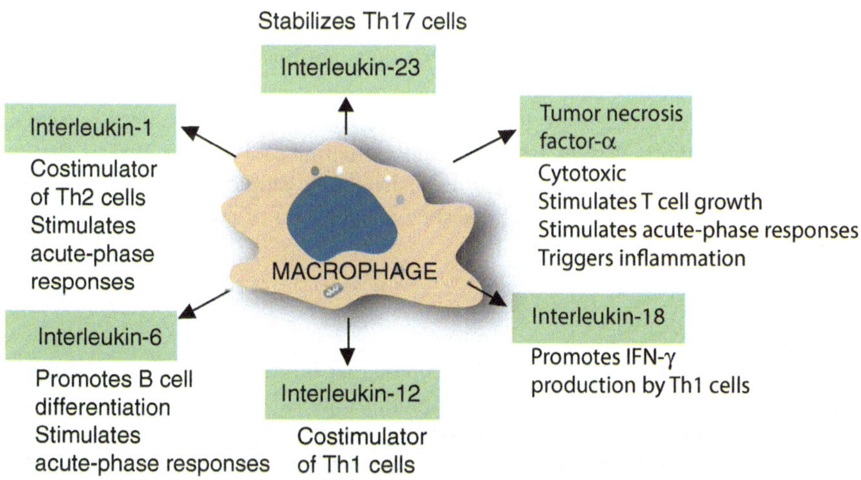

FIGURE 7.7

The production of cytokines by activated macrophages.

In rodents, M1 cells produce greatly increased amounts of nitric oxide synthase 2 (NOS2). This, in turn, generated antibacterial nitric oxide. The nitric oxide generated can destroy nearby tumor cells and intracellular bacteria such as *L. monocytogenes*. However, not all mammals employ this pathway. The available evidence suggests that in the horse, neither bone marrow-derived macrophages nor alveolar macrophages generate nitric oxide. Nor do they express NOS2 mRNA (Karagianini et al., 2013, 2017; Young et al., 2018).

M2 macrophages

M2 macrophages differ from M1 cells in their receptor expression, cytotoxic function, and cytokine production. They are generated by exposure to M-CSF, IL-4, and IL-13. M2 cells do not produce NO but instead convert arginine to ornithine using the enzyme arginase. M2 cells upregulate their production of IL-8, IL-10, IL-1RA, and CCL2 (MCP-1). M2 cells are regulatory and anti-inflammatory, and they promote the resolution of inflammation and wound repair. They are protective against some parasitic diseases by assisting in walling off parasitic larvae (Chow et al., 2016).

TGF-β from M2 cells stimulates extracellular matrix (ECM) production by fibroblasts. M2 cells also secrete the matrix component fibronectin. They also secrete transglutaminase, which promotes ECM cross-linking, and osteopontin, which promotes cell-binding to the ECM. Arginase is involved in proline and polyamine synthesis. Proline is required for ECM construction, whereas polyamines are required for cell proliferation. M2 cells secrete platelet-derived growth factor (PDGF), insulin-like growth factor (IGF), and TGF-β, all of which promote cell proliferation. They also secrete fibroblast-like growth factor-β (FGF-β), TGF-α, and vascular endothelial growth factor (VEGF), which promote angiogenesis. Thus, the cytokines produced by M2 cells promote resolution of inflammation and wound repair and have anti-inflammatory, fibrotic, proliferative, and angiogenic properties.

M2 macrophages are also unique in that they can fuse with other macrophages and, as a result, differentiate into multinuclear osteoclasts in bone. They can also fuse with other macrophages to form multinucleated giant cells in other tissues. Giant cells play important roles in chronic inflammation and the removal of foreign bodies (>45 μm) that are too large to be destroyed by single cells. Langhans giant cells are a subtype that contains a horseshoe-shaped ring of nuclei and are found in chronic granulomas such as tubercles.

CD163

CD163 is a high-affinity macrophage receptor that binds haptoglobin-hemoglobin complexes and hence acts to reduce hemoglobin-induced damage in injured tissues. CD163 is also a member of the Scavenger Receptor Cysteine-Rich (SRCR) family (Etzerodt & Moestrup, 2013). CD163 has nine SRCR domains, with a transmembrane segment and a short cytoplasmic tail. It is expressed on equine tissue macrophages, a subset of monocytes, and on DCs. Its expression is upregulated at inflammatory sites where it acts to remove proinflammatory hemoglobin (Etzerodt & Moestrup, 2013). It is also released into the circulation by inflammatory macrophages. There are three known types of CD163 molecules: CD163a, CD163b, and CD163c-a. CD163c-a and CD163A are expressed not only on some T cells but also on multiple other cell types (Hsu et al., 2011). CD163 can also act as a pattern recognition receptor that can bind to Gram-positive or Gram-negative bacteria and trigger cytokine production.

CD163 is expressed in large quantities in equine exuberant granulation tissue. This is a wound healing disorder where a persistent inflammatory response persists beyond that necessary to heal a wound properly. The reasons for this are unknown; however, there are very high numbers of CD163-positive macrophages in the fibrotic regions of the granulation tissue (Du Cheyne et al., 2021). CD163 macrophages are also present in large numbers throughout the equine gastrointestinal tract from the stomach to the colon. Their functions are unknown. They tend to be closely associated with the myenteric plexus and intestinal neurons. It has been suggested that they play a role in regulating gut motility (Lisowski et al., 2020). They are also present in the uveal tract, especially the ciliary body of the equine eye (Sano et al., 2016).

B cells

In addition to their role as antibody producers, B cells are also effective antigen-presenting cells. Following antigen binding, the antigen receptor (BCR) is internalized and either degraded or transported to an intracellular compartment, where MHC class II molecules and antigen fragments combine. These antigen-MHC class II complexes are then carried to the B cell surface and presented to helper T cells. If an antigen presented by an APC binds to a BCR, the antigen may be extracted from the presenting cell and endocytosed by the B cell. This antigen is delivered to endosomes where it also complexes with MHC class II molecules. Since all the antigen receptors on a single B cell are identical, each B cell can bind only a single antigen. This makes them much more efficient antigen-presenting cells than macrophages, which must present any foreign material that comes their way. This is especially true in primed animals, in which large numbers of B cells can bind and efficiently present a specific antigen. As a result, B cells can activate helper T cells with 1/1000 of the dose of antigen required to activate macrophages (Batista & Harwood, 2009).

Other antigen-processing cells

T cells may also be activated by antigens presented by many different "non-professional" cell types. These include neutrophils, eosinophils, basophils, T cells, endothelial cells, fibroblasts, NK cells, smooth muscle cells, microglial cells, and thymic epithelial cells. Their effectiveness depends on the local environment. Thus, fibroblasts may be very effective antigen-processing cells when located within granulomas. Presumably, co-stimulation can come from other nearby cells in this cytokine-rich environment. Vascular endothelial cells can also take up antigens, synthesize IL-1β, and under the influence of IFN-γ, express MHC class II molecules. Even skin keratinocytes can secrete IL-1β, express MHC class II molecules, and present antigens to T cells.

Antigen processing

The MHC class II pathway

The presentation of exogenous antigens to T cells is mediated by MHC class II molecules of the ELA system. These are cell surface receptors that bind processed peptide fragments. Although many cells can phagocytose foreign antigens, only those that can express antigen fragments bound to MHC class II molecules can trigger a T cell response. As described previously, the most efficient antigen-processing cells are thus mature MHC class II^+ DCs (Watts, 2005). MHC class II molecules bind peptides from processed antigens and present them to helper T cells. The helper cells will recognize and respond to these peptides only if the peptides are bound to MHC class II molecules. If a peptide is presented to T cells in the absence of MHC class II, the T cells will be turned off or die, and tolerance may result (Pishesha et al., 2022).

Exogenous antigen processing involves multiple steps. First, the antigen must be endocytosed by DCs or macrophages and taken into phagosomes. These phagosomes then fuse with lysosomes. The ingested proteins are then broken up by lysosomal proteases into peptide fragments of varying sizes. The endosomes containing these peptide fragments then fuse with other endosomes carrying newly synthesized MHC class II molecules to form the lysosome-MHC class II compartment (MIIC). An MHC class II antigen-binding groove can hold a foreign peptide of 12–24 amino acids as a straight, extended chain that projects out of both ends of the binding groove. Side chains from the peptide bind in pockets on the walls of the binding groove (Fig. 9.3). Unlike most new transmembrane proteins that are expressed minutes after assembly, MHC class II molecules are retained inside the cell for several hours until they are needed. Once the foreign peptide binds to an MHC molecule, the MIIC vesicle moves toward the cell surface. When it reaches the surface, the MHC-peptide complex is exposed and available for inspection by any passing T cell (Fig. 7.8).

It has been calculated that an antigen-processing DC can express up to 2×10^5 MHC class II molecules that can present peptide fragments to T cells. If co-stimulation is provided, a single T cell can be activated by exposure to as few as 200–300 of these peptide-MHC complexes. It is therefore possible for a single antigen-processing dendritic cell to present many different peptides to different T cells simultaneously.

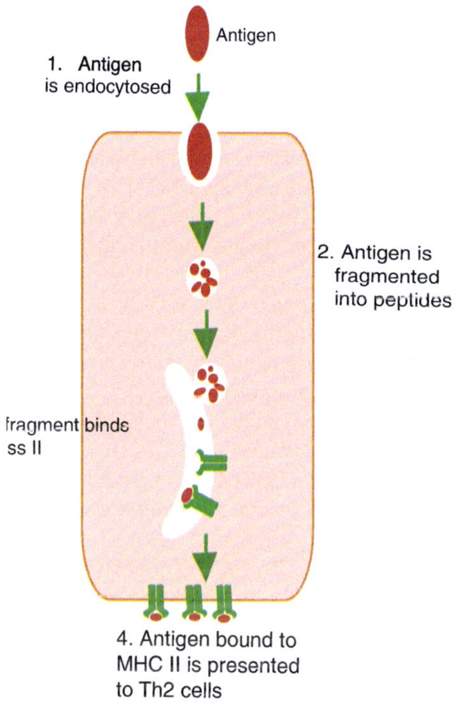

FIGURE 7.8 The processing of exogenous antigen by an antigen-presenting cell.

Ingested antigens are taken into phagosomes where they are fragmented by proteases. Peptides are then carried to the endosomal compartments, where the antigenic peptides are placed in the binding grooves of MHC class II molecules. The antigen-MHC complexes are then transported to the cell surface where they are presented to helper T cells.

Histiocytosis and histiocytomas

Histiocytic tumors in horses are very uncommon. When they do occur, however, they tend to be highly aggressive and frequently metastasize. The cells are intermediate in morphology between monoblasts and tissue histiocytes. There has been a single report in an Arabian filly (Paciello et al., 2013).

References

Aharonson-Raz, K., Lohmann, K. L., Townsend, H. G., Marques, F., & Singh, B. (2012). Pulmonary intravascular macrophages as proinflammatory cells in heaves, an asthma-like equine disease. *American Journal of Physiology - Lung Cellular and Molecular Physiology, 303*, L189–1198.

Aharonson-Raz, K., & Singh, B. (2010). Pulmonary intravascular macrophages and endotoxin-induced pulmonary pathophysiology in horses. *Canadian Journal of Veterinary Research, 74*, 45–49.

Batista, F. D., & Harwood, N. E. (2009). The who, how and where of antigen presentation to B cells. *Nature Reviews Immunology, 9*(1), 15–27.

Bennett, W. E., & Cohn, Z. A. (1965). The isolation and selected properties of blood monocytes. *Journal of Experimental Medicine, 123*, 145–159.

Berczi, I., Bertok, L., & Bereznai, T. (1966). Comparative studies on the toxicity of *Escherichia coli* lipopolysaccharide endotoxin in various animal species. *Canadian Journal of Microbiology, 12*, 1070–1071.

Bowlby, C. M., Purmessur, D., & Durgam, S. S. (2023). Equine peripheral blood CD14+ monocyte-derived macrophage in vitro characteristics after GM-CSF pretreatment and LPS+ IFN -γ or IL-4 + IL-10 differentiation. *Veterinary Immunology and Immunopathology*. https://doi.org/10.1016/vetimm.2022.110534

Burrows, G. E. (1981). Dose-response of ponies to parenteral *Escherichia coli* endotoxin. *Canadian Journal of Comparative Medicine, 45*, 207–210.

Chitko-McKown, C. G., & Blecha, F. (1992). Pulmonary intravascular macrophages: A review of immune properties and functions. *Annales de Recherches Veterinaires, 23*, 201–214.

Chitko-McKown, C. G., Chapes, S. K., Brown, R. E., Phillips, R. M., et al. (1991). Porcine alveolar and pulmonary intravascular macrophages: Comparison of immune functions. *Journal of Leukocyte Biology, 50*, 364–372.

Chow, K. V., Lew, A. M., Sutherland, R. M., & Zhan, Y. (2016). Monocyte-derived dendritic cells promote Th polarization, whereas conventional dendritic cells promote Th proliferation. *Journal of Immunology., 196*(2), 624–636.

Du Cheyne, C., Martens, A., & De Spiegelaere, W. (2021). High numbers of CD163-positive macrophages in the fibrotic region of exuberant granulation tissue in horses. *Animals*. https://doi.org/10.3390/ani11092728

Etzerodt, A., & Moestrup, S. K. (2013). CD163 and inflammation: Biological, diagnostic and therapeutic aspects. *Antioxidants and Redox Signaling, 18*, 2352–2363.

Hamada, M., Takechi, M., & Itakura, C. (1992). Langerhans' cells in equine cutaneous papillomas and normal skin. *Veterinary Pathology Online, 29*, 152–160.

Hodge, A. L., Baxter, A. A., & Poon, I. K. H. (2022). Gift bags within the sentinel cells of the immune system: The diverse role of dendritic cell-derived extracellular vesicles. *Journal of Leukocyte Biology, 111*, 903–920.

Hsu, H., Cheng, C., Baldwin, C., & Telfer, J. C. (2011). CD163/WC1 functions as a pattern recognition receptor and co-receptor for the γδ TCR. *Journal of Immunology*. https://doi.org/10.4049/jimmunol.186.Supp.113.18

Kang, H., Lee, G. K. C., Bienzle, D., Arroyo, L. G., et al. (2023). Equine alveolar macrophages and monocyte-derived macrophages respond differently to an inflammatory stimulus. *PLoS One*. https://doi.org/10.1371/journal.pone.0282738

Karagianni, A. E., Kapetanovic, R., McGorum, B., Hume, D. A., & Pirie, S. R. (2013). The equine alveolar macrophage: Functional and phenotypic comparisons with peritoneal macrophages. *Veterinary Immunology and Immunopathology, 155*, 219–228.

Karagianni, A. E., Kapetanovic, R., Summers, K. M., McGorum, B., et al. (2017). Comparative transcriptome analysis of equine alveolar macrophages. *Equine Veterinary Journal, 49*, 375–382.

Karagianni, A. E., Lisowski, Z. M., Hume, D. A., & Pirie, R. S. (2020). The equine mononuclear phagocyte system: The relevance of horse as a model for understanding human innate immunity. *Equine Veterinary Journal*. https://doi.org/10.1111/evj.13341

Kurotaki, T., Narayama, K., Arai, Y., Arai, S., et al. (2002). Langerhans cells within the follicular epithelium and the intradermal sweat duct in equine insect hypersensitivity "Kasen. *Journal of Veterinary Medical Science, 64*(6), 539–541.

Lee, Y., Kiupei, M., Soboll, & Hussey, G. (2017). Characterization of respiratory dendritic cells from equine lung tissues. *BMC Veterinary Research*. https://doi.org/10.1186/s12917-017-1240-z

Lesbats, J., Brillac, A., Reisz, J. A., Mukherjee, P., et al. (2025). Macrophages recycle phagocytosed bacteria to fuel immunometabolic responses. *Nature*. https://doi.org/10.1038/s41586-025-08629-4

Lisowski, Z. M., Sauter, K. A., Waddell, L. A., Hume, D. A., et al. (2020). Immunohistochemical study of morphology and distribution of CD16e +ve macrophages in the normal adult equine gastrointestinal tract. *Veterinary Immunology and Immunopathology*. https://doi.org/10.1016/j.vetimm.2020.110073

Liu, W. H., Liu, J. J., Wu, J., Zhang, L. L., et al. (2013). Novel mechanism of inhibition of dendritic cells maturation by mesenchymal stem cells via interleukin-10 and the JAK1/STAT3 signaling pathway. *PLoS One, 8*(1), Article e55487.

Longworth, K. E., Jarvis, K. A., Tyler, W. S., Steffey, E. P., & Staub, N. C. (1994). Pulmonary intravascular macrophages in horses and ponies. *American Journal of Veterinary Research, 55*(3), 382–388.

Lopez, B. S., Hurley, D. J., Giancola, S., Giguere, S., et al. (2020). Phenotypic characterization of equine monocyte-derived dendritic cells generated ex vivo using commercially available serum-free medium. *Veterinary Immunology and Immunopathology, 222*, Article 110036.

Mauel, S., Steinbach, F., & Ludwig, H. (2006). Monocyte-derived dendritic cells from horses differ from dendritic cells of humans and mice. *Immunology, 117*, 463–473.

Morris, D. D., Crowe, N., Moore, J. N., & Moldawer, L. L. (1992). Endotoxin-induced production of interleukin 6 by equine peritoneal macrophages in vitro. *American Journal of Veterinary Research, 53*(8), 1298–1301.

Mosser, D. M., & Edwards, J. P. (2008). Exploring the full spectrum of macrophage activation. *Nature Reviews Immunology, 8*, 958–969.

Moyo, N. A., Marchi, E., & Steinbach, F. (2013). Differentiation and activation of equine monocyte-derived dendritic cells are not correlated with CD206 or CD83 expression. *Immunology, 139*, 472–483.

O'Neill, H. C., & Quah, B. J. C. (2008). Exosomes secreted by bacterially infected macrophages are proinflammatory. *Science Signaling, 1*, 1–5.

Paciello, O., Passantino, G., Costagliola, A., Papparella, S., & Perillo, A. (2013). Histiocytic sarcoma of the nasal cavity of a horse. *Research in Veterinary Science, 94*, 648–650.

Patel, R. S., Tomlinson, J. E., Divers, T. J., Van der Walle, G. R., & Rosenberg, B. R. (2021). Single-cell resolution landscape of equine peripheral blood mononuclear cells reveals diverse cell types including T-bet^{+} B cells. *BMC Biology, 19*(1), 13. https://doi.org/10.1186/s12915-020-00947-5

Pishesha, N., Harmand, T. J., & Ploegh, H. L. (2022). A guide to antigen processing and presentation. *Nature Reviews Immunol, 22*, 751–764.

Porcheray, E., Viaud, S., Rimaniol, A.-C., et al. (2005). Macrophage activation switching: An asset for the resolution of inflammation. *Clinical and Experimental Immunology, 142*, 481–489.

Reizis, B. (2019). Plasmacytoid dendritic cells: Development, regulation and function. *Immunity, 50*, 37–50.

Rzepecka, A., Zmigrodzka, M., Witkowska-Pitaszewicz, O., et al. (2019). CD4 and MHCII phenotypic variability of peripheral blood monocytes in dogs. *PLoS One*. https://doi.org/10.1371/journal.pone.0219214

Sano, Y., Matsuda, K., Okamoto, M., Takehana, K., et al. (2016). Distribution of CD163-positive cell and MHC class II positive cell in the normal equine uveal tract. *Journal of Veterinary Medical Science, 78*(2), 287–291.

Siedek, E., Little, S., Mayall, S., Edington, N., & Hamblin, A. (1997). Isolation and characterization of equine dendritic cells. *Veterinary Immunology and Immunopathology, 60*, 15–31.

Singh, R., Pearce, J. W., Gamage, L. N., Janardhan, K., & Caldwell, S. (2004). Depletion of pulmonary intravascular macrophages inhibits acute lung inflammation. *American Journal of Physiology - Lung Cellular and Molecular Physiology, 286*, L363–L372.

Summerfield, A., Auray, G., & Ricklin, M. (2015). Comparative dendritic cell biology of veterinary mammals. *Annual Review of Animal Biosciences*. https://doi.org/10.1146/annurev-animal-022114-111009

Tan, B. H., Meinken, C. C., Bastian, M., et al. (2006). Macrophages acquire neutrophil granules for antimicrobial activity against intracellular pathogens. *Journal of Immunology, 177*, 1864–1871.

Watts, C. (2005). Phagosome neutrality in host defense. *Cell, 126*, 17–19.

Werners, A. H., Bull, S., Fink-Gremmels, J., & Bryant, C. E. (2004). Generation and characterization of an equine macrophage cell line (e-CAS cells) derived from equine bone marrow cells. *Veterinary Immunology and Immunopathology, 97*(1–2), 65–76.

Wilson, M. E., McCandless, E. E., Olszewski, M. A., & Robinson, N. E. (2020). Alveolar macrophage phenotypes in severe equine asthma. *The Veterinary Journal*. https://doi.org/10.1016/j.tvjl.2020.105436

Young, R., Bush, S. J., Lefevre, L., McCulloch, M. E. B., et al. (2018). Species-specific transcriptional regulation of genes involved in nitric oxide production and arginine metabolism in macrophages. *ImmunoHorizons*. https://doi.org/10.4049/immunohorizons.1700073

Ziegler, A., Marti, E., Summerfield, A., & Baumann, A. (2016). Identification and characterization of equine blood plasmacytoid dendritic cells. *Developmental and Comparative Immunology, 65*, 352–357.

CHAPTER

The equine lymphoid system

8

Although antigens are trapped and processed by dendritic cells, macrophages, and B cells, adaptive immune responses are actually mounted by lymphocytes. Lymphocytes are responsible for the production of antibodies as well as for mediating cell-mediated immune responses. The lymphoid organs have therefore evolved to provide an environment for efficient interactions among lymphocytes, antigen-presenting cells, and foreign antigens as well as sites where lymphocytes can respond optimally to processed antigens (Fig. 8.1).

Sources of lymphocytes

Lymphocytes are first detected in the fetal foal's thymus, mesenteric lymph nodes and the intestinal wall. In older fetuses and adult horses, their stem cells are mainly located in the bone marrow.

Bone marrow

The bone marrow has multiple functions in adult horses and donkeys. It is a hematopoietic organ containing the precursors of all blood cells, including lymphocytes. It is also a primary lymphoid organ (a site where newly produced lymphocytes can mature). Like the spleen, liver, and lymph nodes, the bone marrow is also a secondary lymphoid organ where circulating antigens can be trapped by dendritic cells and macrophages. It is lined by a layer of cells covering the bone surface, endosteum, and this layer contains aggregates of osteoblasts and osteoclasts. The bone marrow also contains large numbers of antibody-producing plasma cells and is therefore a significant source of serum antibodies.

In foals, the hematopoietic bone marrow is primarily found within their long and flat bones. However, as the animals age, their medullary cavities become progressively filled with adipocytes, and the hematopoietic tissue tends to be confined to the trabecular cavities of flat bones as well as the epiphysis and metaphysis of the long bones.

Bone marrow is abundant in the sternum, ileum, and ribs of the horse. It contains both hematopoietic stem cells and adipocytes. The progenitors of lymphocytes are produced in the bone marrow under the influence of growth factors. These

The Immunology of Horses and Donkeys. https://doi.org/10.1016/B978-0-443-44863-8.00020-X

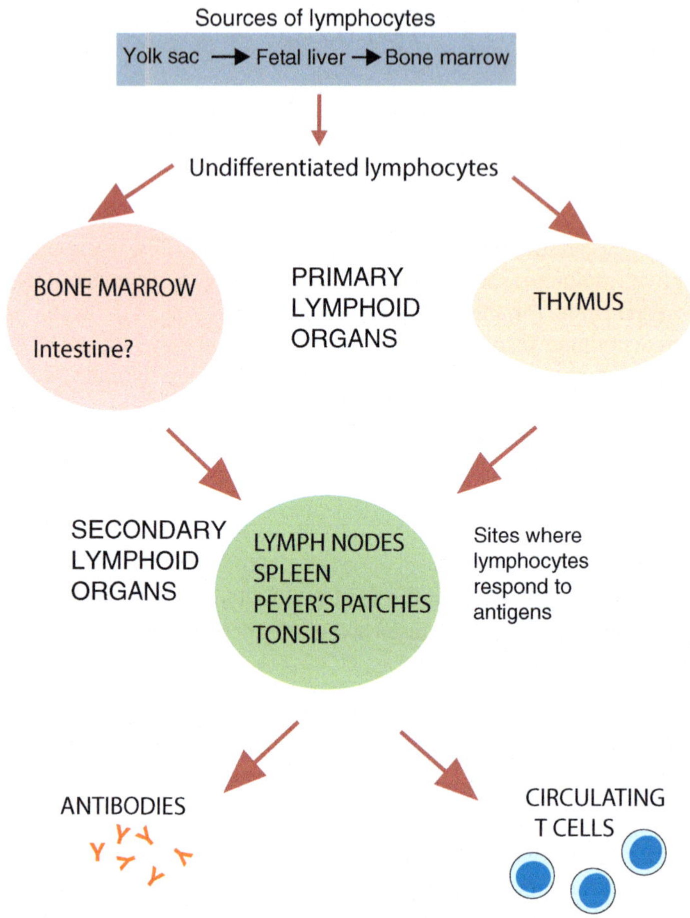

FIGURE 8.1 The functions of the major horse lymphoid organs.

progenitors ultimately give rise to NK, B, and T cells. These stem cells are generally found close to the endosteum, but as the cells differentiate, they spread throughout the marrow before migrating to the other primary lymphoid organs.

Because of its multiple functions, the bone marrow can be divided into hematopoietic and vascular compartments. The hematopoietic compartment contains stem cells for all the blood cells, in addition to macrophages, dendritic cells, and lymphocytes. It is enclosed by a layer of adventitial cells. In older horses, these adventitial cells may become so loaded with fat that the marrow may have a fatty yellow appearance. There is no exclusive B cell development site in the equine bone marrow, although it is suggested that precursor B cells develop at the outer edge of the marrow and migrate to the center as they mature and multiply.

Primary lymphoid organs

As foals develop in utero, newly produced, immature lymphocytes emigrate from the bone marrow to the primary lymphoid organs where they complete their development. Thus, T cells and B cells are initially differentiated based on the primary organ in which they mature. All T cells mature in the thymus. Equine B cells, in contrast, complete their development within the bone marrow and the gastrointestinal lymphoid tissues.

Thymus

The developing thymus is first seen in the fetal foal at 11–12 weeks post-conception (MacKenzie, 1975). However, it grows rapidly in late pregnancy and for the first months after a foal is born. Most of the thymus in the newborn foal is located in the anterior mediastinum, ventral to the trachea and the large thoracic blood vessels. It consists of two grayish-pink lobes on each side of the thoracic cavity. divided into lobules held together by connective tissue, together with some adipose tissue. The thymic lobes extend as a chain of lobules up the neck between the trachea and carotid arteries, sometimes extending as far as the thyroid gland. The cervical part of the equine thymus is very variable. It may extend from either both lobes or from a single lobe and subsequently bifurcate. There is no clear distinction between the right and left lobes, even though they develop separately from the third guttural pouches (Sisson & Grossman, 1953).

The overall histologic structure of the equine thymus is similar to that seen in other mammals, multiple lobes each with a distinct cortex and medulla. As the animal ages, the thymic parenchyma progressively shrinks, but the extra parenchymal components do not. An unusual feature is the occurrence of prominent nonlymphoid hematopoiesis, including the production of eosinophils, mast cells, and plasma cells in the equine thymus (Contreiras et al., 2004). Lymphatic vessels full of lymphocytes are especially prominent and presumably serve as the routes by which selected T cells leave the organ once fully functional.

The size of the thymus changes as foals age. Its relative size is greatest in foals about 2 months of age. Between 6 and 18 months of age, it begins to involute. Note that this is well before puberty. Initially, the involution involves only the thymic cortex. The lymphocytes eventually disappear, leaving only the epithelial cells. Subsequently, epithelial cell numbers drop, leaving just mast cells and plasma cells (Contreiras et al., 2004). The number of epithelial cells drops progressively, leaving the thymic capsule and septae largely intact. There is also a progressive increase in

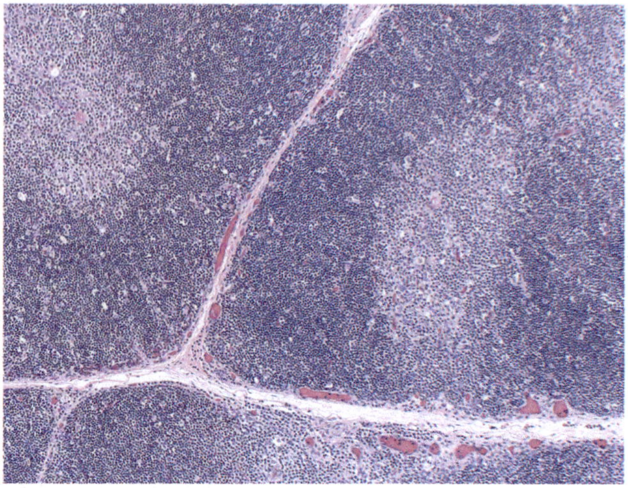

FIGURE 8.2 The histology of the foal thymus.

Observe how it is divided into lobules, each with a darker staining cortex and a paler staining medulla in each lobule. Original magnification ×10.

- Courtesy of Dr Brian Porter.

the amount of adipose tissue in the thymus. As a result, by the time the horse reaches 3 years of age, it has largely been replaced by adipose tissue (Contreiras et al., 2004). A thin remnant of thymic tissue usually persists in the anterior mediastinum (Fig. 8.2).

The maternal thymus also undergoes involution during pregnancy (Laan et al., 2016). There is a reduction in all the thymic cell populations, both lymphoid and epithelial. This may play a role in promoting maternal tolerance of her fetus. The mares thymus recovers post-partum; usually by the end of lactation.

Structure

The thymus consists of lobules of loosely packed epithelial cells, each covered by a connective tissue capsule and separated by septa. The outer part of each lobule, the cortex, is densely infiltrated with lymphocytes (thymocytes). It is distinct from the inner medulla, which contains fewer lymphocytes, and the epithelial cells are more obvious (Fig. 8.2). These thymic epithelial cells possess abundant cytoplasm as well as extensive cytoplasmic processes. These processes come into close contact with thymocytes (Fig. 8.3).

Within the medulla are also found round, layered bodies called Hassall's corpuscles. These are heterogeneous structures that vary greatly in size and may have a central cavity or cyst lined by pseudostratified or glandular epithelial cells. They are present in the fetal thymus and become more obvious as the thymus atrophies (MacKenzie, 1975). The remains of a small blood vessel may be found at their

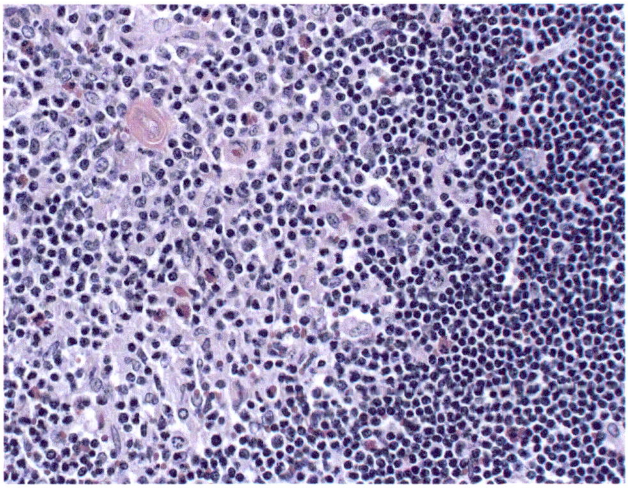

FIGURE 8.3 A high power view of a section of foal thymus.

Note the Hassall's corpuscle in the top left. There are also significant numbers of eosinophils present. Original magnification, ×40.

- Courtesy of Dr Brian Porter.

center. Keratinization of the Hassall's corpuscles is especially evident. An abnormally thick basement membrane and a continuous layer of epithelial cells surround the capillaries that supply the thymic cortex. This barrier prevents circulating foreign antigens from entering the cortex.

A feature of the equine thymus is the presence of prominent lymphatic vessels full of lymphocytes. These are efferent lymphatics through which the newly produced T cells reach the secondary lymphoid organs and the bloodstream. The thymus also contains high endothelial venules that become obvious after 9 months of age.

Function

The neonatal thymus is the source of T cells. T-cell precursors originate in the fetal bone marrow and then enter the thymus. Once within the thymus, these newly arrived thymocytes divide rapidly. Of the new cells produced, most soon die by apoptosis, whereas the survivors, 5%–25%, remain in the thymus for 4–5 days before leaving and colonizing the secondary lymphoid organs.

T cells that enter the thymus have two conflicting tasks. They must recognize foreign antigens, but at the same time, must not respond to normal body constituents. A two-stage selection process in the thymic medulla accomplishes this feat. Thus, T cells with receptors that bind self-antigens strongly and that could therefore cause autoimmunity undergo death by apoptosis. Likewise, T cells with receptors that cannot bind any major histocompatibility complex (MHC) class II molecules and are thus unable to react to any processed foreign antigens are also killed. The T cells that survive this "negative selection" process can still recognize specific MHC class II–antigen complexes with moderate affinity and are therefore stimulated to grow and mature—a process called positive selection. These selected T cells eventually leave the thymus, circulate in the bloodstream, and subsequently colonize the secondary lymphoid organs.

Thymic nurse cells are very large epithelial cells located within the thymic cortex that may contain up to 50 thymocytes within specialized cytoplasmic vesicles. It is unclear just what their function is, but the intracellular environment may be a site for positive thymocyte selection (Contreiras et al., 2004; Hendrix et al., 2010).

The autoimmune regulator (AIRE)

Medullary thymic epithelial cells (mTECs) are unique since they collectively express thousands of protein-coding genes. In addition, these cells have a very high level of autophagy. As a result, they present developing T cells with an enormous diversity of normal cellular proteins. Thymic epithelial cells and dendritic cells within the medulla use a unique transcription factor called the autoimmune regulator (AIRE). Equine AIRE is a protein of 564 amino acids (59.2 KDa) containing 584 amino acids encoded on chromosome ECA26. It binds to histones and regulates gene transcription in such a way that a huge diversity of self-proteins can be expressed by a single mTEC. Thus AIRE effectively promotes promiscuous gene transcription. As a result, mTECs can collectively present the developing T cells with many of the normal proteins that they are likely to encounter when they leave the thymus and circulate through the body. In this way, the mTECs ensure that self-reactive T cells are exposed to diverse normal tissue antigens and, as a result, most self-reactive cells are eliminated. This system ensures that T cells leaving the thymus cannot recognize or respond to most normal body components.

Other functions

The equine thymus has other functions in addition to selecting T cells. For example, it contains large numbers of eosinophils. These eosinophils are mainly found in the perivascular spaces and within the cortex (Figs. 8.3). Eosinophilopoiesis is very active in this organ until the horse reaches about 30 months of age. Their numbers then decline progressively (Contreiras et al., 2004). (It is suggested that they are attracted by interleukin-5 produced within the thymus. Alternatively, it has been suggested that their presence may be a consequence of an infestation with the nematode parasite *Strongyloides* spp. (Katkiewicz & Zajac, 2008). Mature eosinophils are obvious in the medulla surrounding the Hassall's corpuscles. Mast cells are also prominent in the thymic cortex. Plasma cells are very obvious in the involuting organ, often located close to eosinophils and mast cells. Erythropoietic foci can also be found within the thymus of horses up to 9 years of age.

Secondary lymphoid organs

In contrast to the bone marrow and thymus, the secondary lymphoid organs of the horse arise late in fetal life and persist in adults. Examples of secondary lymphoid organs include the spleen, the lymph nodes, and the tonsils, as well as lymphoid aggregates in the intestinal, respiratory, and urogenital tracts. These organs contain dendritic cells that trap and process antigens and lymphocytes that mediate the immune responses. The structure and location of these organs facilitate antigen trapping and provide an optimal environment for the initiation of immune responses. Secondary lymphoid organs are connected to both the blood and lymphoid systems, thus allowing them to encounter and respond to any circulating antigens.

Lymph nodes

Structure

Unlike other mammals with large single lymph nodes, horses and donkeys employ lymphocenters; clusters of small lymph nodes, 1–20 mm in size (Fig. 8.4).

For example, the axillary lymphocenter contains 12–20 lymph nodes; the cubital lymphocenter contains 5–20 nodes, while the popliteal lymphocenter contains 3–12 nodes (Khalil et al., 2022; Sisson & Grossman, 1953). As a result, it has been estimated that horses possess a total of about 8000 lymph nodes. Thousands of these small nodes filter lymph from the intestine, especially the cecum and colon (Kainer & McCracken, 1998) (Fig. 8.5).

Lymph nodes are round bean-shaped filters placed on lymphatic vessels in such a way that they can trap antigens carried in the lymph. Each node is surrounded by a capsule beneath which is a reticular network filled with lymphocytes, macrophages, and dendritic cells, and through which lymphatic sinuses penetrate. A subcapsular sinus is located immediately under the connective tissue capsule. Other sinuses pass through the body of the node but are most prominent in the medulla. The sinus network appears to be much more extensive in equine lymph nodes than in other mammals. Afferent lymphatics enter each node around its circumference, and efferent lymphatics leave from a depression or hilus on one side. The blood vessels supplying a lymph node also enter and leave through the hilus (Fig. 8.6).

The interior of lymph nodes is divided into a peripheral cortex and a central medulla, separated by a paracortex. B cells predominate in the cortex, where they are arranged in lymphoid follicles. In lymph nodes that have been stimulated by an antigen, some of these follicles form germinal centers. Germinal centers are round, ovoid clusters of cells divided into a light and dark zone. Germinal centers develop when a few antigen-specific B cells enter a follicle and then divide rapidly to become the centroblasts - these form the dark zone. This is the site where B cells proliferate and undergo somatic mutation. The centroblasts eventually produce non-dividing lymphocytes that migrate to the light zone. The light zone is the site where

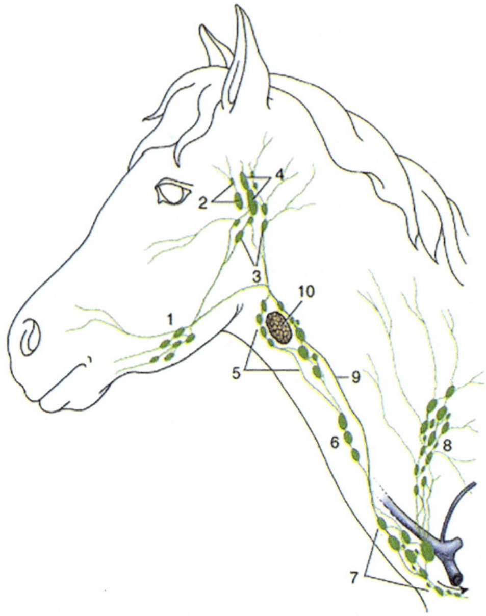

FIGURE 8.4 The lymphatic structures of the head and neck of a horse.

(1) Mandibular lymph nodes; (2) Parotid lymph nodes; (3) Medial retropharyngeal lymph nodes; (4) Lateral retropharyngeal lymph nodes; (5–7) Cranial, middle and caudal deep cervical lymph nodes; (8) Superficial cervical lymph nodes; (9) Tracheal duct; (10) Thyroid gland.

- With permission Dyce et al. (2009).

immunoglobulin class-switching and memory B cell formation occur. Light zones are rich in antigen-trapping follicular dendritic cells (fDCs) and CD4$^+$ T cells.

T cells and dendritic cells predominate in the paracortex. The cells are arranged in cords between the lymphatic sinuses. At the center of each paracortical cord is a high endothelial venule (HEV). These vessels are lined with tall, rounded endothelial cells quite unlike the flattened endothelium found in conventional blood vessels. HEVs are surrounded by concentric layers of fibroblastic reticular cells and a narrow space called the perivenular channel. The lymph node medulla contains lymphatic sinuses separated by medullary cords containing many plasma cells, macrophages, and memory T cells. Secondary lymphoid nodules are often present in the outer cortex and surrounded by a network of lymph sinuses (Heath & Nikles, 1991).

Lymph nodes are very busy organs with cells migrating in and out in response to a multitude of chemical signals. These signals are delivered through the reticular fibers that provide the structural scaffolding of the lymph node. These fibers are hollow and serve as conduits for the rapid transmission of signaling molecules. The

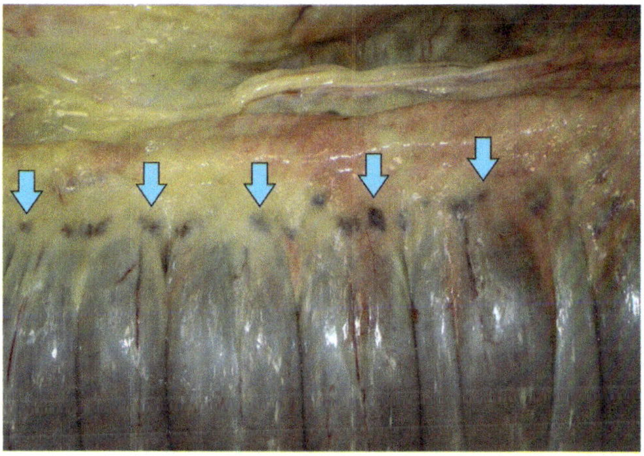

FIGURE 8.5

A chain of multiple small lymph nodes (Arrows) filter the lymph draining the equine colon.

- Courtesy of Dr Laura Bryan.

conduits consist of bundles of collagen fibers ensheathed by fibroreticular cells (Roozendaal et al., 2009). The fibroreticular cell wall is not continuous, so that dendritic cells can insert their dendrites through the gaps and sample the antigens within the lymphatic fluid. The conduits provide for the rapid delivery of soluble antigens from the afferent lymph to the lumen of HEVs and enable these antigens to reach deep into a node (Harwood & Batista, 2009).

Afferent lymphatics enter lymph nodes either into the subcapsular sinus or directly into sinuses deep within the node (Heath & Perkins, 1989). They connect with these sinuses through oval or round holes. Efferent lymphatics receive the lymph from the medulla through multiple holes. They are supported by luminal strands that prevent the sinuses from collapsing when the lymph nodes swell.

Function

Lymph nodes act as filters that trap antigens and facilitate the interactions between antigen-presenting cells and antigen-sensitive T and B cells. Each cell must be guided to its appropriate contacts with great precision. A complex mixture of chemokines directs these cells. Thus, chemokines drive the emigration of lymphocytes from HEVs into the lymph node. Dendritic cells, once they encounter and orocess an antigen, are also guided into lymph nodes by chemokines. For example, dendritic cells are attracted to the paracortex, where they present their processed antigens to T cells.

Lymph nodes also contain innate lymphoid cells that are located close to the macrophages lining the lymphatic sinuses. They are thus exposed to IL-18 released when the macrophages encounter invaders. The activated innate lymphocytes, in

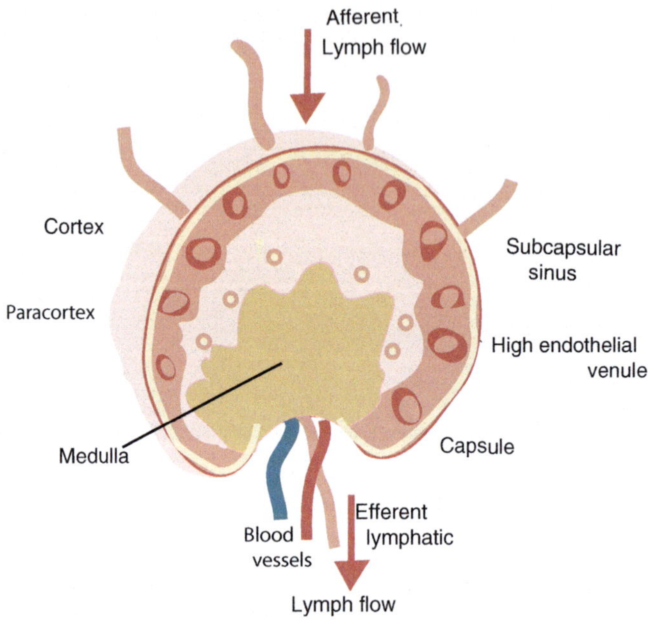

FIGURE 8.6 The structure of an equine lymph node.

These are found in linked clusters called lymphocenters.

turn, rapidly increase IFN-γ secretion that activates the macrophages still further and enhances their phagocytic and antimicrobial activities.

Both B and T cells are highly active and motile. The T cells in the paracortex and the B cells in the cortex are guided by follicular dendritic cells. Chemokines control the relocation and recirculation of lymphocytes and ensure that they end up in the right place. For example, T cells are attracted to the perifollicular area of the cortex. B cells, on the other hand, are attracted to the interior of germinal centers. When T cells are activated, they too may enter germinal centers where they "help" B cells respond to antigens. Other secondary lymphoid organs employ different homing receptors. For example, mucosal addressin cell adhesion molecule-1 (MAdCAM-1) is a homing receptor restricted to blood vessels within Peyer's patches and in the mesenteric lymph nodes of horses. Lymphocytes that recirculate to the intestine express high levels of the MAdCAM 1 ligand.

Soluble antigens entering the node through its afferent lymphatics first pass into the subcapsular sinus. From there, they enter the conduit network and are carried into the cortex. Antigenic particles such as bacteria, are captured by macrophages within the subcapsular sinus. These macrophages carry the bacterial antigens through the sinus floor and directly present them to B cells in the underlying follicles. The B cells then migrate to the T cell-B cell boundary, where they receive specific T cell help. B cells can also enter the paracortex directly from HEVs. There is also a specialized population of follicular dendritic cells clustered around these blood vessels so that immigrating B cells can survey any antigens they may be carrying. This is also a perfect location to receive T cell help.

When bacteria invade tissues, the resident dendritic cells are activated and migrate to the draining lymph nodes, where they accumulate in the paracortex and cortex. These dendritic cells form a web through which antigens must pass. Captured antigens are presented by the dendritic cells to T cells. T cells are initially activated in the paracortex, whereas the B cells remain randomly dispersed in the primary follicles. Both cell populations then migrate to the edges of the follicles, where they interact. Once antibody production is initiated, the progeny of these B cells move to the medulla and begin to secrete antibodies. Some of these antibody-producing cells escape into the efferent lymph and colonize downstream lymph nodes and the bone marrow. Several days after antibody production is first observed in the medulla, germinal centers appear in the cortex.

Adherence to follicular dendritic cells is the predominant means of antigen trapping once an animal has been sensitized by previous exposure to an antigen. In a secondary response, the germinal centers become less obvious as activated memory cells emigrate into the efferent lymph. Once this stage is completed, the germinal centers redevelop.

Several thousand small lymph nodes filter the lymph that drains from the equine gastrointestinal tract (Figs. 8.4). Afferent lymphatic vessels branch before entering the nodes and then connect to an extensive network of subcapsular and trabecular sinuses. This network of sinuses can accommodate major changes in lymph flow originating in the intestinal wall (Nikles & Heath, 1992).

Lymphocyte circulation

Lymphocytes, especially T cells, are highly mobile. They migrate from the bone marrow to the thymus and secondary lymphoid organs; they circulate around the body in blood and lymph and move from lymphoid organs to sites of microbial invasion. T cells constantly circulate and are the predominant lymphocytes in equine blood. As they travel, they survey the body for foreign antigens and preferentially home to sites of microbial invasion and inflammation.

Circulating T cells leave the bloodstream by two routes. T cells that have not previously encountered antigens ("naïve" T cells) bind to HEVs in lymph nodes. The high endothelial cells in these vessels are not joined by tight junctions but are linked by discontinuous "spot-welded" junctions. This means that lymphocytes can easily migrate between the high endothelial cells. Circulating lymphocytes can adhere to these high endothelial cells and then migrate into the paracortex. The emigration of lymphocytes from HEVs resembles that of neutrophils in inflamed blood vessels. Thus, the cells initially roll along the endothelial surface, binding to selectins. As they roll, they become activated and express integrins. As a result, they decelerate, stop, and then emigrate. The number and length of HEVs are variable and controlled by local immune activity. Thus, stimulation of a lymph node by the presence of antigens results in a rapid increase in the length of its HEVs. If, however, a lymph node is protected from antigens, its HEVs shorten.

In contrast to naïve T cells, memory T cells leave the bloodstream through conventional blood vessels in tissues and are then carried to lymph nodes through afferent lymphatics. They leave the lymph nodes through the efferent lymphatics. These efferent lymphatics eventually join together to form large lymph vessels. The largest of these lymph vessels is the thoracic duct, which drains the lymph from the lower body and the intestine and empties it into the anterior vena cava. The tributaries of the thoracic duct include two lumbar trunks that drain the lumbar glands and the intestinal trunks and then connect through a dilated sac, the cisterna chyli. The head, neck, and thorax of the horse (and donkey) are drained by the right lymphatic duct. It is possible to map the regions (lymphosomes) drained by each lymph node based on the tracing of injected colored dyes. Thus, the lymphatic vessels draining a specific region of the body all converge on the same cluster of regional lymph nodes.

Spleen

The spleen of the horse has the largest blood storage capacity among mammals. It has been estimated that it can store between 6 and 12 L of blood at rest (Freeman et al., 2022). This stored blood is estimated to occupy 66% of the splenic volume in the horse (Roriz et al., 2013).

The spleen is the largest secondary lymphoid organ in the horse. It is located in the anterior left side of the abdominal cavity between the stomach and the rib cage. The body of the spleen is attached to the stomach by the splenic ligament. Accessory spleens are rarely encountered in the horse. The horse spleen is of the non-sinusal type and thus can store a large amount of blood for quick release in emergencies (Udroiu, 2006). These emergencies include intense exercise such as racing or escaping from predators. The spleen can contract rapidly under the influence of the sympathetic nervous system acting through the splenic nerve (Udroiu, 2017). It is therefore classified as a storage spleen. Storage spleens are found in perissodactyls and carnivores. Both require a reserve of red cells to be readily available while escaping or hunting. They have a thick muscular outer capsule with many well-developed trabecule made of smooth muscle penetrating the splenic parenchyma. This smooth muscle may contract the spleen so that, if necessary, it can provide the horse with a significantly increased blood supply. A useful feature when galloping at high speed.

A thick splenic capsule and trabecule rich in smooth muscle cells are therefore a feature of equids - horses and donkeys. The capsule is bilayered, with the inner layer and the trabecule composed of elastic fibers and smooth muscle cells. In these species, the trabecule can constitute as much as 25% of the splenic volume, and these are very much storage spleens. Within the capsule is contained the splenic red and white pulp (Fig. 8.7).

The capsule consists of elastic tissue fibers with abundant smooth muscle cells that take up about two-thirds of the thickness of the capsule. There are many thick trabecule that are also rich in smooth muscle fibers. It contains a few elastic fibers (Udroiu & Sgura, 2017).

The white pulp

The spleen can be considered a specialized filter for blood-borne antigens. The filtering process removes particles such as microorganisms, cellular debris, and aged blood cells. This filtering function, together with highly organized lymphoid tissue, makes the spleen an important component of the mammalian immune defenses (Figs. 8.6).

Arteries entering the spleen pass through the muscular trabecule before entering the white pulp and branching into arterioles. Immediately on leaving the trabecule, each arteriole is surrounded by a periarteriolar lymphoid sheath. The central arteriole eventually leaves this sheath and branches into penicillary arterioles (Fig. 8.8).

The white pulp is abundant (although less prominent than in humans), and sinusoids are obvious within the marginal zone. The stroma is formed by reticular fibers. The white pulp contains both B and T cells, which accumulate in their specific zones under the influence of chemokines. They aggregate around the splenic arterioles to form the periarteriolar lymphoid sheaths that consist largely of T cells. Within these sheaths, the T cells interact with dendritic cells and passing B cells. The B cell areas, in contrast, consist of round primary follicles scattered through the sheaths. These follicles are sites where germinal center formation, clonal expansion, isotype switching, and somatic hypermutation occur.

The white pulp is separated from the red pulp by a marginal sinus, a reticulum sheath, and a marginal zone of cells. This marginal zone is an important transit

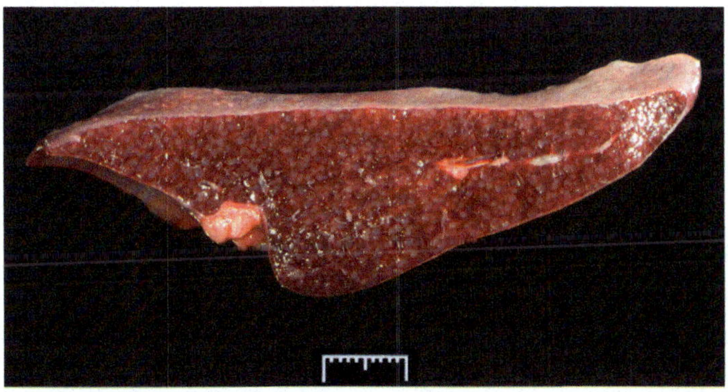

FIGURE 8.7 A cross-section of a foal spleen.

Notice the numerous pale follicles that constitute the white pulp as well as the obvious capsule.

- Courtesy of Dr Brian Porter.

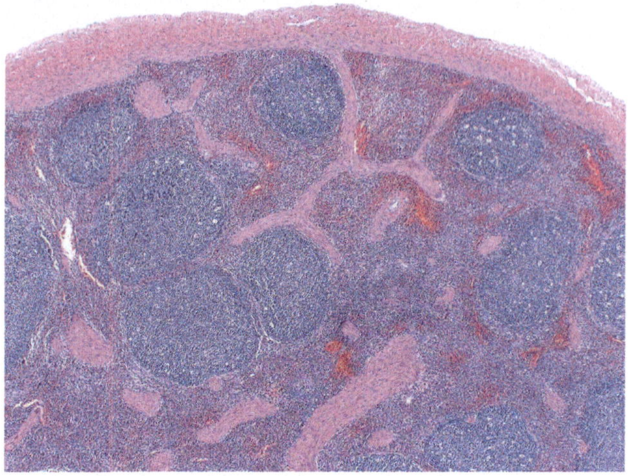

FIGURE 8.8 A section of a normal horse foal spleen.

Note the thick muscular capsule and trabecule. The nuclei of the lymphoid cells in the white pulp are very obvious in this young animal. Original magnification ×4.

- Courtesy of Dr Brian Porter.

area for leukocytes moving between the blood and the white pulp. It is also rich in macrophages, dendritic cells, and B cells. Most of the blood that enters the spleen flows into the marginal sinus and through the marginal zone before returning to the circulation through venous sinuses. This flow pattern ensures that these antigen-presenting cells can capture any blood-borne antigens and deliver them to the B cells in the marginal zone. The white pulp is involved in adaptive immune responses, whereas cells of the marginal zone can participate in both innate and adaptive responses. Splenic white pulp does not contain HEVs. Instead, lymphocytes enter the white pulp through the marginal zone, although the route by which they leave is unclear.

While the spleen is an important lymphoid organ, as pointed out in the previous chapter, however, horses employ pulmonary intravascular macrophages to capture a much larger proportion of blood-borne foreign particulates in their lungs.

The red pulp

In addition to its immune functions, the spleen also stores red cells and platelets. It recycles iron and undertakes red cell production in the fetus. Macrophages in the red pulp specialize in removing aged red blood cells and so regulate iron recycling.

The red pulp consists of a three-dimensional mesh of venous sinuses and splenic cords that occupies about two-thirds of the spleen volume (Roriz et al., 2013). The cords contain large numbers of lymphocytes, macrophages, plasma cells, and erythrocytes (Udroiu, 2017). The red pulp and marginal zone of the spleen contain

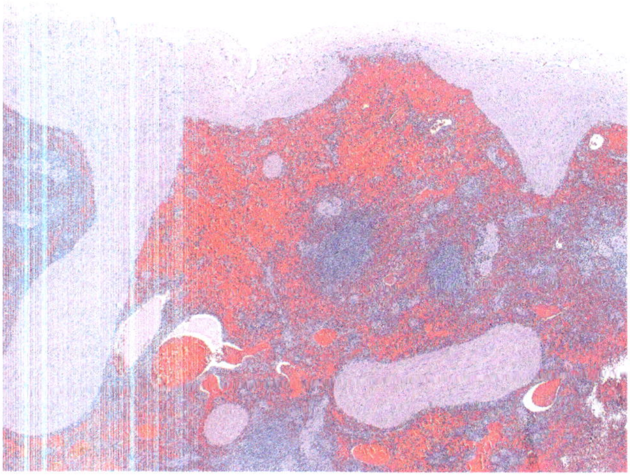

FIGURE 8.9 A section of the spleen from a miniature donkey.

Note the thick muscular capsule at the top. The red pulp is more obvious in this adult animal when compared to the horse foal spleen in the previous figure. Original magnification ×4.

- Courtesy of Dr. Brian Porter.

ellipsoids and penicillary arteries. The arterial capillaries open directly into these venous sinusoids. This is a similar pattern to that observed in the human spleen. Ellipsoids are found in both the marginal zone and red pulp. They are spherical or elliptical structures surrounded by two or three sinuses. These specialized capillary segments surround the penicillary arteries within the red pulp. They contain macrophages and serve as highly efficient filters. Thus, they can capture particles such as fat droplets, bacteria, and immune complexes (Sorby et al., 2005). Heavy granular deposits of the breakdown product, hemosiderin may be present in the spleens of old horses. The structure of the donkey spleen is very similar to that of the horse (Fig. 8.9).

The respiratory tract

Because of its large size and the volume of air that passes through the airways with every breath (100,00L/24 hours), the horse may be considered more vulnerable to inhaled respiratory pathogens than smaller, slower mammals. Especially when stabled, it is constantly exposed to airborne particles that are trapped in the nasal mucus and then carried into the oropharynx by ciliary action. Histology shows that lymphocytes are present in the respiratory lamina propria from the nasal cavity to small bronchioles, under 5 mm in diameter. There are also isolated lymphoid patches, some with follicles associated with these bronchioles. Their abundance varies between individual horses, possibly reflecting their level of exposure to inhaled antigenic particles. Lymphoid follicles are dispersed within the mucosae of the nasal tract, the nasopharynx, and close to the auditory meatus. Laryngeal and tracheal lymphoid tissues are also present. All these lymphoid sites contain both primary and secondary follicles, separated by a parafollicular area and covered by a dome epithelium (Mair et al., 1987).

Bronchus-associated lymphoid tissue (BALT) is not present before birth in the foal. Surveys have shown that BALT is present in less than half of the horses surveyed. It has been suggested that species like horses with a well-developed lymphoid tissues in their pharynx and larynx have less need for bronchial lymphoid tissues. This, of course, probably depends upon the cleanliness of the inhaled air. Air from a dusty stable is very different from the air in an open pasture. When BALT does develop, it is located in bronchioles at bifurcations, where inhaled material is most likely to impact the epithelium (Liebler-Torino and Pabst, 2006) (Figs. 8.5).

The tonsils

The horse has a set of well-developed lymphoid tonsils that surround its pharyngeal region. They are collectively known as Waldeyer's ring and serve to trap inhaled and ingested pathogens.

Thus, there is a lingual tonsil located at the root of the tongue. There is also a prominent tonsil located on the oral side of the soft palate. This palatine tonsil consists of a central crypt surrounded by primary and secondary lymphoid follicles and interfollicular lymphoid tissue (Casteleyn et al., 2011) (Fig. 8.10).The palatine tonsil extends from the base of the tongue to the base of the epiglottis and laterally to the glossoepiglottal fold. Its epithelial cover forms crypts and is heavily infiltrated with lymphocytes. Langerhans cells are interspersed between the epithelial cells. Compared to the lingual tonsil, $CD4^+$ T cells are more numerous, whereas $CD8^+$ cells are less numerous. B cells and macrophages are also present in large numbers. M cells are not present in the epithelium. HEVs are also present within these tonsils (Kumar & Timoney, 2005).

M cells are specialized antigen-trapping epithelial cells that possess multiple short microfolds on their apical surface. They provide a route by which antigens can be passed from their apical surface to the basal surface and subsequently presented to lymphocytes and macrophages.

Horses also have two nasopharyngeal tonsils in the dorsal nasopharynx at the end of the nasal septum. These are not well defined and difficult to see macroscopically. As in other species, there are also diffuse lymphoid tissues and isolated follicles located around the opening of the auditory tube – the tubal tonsils. These are continuous with the nasopharyngeal tonsils. The follicle-associated epithelium overlying these tonsils contains M cells. The central follicular areas are composed largely of B cells, but the dome and parafollicular areas contain both $CD4^+$ and $CD8^+$ T cells (Kumar et al., 2001). The nasopharyngeal tonsils are especially important in the horse since they are strategically located at the entrance to both the respiratory

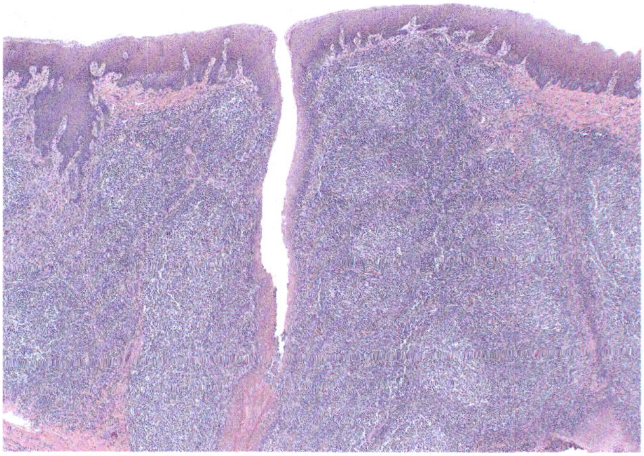

FIGURE 8.10 A section of an equine palatine tonsil.

Note the obvious tonsilar crypt and the absence of a protective epithelial cell layer at its base. This is a site that is vulnerable to microbial invasion. Original magnification ×4.

- Courtesy of Dr Brian Porter.

and digestive tracts. Follicle-associated epithelium overlies the lymphoid tissues of the nasopharyngeal tonsil caudal to the pharyngeal opening of the guttural pouch. This epithelium also contains a population of M cells. $CD4^+$ lymphocytes are scattered throughout the lamina propria, and they also form subepithelial dense aggregates. The central area of the tonsil is rich in B cells, while the dome and parafollicular areas contain both $CD4^-$ and CD8-positive T cells. CD8-positive cells are also present within the epithelium (Kumar et al., 2001).

The digestive tract

Lymphocytes are present in large numbers in the walls of the gastrointestinal tract. They are located within the epithelial cell layer (intraepithelial lymphocytes) as well as within the lamina propria. They include both B and T cells as well as plasma cells. However, large numbers are also present within the organized lymphoid tissues of the intestinal wall.

Peyer's patches

The small intestine

Peyer's patches are present in both the jejunum and ileum. These structures develop during gestation, and 245–320 Peyer's patches have been counted in the jejunum of the newborn foal. Many disappear as the animal ages, and their numbers drop to 100–200 in adult horses. In the terminal ileum of the newborn foal, however, there is a large aggregated lymphoid patch. It persists and increases in size until sexual maturity, but eventually disappears in older horses (Liebler-Torino & Pabst, 2006).

Peyer's patches (PPs) are located in the walls of the small intestine. They fom round or oval raised plaques in the duodenum and jejunum but elongate toward the ileum and vary in size from 2 × 10 to 36 × 14 mm. They are randomly distributed along the small intestine. Those in the terminal ileum merge to form a single, very large ileal PP about 25–35 cm long that forms a continuous structure that extends forward from the ileocecal junction. It is about 10 mm wide at the anterior end but widens until it involves the full circumference of the ileum at the ileocecal junction. Within these lymphoid patches, there is some structural diversity. Thus, they can form follicle/dome structures, or they can consist of follicles within the lamina propria, or they can form lymphoglandular complexes.

In the PPs that consist of follicles and domes, the follicles are located in the submucosa and penetrate the muscularis mucosae, where they are covered by the dome epithelium (Lowden & Heath, 1995). Isolated follicles may be present in the submucosa lamina propria. In the lymphoglandular complexes, the follicles are present in the submucosa and are associated with an epithelial invagination that extends through the muscularis mucosa. The follicle-associated epithelium consists of enterocytes, M cells, and an embedded population of intraepithelial lymphocytes and goblet cells (Fig. 8.11).

The lymphoid follicles consist of germinal centers, each consisting of densely packed small lymphocytes. Each germinal center has a central light zone and a basal dark zone. The light zone contains lymphoblasts, reticulum cells, and macrophages. The dark zone consists of lymphocytes and lymphoblasts. The jejunal PPs are similar in structure to the duodenal PPs, although their lymphoid nodules are more elongated. The duodenal PPs also have invaginations in the dome epithelium that are absent from the jejunal patches (Pabst et al., 2005). These extend into the submucosa, where they are surrounded by solitary lymphoid nodules. While surrounded by IgA^+ plasma cells, there are very few of these cells within the germinal centers themselves. T cells are largely restricted to the interfollicular areas and the corona immediately covering the follicles.

The large aggregated ileal PP has small, elongated domes and poorly developed interfollicular areas separating very large follicles. Their coronas are thinner and less obvious. The domes of only a few follicles extend into the mucosa. T cells are present in the corona, the interfollicular areas, with fewer in the domes and the germinal centers. The ileal PPs contain fewer T cells than the jejunal PPs.

The large intestine

In the equine large intestine, multiple lymphoid follicles are distributed from the cecum to the rectum. Their concentration is greatest in the cecum. They may form a circular accumulation at the cecal apex. In the pelvic flexure, and along

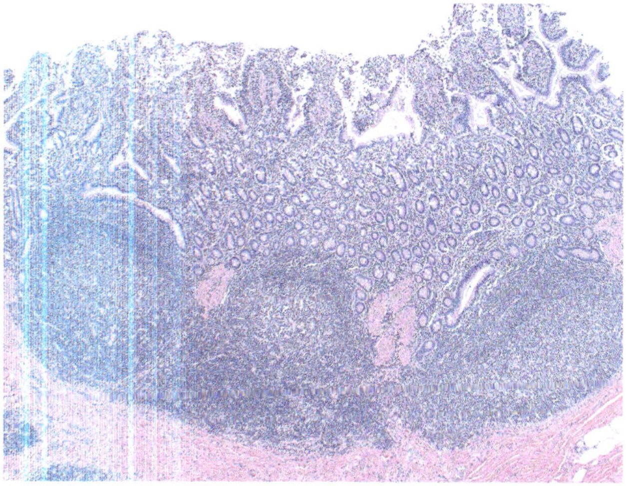

FIGURE 8.11 The submucosal lymphoid tissue in a horse intestinal wall.

Note the multiple submucosal lymphoid follicles, with germinal centers. Original magnification ×4.

- Courtesy of Dr Brian Porter.

the anal ring. It has been calculated that on average, the cecum in young horses contains about 25,000 lymphoid follicles (Liebler-Torino & Pabst, 2006).

Lymphoglandular complexes

Lymphoglandular complexes are also present in the wall of the equine large intestine and cecum. These consist of submucosal masses of lymphoid tissue penetrated by radially branching extensions of mucosal glands. These glands penetrate both the submucosa and the lymphoid nodule. They are lined by intestinal columnar epithelium containing goblet cells, intraepithelial lymphocytes, and M cells. Their function is unknown, but they contain many plasma cells, suggesting that they are sites of antibody production.

Other secondary lymphoid organs

Secondary lymphoid organs of the horse include not only the spleen, tonsils, and lymph nodes but also the bone marrow and lymphoid tissues scattered throughout the body, most notably in the digestive, respiratory, and urogenital tracts. The lymphoid tissues of the intestinal tract constitute the largest pool of lymphocytes in the body, but the bone marrow also contains very large numbers of lymphocytes. Fat-associated lymphoid clusters are small secondary lymphoid nodules within adipose tissues underlying serosal membranes such as the mesentery. Bronchus-associated lymphoid tissue in the form of bronchial lymphoid aggregates is found in the bronchial submucosa, in some horses. Apart from the nasopharyngeal tonsils, there are no organized lymphoid tissues within the equine nasal cavity. However, the nasal mucosa contains many isolated lymphoid cells, especially IgA-positive plasma cells.

References

Casteleyn, C., Breugelmans, S., Simoens, P., & Van den Broeck, W. (2011). The tonsils revisited: Review of the anatomical localization and histologic characterization of the tonsils of domestic and laboratory animals. *Journal of Immunology Research.* https://doi.org/10.1155/2011/472-460

Contreiras, E. C., Lenzi, H. L., Meirelles, M. N. L., Caputo, L. F. G., et al. (2004). The equine thymus microenvironment: A morphological and immunohistochemical analysis. *Developmental & Comparative Immunology, 28*, 251–264.

Freeman, K. P., Farr, A. J., & Barrelet, A. (2022). *Hematology of equids.* Wiley Blackwell (Chapter 10). Schalm's Veterinary Hematology. 7th ed.

Harwood, N. E., & Batista, F. D. (2009). The antigen expressway: Follicular conduits carry antigen to B cells. *Immunity, 30*, 177–179.

Heath, T. J., & Nikles, S. J. (1991). Relationship between lymphoid nodules and lymph sinuses in lymph nodes: A study in horses. *Journal of Anatomy, 178*, 39–43.

Heath, T. J., & Perkins, N. R. (1989). Pathways between lymph vessels and sinuses in lymph nodes: A study in horses. *The Anatomical Record, 223*, 420–424.

Hendrix, T. M., Chilukuri, R. V. E., Martinez, M., Olushoga, Z., et al. (2010). Thymic nurse cells exhibit epithelial progenitor phenotype and create unique extracytoplasmic membrane space for thymocyte selection. *Cellular Immunology, 261*(2), 81–92.

Kainer, R. A., & McCracken, T. O. (1998). *The coloring atlas of Horse Anatomy.* Dogwise Publishing.

Katkiewicz, M., & Zajac, S. (2008). Thymitis eosinophilica in clinically healthy horses from 2 months to 7 years of age. *Medycyna Weterynaryjna, 64*(8), 995–997.

Khalil, A. H., Sayed-Ahmed, A., Kandiel, M. M. M., Nasr, M. A., & Abd-Algalil, A. S. A. (2022). Ultrasonographic and gross anatomical characterization of superficial lymph nodes in donkey (*Equus asinus*). *Benha Veterinary Medical Journal, 42*, 128–133.

Kumar, P., & Timoney, J. F. (2005). Histology, immunohistochemistry and ultrastructure of the equine palatine tonsil. *Anatomia Histologia Embryologia, 34*, 192–198.

Kumar, P., Timoney, J. F., & Sheoran, A. S. (2001). M cells and associated lymphoid tissue of the equine nasopharyngeal tonsil. *Equine Veterinary Journal, 33*(3), 224–230.

Laan, M., Haljasorg, U., Kisand, K., Salumets, A., & Peterson, P. (2016). Pregnancy-induced thymic involution is associated with suppression of chemokines essential for T-lymphocyte progenitor homing. *European Journal of Immunology, 46*, 2008–2017.

Liebler-Torino, E., & Pabst, R. (2006). MALT structure and function in farm animals. *Veterinary Research, 37*(3), 257–280. https://doi.org/10.1051/vetres.2006001

Lowden, S., & Heath, T. (1995). Lymphoid tissues in the ileum of young horses: Distribution, structure and epithelium. *Anatomy and Embryology, 192*, 171–179.

MacKenzie, C. D. (1975). Histological development of the thymic and intestinal lymphoid tissue of the horse. *Journal of the South African Veterinary Association, 46*(1), 47–55.

Mair, T. S., Batten, E. H., Stokres, C. R., & Bourne, F. J. (1987). The histological features of the immune system of the equine respiratory tract. *Journal of Comparative Pathology, 97*, 575–586.

Nikles, S. A., & Heath, T. J. (1992). Pathways of lymph flow through intestinal lymph nodes in the horse. *The Anatomical Record, 232*, 126–132.

Pabst, O., Herbrand, H., Worbs, T., Feiedrichsen, M., et al. (2005). Cryptopatches and isolated lymphoid follicles. Dynamic lymphoid tissues dispensable for the generation of intraepithelial lymphocytes. *European Journal of Immunology, 35*, 98–107.

Roozendaal, R., Mempel, T. R., Pitcher, L. A., et al. (2009). Conduits mediate transport of low molecular weight antigen to lymph node follicles. *Immunity, 30*, 264–276.

Roriz, G. D., Barreto-Vianna, A. R. C., Leonardo, A. S., Castro, M. B., et al. (2013). Histomorpho quantitative characterization of spleen in horses. *Australian Journal of Basic and Applied Sciences, 7*(11), 83–86.

Sørby, R., Wein, T. N., Husby, G., Espenes, A., & Landsverk, T. (2005). Filter function and immune complex trapping in splenic ellipsoids. *Journal of Comparative Pathology, 132*, 313–321.

Sisson, S., & Grossman, J. D. (1953). *The anatomy of the domestic animals* (4ed.). Philadelphia: Saunders.

Udroiu, I. (2006). Evolution of sinusal and non-sinusal spleens of mammals. *Hystrix the Italian Journal of Mammalogy, 17*(2), 99–116.

Udroiu, I. (2017). Storage of blood in the mammalian spleen: An evolutionary perspective. *Journal of Mammalian Evolution, 24*, 243–260.

Udroiu, I., & Sgura, A. (2017). The phylogeny of the spleen. *The Quarterly Review of Biology, 92*(4), 411–443.

CHAPTER

9 ELA—The equine major histocompatibility complex

Resistance to infectious diseases is one of the most strongly inherited disease traits. After all, a lethal infection effectively removes susceptible individuals from the gene pool. "Survival of the fittest" applies most strongly to individuals that successfully defend themselves against microbial infections. As a result, many genes influence immunity and resistance to infection. The most important of these genes are those encoding the cell surface glycoproteins that constitute the major histocompatibility complex (MHC) and serve as antigen-presenting receptors that trigger adaptive immune responses.

Antigen processing

In order to trigger an adaptive immune response, antigen molecules must first be processed. They are phagocytosed, broken up inside cells such as dendritic cells, and the resulting fragments bound to appropriate cell-surface receptors. These receptors belong to a large family of glycoproteins encoded by genes clustered together to form the major histocompatibility complex (MHC). These receptors are therefore called MHC molecules. Antigens can only trigger an adaptive immune response after binding to MHC molecules. The MHC molecules present their attached antigens to helper T cell antigen receptors and, if they are recognized by the T cell, they trigger a response. Since MHC molecules act as antigen-presenting receptors, the genes encoding them effectively determine which antigens can be bound and so trigger adaptive immunity. Thus, the MHC can be considered a cluster of genes that control antigen presentation and, as a result, determine resistance or susceptibility to infectious diseases. The ability of pathogens to evade, escape, or subvert immune defenses has placed strong selection pressures on MHC genes and has resulted in their rapid evolution and unique diversity (Nei et al., 1997).

All mammals possess an MHC. Each MHC contains about 200 expressed genes divided into three classes (I, II, and III). Each class is clustered in its own genetic region. The class I region contains genes coding for MHC molecules expressed on most nucleated cells. Class I genes can be subdivided into those that are highly polymorphic (class Ia genes) and those that show very little polymorphism (class Ib genes). (Polymorphism refers to structural variations between proteins.) Some class I genes may also be located outside the MHC on a different chromosome. The genes in MHC class II regions encode polymorphic MHC molecules, usually restricted to

The Immunology of Horses and Donkeys. https://doi.org/10.1016/B978-0-443-44863-8.00002-8

the professional antigen-presenting cells such as dendritic cells, macrophages, and B cells. The genes located within the MHC class III region have a very different function. They encode diverse proteins, many of which are important in innate immunity, such as complement components and some cytokines. Although each mammalian MHC contains all three gene regions, their gene content and arrangements vary among species (Kumanovics et al., 2003) (Fig. 9.1).

MHC class I-bound antigens of intracellular origin, such as viral antigens, stimulate type 1 helper T cells and so trigger cell-mediated immune responses. Class II-bound antigens of extracellular origin, such as antigens from phagocytosed bacteria, stimulate type 2 helper T cells and so trigger antibody-mediated immune responses.

Every mammalian MHC contains class I, class II, and class III gene regions. When the MHCs of different mammals are compared, some regions, such as class III, are conserved, whereas others are highly diverse. In general, genes within the class II and class III regions possess obvious orthologs in all species. That is, they are clearly derived from a single mammalian ancestor and have not been subjected to major rearrangements during evolution. MHC class I genes, in contrast, have evolved so frequently and been reorganized many different times by deletions and duplications so that their amino acid sequences differ widely, and it is very difficult to compare class I genes between different species. They are said to be paralogous.

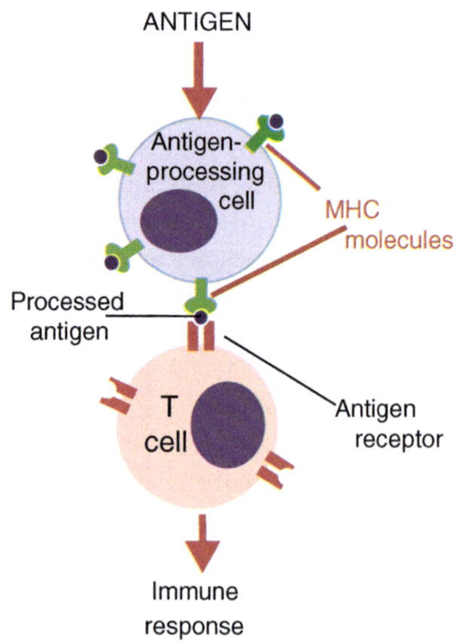

FIGURE 9.1 The key initial step in any immune response is the presentation of antigens by antigen-processing cells to antigen-sensitive cells.

This step is mediated by MHC molecules located on the surface of antigen-processing cells. The complex is recognized by the T cell antigen receptors.

The equine major histocompatibility complex

The collective name given to the proteins encoded by MHC genes depends on the species. In humans, these molecules are called human leukocyte antigens (HLA); in horses they are called equine leukocyte antigens (ELA), and in the donkey they are called, MHC-Eqas. The complete set of alleles found within an individual animal's MHC is called its MHC haplotype.

The overall structure of the equine MHC was first established by identifying and sequencing bacterial artificial chromosomes (Gustafson et al., 2003). The MHC complex is located on chromosome EAC20q14-22. The class I region is proximal to the centromere, the class II region is distal, and the class III region is located in between the class I and class II regions. Subsequent high-resolution genotyping has revealed the unique features of the ELA-MHC complex, including breed diversity and extreme polymorphism (Vasoya et al., 2023).

ELA class I molecules

ELA-MHC class I molecules are receptors for endogenous antigens such as viruses. As a result, they are expressed on most nucleated cells. In horses, for example, class I molecules can be detected on lymphocytes, platelets, granulocytes, hepatocytes, kidney cells, and sperm. They are not usually found on red cells, gametes, neurons, or trophoblast cells. Some cells, such as myocardial and skeletal muscle, may express very few class I molecules. Class I genes can be subdivided into highly polymorphic, "classical" (Class Ia) and nonpolymorphic "nonclassical" (Class Ib) genes. Their products differ in their tissue distribution and functions. The nonclassical class Ib genes have a similar structure to the class Ia genes. They may be truncated in their cytoplasmic domain at the 3′ end. They also tend to have restricted tissue distribution and bind a small number of specific ligands. Conversely, the function of the MHC class Ia molecules is to present an enormous diversity of processed endogenous antigenic peptides to Th1 helper cells and $CD8^+$ cytotoxic T cells. In addition, as described in the next chapter, they must interact with the cell surface receptors that control natural killer cell cytotoxic activities.

Structure

ELA class I molecules consist of paired glycoprotein chains (heterodimers). An α-chain (45 kDa) is attached to a much smaller invariant chain called β_2-microglobulin ($ß_2$M) (12 kDa). The α-chain is inserted into the cell membrane. It consists of five domains: three extracellular domains called α_1, α_2, and α_3, each about 100 amino acids long; a transmembrane domain; and two cytoplasmic domains. The antigen-binding site is formed by the folded α_1 and α_2 domains. The β_2M chain consists of a single domain and serves to stabilize the structure (Fig. 9.2).

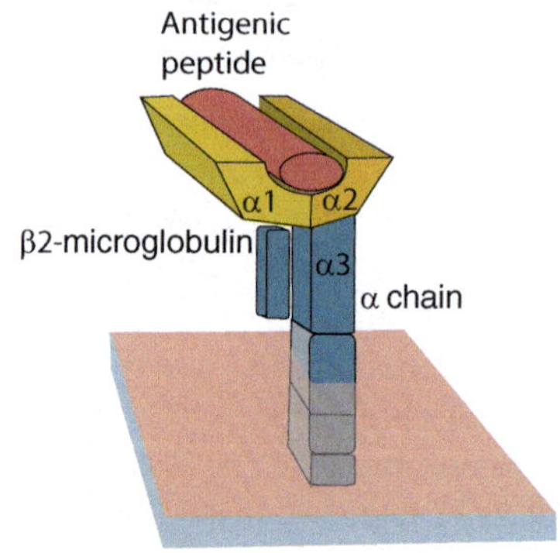

FIGURE 9.2 A schematic structure of a class Ia MHC molecule on a cell membrane.

Its antigen-binding site is formed by the folding of both its α_1 and α_2 domains. The β2M molecule serves to stabilize the structure.

The α_1 and α_2 domains of MHC class I molecules fold together to form an open-ended groove. A flat β sheet forms the floor of this groove, and its walls are formed by two α-helices. This groove can bind antigenic peptides that are 8–10 amino acids long. The variable sequences located along the walls of this groove determine its shape. The shape of the groove, in turn, determines which peptides can be bound and so used to trigger immune responses (Hulpke & Tampe, 2013) (Fig. 9.3).

A complete MHC class I gene thus consists of eight exons encoding a 5′ leader sequence, α1, α2, and α3 domain genes, a transmembrane domain, and two cytoplasmic domains at the 3′ end. It is approximately 4000 bases in length.

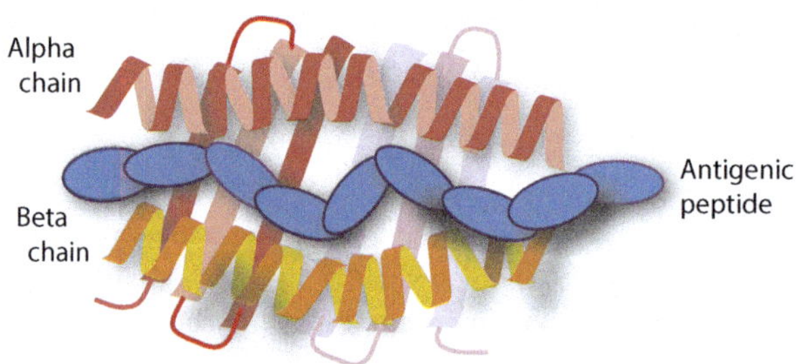

FIGURE 9.3 The MHC class II antigen binding site.

The arrangement of an antigenic peptide chain within the antigen binding site. The MHC class I site is very similar but uses two alpha chain domains. However they are closed at each end.

Gene arrangement

Fifteen different MHC class I genes have been identified in the horse class I region (Tallmadge et al., 2005). Of these, seven appear to be functional. The remaining eight appear to be pseudogenes (Janova et al., 2009).

The ELA class I region is subdivided into three sub-regions, A, B, and C. Region A is a small isolated region that begins at the *BTNL2* gene. Only two MHC class I genes are found within the A region. Region B is at the telomeric end of the class I region between *BAT1* and MIC, and six MHC class I genes are found in this region. Region C is located within the class I region between the *GNL1* and *TRIM26* genes and contains seven MHC class I genes. The nomenclature of these class I loci classifies them as ELA-A1, ELA-A2, etc, up to ELA-A19 (Fig. 9.4).

Most mammalian class I genes appear to have originated in three duplication blocks termed alpha, beta, and kappa, located within the class I region. Horse class I regions B and C generally correspond to the beta and kappa duplication blocks. The alpha block is located at the *BNTL2* end of the class II region, the beta block is located at the junction of the class III and I regions, while the kappa block is located between *GNL1* and *TRIM26* within the class I region. The horse beta block contains two putative nonclassical genes and four pseudogenes. In the horse kappa block, there are four classical genes, one putative nonclassical gene, and two pseudogenes. This isolated alpha block (A region) appears to be unique to the horse (Tallmadge et al., 2010).

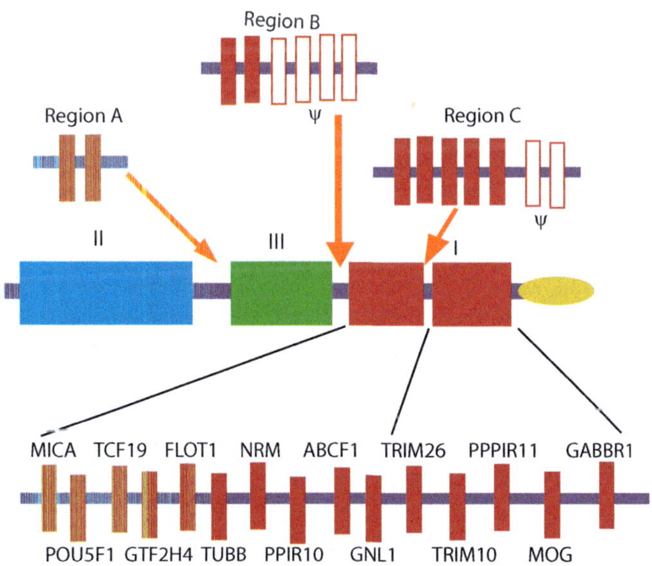

FIGURE 9.4 The arrangement of the equine MHC class I region.

ψ denotes a pseudogene.

- *Data from Tallmadge, R. L., Lear, T. L., & Antczak, D. F. (2005). Genomic characterization of MHC class I genes in the horse. Immunogenetics, 57, 763–774.*

Seven other genes located within the ELA class I region (*POU5F1, TCF19, GNL1, TRIM26, TRIM10, PP1R11*, and *MOG* are highly conserved framework genes. Within the framework scaffold are the duplication blocks (Gustafson et al., 2003).

Polymorphism

The MHC class I genes contain many diverse SNPs that are primarily concentrated in the exons encoding their antigen-binding sites. The number of expressed MHC class I loci varies between individual horse haplotypes. The use of high-resolution genotyping has identified 152 novel MHC class I sequences that collectively represent 86 novel MHC class I allelic groups. Sixty-nine MHC1 alleles have been identified in Thoroughbreds and 83 in Norwegian Fjord horses (Vasoya et al., 2023). This same study identified 33 different MHC class I haplotypes. All but two of the MHC1 haplotypes appeared to be novel. Of the 33 haplotypes, 5 exhibited sequence variation. Another feature of the Thoroughbreds tested was that the number of class I genes expressed ranged from 6 to 16. Many of these alleles were present at very low frequency (0.2%) (Vasoya et al., 2023).

Plasil et al. have identified the exon-2-exon3 alleles in three different horse breeds originating in different geographical regions (Plasil et al., 2023). They examined the class I genes Eqca-1, Eqca-2, Eqca-7, and Eqca-ψ. They found a total of 116 allelic variants, of which 112 were novel. Eqca-1 and -2 were highly polymorphic with 47 and 42 alleles, respectively. Eqca-7, a nonclassical class I locus, had 10 alleles. The pseudogene Eqca-ψ had 17 putative alleles.

The amino acid polymorphism in the MHC class I α_1 and α_2 domains results from variations in the nucleotide sequences between alleles. These sequence variations result from point mutations, reciprocal recombination, and gene conversion. Point mutations are simply changes in individual nucleotides. Reciprocal recombination involves crossing over between two chromosomes. In gene conversion, small blocks of DNA are exchanged between different class I genes in a non-reciprocal fashion. The donated DNA blocks may come from nearby non-polymorphic class I genes, from non-functional pseudogenes, or from other polymorphic class I genes. As a result of all this, class I MHC genes have the highest mutation rate and diversity of any germline genes yet studied. This high mutation rate implies that there must be significant advantages to be gained by having very polymorphic MHC genes and many diverse MHC antigen receptors.

Horses of different breeds have very different polymorphisms within their ELA complex. However, they do appear to share common genetic patterns, especially within the ELA class II region (Moravcikova et al., 2024). Analysis of horses of different haplotypes has identified three to five classical sequences and two to three nonclassical sequences in each homozygous horse. Together with heterozygous horses, they contain a total of 10 MHC haplotypes. However, the horse MHC is characterized by variations in the number of class I genes expressed in different haplotypes in addition to the allelic polymorphism within each locus (Tallmadge et al., 2010).

Another technique that has been successfully employed to characterize equine MHC haplotypes involves the detection of polymorphic microsatellites. Thus, using this technique, 23 microsatellites have been associated with 12 established equine ELA haplotypes in Standardbreds and Thoroughbreds (Tseng et al., 2010). The technique has also proved useful in examining haplotype diversity in Persian Arabian horses. The technique was able to identify 78 new MHC haplotypes in this breed (Sadeghi et al., 2018). In a similar study using polymorphic microsatellites, 79 unique ELA haplotypes were identified in a population of Icelandic horses. This is a breed that has remained isolated from other, introduced breeds for over a 1000 years (Holmes et al., 2019).

Non-polymorphic ELA class I molecules

Horse cells also express multiple non-polymorphic ELA class I molecules—class Ib molecules. Some are encoded by genes found within the MHC class I region, others by genes located on other chromosomes. These class Ib molecules show reduced expression and tissue distribution compared to class Ia molecules, but are part of the MHC complex. They have limited polymorphism, and they probably originated from class Ia precursors by duplication. These genes code for specific receptors expressed on the surface of regulatory and immature lymphocytes and on hematopoietic cells. They are also heterodimers consisting of a membrane-bound α-chain associated with β_2-microglobulin, so their overall shape and antigen-binding groove are similar to those in MHC class Ia molecules. Since they are not polymorphic, however, these MHC class Ib molecules bind only a limited range of ligands. For example, they act as pattern recognition receptors for commonly encountered microbial PAMPs.

ELA class Ic genes also have limited polymorphism and are found within the MHC. Their products include MICA and MICB,—specialized receptors that are involved in signaling to natural killer (NK) cells but do not bind antigenic peptides (Chapter 10).

Class Id genes are non-polymorphic class I-related genes not located on the MHC chromosome. Many of their products contribute to innate immunity since they also bind PAMPs. For example, CD1 molecules are antigen-presenting receptors that bind lipid antigens (Chapter 10). FcRn is the class Id MHC molecule that acts as an antibody (Fc) receptor on epithelial cells. It is expressed on mammary gland epithelium and the enterocytes of newborn foals (Chapter 2).

ELA class II molecules

The ELA-MHC class II region is about 1.2 mb in size. It contains 35 gene loci (Barbis et al., 1994) (Fig. 9.5).

ELA-MHC class II molecules play a key role in the presentation of processed exogenous antigens. Thus, they are usually only expressed on the professional antigen-processing cells (dendritic cells, macrophages, and B cells) but can be

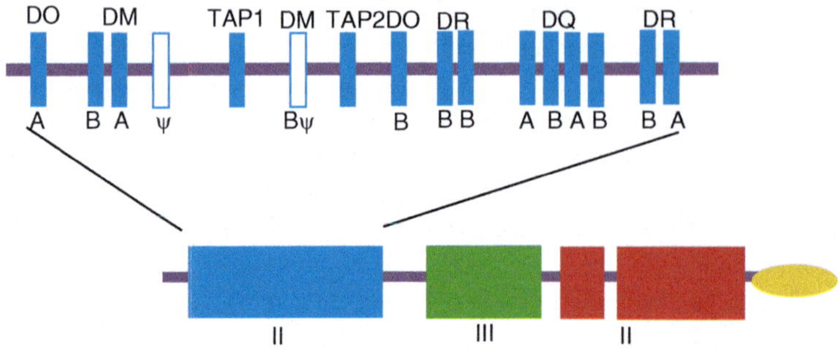

FIGURE 9.5 The arrangement of genes within the equine MHC class II region.

White rectangles are pseudogenes. A genes encode alpha chains whereas B genes encodee beta chains.

- Data from Tallmadge, R. L., Lear, T. L., & Antczak, D. F. (2005). Genomic characterization of MHC class I genes in the horse. Immunogenetics, 57, 763–774.

induced on T cells, keratinocytes, and vascular endothelial cells. In horses, MHC class II molecules are constitutively expressed on nearly all resting adult T cells. The expression of class II molecules is enhanced in rapidly dividing cells and cells treated with IFN-γ. The function of MHC class II proteins is to serve as receptors that present exogenous antigenic peptides to $CD4^+$ helper T cells. This, in turn, triggers a B cell response and antibody formation.

Structure

MHC class II molecules consist of paired peptide chains called α and β. Each chain has two extracellular domains (one constant and one variable), a connecting peptide, a transmembrane domain, and a cytoplasmic domain. A third chain, called the Ii or γ-chain, is required for the assembly of class II molecules within cells and is not expressed on the cell surface (Fig. 9.6).

MHC class II proteins have an antigen-binding groove formed by their α_1 and β_1 domains. Its walls are formed by two parallel α-helices, and its floor consists of a β-sheet. Gene polymorphism results in variations in the amino acids forming the walls of the groove. These variations are generated in the same way as in class Ia molecules. Other genes found within the ELA-MHC class II region code for molecules involved in antigen processing. These include the transporter proteins TAP1 and TAP2 and some proteasome components.

Gene arrangement

At the boundary between the ELA class I and class III regions, there is a large segmental duplication of about 710 kb (Brinkmeyer-Langford et al., 2010). It consists of 11 repeated blocks, 10 of which contain an MHC class I-like sequence and the helicase domain portion of a BAT-1-like sequence. The remaining 11th block contains a full-

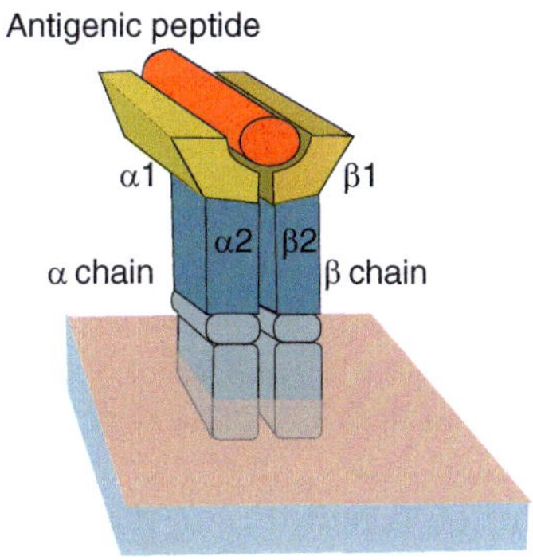

FIGURE 9.6 A schematic diagram showing the structure of an MHC class II heterodimeric receptor expressed on a cell surface.

Note that the antigen-binding site is formed by the variable domains from both α and β peptide chains.

length *BAT1* gene. (BAT-1 encodes an RNA-dependent ATPase that mediates ATP hydrolysis during pre-mRNA splicing.) A similar duplication is found in other Perissodactyls, including the donkey, zebra, and tapir, indicating that this duplication must be of ancient origin, probably originating between 20 and 55 mya. Its persistence and transcription of its open reading frames in equine leukocytes suggest that it is probably functionally important (Brinkmeyer-Langford et al., 2010).

When compared to the MHC class II region in other mammals, this region in horses shows extreme copy number variation, as well as different relative locations and directionality. In an analysis using long-read technology, Viluma et al. identified 23 functional genes m the ELA class II region in addition to 12 pseudogenes (Viluma et al., 2017). The classical MHC II molecules form three groups: DR, DQ, and DP. All three present antigens to T cells. Of the classical MHC class II genes in the ELA, there are six *DRB* loci, of which three are functional. There are also four pairs of *DQA-DQB* genes. The genes *DRB2, DRB3,* and *DQB3* have high sequence conservation (Klumplerova et al., 2020). In contrast, DRB*1* and *DQB1* are highly polymorphic. The nonclassical class II molecules, DO and DM, also have multiple genes. Of these, 20 have undisrupted open reading frames (Viluma et al., 2017) while four are functional: *DOA, DOB, DMA,* and *DMB*.

When comparing these genes to other mammals, significant differences emerge. In the horse, for example, the *DRB* genes are spread across a region spanning 0.7 mb, whereas in humans, mice, cats, pigs, and cattle, they are tightly clustered. In addition, all the other Laurasiatheria—dogs, cats, pigs, and bovines-have a single inverted *DRB* gene, but the horse has five of them. Note that this inverted *DRB* gene is not present in humans or mice. This suggests that the inversion event occurred ~80–100 mya following the separation of the Euarchontoglires but before the divergence of the Laurasiatherian species. This eventually evolved into a separate inverted *ELA-DRB* gene cluster containing both functional genes and pseudogenes (Viluma et al., 2017).

The expression of MHC class II antigens on horse lymphocytes is determined by their MHC haplotype (Barbis et al., 1994). Thus, horses with haplotype H3 have lower levels of MHC class II expression regardless of their age. (Foals also express less MHC class II on their T cells regardless of haplotype).

Polymorphism

As with the class I molecules, recent studies using high-resolution genotyping have altered our views of diversity in the ELA class II region (Vasoya et al., 2023). (In general, as more studies are conducted, more loci and alleles are identified.) Thus, the greatest reported number of identified class II loci is 6 for DRA, 3 for DRB, 2 for DQA, and 2 for DWB. Likewise, the greatest numbers of alleles identified by different investigators are 17 for DRA, 52 for DRB, 27 for DQA and 38 for DQB. These numbers differ greatly between horse breeds. For example, most of these novel alleles were primarily found in Norwegian Fjord horses (102 in Fjords versus 15 in Thoroughbreds). There appear to be at least 41 different MHC class II haplotypes. Eleven of the 41 haplotypes showed multiple sequence variants. In most of these class II haplotypes there were one DRA, two DQA, two DQB, and either two or three DRB loci (Vasoya et al., 2023).

Other studies have identified at least 17 *DRA* alleles, 14 *DRB* alleles, 27 *DQA* alleles, and more than 17 *DQB* alleles in equine class II (Brown et al., 2004; Fraser & Bailey, 1998). Plasil et al. (2023) also investigated these class II genes. They found that the DRA locus consisted of five exon 2 alleles. They also found 15 novel exon 2 alleles in the DQA1 locus.

An analysis of the class II DRB and DQB loci identified three DRB and two DQB loci in the genomes of all equids. The genes DRB2, DRB3, and DQB3 showed high sequence conservation within the species. Polymorphism was much more frequent in DRB1 and DQB1 (Klumplerova et al., 2020). DQB2 was not found in the genome of Asiatic asses (*E. homionus kulan* or *E. h. onager)*. Evidence of gene recombination was found in the DRB1, DRB2, DQB1, and DQB2 genes. Trans-species allele sharing was identified in all genes except DRB1. There was also evidence of positive selection occurring in both the DRB and DQB loci.

Janova et al. have also analyzed the polymorphism of the DRA and DQA genes in the Equidae. There had been 11 previously reported DRA alleles, and they found another 6 (total 17). In addition to 24 pervious DQA alleles, they found an additional 13 (total 37 alleles). Further analysis of the DQA loci has also identified an allele, DQA*1301, located in a second locus (Fraser & Bailey, 1998). This is located not within the ELA system but on chromosome ELA5.

Phylogenetic analysis has also shown evidence of trans-species polymorphisms among the Equidae. The DRA alleles are more often shared by more species. The DQA alleles show strong within-species positive selection (Janova et al., 2009). In another study examining the polymorphism of ELA DRA and DQA in the horse and the plains zebra (*E. quagga*). Kamath and Getz demonstrated a considerable degree of interspecific sharing of alleles. Thus, 3 of 6 DRA alleles examined were also present in the donkey (but none of the DQA alleles). They reported 22 nucleotide sequences and 10 protein sequences in exon 2 of DRA (Kamath & Getz, 2011).

MHC class III molecules

Most of the remaining genes located within the MHC are found in the class III region. This is located centrally between the class I and II regions at ECA20q16 (Deakin et al., 2006). Sequence analysis of the ELA class III region has identified the presence of *C2, Ly6G6c, APOM, RDBP, MSH5,* and *CYP21A2* genes in this region (Gustafson et al., 2003). The gene encoding TNF-α is also present in this region (Bubenikova et al., 2024) (Fig. 9.7).

MHC molecules and disease

Since the function of MHC molecules is to present antigens to the cells of the immune system, MHC genes regulate immune responses. A foreign molecule that cannot be bound to at least one MHC molecule cannot trigger an adaptive immune response. Thus, expression of specific MHC alleles determines resistance to many infectious and autoimmune diseases. Because class Ia and class II MHC molecules are structurally diverse, each MHC allele can bind and present different sets of antigenic peptides. The more diversity within an animal's MHC, the more antigens it can respond to. Thus, an MHC heterozygous animal will express many more alleles and can respond to a greater diversity of antigens than can a homozygous animal (Radwan et al., 2020).

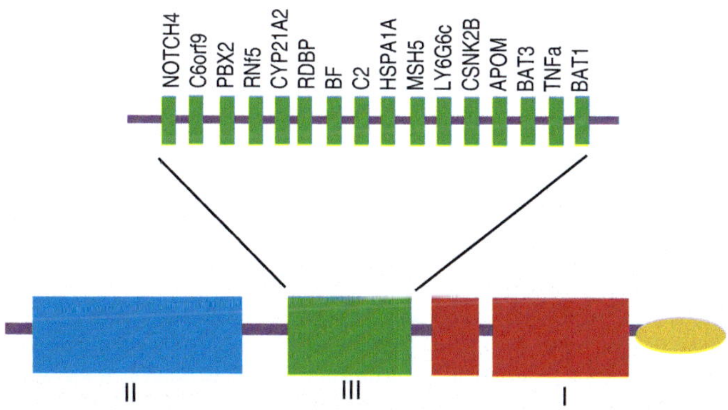

FIGURE 9.7 The arrangement of selected genes within the MHC class III region.

These genes all play a role in innate and adaptive immunity. There are many other genes within this region that have no apparent role in immunity.

- *Data from Gustafson, A. L., Tallmadge, R. L., Ramlachan, N., Miller, D., et al. (2003). An ordered BAC contig map of the equine major histocompatibility complex. Cytogenetic and Genome Research, 102, 189–195.*

This extreme MHC polymorphism is maintained in populations by a process called overdominant selection or heterozygote advantage. Simply put, MHC heterozygotes have a survival advantage because they can respond to a greater diversity of microbial antigens and so are best fitted to resist infectious diseases. The antigen-binding sites of MHC class Ia or II molecules are also very non-specific, and it has been estimated that an average MHC molecule can bind about 2500 different peptides. This is because the MHC groove binds to the peptide backbone of an antigenic protein rather than to its amino acid side chains. Nevertheless, structural constraints limit the efficiency of binding of each allele. As a result, it is likely that only one or two peptides from an average antigenic protein can bind strongly to any given MHC molecule. The ability of MHC molecules to bind antigens is therefore a limiting factor in generating adaptive immunity and resistance to infectious agents. Increasing the diversity of MHC molecules increases the diversity of antigenic peptides that can be bound and so increases resistance to infectious diseases. Because most horses are MHC heterozygotes, each individual normally expresses, about six different class Ia molecules (The number of expressed MHC molecules is not greater because that would increase the risk that the MHC molecules could bind and present more self-antigens. This would require the elimination of many more self-reactive T cells during their development in the thymus.

There are many examples of links between MHC haplotype and resistance to infectious disease. For example, in horses, an allergic response to the bites of *Culicoides* midges is linked to ELA-Aw7 (Viluma et al., 2017). Other studies on *Culicoides* hypersensitivity have indicated that a class II allele, *COR112:274,* is associated with disease susceptibility in both Icelandic horses and Exmoor ponies. Homozygosity across the entire MHC class II region is associated with a significantly higher risk of developing insect bite hypersensitivity (Andersson et al., 2012). The equine MHC has also been shown to influence susceptibility to West Nile Virus infection (Tallmadge et al., 2020). The equine MHC class II haplotype also determines genetic susceptibility to sarcoid tumors caused by bovine papilloma virus (Chapter 21) (Vychodilova et al., 2025) (Box 9.1).

Box 9.1 MHC and sperm count in horses

MHC and sperm count in horses

The MHC locus in mammals such as horses is located close to clusters of genes that encode nasal olfactory receptors. As a result, MHC haplotypes are closely linked to body odors. Mate choice appears to be determined in some species by odor. For example, 12 stallions were exposed to an MHC-similar mare and then to an MHC-dissimilar mare or vice versa for 4 weeks. Blood testosterone levels were determined weekly. Ejaculates were collected at the end of the experiment. Testosterone levels were higher in the stallions exposed to the MHC-dissimilar mare than to the MHC-similar mare. Sperm numbers were correlated to mean testosterone levels and were higher if MHC-dissimilar mares were presented last than if MHC-similar mares were presented last. Thus, MHC-linked olfactory signals influence testosterone levels and sperm counts (Burger et al., 2015).

MHC evolution

An analysis of the MHC class I genes among the different members of the Order Perissodactyla has revealed that they fall into six distinct groups, A to F. Five of these groups (A to E) contain genes and alleles that are found in all equid species. One group, F, is specific to the rhinoceros. Four of the groups contained only a single sequence or very few, suggesting that they were not polymorphic. The single remaining group, group B, contained the great majority of known equid genes. Thus, this diversification among class I genes occurred before the emergence of the Equidae (Holmes & Ellis, 1999). As a result, except for the rhinoceroses, they have a relatively conserved structure (Holmes & Ellis, 1999).

Przewalski's horse *E. ferus przewalskii*, is the only truly wild horse species surviving today. The polymorphism of the DQA, MHC class II locus has been analyzed in this endangered species (Tang et al., 2022). The current population of this species has been derived from 12 founder animals. As a result, only seven alleles were identified in the two existing populations. Thus, their genetic diversity is very limited. Presumably, this loss of diversity occurred when these animals went through an extreme population bottleneck.

In marked contrast to Przewalski's horse, the domestic donkey (*E. asinus*) MHC (Eqas) exhibits a considerable amount of allelic polymorphism (Arbanasic et al., 2013). For example, in a study of 248 donkeys sampled across the Balkan peninsula, ten DRA alleles were identified. In another study examining the DRA locus in Asiatic and African donkeys, the results showed major differences in donkey populations, not only in the number of DRA alleles, but also in expected heterozygosity values. Thus, using the polymorphic microsatellite assay, up to 11 alleles were detected (Vranova et al., 2011). However, further analysis indicated that this DRA polymorphism varied greatly between donkey populations. It also appeared that this had developed relatively recently and that there had been little positive selection at this locus. It appears to be primarily the result of selective breeding of domestic donkeys as well as their different genetic origins.

Antigen processing

The MHC class I pathway

One function of T cell–mediated immune responses is the identification and destruction of cells producing abnormal or foreign proteins. The best examples of such cells are those infected by viruses. Viruses take over the protein-synthesizing machinery of infected cells and use it to make new viral proteins. To control virus infections, cytotoxic T cells must be able to recognize any viral proteins expressed on the surface of infected cells. T cells can indeed recognize and respond to these endogenous antigens, but only if they first are processed and bound to MHC class I molecules.

As described above, MHC class I molecules are cell surface receptors folded in such a way that a large antigen-binding groove is formed. This binding groove, however, differs from that on MHC class II molecules in that it is closed at each end. Overall, however, the antigen-binding sites on class II and class I molecules function in a similar manner.

Living cells continually break up and recycle the proteins they produce. As a result, abnormal proteins are removed, regulatory peptides do not accumulate, and amino acids are recycled. As a first step, the protein must be tagged. To do this, ubiquitin, a small protein found in all eukaryotic cells, attaches to lysine residues in target proteins. Additional ubiquitin molecules then attach to the protein-bound ubiquitin so that multiple ubiquitin molecules are linked like beads on a string. A chain of four ubiquitin molecules appears to be optimal for processing. These polyubiquinated proteins are marked for destruction since they are recognized by enzyme complexes called proteasomes (Fig. 9.8).

Proteasomes are large multi-enzyme complexes whose function is to degrade unwanted intracellular proteins (Finley et al., 2016). They are tubular structures with an inner channel that contains the protease activity and two outer rings that regulate which proteins can enter and be destroyed. Ubiquitinated proteins bind to the outer rings, the tagged protein is unfolded, and the ubiquitin is released and reused (Bohj & Chen, 2009). The unfolded protein is inserted into the inner channel of the proteasome, where it is chopped up into 8- to 15-amino acid long peptides. Most of these peptide fragments are recycled into new proteins. For about 1 in a million molecules, however, the peptides are rescued from further breakup by attachment to transporter proteins. Two transporter proteins are used: TAP-1 and TAP-2 (*TAP* stands for *T*ransporter for *A*ntigen *P*rocessing). TAP-1 and TAP-2 form a heterodimer that binds peptide fragments and transports them into endosomes. Ideally, an 8- to 10-amino acid peptide precisely fits the binding site on the MHC heterodimer. In this case, the peptide is loaded into the TAP dimer, carried to a newly formed MHC, and if it fits the MHC antigen-binding site, it is transferred. Once loaded on the MHC, the MHC-peptide complex is carried to the cell surface by its normal secretory pathway, where it is displayed for many hours.

A cell can express about 10^6 MHC-peptide complexes on its surface at any one time. A minimum of about 200 MHC class I molecules loaded with the same viral peptide is required to activate a cytotoxic T cell. Thus, the MHC-peptide complexes can provide passing T cells with fairly complete information on virtually all the proteins being made by a cell. Analyses of peptide binding indicate that the binding groove of a class I protein can bind over a million different peptides with significant affinity. The number is not unlimited, however, because each MHC type usually shows preferences for peptides with certain structures. In fact, out of the great number of peptides generated from the proteome of a pathogen, only a few "immunodominant" peptides are recognized by most of the host's T cells. Thus, cytotoxic T cells can screen these peptides to determine whether any are "foreign" and bind to their TCRs. If so, the presenting cells are killed along with any viruses inside them.

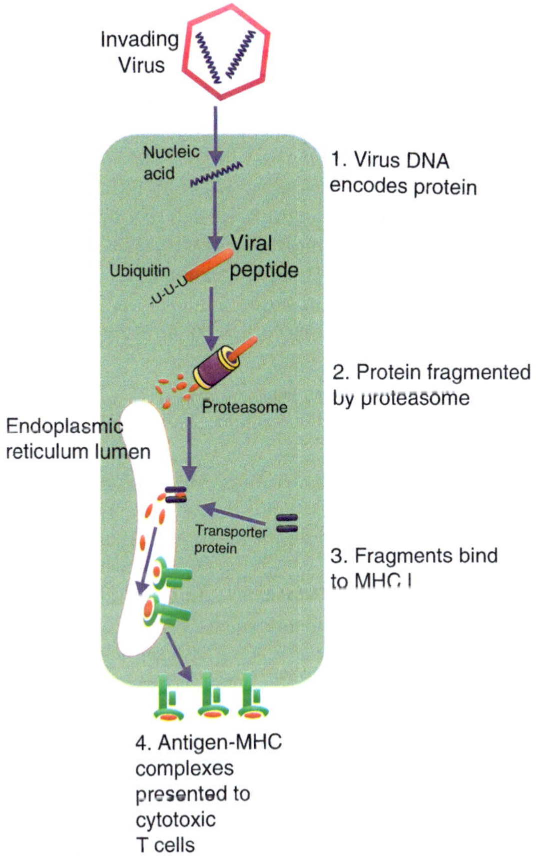

FIGURE 9.8 The MHC class I antigen-processing pathway.

Endogenous protein antigens are fragmented by the proteosome. Only antigen fragments that can bind in the groove of a class I MHC molecule will trigger an immune response. This is called MHC restriction. Thus the genes that code for these MHC molecules will also determine immune responsiveness.

References

Andersson, L. S., Swinbune, J. E., Meadows, J. R. S., Brostrom, H., et al. (2012). The same ELA class II risk factors confer equine insect bite hypersensitivity in two distinct populations. *Immunogenetics, 64*, 201–208.

Arbanasic, H., Galov, A., Ambriovic-Ristov, A., Griselj, J., et al. (2013). Extensive polymorphism of the major histocompatibility complex DRA gene in Balkan donkeys: Perspectives on selection and genealogy. *Animal Genetics*. https://doi.org/10.1111/age.12054

Barbis, D. P., Bainbridge, D., Crump, A. L., Zhang, C. H., et al. (1994). Variation in expression of MHC class II antigens on horse lymphocytes determined by MHC haplotype. *Veterinary Immunology and Immunopathology, 42*(1), 103–114.

Bohj, V. G., & Chen, Z. J. (2009). Ubiquitylation in innate and adaptive immunity. *Nature, 458*, 430–437.

Brinkmeyer-Langford, C. L., Murphy, W. J., Childers, C. P., & Skow, L. C. (2010). A conserved segmental duplication within ELA. *Animal Genetics, 41*(Suppl. 2), 186–195.

Brown, J. J., Thomson, W., Clegg, P., Eyre, S., et al. (2004). Polymorphisms of the equine major histocompatibility complex class II DRA locus. *Tissue Antigens, 64*, 173–179.

Bubenikova, J., Plasil, M., Futas, J., Stejskalova, K., et al. (2024). Diversity of major histocompatibility complex (MHC) and natural killer cell receptor (NKR) genes and their interactions in domestic horses. *HLA*. https://doi.org/10.1111/tan.15387

Burger, D., Dolivo, G., Marti, E., Sieme, H., & Wedekind, C. (2015). Female major histocompatibility complex type affects male testosterone levels and sperm number in the horse (*Equus caballus*). *Proceedings of the Royal Society A: Mathematical, Physical and Engineering Sciences B, 282*, Article 20150407.

Deakin, J. E., Papenfuss, A. T., Belov, K., Cross, J. C. R., et al. (2006). Evolution and comparative analysis of the MHC class III inflammatory region. *BMC Genomics*. https://doi.org/10.1186/1471-2164/7/281

Finley, D., Chen, X., & Walters, K. J. (2016). Gates, channels, and switches: Elements of the proteasome machine. *Trends in Biochemical Sciences, 41*(1), 77–93.

Fraser, D. G., & Bailey, E. (1998). Polymorphism and multiple loci for the horse *DQA* gene. *Immunogenetics, 47*, 487–490.

Gustafson, A. L., Tallmadge, R. L., Ramlachan, N., Miller, D., et al. (2003). An ordered BAC contig map of the equine major histocompatibility complex. *Cytogenetic and Genome Research, 102*, 189–195.

Holmes, E. C., & Ellis, S. A. (1999). Evolutionary history of MHC class I genes in the mammalian order Perissodactyla. *Journal of Molecular Evolution, 49*, 316–324.

Holmes, C. M., Violette, N., Miller, D., Wagner, B., et al. (2019). MHC haplotype diversity in Icelandic horses determined by polymorphic microsatellites. *Genes and Immunity, 20*, 660–670.

Hulpke, S., & Tampe, R. (2013). The MHC I loading complex: A multitasking machinery in adaptive immunity. *Trends in Biochemical Sciences, 38*(8), 412–420.

Janova, E., Matiasovic, J., Vahala, J., Vodicka, R., et al. (2009). Polymorphism and selection in the major histocompatibility complex DRA and DQA genes in the family Equidae. *Immunogenetics, 61*, 513–527.

Kamath, P. L., & Getz, W. M. (2011). Adaptive molecular evolution of the major histocompatibility complex genes, DRA and DQA in the genus equus. *BMC Evolutionary Biology, 11*, 128.

Klumplerova, M., Splichalova, P., Oppelt, J., Futas, J., et al. (2020). Genetic diversity, evolution and selection in the major histocompatibility complex DRB and DQB loci in the family *Equidae. BMC Genomics*. https://doi.org/10.1186/s12864-020-07089-6

Kumanovics, A., Takada, T., & Fischer Lindahl, K. (2003). Genomic organization of the mammalian MHC. *Annual Review of Immunology, 21*, 629–657.

Moravcikova, N., Kasarda, R., Vydrova, H. V., Vostry, L., et al. (2024). Genomic variability of the MHC region: Empirical evidence from five horse breeds. *Livestock Science, 284*, Article 105480.

Nei, M., Gu, X., & Sitnikova, T. (1997). Evolution by the birth-and-death process in multigene families of the vertebrate immune system. *Proceedings of the National Academy of Sciences of the United States of America, 94*, 7799–7806.

Plasil, M., Oppelt, J., Klumplerova, M., Bubenikova, J., et al. (2023). Newly identified variability pf the antigen binding site coding sequences of the equine major histocompatibility complex class I and class II genes. *HLA, 102*, 489–500.

Radwan, J., Babik, W., Kaufman, J., Lenz, T. L., & Winternitz, J. (2020). Advances in the evolutionary understanding of MHC polymorphism. *Trends in Genetics, 36*, 298–311.

Sadeghi, R., Moradi-Shahrbabak, M., Ashtiani, S. R. M., Miller, D. C., & Antczak, D. F. (2018). MHC haplotype diversity in Persian Arabian horses determined using polymorphic microsatellites. *Immunogenetics, 70*, 305–315.

Tallmadge, R. L., Antczak, D. F., & Felippe, M. J. B. (2020). Genetics of immune disease in the horse. *Veterinary Clinics: Equine, 36*, 273–288.

Tallmadge, R. L., Campbell, J. A., Miller, D. C., & Antczak, D. F. (2010). Analysis of MHC class I genes across diverse MHC haplotypes. *Immunogenetics, 62*(3), 159–172.

Tallmadge, R. L., Lear, T. L., & Antczak, D. F. (2005). Genomic characterization of MHC class I genes in the horse. *Immunogenetics, 57*, 763–774.

Tang, Y., Liu, G., Zhao, S., Li, K., et al. (2022). Major histocompatibility cmoplex (MHC) diversity of the reintroduced populations of endangered Przewalski's horse. *Genes*. https://doi.org/10.3390/genes13050928

Tseng, C. T., Miller, D., Cassano, J., Bailey, E., & Antczak, D. F. (2010). Identification of equine major histocompatibility complex haplotypes using polymorphic microsatellites. *Animal Genetics, 41*(Suppl. 2), 150–153.

Vasoya, D., Tzelos, T., Benedictus, L., Karafianni, A. E., et al. (2023). High-resolution genotyping of expressed equine MHC reveals a highly complex MHC structure. *Genes*. https://doi.org/10.3390/genes14071422

Viluma, A., Mikko, S., Hahn, D., Slow, L., et al. (2017). Genomic structure of the horse major histocompatibility complex class II region resolved using PacBio long-read sequencing technology. *Scientific Reports*. https://doi.org/10.1038/srep45518

Vranova, M., Alloggio, I., Qablan, M., Vyskocil, M., et al. (2011). Genetic diversity in the class II major histocompatibility DRA locus in European, Asiatic, and African domestic donkeys. *Infection, Genetics and Evolution*, 1136–1141.

Vychodilova, L., Plasil, M., Futas, J., Kopeka, A., et al. (2025). Genetic susceptibility to srcoid in Arabian horses: Associations with MHC class II and compound MHC class I/KLRA genotypes. *Veterinary Research Communications*. https://doi.org/10.1007/s11259-025-10748-2

CHAPTER

Equine innate lymphoid cells

10

Natural killer (NK) cells are cytotoxic lymphocytes found in normal, unsensitized animals. They are medium to large lymphocytes containing multiple cytoplasmic electron-dense granules that contain granzyme B and perforins. Granzymes are a family of serine proteases found in lymphocyte cytotoxic granules. These cytotoxic cells are produced by bone marrow stem cells and are found in peripheral blood, lymph nodes, spleen, lung, liver, and bone marrow, but not in the thymus. In horses, NK cells consist of diverse subpopulations with different degrees of maturity and activation states. As a result, their cell surface phenotype, as determined by flow cytometry, varies greatly. As their name implies, they are innately cytotoxic. In addition, NK cells are major producers of cytokines, especially interferon-γ and TNF-α. They also produce multiple chemokines (Mace, 2023). Their prime function is the identification and removal of virus-infected or otherwise abnormal cells. They also play a key role in the initial defensive responses against bacterial and parasitic infections.

Unlike T and B cells that circulate as resting cells and so require several days to become fully activated, NK cells are "on call" and can be rapidly activated by interferons released from virus-infected cells or by IL-12 from stimulated macrophages. As a result, NK cells promptly attack tumor and virus-infected cells. They participate in innate defenses within hours, long before antigen-specific primary adaptive responses can be generated. Because they produce numerous cytokines and chemokines, they also modulate other aspects of the immune system.

NK cells kill some tumor cells, foreign cells, and virus-infected cells. NK cells can also destroy some cultured tumor cells, and there is a positive correlation between this activity in vitro and resistance to tumors in vivo. Stressors such as surgery may depress NK activity and so promote tumor growth. Uterine NK cells also play an important role in the maintenance of pregnancy (Chapter 2).

Equine NK cells

Foals suffering from an inherited severe combined immunodeficiency are unable to mount either T or B cell responses (Chapter 23). However, they still possess a population of large granular lymphocytes in their bloodstream. Following exposure to interleukin-2, this cell population demonstrated a consistently high level of cytotoxic activity against YAC-1 lymphoma or K562 erythroleukemia target cells.

The Immunology of Horses and Donkeys. https://doi.org/10.1016/B978-0-443-44863-8.00026-0

(These are typical experimental NK cell targets.) (Magnuson et al., 1987). These natural killer cells appear to account for about 5% of peripheral blood mononuclear cells in normal healthy horses.

NK cells can also be identified by their expression of a key activating receptor molecule, NKp46 (CD335). This is a receptor capable of triggering NK cell cytotoxicity. It appears to be well-conserved among the domestic mammals. Thus, the use of a fluorescent-labeled monoclonal antibody against NKp46 labeled between 0.8% and 2.1% (mean, 1.3%) of equine peripheral blood lymphocytes (Noronha, Harman, et al., 2012). Flow cytometry showed that these positive cells had a size and side-scatter (granularity) similar to that seen in NKp46$^+$ cells in humans and cattle. They were also differentiated from T cells by not expressing the TCR signaling component CD3 (Noronha, Harman, et al., 2012). While these are mainly NK cells, they also include some related innate cells such as NKT and LAK cells.

An alternative NK cell marker is termed NK-5C6. This is a highly conserved protein that is expressed on the NK cells of many different species, including horses (Harris et al., 1993). It is present on approximately 10% of equine peripheral blood lymphocytes (Vivieros & Antczak, 1999). These cells are CD3$^-$, CD4$^-$, and CD8$^-$ but express MHC class I as well as LFA-1 molecules. A cell population enriched in these NK-5C6$^+$ cells showed enhanced cytotoxicity against an MHC-deficient NK target cell line. They did not kill MHC-positive target cells. These NK cells could be distinguished from another population of cytotoxic cells whose activity was stimulated by the presence of interleukin-2. These lymphokine-activated killers (LAK cells) were cytotoxic for both MHC$^-$ and MHC$^+$ cellular targets and thus readily distinguishable from true NK cells (Vivieros & Antczak, 1999).

A subpopulation of equine peripheral blood mononuclear cells has therefore been shown to have NK cell functionality by several different measures. They have NK-type cytotoxicity against both allogeneic and xenogeneic targets (Chong et al., 1992). Their most susceptible target is the human tumor cell line,—Chang liver cells. Other susceptible targets included rabbit kidney cells (RK-13), equine sarcoid cells, and embryonic equine kidney (EEK) cells. Embryonated equine lung cells (EEL) and mouse YAC-1 T-cells are also susceptible targets. Horse mononuclear cells exhibit high levels of NK activity against EEK. EEL and RK-13 cells that are infected with equine herpesvirus-1 (EHV-1). Similarly, they can kill EEK and EEL cells infected with Semliki Forest virus. Cytotoxicity against these vulnerable targets developed between 4 and 8 h of incubation and reached a maximum 24 h later. Immunization of foals with live EHV-1 did not induce significant changes in NK toxicity against Chang liver cells and EHV-1-infected targets when compared to the cells of a healthy adult horse. Equine NK cells are also cytotoxic for MHC-class I-deficient target cells (Vivieros & Antczak, 1999).

As in humans, equine NK cells play an important role in remodeling the placenta as it grows, and the fetal foal develops in utero. As discussed in Chapter 2, the interaction zone between the endometrial cups and the uterus is a site of both immune activity and rigorous immune regulation. There are dense infiltrations of lymphocytes surrounding the endometrial cup structures in the horse placenta during early pregnancy (Noronha, Huggler, et al., 2012). It has been shown that there is a significant enrichment in the uterine NK cell populations in the mare's placenta during pregnancy. In addition, there is a large population of NK cells present in the endometrium of cycling mares (Jaworska et al., 2022). Using anti-NKp46, approximately 6% of the endometrial lymphocytes stained positively for this receptor, irrespective of the stage of the estrus cycle. Presumably, these NK cells are also required to play a defensive role following mating (Figs. 10.2 and 10.3).

NK cell MHC receptors

NK cells do not make the enormous diversity of antigen-specific receptors employed by T and B cells. Instead, they use two types of receptors to distinguish normal from abnormal cells. One type detects the presence of MHC class I antigens on target cells; the other detects "stress" molecules expressed on unhealthy cells, such as tumors or virus-infected cells. NK cells thus recognize abnormal cells using two different strategies. One is a "missing self" strategy by which NK receptors bind MHC class I molecules expressed on healthy cells, and as a result, this inhibits NK cell killing. If, however, a cell fails to express MHC class I, these inhibitory signals are not generated, the T cell is activated and the target cell will be killed. This occurs, for example, when a virus suppresses cellular MHC class I expression to avoid destruction by cytotoxic T cells. Likewise, tumor cells that fail to express MHC class I are also killed by NK cells (Schwartz et al., 2017) (Fig. 10.1).

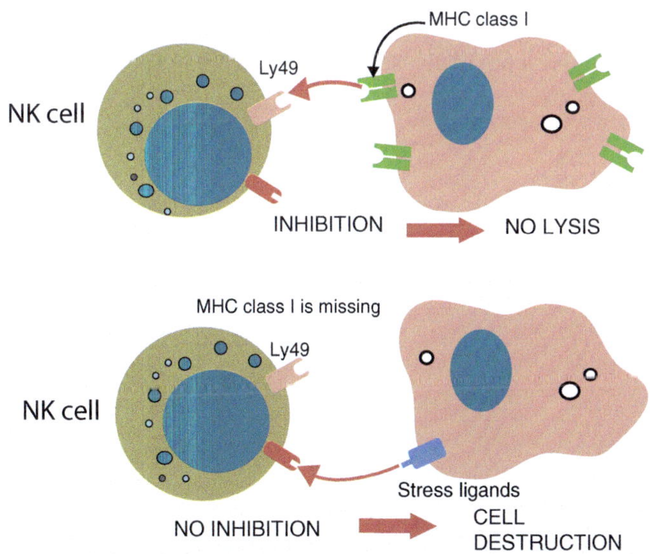

FIGURE 10.1 The two triggers that activate equine NK cells.

One is the absence of expression of MHC molecules and the second is the expression of cellular stress proteins.

The second NK cell activation strategy employs receptors that recognize the presence of stress-induced proteins on targeted cells. When the NK cells detect these stress proteins, an activating signal is generated, and the NK cells kill the stressed cells. Cells infected by viruses and intracellular bacteria, as well as some cancer cells, express these stress proteins (Hao et al., 2006).

The NK receptor (NKR) complex

Mammals employ two different types of receptors for MHC antigens on their NK cells. Most are inhibitory and serve to prevent excessive NK cell killing. Some, however, are activating and will trigger NK cell cytotoxicity. Rodents employ members of the Ly49 family as natural killer receptors. These are a family of C-type lectin-like cell-membrane-associated proteins. (The Ly numbering system was an early attempt to classify the antigenic proteins on the surface of mouse lymphocytes.) Other mammalian families employ members of the killer cell immunoglobulin-like receptor (KIR) family—except the Equidae. In marked contrast to the other non-rodent mammals, the domestic horse and other members of the Equidae employ multiple inhibitory Ly49-like receptors. This is a result of a significant expansion of the *LY49* gene locus, presumably by repeated gene duplication (Futas & Horin, 2013; Takahashi et al., 2004). These *LY49* genes are located on chromosome ECA 6q13 (Fig. 10.2).

Ly49 receptors

The *LY49* and *KIR* gene families have been analyzed in the Equidae. Genomic analysis has shown the presence of at least six highly conserved polymorphic *LY49* genes

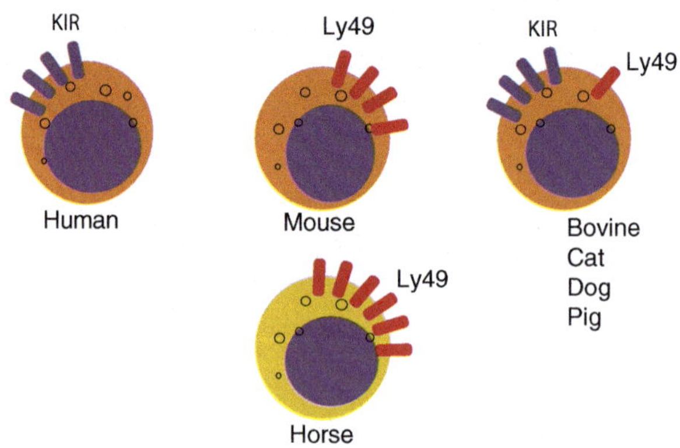

FIGURE 10.2 The receptors that activate NK cells in mammals belong to multiple protein families.

Equids are unique in that, like rodents, their NK cells respond almost exclusively to ligands that bind their Ly49 receptors.

in the NK gene complex of horses, asses, and zebras (Futas & Horin, 2013). They are, in order:

5'—LY49F- LY49A-LY49B-LY49C-LY49E-LY49D-3″

Five of their products have a conserved immunotyrosine inhibitory motif (ITIM) motif while one has an arginine in its transmembrane region and may not be functional (Takahashi et al., 2004). All five of these functional *LY49* genes are present across the entire perissodactyl family, including not only the equids, but also rhinos and tapirs (Futas & Horin, 2013).

Some variants of equine Ly49A and Ly49 B with truncated C-type lectin domains are unlikely to be functional; however, the remaining Ly49 genes all appear to encode fully functional receptors. Thus, Ly49A, Ly49B, Ly49D, Ly49E, and Ly49F appear to be functional inhibitory receptors. On the other hand, Ly49C probably acts as an activating receptor. The presence of multiple transcribed Ly49 sequences suggests that, horses employ these as their primary MHC class I receptors (Gagnier et al., 2003).

Equine Ly49 F has been cloned and sequenced. It is a single-pass type II membrane protein containing 294 amino acids and a molecular weight of 33.7 kDa. It forms functional disulfide-bonded homodimers. The *LY49* genes are located on chromosome ECA6q13 (Horecky et al., 2014, pp. 490–493).

The leukocyte receptor complex

Other mammals employ KIRs to bind MHC molecules. Several KIR-like gene sequences have also been detected in the equine genome, although only one, *KLRA3*, appears likely to encode a functional NK cell receptor (Futas & Horin, 2013). It is located on chromosome ECA10p12 (Takahashi et al., 2004). The other KIR genes contain premature stop codons or frameshift mutations. Two of them have mutated ITIM motifs. There is also a non-functional KIR-immunoglobulin-like transcript fusion gene (*KIR-ILTA*) present in horses, donkeys, and plains zebra (*E. quagga*). There are two probable pseudogenes (*KIRP1* and *KIRP2*) with premature stop codons or frameshift mutations, and a *KIR3DL*-like sequence has also been identified. This protein contains a single non-mutated immune-tyrosine-based inhibition motif (ITIM) and is potentially functional.

It has been found that associations exist between specific combinations of MHC/NKR haplotypes. and different equine diseases. This suggests that these gene complexes did not evolve independently. For example, in a study investigating the Camargue, African, and Romanian horse breeds, significant associations were found between the variable *KLRA3* gene, its haplotypes, and the equine MHC class I loci, *EQCA-1* and *EQCA-2* genes. This suggests that KLRA3 is probably a significant MHC receptor (Bubenikova et al., 2024). There is also an association between some *KLRA* genes and susceptibility of Arabian horses to sarcoid tumors, implying a role for NK cells in controlling this cancer (Chapter 21) (Vychodilova et al., 2025).

Other equine NK cell receptors

LILR receptors

Leukocyte immunoglobulin-like receptors (LILR) are expressed on innate immune cells and regulate both innate and adaptive immune responses. They each consist of a single peptide chain containing two to four immunoglobulin domains. Horses have three *LILR* genes located on chromosome ECA10 close to the other KIR-related genes. They all contain inhibitory ITIM motifs (Futas & Horin, 2013).

NKG2/CD94 receptors

Equine NK cells also express NKG2D (Natural Killer Group 2, member D). NKG2D is an activating homodimeric receptor expressed on equine NK and $CD8^+$ T cells. It associates with signaling adaptors such as DNA activation proteins of 10 kDa (DAP10) and 12 kDa (DAP12). Horse NK cells have also been shown to express CD94 which forms one chain of the NKG2D heterodimer (Noronha, Harman, et al., 2012) (Fig. 10.3).

NKG2D is expressed on NKp46 (CD355)-positive cells in peripheral blood, mesenteric lymph nodes, and intraepithelial lymphocytes. When its ligands bind to NKG2D, they override the inhibitory effects of conventional MHC class I molecules and trigger NK cytotoxicity. NKG2D is also expressed on activated T cells, suggesting that they also play a role in innate immunity (Fig. 10.4).

The two important NKG2D ligands in humans are polymorphic MHC class I-like molecules called MIC-A (major histocompatibility complex, class I chain-related A) and MIC-B, coded for by MHC class I genes. Unlike conventional class I molecules, these do not bind antigenic peptides. While minimally expressed on normal, healthy cells, MIC-A and MIC-B are expressed in large amounts by stressed cells. These stresses may include DNA damage due to ionizing radiation or alkylating agents, heat shock, and oxidative stress. They are also overexpressed in tumor cells and virus-infected cells.

The four equine MHC class I chain-related (MIC) genes are located within the ELA class I region. The four genes are labeled, *MIC1* to *MIC4*. Some of these MIC genes are polymorphic and their presence varies with haplotype, although the *MIC4* gene is consistently present in all haplotypes. The presence of the other

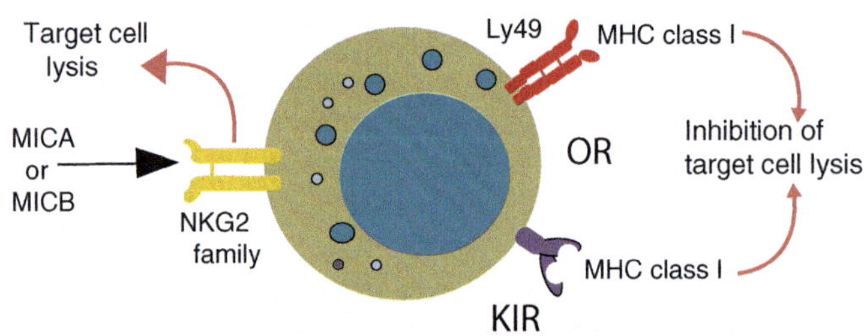

FIGURE 10.3

The major receptors expressed on equine NK cells and their ligands.

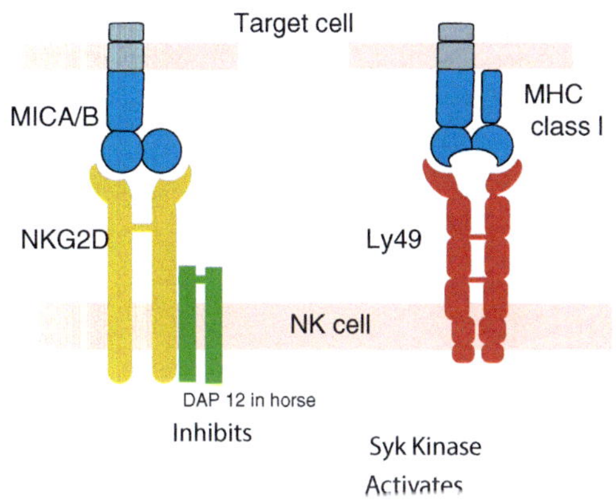

FIGURE 10.4

The structure and functions of the major equine NK cell receptors.

three is variable. MIC4 is an NKG2D ligand and probably plays a similar role to human MIC-A and MIC-B. CD94 (also called KLRD-1) is a C-type lectin that serves as one chain of the NKG2A heterodimer. It binds to its ligands, MIC1 and MIC4. In vitro cultivation of NKp46$^+$ cells with soluble MIC1 or MIC4 results in increased IFN-γ production.

ULBP proteins

In humans, two proteins bind to the cytomegalovirus UL16 protein. These UL-binding proteins (ULBP) also interact with the NKG2D receptor and cause its activation. (The cytomegalovirus UL16 disrupts this interaction.) ULBP proteins belong to the MHC class I superfamily. They are cell surface proteins with α1 and α2 domains but no α3-like domains. Equine UL16 binding protein-1 has been cloned and characterized. It is a protein of 27.9 kDa whose gene is located on chromosome ECA31.

Natural cytotoxicity receptors

As pointed out above, NKp46 (also called NCR1) is a marker of equine NK cells. This is a protein of 305 amino acids. and 34.7 kDa, whose gene is located on chromosome ECA10. Together with NKp44 and NKp30, NKp46 forms a family of receptors that recognize ligands on tumor cells, virus-infected cells, and also foreign cells (Noronha, Huggler, et al., 2012).

Fc receptors

In addition to the receptors listed above, equine NK cells can also recognize and kill target cells using an antibody-dependent pathway employing the low-affinity immunoglobulin receptor, CD16 (FcγRIII). CD16 is a 38-kDa transmembrane protein. When antibodies bind to target cells, the bound antibody links to NK cell CD16, triggering a cytotoxic response, andas a result, the target cells are killed. NK cells can spontaneously release their CD16 so that the NK cell can detach from an antibody-coated target cell after it has delivered its lethal hit. Many NK cells thus participate in antibody-dependent cellular cytotoxicity (ADCC). CD16 is also expressed at high levels on a subset of monocytes and lymphocytes. The CD16-positive lymphocytes are T cells ($CD3^+$ $CD8^+$ $CD5^{dim}$ $\alpha/\beta TCR^+$), and NK cells ($CD3^-$ $CD5^-$ $CD94^+$).

Effector mechanisms

Although NK cells are active in non-immune horses, virus infections or interferon inducers enhance their activity. NK cells require priming to become fully responsive. Thus, infections attract NK cells to lymph nodes where they are activated. Like other immune cells, NK cell activities are regulated by multiple cytokines. For example, IL-2 and IL-4 enhance their cytotoxicity, whereas IL-3 promotes NK survival. When macrophages phagocytose invading organisms and produce TNF-α and IL-12, these cytokines then induce IFN-γ production by NK cells. The IFN-γ enhances NK activity further by promoting the rapid differentiation of pre-NK cells.

Target cell recognition

NK cells can act as "serial killers," and a single NK cell can kill multiple target cells. Once activated, the NK cells kill their targets through either the perforin/granulysin/NK-lysin pathway or through contact-dependent death receptors. These include Fas-Fas ligand (CD95L) and TRAIL-R1/R2 on target cells. Cytotoxic granules are stored preformed in resting NK cells (in contrast to cytotoxic T cells, which only produce theirs on demand). Once an NK cell encounters a target cell, a synapse forms at the contact site. Activating KIRs cause the MHC molecules to form a ring around a cluster of adhesion molecules. At the center of the synapse, there is a supramolecular activation cluster (SMAC) through which the NK cell lytic granule contents can pass into the target cell. Receptors and signaling molecules also segregate in the central SMAC, whereas adhesive integrins accumulate in the peripheral SMAC.

Equine NK-lysin has been cloned and sequenced (Davis et al., 2005). It is a protein of 83 amino acids that is 53% identical to the NK-lysin of the bovine and 41% identical in its amino acid sequence to equine granulysin. It is highly positively charged. It has powerful antibacterial activity as well as being lethal for NK target cell lines. In addition to NK cells, it is expressed in $CD4^+$ and $CD8^+$ T cells in the horse. The cytotoxic proteins, perforin and granulysin, are also found in NK cell granules, and their expression is increased by exposure to IL-2 and IL-12. Perforin is a protein of 70–72 kDa that produces small (5–7 nm dia) channels in target cell surfaces. Presumably, granzymes are injected into the target cells through these perforin channels (Netea et al., 2016).

NK cells can kill bacteria, fungi, and protozoan parasites in addition to the abnormal cells described above. Thus, NK cells are cytotoxic for fungi such as Cryptococcus or Aspergillus. This cytotoxicity is mediated by secreted perforins. NK cells can also bind bacteria through cell surface receptors such as NKp46 and

NKG2D. Their perforins and granzymes can kill bacteria such as *Mycobacterium tuberculosis, Pseudomonas aeruginosa, E. coli, Staph aureus*, and *L. monocytogenes* (Mody et al., 2019). Equine granzyme B has been isolated and characterized (Piuko et al., 2007). Granzyme B is a protease that can activate a cell death program in many bacteria by cleaving vital conserved biosynthetic and metabolic enzymes. As a result, it disrupts bacterial protein synthesis, folding, and degradation. Because it destroys so many proteins, bacteria are unlikely to develop resistance to NK cell attack (Dotiwala et al., 2017).

In addition to attacking target cells by direct cell-cell contact and cytotoxicity, NK cells also produce extracellular vesicles. These exosomes are taken up by target cells via micropinocytosis and so deliver cytotoxic molecules directly to their targets (Enomoto et al., 2022).

Trained immunity

Blood monocytes and NK cells increase in number and activity in response to infections. They decline once invaders have been eliminated. Some of these activated cells may, however, persist, develop a "memory" and mount a form of secondary response when they encounter a similar stimulus again. For example, in mice, NK cells bearing a KIR specific for cytomegalovirus can expand their numbers in response to viral antigens. These NK "memory" cells can persist in both lymphoid and non-lymphoid tissues for several months. These self-renewing memory cells can be reactivated on re-exposure to the viral antigen. Adoptive transfer of these reactivated NK cells leads to a rapid expansion of their numbers and protective immunity to cytomegalovirus in recipients.

As described previously, NK cells employ multiple activating receptors with different specificities (Moorlag et al., 2018). Thus, an NK cell initially activated through one receptor may well be reactivated through a different receptor. For example, NK cells initially activated through Ly49 may be reactivated through NKG2D. This NK "memory" response could therefore be more accurately described as "training" rather than memory (Hu et al., 2022). There is also some evidence that this trained immunity may be vertically transmitted from a mother to her offspring (Katzmarski et al., 2021).

Innate immune memory is not restricted to NK cells. In vivo, 24 h, treatment of cultured blood monocytes with PAMPs that target dectin-1, TLR2, or TLR4 was followed 6 days later with an immune challenge with bacterial LPS or an immunostimulating peptide (Pam3CysSerLys4). TNF-α production was measured. The monocytes previously "trained" by exposure to a β-glucan produced significantly more ($30\times$) TNF-α than naive cells. The trained cells also produced increased amounts of IL-6 and IL-1β. The "training" also resulted in increased reactive oxygen species production as well as improving the phagocytic activity of the macrophages.

In other situations, β-glucans can act on hematopoietic stem cells through GM-CSF to induce persistent myelopoiesis following a secondary challenge with lipopolysaccharide or infection. In vitro, monocytes can be treated with beta-glucans.

After several days' rest, they can be restimulated, and their production of cytokines and reactive oxygen species measured. Cells primed in this way showed enhanced stimulation after exposure to unrelated stimuli, as shown by increased production of reactive oxygen species. This trained immunity is dependent upon epigenetic remodeling and rewiring of cellular metabolic pathways, resulting in a persistent inflammatory phenotype. This is reflected by increased expression of the insulin-like growth factor-1 receptor and the accumulation of intracellular mevalonate (Bekkering et al., 2018).

NKT cells

Natural killer T cells (NKT cells) are a cell population that combines the properties of NK cells and T cells. They are innate-like T cells that express both NK cell markers and a TCR. NKT cells express a TCR consisting of an invariant α-chain associated with variable β-chains. NKT cells respond specifically to lipid, lipopeptide, and glycolipid antigens presented to them by a family of MHC class I-like molecules called CD1. Morphologically, NKT cells are large lymphocytes containing electron-dense granules. They promote immunity in response to lipid antigens from infectious agents and tumor cells. They are found in the liver, spleen, blood, and especially in adipose tissue (Bentley et al., 2019). Many are found in the sinusoids of the liver.

NKT cells play an important role in combating mycobacterial infections. Thus, when purified lipids from *Myco. bovis* such as their phosphatidyl mannosides are added to a purified mononuclear cell preparation in vitro, some of the cells respond by proliferating significantly. These proliferating cells have been characterized and shown to be $CD3^{+}$ $NKp46^{+}$ NKT cells. These $NKp46^{+}$ $CD8^{+}$ NKT cells are also recruited to the nasal mucosa of the upper respiratory tract during equine herpesvirus-1 infections.

In the absence of prior antigenic stimulation, NKT cells respond more rapidly than conventional T cells. They produce pro-inflammatory cytokines such as IFN-γ and TNF-α as well as anti-inflammatory cytokines such as IL-4 and IL-10. As a result, they can modulate immunity in a broad spectrum of diseases. NKT cells trigger chemokine and cytokine release, enhance NK function, and promote dendritic cell maturation and B cell responses. NKT cells inhibit the development of Th17 cells and regulate IL-17 production. NKT cells also secrete IL-12 that acts on neutrophils to decrease their production of IL-10. They play a role in allergies, antitumor immunity, autoimmunity, and antimicrobial immunity, especially to mycobacteria. Thus, they link the T-cell system with the innate NK cell system.

Some NKT cells (type 1) also express receptors for inflammatory cytokines produced by antigen-presenting cells. They can be activated either in combination with TCR-mediated signals or even without such signals.

A subpopulation of NKT cells (type II) use diverse TCRs where both α- and β-chains contribute equally to antigen binding. Their functions are predominantly anti-inflammatory, and they recognize diverse hydrophobic antigens. The type II cells also suppress the type I NKT cells, suggesting that they have an immunoregulatory role (Dhodapkar & Kumar, 2017).

NKT cells and CD1

CD1 proteins are non-polymorphic ELA class I proteins expressed on professional antigen-presenting cells such as epidermal Langerhans cells, other dendritic cells, and macrophages. They have a similar overall structure to other MHC class I molecules with an alpha-heavy chain paired with β2 microglobulin. They have an antigen-binding groove formed by two parallel alpha-helices (Wegrecki, 2023). They serve as lipid-specific, antigen-presenting receptors (Porcelli & Modlin, 1999). The CD1 system therefore allows the immune system to respond to antigenic lipids, glycolipids, and lipoproteins such as bacterial lipopeptides (Fig. 10.5). It thus complements the MHC-peptide presentation system. Some CD1 proteins present lipid antigens to conventional T cells while others present lipids to NKT cells (Zajonc, 2016). These diverse CD1 proteins differ in their antigen-binding domains as well as in their cytoplasmic domains. Thus, they may recognize different lipid antigens and traffic differently.

CD1-restricted invariant NKT cells have been identified in humans and mice, pigs, and horses (Van Beeck et al., 2009). Using an invariant T cell α chain, these

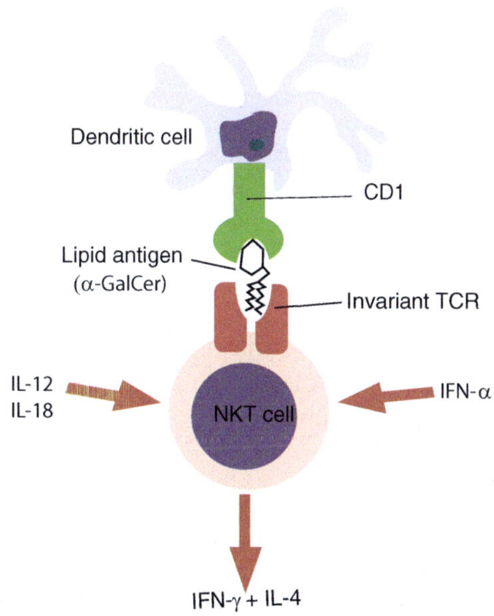

FIGURE 10.5 The NKT/CD1 system.

NKT cells use an invariant T cell receptor to bind lipid antigens presented by the invariant MHC class I molecule CD1.

cells can usually be activated by the glycolipid ligand α-galactosylceramide (α-GalCer) presented by a CD1 molecule. The CD1 gene family consists of a group of nonpolymorphic MHC class Ib molecules that specifically present lipid antigens to T cells. The presence of a functional CD1 system appears to be critical for equine health. In the horse, for example, CD1 has been shown to present lipids from the major pathogen, *Rhodococcus equi,* to cytotoxic T cells. The equine genome contains 13 complete CD1 genes located in a 918 kb region on chromosome ECA5. Of these genes, seven are homologous to human CD1a, two to CD1b, one each to CD1c and CD1d, and two to CD1e. The genome also contains five non-functional pseudogenes. This is one of the largest CD1 gene families yet recorded in mammals. Twelve of these CD1 molecules have been shown to be expressed on antigen-presenting cells, including monocytes, macrophages, and dendritic cells. The polymorphism within the CD1 family is restricted to the antigen-binding α1 and α2 domains, suggesting that multiple different lipid antigens can be presented and recognized. Lacking a tyrosine sorting motif, these eqCD1 molecules are predicted to colocalize with *R. equi* in intracellular vesicles (Dossa et al., 2014).

Although horses clearly possess functional NKT cells as well as a large CD1 gene family, they also differ in some respects from other mammals. For example, while α-GalCer is a potent NKT cell stimulator in most species examined, it is not, however, an immunostimulatory NKT cell agonist in the horse (Dossa et al., 2015). This lack of response to α-GalCer immunization has caused some investigators to question whether equine NKT cells are functional. Analysis, however, suggests that α-GalCer may simply be too long for the equine CD1 antigen binding site.

LAK cells

When peripheral blood mononuclear cells are activated by the presence of interleukin-2 (IL-2) a population of cytotoxic T cells develops. These are known as lymphokine-activated killer (LAK) cells. They exert their cytotoxic activity only on equine target cells (Hormanski et al., 1992). LAK cells appear to originate from $CD8^+$ T cells and depend upon CD8 for their cytotoxicity (Lunn et al., 1996). Equine LAK cells produce granzyme B and use this to induce apoptosis in an equine tumor cell line (EqT8888) (Liu et al., 2011). In addition to their cytotoxic activity, LAK cells also produce IFN-γ. LAK activity in young (~1-year-old) horses is much less than in older (~10-year-old) animals.

MAIT-MR1 cells

Mucosal-associated invariant T (MAIT) cells are another equine T cell population that interfaces between conventional T cells and NK cells. They express semi-invariant TCRs that recognize non-peptide antigens. They are CD4/CD8 double-negative cells. MAIT cells appear to be multifunctional and are engaged in both antibacterial and antiviral host defense. They appear to be present in all mammals (Harly et al., 2022). They are also highly conserved in the mammals analyzed to date (Edmans et al., 2024). MAIT cells have an effector memory phenotype that is independent of their location, and they employ the transcription factors PLZF (promyelocytic leukemia zinc finger) and EOMES (eomesodermin) (Edmans et al., 2024). They are found in peripheral blood and are CD8α^+. They also express high levels of CD23 (FcεRII). Their lack of expression of CD8β suggests that they are innate T cells. They express TRBV25-1, TRBV28, and CXCR6, and have a highly restricted TCR repertoire—a phenotype typical of MAIT cells in other species. MAIT-like cells, like NKT cells, have an elongated receptor alpha chain (TRA). They express an orthologous TRAV1-TRAJ33 TCR α chain.

Horses have a single MHC class I-related (MR1) gene (Reinink & Van Rhijn, 2016). MR1 is a heterodimer with a variable β and a constant α chain. MAIT cells recognize and respond to antigens presented by MR1. On activation, they produce IL-4 and IL-17. The antigens involved in this process are metabolites derived from the synthesis of riboflavin by bacteria and fungi. As a result, MAIT cells are engaged in the immunity to infections caused by Mycobacteria, Salmonella, and *E. coli*.

Innate helper cells

Some innate lymphocytes serve as environmental sensors and defenders of body surfaces. As such, they interact with the microbiota and can respond to foreign antigens immediately after they are produced. These innate lymphoid cells (ILCs) are critical components of the immune defenses. Many of these ILCs are helper cells that regulate immune responses to the intestinal microbiota and play important roles in allergic disease, autoimmunity, and obesity (Fig. 10.6).

Innate lymphoid cells, in their role as helper cells, play an important part in the very early stages of antimicrobial immune responses. They also contribute to tissue repair and defense as well as the maintenance of epithelial integrity on body surfaces (Colonna, 2018). These "helper" ILCs are classified into three types. Type 1 defends against viruses, intracellular bacteria, and parasites. Type 2 defends against

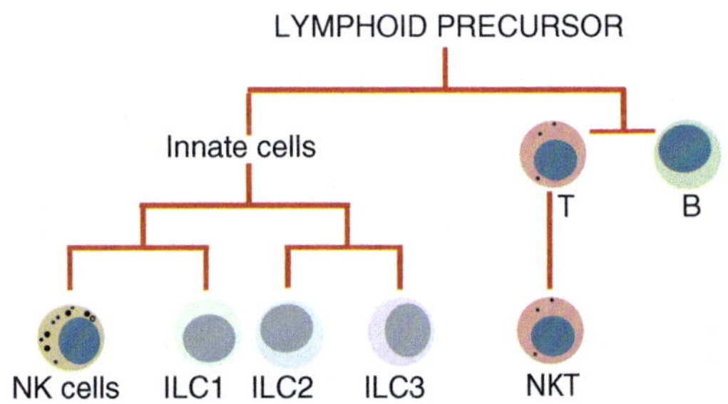

FIGURE 10.6

The diversity of different innate lymphoid cells in horses.

helminths, and type 3 cells promote immunity to extracellular bacteria (Artis & Spits, 2015).

Type 1 innate lymphoid cells

Type 1 ILCs are found in the liver as well as under body surfaces, such as beneath the surface of the intestinal mucosa, where they are scattered through the lamina propria. They develop from lymphoid stem cells through the use of the transcription factor T-bet. When stimulated, type 1 ILCs produce large amounts of the Th1-associated cytokines, interferon-γ and TNF-α. They do this in response to activation by IL-12, IL-15, and IL-18 from dendritic cells (DC1 cells). As a result, they can activate macrophages and trigger type 1 immune responses (Fig. 10.7). ILC1 cells differ from NK cells in that they do not produce perforins and so are not cytotoxic. ILC1 cells are however, essential for defense against many viruses, intracellular bacteria, and protozoa, and some cancers. They also antagonize type 2 immune responses (Nabekura & Shibuya, 2020). ILC1 cells can be converted into ILC3 cells by exposure to IL-23, IL-1β, and retinoic acid. Conversely, ILC3 cells may turn into ILC1 cells under the influence of IL-12, IL-15, and IL-18. NK cells are closely related to type 1 ILCs since they also produce IFN-γ and rely on T-bet for gene transcription. NK cells can be converted to ILC1 cells by exposure to TGF-β.

Type 2 ILCs

Type 2 ILCs are found in the lungs, skin, bone marrow, liver, mesenteric fat, and small intestine (Splits & Mjosberg, 2022) (Fig. 10.8). They arise from lymphoid

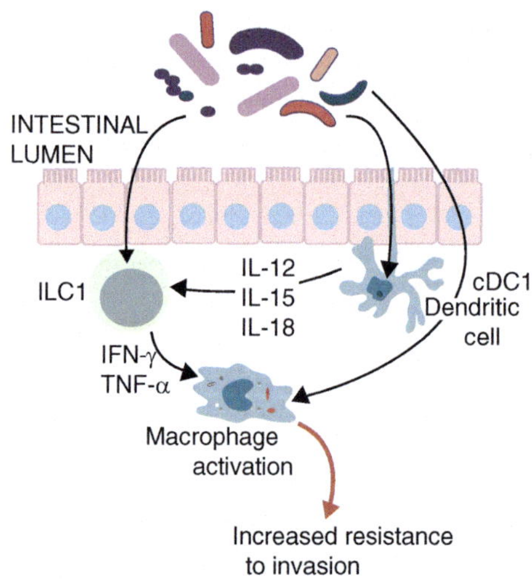

FIGURE 10.7

The functions of ILC-1 cells in protecting body surfaces.

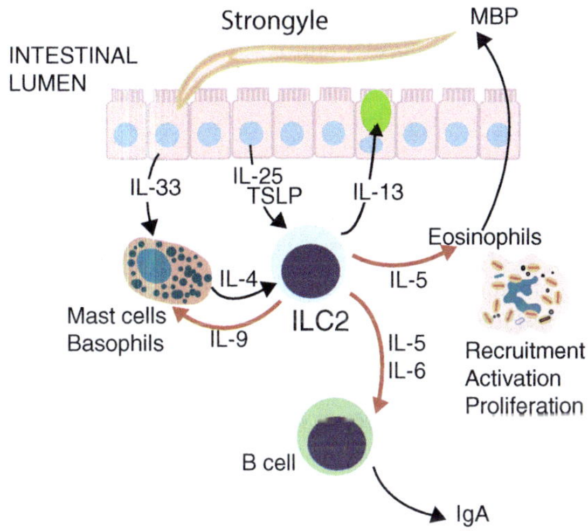

FIGURE 10.8

The functions of ILC2 cells and their role in antiparasite immunity.

stem cells through the use of two unique transcription factors, GATA-binding protein-3 (GATA3) and retinoic acid receptor-related orphan receptor-α (ROR-α). ILC2s produce large amounts of the Th2-associated cytokines IL-5 and IL-13 and smaller amounts of IL-4 and IL-9 in response to thymic stromal lymphopoietin (TSLP), IL-25, and IL-33 from epithelial cells. As such, they regulate the activities of Th2 cells, M2 macrophages, and eosinophils. ILC2 cells are required for the development of early innate immunity to parasitic helminths such as the equine Strongyles. (ILC2s are the major source of IL-13 during helminth infections) as well as regulating type 2 immune responses, such as asthma and allergic disease. ILC2s play a key role in regulating type 2 immunity. Thus, they control eosinophil production and so can induce an eosinophilia. They also promote mucus production by goblet cells, alternative activation of macrophages, and tissue repair (Jarick et al., 2022). ILC2s can be readily converted into ILC1s by IL-12, and this can be reversed by IL-4 (Belz, 2016). They express the characteristic ILC phenotype, $CD45^+$, $CD11b^-$, $CD5^-$, $CD21^-$, and $CD25^+$. ILC2 cells play a key role in the pathogenesis of equine Culicoides hypersensitivity (Chapter 19).

Type 3 ILCs

Type 3 ILCs are primarily involved in the defense of body surfaces. They are found in the mucosa of the gastrointestinal tract (lamina propria, tonsils, and Peyer's patches) as well as in the lungs and skin. They use RORγt as their transcription factor. ILC3s produce IL-17 and IL-22 in response to stimulation by TSLP and IL-23 and thus resemble Th17 cells in their cytokine profile. They play a central role in immunity on mucosal surfaces by responding to extracellular bacteria and fungi.

They do this by producing IL-22. On exposure to IL-22, enterocytes produce defensins that protect the intestinal epithelium. ILC3-derived IL-22 also inhibits T cell-mediated intestinal inflammation by suppressing those cells that respond to antigens from commensal bacteria. IL-22 from ILC3s also inhibits the growth of segmented filamentous bacteria (Chapter 14) (Valle-Noguera et al., 2021). They also play an important role in resistance to intestinal nematode infestations (Chapter 19).

Because they are required for the development of lymph nodes, Peyer's patches, and isolated lymphoid follicles, ILC3s also function as lymphoid tissue inducer (LTi) cells. In this role, they regulate the differentiation of B cells. They activate dendritic cells and so influence IgA class switching on surfaces. In the spleen, ILC3s express the B cell growth factors BAFF, APRIL, and CD40L and stimulate IgM production (Lane et al., 2009; Withers, 2011). There is also evidence for the presence of a population of innate regulatory cells (ILCregs) in the intestines that control inflammatory responses through the release of IL-10 (Wang et al., 2017).

References

Artis, D., & Spits, H. (2015). The biology of innate lymphoid cells. *Nature, 517*, 293–301.

Bekkering, S., Arts, R. J. W., Novakovic, B., et al. (2018). Metabolic induction of trained immunity through the mevalonate pathway. *Cell, 172*, 135–146.

Belz, G. T. (2016). ILC2s masquerade as ILC1s to drive chronic disease. *Nature Immunology, 17*, 611–612.

Bentley, E. G., Pugh, G., Gledhill, L. R., & Flynn, R. J. (2019). An analysis of the immune compartment within bovine adipose tissue. *Developmental & Comparative Immunology.* https://doi.org/10.1016/j.dci.2019.103411

Bubenikova, J., Plasil, M., Futas, J., Stejskalova, K., et al. (2024). Diversity of major histocompatibility complex (MHC) and natural killer cell receptor (NKR) genes and their interactions in domestic horses. *HLA.* https://doi.org/10.1111/tan.15387

Chong, Y. C., Duffus, W. P. H., & Hannant, D. (1992). Natural killer cells in normal horses and specific-pathogen-free foals infected with equine herpesvirus. *Veterinary Immunology and Immunopathology, 33*, 103–113.

Colonna, M. (2018). Innate lymphoid cells: Diversity, plasticity, and unique functions in immunity. *Immunity, 48*, 1104–1117.

Davis, E. G., Sang, Y., Rush, B., Zhang, G., & Blecha, F. (2005). Molecular cloning and characterization of equine NK-lysin. *Veterinary Immunology and Immunopathology, 105*, 163–169.

Dhodapkar, M. V., & Kumar, V. (2017). Type II NKT cells and their emerging role in health and disease. *Journal of Immunology, 198*, 1015–1021.

Dossa, R. G., Alperin, D. C., Garzon, D., Mealey, R. H., et al. (2015). In contrast to other species, α-galactosylceramide (α-GalCer) is not an immunostimulatory NKT cell agonist in horses. *Developmental & Comparative Immunology, 49*, 49–58.

Dossa, R. G., Alperin, D. C., Hines, M. T., & Hines, S. A. (2014). The equine CD1 gene family is the largest and most diverse yet identified. *Immunogenetics, 66*, 33–42.

Dotiwala, F., Santara, S. S., Binker-Cosen, A. A., Li, B., et al. (2017). Granzyme B disrupts central metabolism and protein synthesis in bacteria to promote an immune cell death program. *Cell, 171*, 1125–1137.

Edmans, M. D., Connelley, T. K., Morgan, S., Pedilongco, T. J., et al. (2024). MAIT cell-MR1 reactivity is highly conserved across multiple divergent species. *Journal of Biological Chemistry.* https://doi.org/10.1016/j.jbc.2024.107337

Enomoto, Y., Li, P., Jenkins, L. M., Anastasakis, D., et al. (2022). Cytokine-enhanced cytolytic activity of exosomes from NK cells. *Cancer Gene Therapy, 29*, 734–749.

Futas, J., & Horin, P. (2013). Natural killer cell receptor genes in the Family Equidae: Not only Ly49. *PLoS One*. https://doi.org/10.1371/journal.pone.0064736

Gagnier, L., Wilhelm, B. T., & Mager, D. L. (2003). Ly49 genes in non-rodent mammals. *Immunogenetics, 55*, 109–115.

Hao, L., Klein, J., & Nei, M. (2006). Heterogeneous but conserved natural killer receptor gene complexes m four orders of mammals. *Proceedings of the National Academy of Sciences of the United States of America, 103*(9), 3192–3197.

Harly, C., Robert, J., Legoux, F., & Lantz, O. (2022). γδT, NKY, and MAIT cells during evolution: Redundancy or specialized functions? *Journal of Immunology, 209*, 217–225.

Harris, D. T., Camenisch, T. D., Jaso-Friedmann, L., & Evans, D. L. (1993). Expression of an evolutionarily conserved function-associated molecule on sheep, horse, and cattle natural killer cells. *Veterinary Immunology and Immunopathology, 38*, 273282.

Horecky, C., Horecka, E., Horin, P., & Knoll, A. (2014). *NKR genes region and their genetic diversity in horses* (pp. 490–493). MendelNet.

Hormanski, C. E., Truax, R., Pourciau, S. S., Folsom, R. W., & Horohov, D. W. (1992). Induction of lymphokine activated killer cells of equine origin: Specificity for equine target cells. *Veterinary Immunology and Immunopathology, 32*, 25–36.

Hu, S., Xiang, D., Zhang, L., Wang, S., et al. (2022). The mechanisms and cross-protection of trained innate immunity. *Virology Journal*. https://doi.org/10.1186/s12985-022-01937-5

Jarick, K. J., Topczewska, P. M., Jakob, M. O., Yano, H., et al. (2022). Non-redundant functions of group 2 innate lymphoid cells. *Nature, 611*, 794–799.

Jaworska, J., de Mestre, A. M., Wisniewska, J., Wagner, B., et al. (2022). Populations of NK cells and regulatory T cells in the endometrium of cycling mares—A preliminary study. *Animals*. https://doi.org/10.3390/ani12233373

Katzmarski, N., Dominguez-Andres, J., Cirovic, B., Renieris, G., et al. (2021). Transmission of trained immunity and heterologous resistance to infections across generations. *Nature Immunology, 22*(11), 1382–1390.

Lane, P. J. L., McConnell, F. M., Withers, D., Gaspal, F., et al. (2009). Lymphoid tissue inducer cells: Bridges between the ancient innate and the modern adaptive immune systems. *Nature Immunology, 2*(6), 472–477.

Liu, C., Betancourt, A., Cohen, D. C., Adams, A. A., et al. (2011). Granzyme B-mRNA expression by equine lymphokine-activated killer cells is associated with the induction of apoptosis in target cells. *Veterinary Immunology and Immunopathology, 143*, 108–115.

Lunn, D. P., Schram, B. R., Vagnoni, K. E., Schobert, C. S., et al. (1996). Positive selection of EqCD8+ precursors increases equine lymphokine-activated killing. *Veterinary Immunology and Immunopathology, 53*, 1–13.

Mace, E. M. (2023). Human natural killer cells: Form, function and development. *The Journal of Allergy and Clinical Immunology, 151*(2), 371–385.

Magnuson, M. S., Perryman, L. E., Wyatt, C. R., Mason, P. H., & Talmadge, J. E. (1987). Large granular lymphocytes from SCID horses develop potent cytotoxic activity after treatment with human recombinant interleukin 2. *Journal of Immunology, 139*(1), 61–67.

Mody, C. H., Ogbomo, H., Xiang, R. F., Kyei, S. K., et al. (2019). Microbial killing by NK cells. *Journal of Leukocyte Biology, 105*, 1285–1296.

Moorlag, S., Roring, R. J., Joosten, L. A. B., & Netea, M. G. (2018). The role of the interleukin-1 family in trained immunity. *Immunological Reviews, 281*, 28–39.

Nabekura, T., & Shibuya, A. (2020). Type I innate lymphoid cells: Soldiers at the front line of immunity. *Biomedical Journal, 44*(2), 115–122.

Netea, M. G., Joosten, L. A., Latz, E., Mills, K. H., et al. (2016). Trained immunity: A program of innate immune memory in health and disease. *Science, 352*, aaf1098.

Noronha, L. E., Harman, R. M., Wagner, B., & Antczak, D. F. (2012). Generation and characterization of monoclonal antibodies to equine NKp46. *Veterinary Immunology and Immunopathology, 147*(1–2), 60–68.

Noronha, L. E., Huggler, K. E., de Mestre, A. M., Miller, D. C., & Antczak, D. F. (2012). Molecular evidence for natural killer-like cells in equine endometrial cups. *Placenta, 33*, 379–386.

Piuko, K., Bravo, I. G., & Muller, M. (2007). Identification and characterization of equine granzyme B. *Veterinary Immunology and Immunopathology, 118*, 239–251.

Porcelli, S. A., & Modlin, R. L. (1999). The CD1 system: Antigen-presenting molecules for T cell recognition of lipids and glycolipids. *Annual Review of Immunology, 17*, 297–329.

Reinink, P., & Van Rhijn, I. (2016). Mammalian CD1 and MR1 genes. *Immunogenetics, 68*, 515–523.

Schwartz, J. C., Gibson, M. S., Heimeier, D., & Koren, S. (2017). The evolution of the natural killer complex: A comparison between mammals using new high-quality genome assemblies and targeted annotation. *Immunogenetics, 69*, 255–269.

Splits, H., & Mjosberg, J. (2022). Heterogeneity of type 2 innate lymphoid cells. *Nature Reviews Immunology, 22*, 701–712.

Takahashi, T., Yawata, M., Raudsepp, T., et al. (2004). Natural killer cell receptors in the horse: Evidence for the existence of multiple transcribed *LY49* genes. *European Journal of Immunology, 34*, 773–784.

Valle-Noguera, A., Ochoa-Ramos, A., Gomez-Sanchez, M. J., & Cruz-Adalia, A. (2021). Type 3 innate lymphoid cells as regulators of the host-pathogen interaction. *Frontiers in Immunology*. https://doi.org/10.3389/fimmu.2021.748851

Van Beeck, F. A. L., Reinink, P., Hermsen, R., Zajonc, D., et al. (2009). Functional CD1d and/or NKT invariant chain transcript in horse, pig, African elephant, and Guinea pig, but not in ruminants. *Molecular Immunology, 46*, 1424–1431.

Vivieros, M. M., & Antczak, D. F. (1999). Characterization of equine natural killer and IL-2 stimulated lymphokine activated killer cell populations. *Developmental & Comparative Immunology, 23*, 521–532.

Vychodilova, L., Plasil, M., Futas, J., Kopeka, A., et al. (2025). Genetic susceptibility to sarcoid in Arabian horses: Associations with MHC class II and compound MHC class I/KLRA genotypes. *Veterinary Research Communications*. https://doi.org/10.1007/s11259-025-10748-2

Wang, S., Xia, P., Chen, Y., Qu, Y., et al. (2017). Regulatory innate lymphoid cells control innate intestinal inflammation. *Cell, 171*, 201–216.

Wegrecki, M. (2023). CD1a-mediated immunity from a molecular perspective. *Molecular Immunology, 158*, 43–53.

Withers, D. R. (2011). Lymphoid tissue inducer cells. *Current Biology, 21*(10), RR381–R382.

Zajonc, D. M. (2016). The CD1 family: Serving lipid antigens to T cells since the Mesozoic era. *Immunogenetics, 68*(8), 561–576.

CHAPTER

The equine B cell system 11

B cells are the lymphocytes whose function is to synthesize and secrete antibodies in response to antigens. In order to recognize antigens, they express specific antigen receptors on their surface (BCRs). B cells must first be activated by the binding of a specific antigen to these receptors, and at the same time receive appropriate assistance from cytokines produced by helper T cells. Provided the B cell receptors can bind to the presented antigen and they receive appropriate costimulation, the B cells will multiply repeatedly, and differentiate into plasma cell and memory cell populations. The plasma cells eventually secrete large quantities of specific antibodies. Antibodies are immunoglobulins that have the ability to bind strongly to specific foreign antigens. These bound antibodies then promote complement activation, virus and toxin neutralization and phagocytosis leading ultimately to the elimination of any invaders.

Immunoglobulin structure

Immunoglobulins are glycoproteins of about 160 kDa consisting of four linked peptide chains. These chains consist of two identical pairs: two heavy chains, each about 55 kDa in size, and two light chains, of about 25 kDa. The light chains are linked by disulfide bonds to the heavy chains so that the complete molecule forms the letter Y. The tail of the Y (called the Fc region) is formed from the paired heavy chains and attaches to the B cell surface. The arms of the Y (called the Fab regions) are formed by paired light and heavy chains, and they bind antigens. The antigen-binding sites are formed by the grooves between the light and heavy chains. When expressed on B cell surfaces they serve as antigen receptors. TThus, each B cell antigen receptor (BCR)/immunoglobulin molecule has two identical antigen-binding sites (Fig. 11.1).

Light chains

Immunoglobulin light chains are constructed from two domains, each containing about 110 amino acids. The amino acid sequences in the light chain C-terminal domains in the BCRs from different B cells are identical and are called constant domains (C_L). In contrast, the sequences in the N-terminal domains differ in each B cell and so form variable domains (V_L). Horses make two types of light chains,

The Immunology of Horses and Donkeys. https://doi.org/10.1016/B978-0-443-44863-8.00011-9

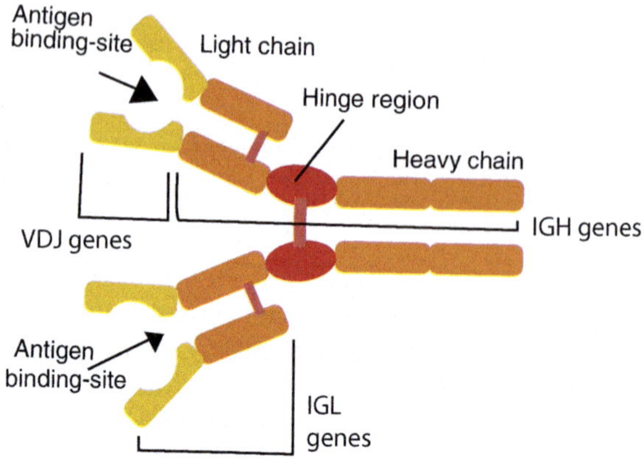

FIGURE 11.1 The structure of equine IgG and the regions coded for by specific genes.

Unlike other proteins, immunoglobulins are encoded by multiple genes. The antigen binding sites are encoded by V, D. and J genes. The remainder of the molecule is encoded by light and heavy chain constant region genes.

called κ (kappa) and λ (lambda). Although their amino acid sequences are different, they are functionally identical. The ratio of κ to λ chains in BCRs varies among the mammals. Horses employ 92% λ chains.

Heavy chains

Immunoglobulin heavy chains are constructed from four or five protein domains, each of about 90–100 amino acids. The N-terminal domain is the variable (V_H) domain. The remaining three or four domains show few sequence differences and thus are constant (C_H) domains.

Equine B cells make five different classes of heavy chains that differ in their heavy chain sequence and domain structure. As a result, each antibody class has a different biological activity. The five different immunoglobulin heavy chains are called α, γ, δ, ε, and μ. These heavy chains determine the immunoglobulin class (or isotype). Thus, immunoglobulin molecules that use α heavy chains are called immunoglobulin A (IgA), and those that use γ chains are called IgG; μ chains are used in IgM, δ chains in IgD, and ε chains in IgE.

Variable domains

Immunoglobulin variable region domains are each encoded by three genes, called variable (V), diversity (D) and joining (J), genes. They are attached to the constant region gene (C). The combination of the 4 V, D, J, and C genes requires three joining sites. These sites encode the amino acid sequences where antigens bind. Because their shapes must match that of the antigen, they are termed complementarity-determining regions (CDRs) and are numbered from 1 to 3. When the sequences of the V domains from light and heavy chains are examined in detail, two features become apparent. First, their sequence variation is largely confined to the three CDRs, each containing 6 to 10 amino acids, within the variable domain. These CDR regions are said to be hypervariable. Between the three hypervariable regions are relatively constant sequences called framework regions. The hypervariable regions in the paired light and heavy chains determine the shape of the antigen-binding site and thus the specificity of antigen binding. Each V-domain is folded in such a way that its three CDRs come into close contact with the bound antigen (Fig. 11.2). In general, CDR3 contributes most to antigen-binding.

Constant domains

Mammals employ different antibody molecules for different tasks. These differences are determined by the shape, size, and functionality of their heavy chains. For example, the number of constant domains differs between immunoglobulin heavy chain classes. There are three constant domains in a γ heavy chain; they are labeled, from the N-terminal end, as C_H1, C_H2, and C_H3. Three constant domains are also found in α and most δ chains, whereas μ and ε chains have a fourth constant domain called C_H4.

Since heavy chains are paired, the domains in each chain come together to form structures by which antibody molecules can exert their biological functions. Thus, the paired V_H and V_L domains together form the antigen-binding site, while the

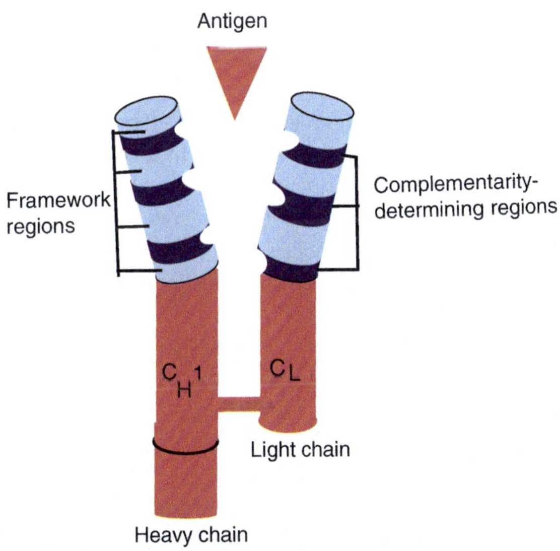

FIGURE 11.2

How paired light and heavy chains come together so that their complementarity determining regions form the antigen binding site immunoglobulins possess two of these.

C_H1 and C_L domains together stabilize the antigen-binding site. The paired C_H2 domains of IgG contain a site that activates the classical complement pathway (Chapter 3) and a site that binds to Fc receptors on phagocytic cells. The paired domains on the heavy chains also regulate the transfer of IgG into colostrum and antibody-mediated cellular cytotoxicity. When immunoglobulin molecules act as B cell receptors, their Fc region is embedded in the B cell surface membrane. These cell-bound immunoglobulins differ from the secreted form in that they have a small transmembrane domain attached to their C-terminus. This contains the hydrophobic amino acids that link it to the B cell-membrane lipids.

The Hinge region

One important feature of immunoglobulin molecules is that their Fab regions can swing freely around the center of the molecule as if hinged. This hinge consists of a short domain of about 12 amino acids located between the C_H1 and C_H2 domains. The hinge region contains many hydrophilic and proline residues that cause the peptide chain to unfold and make this region readily accessible to proteases. This region also contains the interchain disulfide bonds that bind the four peptide chains together. Proline, because of its configuration, produces a 90-degree bend when inserted in a polypeptide chain. Because amino acids can rotate around peptide bonds, the effect of closely spaced proline residues is to produce a flexible joint around which the immunoglobulin chains can swing freely. The μ chains of horse IgM do not possess a hinge region.

Heavy chain genes

The horse immunoglobulin heavy chain gene locus (IGH) is about 190 kb in size and is located on chromosome ECA 24q. It is arranged in reverse orientation. It contains the genes containing the variable regions in addition to eleven genes encoding all the heavy chains. Repeated duplication of the IGHG heavy chain loci has resulted in the production of seven functional IgG subclass genes in the horse (Wagner et al., 2004). All seven of these G genes are expressed, in addition to the four other heavy chain genes, M, D, A, and E (Wagner, 2009) (Fig. 11.3).

The seven IgG subclasses are designated IgG1 through IgG7. The order of the seven IGHG genes in the horse is 5′-G1-G2- G3- G7-G4-G6-G5-3’. This nomenclature is relatively recent. Previously, the IgG subclasses were labeled by letters, e.g., a, b, c, and T (Table 11.1).

IgG1: This major immunoglobulin subclass is the only one produced in the fetal foal. It is present in serum, colostrum and milk at moderately high concentrations. IgG1 acts like IgM in primary immune responses and appears to participate in both Th1 and Th2-mediated antibody responses (Wagner, 2024).

IgG2 is a minor subclass present in very low concentrations in normal horse serum and very little is known about its biological properties (Wagner, 2006).

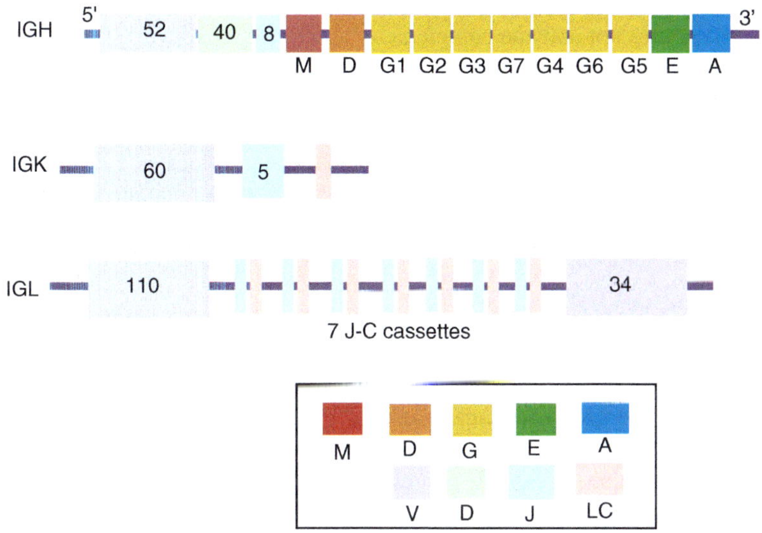

FIGURE 11.3 The organization of the equine immunoglobulin gene loci.

Both horses and donkeys possess seven IgG heavy chain genes.

Table 11.1 Horse IgG nomenclature.

New name	G1	G2	G3	G4	G5	G6	G7
Old name	IgGa	–	IgG(T)	IgGb	IgG(T)	IgGc	IgGb

IgG3 and IgG5 are very closely related. These were originally considered a single subclass classified as IgG(T). Much of the available literature does not distinguish between IgG3 and IgG5 so they are commonly referred to as IgG3/5. IGG3 has a longer hinge region than the other IgG subclasses. IgG5 shares some functional similarity with IgG3. For example both can readily activate the leukocyte respiratory burst through their Fc receptors. IgG3 is a potent activator of the classical complement pathway (Lewis, Meehan, et al., 2008).

IgG7 is adjacent to and closely related to IgG4 and likely resulted from a recent duplication ofthe IGHG4 gene. They share 96% sequence homology, and the major sequence difference is in their hinge region. Because they are so closely related, they cannot be distinguished serologically (hence their original classification was IgGb and they are now IgG4/7. The relative expression ratio of IgG7 to IgG4 is 1:1.6. This duplication event has been detected in all horse breeds examined to date, including both Thoroughbred horses and the isolated population of Icelandic horses (Wagner et al., 2004). Thus, the IGHG4/7 duplication event occurred more than 1000 years ago (Lewis, Meehan, et al., 2008).

IgG6 is a minor isotype present in low concentrations in normal horse serum and colostrum. It does not activate complement or activate leukocytes (Lewis, Wagner, & Woof, 2008).

Horses also express the four other immunoglobulin classes, IgM, IgD, IgA, and IgE. The equine IgM locus spans 1472 bp and encodes 451 amino acids. Its C_H3 and C_H4 exons are highly conserved. The horse IGHD gene is located 5 kb downstream from IGHM. It spans about 9.1 kb and contains eight exons that are very similar in sequence to human IgD, namely,

$$-C_H1\text{-}H1\text{-}H2\text{-}C_H2\text{-}C_H3\text{-}\ S\text{-}M1\text{-}M2\text{-}$$

Overall, equine IgD shows 64% homology with the human IgD gene (Wagner et al., 2004). As in humans, no switch region has been detected upstream of the IGHD gene. Thus, IGHD is located very close to the IGHM gene, and it is possible that long pre-messenger transcripts might be generated first and then subjected to alternative splicing or processing. IgD appears to be expressed at least at the mRNA level in equine B cells. If expressed at the protein level, equine IgD levels are probably very low.

The equine IgE locus is similar to the IgM locus in that there is no separate hinge region for IgE, and flexibility is conferred by the C_H2 domain. Interestingly, IgE concentrations in the bloodstream are about 1000-fold higher in normal horses than in normal humans (Wagner et al., 2004).

The horse IgA locus contains three exons. These encode two constant domains and a single hinge region. The hinge region is an extension of the $C\alpha 2$ domain. IgA is found in horse serum as well as in the mucosal secretions, as in other mammals (Wagner, 2009). The IgA in mucosal secretions is produced in the form of secretory IgA. That is a dimer connected by a 17 kDa joining (J) chain. It is transported onto mucosal surfaces by the polymeric Ig receptor (pIgR), a type I transmembrane glycoprotein. The extracellular component of the pIgR is cleaved off to form secretory component, which then protects the IgA against destruction by bacterial proteases. Both the equine J chain and pIgR have been characterized. The J chain contains four exons while pIgR contains 11. Their genes have been mapped to equine chromosomes ECA3 and ECA5 respectively (Lewis et al., 2010). Many of the functions of IgA are mediated through its specific receptor, FcαR, also called CD89. This receptor has been identified and characterized in the horse, where its gene is located on chromosome ECA10 (Morton et al., 2005). The genes encoding the other immunoglobulin Fc receptors are located on equine chromosome ECA5.

Variable region genes

As in other mammals, the antigen-binding immunoglobulin variable domains are encoded by three separate genes; variable (V), diversity (D), and joining (J) (Vadnais et al., 2017). These are joined in the order V-D-J and then connected to the appropriate constant (C) region genes. The IGH locus in the horse contains a total of 57 IGHV genes, 46 IGHD genes, and 9 IGHJ genes. IGMT) (Sinkora et al., 2022).

IGHV

The 57 IGV genes in the equine IGH locus can be classified into seven subfamilies based on sequence similarities. These horse IGHV subfamilies belong to all three mammalian clans (Sun et al., 2010). Thus, subfamilies 1 and 5 belong to clan I; subfamilies 2, 4, 6, and 7, to clan II, and subfamily 3 belongs to clan III. Note that clan III IGHV segments are found in all mammals, including camels, rabbits, platypus, opossums, and pigs. In humans and mice, clan III is preferentially expressed during fetal life, so these IGHV genes may play a role in the development of the foal's immune system. While horse subfamily 3 has at least 10 members, none appear to be functional (Kirkham et al., 1992). Examination of the equine B cell repertoire indicates that horses prefer to use the IGHV2 subfamily which is expressed in 92.49% of B cells and IGLV8, which is found in 8.25% of them. A CDR3 extended loop structure also predominates in the horse (Manso et al., 2018).

IGHD

There are 46 IGHD genes in the IGH locus, of which 16 are functional. 28 are open reading frames (ORFs). (ORFs are gene sequences that begin with a start codon and end with a stop codon. Their sequences probably encode a gene and interestingly, none are yet considered pseudogenes.) The 46 identified D genes are among the largest number recorded in mammals (although elephants have 87) (Walther et al., 2015). The horse IGHD genes range from 18 to 48 bp in length. This is longer than in humans (11–37 bp) but significantly shorter than in cattle. Horses, therefore, predominantly employ gene recombination.

IGHJ

Of the nine equine IGHJ genes, six are functional while three are open reading frames.

Light chain genes

As pointed out above, horses employ 92% lambda light chains and only 8% kappa light chains. The ratio of Vλ to Vκ genes corresponds to the preponderance of lambda chain use in horse serum, where the ratio is 19:1 (Walther et al., 2015). As a result, the kappa chains are much less diverse than the lambda chains. For example, the equine kappa light chain gene locus (IGK) contains 60 IGKV, five IGKJ, and one IGKC genes. It is arranged in a single cluster of 820 kb. On the other hand, the lambda light chain locus (IGL) contains seven IGLC genes, each preceded by a single IGLJ gene and 144 IGLV genes divided into two clusters, both upstream and downstream of the J-C cluster. They extend for 1310 kb on chromosome ECA8. Each of the seven lambda J gene segments is associated with a constant gene (Walther et al., 2015). Horses preferentially use IGLV8.

The two clusters of V lambda genes are arranged in opposite transcriptional orientations. Within each cluster, there are both functional genes and pseudogenes. There are many more open reading frames (ORFs) and pseudogenes than functional IGLV genes. However, allotypic and allelic variants are seen in IGLC1, IGLC5, and IGLC6/7. Two IGLV pseudogenes are also transcribed. These pseudogenes may also be used for gene conversion. V gene usage appears not to change throughout the animal's life, although sequence diversity increases as foals develop from fetuses to adults (Tallmadge et al., 2013).

B cell antigen receptors

As described in Chapter 2, B cells expressing IgM receptors for foreign antigens can be found in the spleen of fetal foals as early as 90 days of gestation. Eventually, the primary site of B-cell lymphogenesis switches to the bone marrow. Here, the B cells undergo diversification and selection. They undergo preliminary diversification, where the appropriate genes are joined together to encode complete heavy chains. A significant increase in immunoglobulin diversity occurs during the long fetal life in the horse, especially through the last two-thirds of gestation, despite the absence of stimulation by foreign antigens. This diversity begins increasing about day 120 of gestation and is focused on the third heavy chain complementarity-determining region (CDR3). In neonatal foals, the diversity increases in the second CDR as well. In adult animals, variation in the first CDR increases belatedly, although it is usually much less diverse than are CDRs 2 and 3. This increase in diversity results from the differential usage of the three V-region genes. Some V, D, and J genes are used predominantly throughout life, and changes in relative gene usage do not occur as horses age (Walther et al., 2015).

Receptor diversity

The most obvious way to generate immunoglobulin V-region diversity is to select 1 V gene segment at random from the available pool and join it to one randomly selected J segment; a process called recombination. Since many V and J segments are available, the number of possible combinations can be very large. For example, if there are 57 V segments, 46 D segments, and 9 J segments, then $57 \times 46 \times 9 = 23{,}598$ different V region configurations can be constructed simply by random selection.

Although random recombination of two or three gene segments generates much V-region diversity, additional mechanisms increase this diversity still further. This process is called somatic hypermutation. For example, endonucleases can remove nucleotides randomly from the cut ends of the genes before they rejoin. This results in changes in their nucleotide sequence at the splice site and variations in the amino acid sequence in the V region. Alternatively, multiple additional nucleotides may be inserted at the splice site and so greatly increase junctional diversity.

Analysis of the diversity of equine B cells has revealed 248,169 unique IgM clones and 66,141 unique IgG clones from four adult horses. These appeared to account for about 50%–80% of their total IgM and IgG (Navas et al., 2022). However, about 80% of these antibodies used only three IGHV genes! and 55% used only one IGHJ gene segment. This limited VJ diversity is compensated for by the junctional diversity in these regions. The length of the J region is longer in horses than in other domestic mammals, and nucleotide addition ranges from 0 to 111 nucleotides! Around 45% of the antibody clones have more than 10 nucleotides inserted in the junctional region. Thus, junctional diversity is critically important in the horse.

The degree to which a B cell responds to an antigen is directly related to the strength (affinity) with which its receptors bind that antigen. The better the fit between the antigen and its receptor, the greater will be the stimulus received by the B cell. If a BCR cannot bind an antigen, the B cell will not be stimulated and will die. In contrast, those B cells whose receptors bind antigens with a high affinity survive and proliferate. Thus, as B cells respond to an antigen, successive cycles of mutation and selection of the highest-affinity receptors eventually generate populations of B cells producing very-high-affinity antibodies. Somatic hypermutation does not, however, begin until after B cells have switched from making IgM to making either IgG or IgA. This suggests that the mutation mechanism is not activated until after a responding B cell has committed to utilizing a specific heavy chain V gene. As a result, the affinity of IgM antibodies does not increase during a primary immune response, whereas the affinity of IgG antibodies does.

As foals develop and encounter a universe of foreign antigens, their immunoglobulin repertoire must expand accordingly. Studies on these changes in the repertoire suggest that there is similar usage of IGHV, IGHD, and IGHJ genes throughout life. However, some genes are more favored than others. Thus, the segments predominantly used include IGHV2S3, IGHD18S1, and IGHJ1S5. heavy chain CDR3 lengths do not change significantly either. As expected, immunoglobulin diversity increases significantly during the transition from fetal to newborn stages at a time when a foal is undergoing microbial colonization (Tallmadge et al., 2013).

B cell origins

Lymphoid stem cells first appear in the fetal omentum, liver, and yolk sac of the developing foal. In older fetuses and adult horses, these stem cells move to the bone marrow. The bone marrow has multiple functions in adult mammals. It is a hematopoietic organ containing the precursors of all blood cells, including lymphocytes. It is also a primary lymphoid organ (a site where newly produced lymphocytes can mature). For example, in the horse, it contains B cell precursors as well as immature forms of these cells. The marrow is fully functional in adult horses, and B-cell lymphogenesis occurs there throughout their adult life. Equine B cells are mainly derived from $CD34^+$ stem cells located in the bone marrow (Schwab et al., 2017).

While equine B cells are mainly derived from bone marrow stem cells, a second source of B cells is the developing thymus, which contains a significant plasma cell population. Small numbers (~1%) of immunoglobulin-positive B cells are present in the developing horse thymus. Thus, the first immunoglobulin-secreting cells can be found in the fetal thymus at 67 days of gestation. Unlike fetal splenic B cells that only produce IgM, these thymic cells undergo spontaneous class switching (Chapter 8).

The ileal Peyer's patches do not appear to be a significant source of B cells in the horse, unlike the situation in the artiodactyls. (Their surgical removal resulted in no reduction in serum immunoglobulin levels.) The early pre-immune antibody repertoire in foals is relatively limited, with only 224 VH genes accounting for more than 90% of the immunoglobulin variation. Most of this initial diversity is accounted for by heavy chain V gene recombination, but is subsequently greatly expanded by somatic hypermutation (Faili et al., 2002; Papavasiliou & Schatz, 2002).

The presence of the intestinal microbiota significantly promotes the development and diversity of equine B cells, whose numbers within the gastrointestinal tract, especially the ileal Peyer's patch, increase greatly during the first 2 weeks of age. However, B cell receptor diversity may not increase significantly until 4–6 weeks of age.

Equine B cells express CD20 and MHC class II molecules in addition to their antigen receptors. The majority of equine peripheral blood B cells are unusual in that they also express the transcription factor, T-bet (T box expressed in T cells) (Patel et al., 2021). T-bet expression evolved long before the emergence of the adaptive immune system. It is normally expressed in helper T cells where it plays a role in regulating the expression of IFN-γ (Lazarevic et al., 2013). T-bet expression is usually associated with chronic infections and inflammation in humans and mice. In humans, when T cells proliferate and mutate in response to antigenic stimulation, T-bet$^+$ memory B cells develop and promote B cell survival by regulating the transcription of the mature B cell receptor and thus regulating immunoglobulin class switching. T-bet also drives the migration of some B cells to sites of inflammation. In horses, about half of these T-bet$^+$ B cells express IgM, a quarter express IgG, while the remainder express neither (Lazarevic et al., 2013).

B cell activation

The immunoglobulin components of antigen receptors cannot signal directly to their B cell since their cytoplasmic domains contain only three amino acids. However, their C_H4 and transmembrane domains are linked to two glycoprotein heterodimers formed by pairing CD79a (Ig-α) with CD79b (Ig-β). These CD79 heterodimers act as signal transducers (Figure 11.4). The CD79β chains are identical in all BCRs (Clark et al., 1992). Antigen binding and cross-linking of two antigen receptors expose immunoreceptor tyrosine-based activating motifs (ITAMs) on both CD79α and CD79β. Phosphorylation of these ITAMs by src kinases leads to

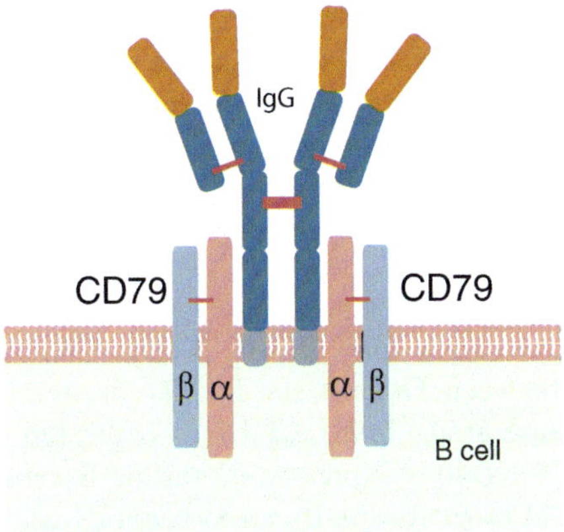

FIGURE 11.4

The structure of the BCR antigen receptor and its signal transduction component CD79.

phosphorylation of phospholipase C and a G-protein. Subsequent hydrolysis of phosphatidylinositol and calcium mobilization generates protein kinase C and calcineurin and activates the transcription factors NF-κB and NF-AT (Tedder et al., 1994). This eventually results in B cell mitosis and immunoglobulin production,—provided the B cell also receives appropriate costimulation from other sources (Gold, 2002).

Costimulation

Although the binding of an antigen to a B cell receptor is an essential first step in B cell activation, this alone is insufficient to fully activate B cells. Complete activation of a B cell also requires multiple signals from other sources. Thus, it requires costimulation by helper T cells and their cytokines; by complement; and by TLRs.

T cell help

When helper T cells provide "help" to B cells, they signal through multiple pathways to promote B cell functions. These signals result in increased B cell expression of BCRs and MHC class II molecules, as well as the receptors for IL-4, IL-5, IL-6, tumor necrosis factor-α (TNF-α), and transforming growth factor-β (TGF-β). They initiate the process that leads to B cell division and differentiation into antibody-secreting plasma cells. The helper T cells provide B cells with signals from secreted cytokines as well as through interacting receptor pairs. T-cell signals also trigger B-cell somatic mutation and immunoglobulin class switching within germinal centers and thus eventually increase antibody binding affinity (Willis-Karp & Finkelman, 2015).

Type 2 helper T (Th2) cells produce multiple cytokines that activate B cells. The most important of these are interleukin-4 (IL-4), IL-5, IL-6, IL-13, and IL-21. To provide these signals, however, the helper T cells must themselves be stimulated by the antigen. This antigen can be presented to them by the professional antigen-presenting cells, such as dendritic cells, macrophages, or even by B cells. Thus, a B cell can capture and process an antigen, present it to a T cell, and then receive co-stimulation from the same T cell.

Cell-cell signaling

Cytokine signaling alone cannot fully activate B cells. Complete activation also requires direct contact between Th cells and B cells through receptor pairs such as CD40 and CD154 (Durie et al., 1994). CD154 is expressed on activated helper T cells, while its receptor CD40 is expressed on resting B cells. CD40 must receive a signal from CD154 in order for the B cell to begin its cell cycle and upregulate its expression of IL-4 and IL-5 receptors. The signals from CD154 then synergize with those from IL-5 receptors to drive B cell activation, memory cell development, and immunoglobulin class switching. Another cell surface molecule, CD28, also found on helper T cells, must also provide co-stimulation by signaling through CD86 on activated B cells. Cross-linking of two IgM BCRs by an antigen will also promote B cell activation (Figure 11.5).

Equine CD40 is a protein of 280 amino acids encoded by a gene located on chromosome ECA22. Its ligand, CD154, consists of 261 amino acids and is encoded by a gene on the X chromosome. CD28 is a cell membrane glycoprotein of 220 amino acids, encoded by a gene on ECA 18. CD86 is a protein encoded by a gene on chromosome ECA11.

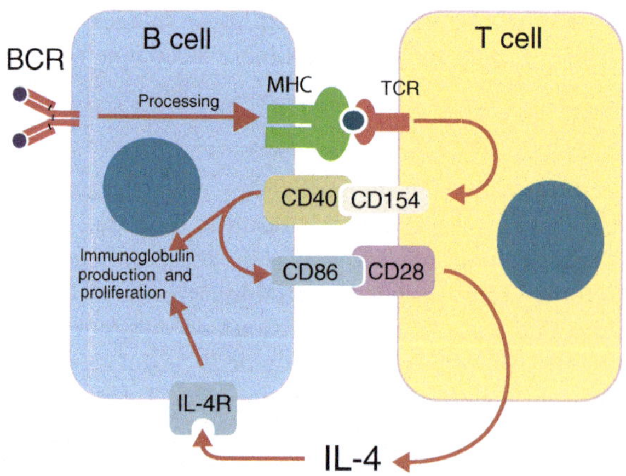

FIGURE 11.5

The multiple conversations and interactions between a helper T cell and a B cell that are required to trigger the B cell response.

Complement help

Effective co-stimulation of B cells also requires signals from the complement system transmitted through the receptor complex CD21/CD19 expressed on the B cell surface. CD21 is a receptor (CR2) whose ligand is C3d. CD19 is its accompanying signaling component. If an antigen with C3d attached binds to CD21, a signal is transmitted through CD19 to the B cell. Stimulation of a BCR plus CD19/CD21 effectively lowers the threshold for B cell activation 100-fold (Figure 11.6).

Toll-like receptor help

Although BCR-antigen-binding plus T cell co-stimulation triggers initial B cell division, this alone cannot induce a prolonged, self-sustaining B cell response. Complete and prolonged activation of B cells also requires coordinated signals from their toll-like receptors (TLRs) (Hayashi et al., 2005). The B–cell–stimulating ligands include flagellins, lipopolysaccharides, and CpG DNA. Signaling through TLR4 enhances B cell antigen presentation, promotes germinal center formation, and is required for optimal antibody production against T-dependent antigens. TLR signaling to memory B cells increases antibody production, but it does not appear to be required for IgA or IgE production. Thus, TLR signaling can substitute in part for T cell help (Pasare & Medzhitov, 2005). The B cell expression of TLRs does, however, differ between subpopulations. For example, TLR2, TLR7, and TLR9 are expressed on all B cell subsets. TLR3 is only expressed on B1-like cells, while TLR4 is expressed only on conventional (B2) cells.

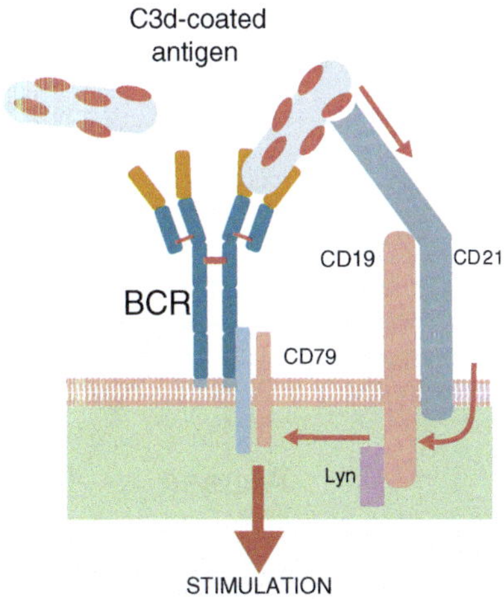

FIGURE 11.6 The role of complement in stimulating B cell responses.

Antigen-bound C3d acts through the CD21⁻CD19 receptor complex.

B cell inhibition

The B cell Fc receptor, FcγRIIb, is a negative regulator of B cell function. When an IgG molecule binds and links this receptor to a BCR through an antigen, it inhibits the B cell response and antibody formation. This acts as a negative feedback system that prevents an excessive and unnecessary antibody response. This also has important practical consequences when vaccinating young animals in the presence of maternal antibodies (Chapter 2). Maternal antibodies block foal antibody responses including those induced by vaccines. Vaccination must be delayed until maternal antibodies have gone.

B cell responses

Once it receives the appropriate stimuli from the multiple sources described above, the B cell is triggered to respond by dividing repeatedly and differentiating into plasma cells and memory cells (Figure 11.7).

The activated B cell antigen receptor produces a tunable signal. That is, it generates signals whose intensity depends on the antigen binding affinity and the degree of co-stimulation received. The affinity of a BCR for its antigen thus greatly influences B cell proliferation and antibody secretion. On the other hand, receptor occupancy influences MHC class II expression and signal transduction. The direction of the immunoglobulin class switch also depends on signals received from Th1 or Th2 cytokines.

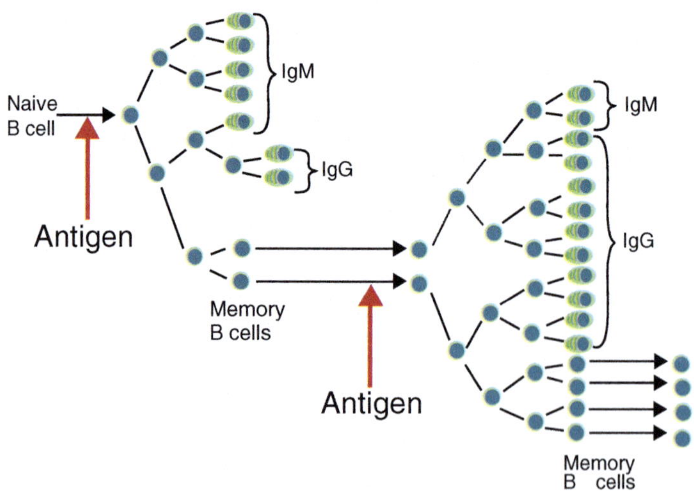

FIGURE 11.7 A typical antigen-driven B cell response.

It generates both antibody producing plasma cells as well as memory cell populations.

Certain antigens can provoke antibody formation in the absence of helper T cells. These so-called T-independent antigens are usually simple repeating polymers such as bacterial lipopolysaccharides and polymerized Salmonella flagellin. These T-independent antigens can bind directly to B-cell TLRs and cross-link multiple BCRs, thus providing a sufficient signal for B-cell proliferation. Characteristically, T-independent antigens only trigger IgM responses and fail to generate memory cells.

It is appropriate to emphasize at this stage that the BCR has the same antigen-binding ability as antibody molecules. Thus, antibodies can bind free intact antigens in solution. This is very different from the α/β T cell receptor, which can only bind processed antigen fragments bound to an MHC molecule. This difference in the antigen-binding ability of B and T cells is significant in that B cells can respond to a greater variety of antigens than T cells. Likewise, antibodies are directed, not against fragments of antigens, but against intact antigen molecules. Antigen-antibody interactions usually depend on the maintenance of the conformation of an antigen if the invader is to be bound and effectively neutralized.

The term clonotype is used to describe a clone of B cells expressing a BCR capable of responding to a single epitope. A newborn foal with few B cells has available only a limited variety of clonotypes, but their diversity increases with age and antigen exposure as a result of increased use of alternative sets of V genes and of somatic hypermutation. This increase in diversity is also stimulated by signals from the intestinal microbiota. In an adult horse, the number of B cells within a given clonotype depends on their exposure to different antigens over the animal's lifetime. Thus, the most used clonotypes will increase greatly in number. Conversely, a completely novel antigen may encounter very few responsive B cells in the spleen or bone marrow of a naive adult horse.

When appropriately stimulated and co-stimulated, B cells undergo repeated division. The B cell division that results from this is asymmetric, since the daughter cell at one pole binds a lot of antigen, while the daughter cell at the opposite pole binds very little or none. The cell that binds the antigen then differentiates into a plasma cell. The daughter cell at the opposite pole that binds very little antigen continues the cycle of dividing and mutating and eventually becomes a memory cell. The cells destined to become plasma cells develop a rough endoplasmic reticulum, increase their rate of protein synthesis, and secrete large quantities of immunoglobulins. Within a few days, these responding cells switch from making IgM to making another immunoglobulin class. This switch occurs within the germinal center and leads to the production of IgG subclasses, IgA, or IgE. This class switch results from the deletion of unwanted heavy chain genes and the joining of variable-region genes to the next available heavy chain genes. The V region and hence the specificity of the antibody produced remains unchanged.

In humans and other domestic mammals, B cell class switching is primarily controlled by IL-4 (Cerutti et al., 2005). For example, IL-4 from Th2 cells directs mouse B cells to produce IgG1 and IgE, whereas it directs human B cells to produce IgG4 and IgE. Other cytokines, such as TGF-β promote the switch to IgA production on body surfaces. As described previously, signals from IL-5 and IL-6 also contribute to class switching. In horses, IL-2 from Th1 cells may also determine which IgG subclass is produced.

As in other mammals, equine B cell functions are also dependent upon the activities of two essential growth factors, BAFF and APRIL. For example, the B cell Activating Factor (BAFF, CD257) is a cytokine required for B cell survival and maturation. Equine BAFF is a homotrimeric glycoprotein containing 233 amino acids and a predicted molecular weight of 26 kDa. Its amino acid sequence is 93% homologous to human BAFF. It can be found on the surface of cells as a type II transmembrane protein or as a soluble protein. BAFF is produced by monocytes, dendritic cells, T cells, and neutrophils. BAFF acts through a key receptor, BAFF-R whose gene is located on chromosome ECA 28 (Wu et al., 2013).

A PRoliferation-Inducing Ligand (APRIL) is also a member of the TNF family of cytokines. It also plays a key role in B-cell development. In the horse, APRIL is a glycoprotein of 16.5 kDa and contains 280 amino acids. (Recombinant protein) produced by monocytes, dendritic cells, T cells, and intestinal epithelial cells. APRIL functions as a soluble cytokine. It promotes B cell division and inhibits their apoptosis. It shares receptors with BAFF. The equine APRIL gene is located on chromosome ECA 11 (Wu et al., 2016).

Plasma cells

A large subset of antigen-stimulated B cells differentiate into plasma cells (Figure 11.8).

Plasma cells are mainly located in the secondary lymphoid organs. Early plasma cells (plasmablasts) can be identified in the cortex and paracortex of lymph nodes and in the marginal zone in the spleen. As the B cells differentiate, the plasma cells emigrate from these areas to the splenic red pulp, the medulla of lymph nodes, and especially to the bone marrow. The bone marrow provides a cytokine environment where plasma cells can survive for long periods. This is probably due to the activities of the stimulating cytokines, BAFF and APRIL.

Plasma cells are ovoid cells, 8–9 μm in diameter. They have a round, eccentrically placed nucleus with unevenly distributed chromatin. They have an extensive cytoplasm that is rich in rough endoplasmic reticulum and stains strongly with basic dyes and pyronin. They have a large, pale-staining Golgi apparatus. Plasma cells can secrete up to 10,000 molecules of immunoglobulin per second. The immunoglobulin produced by a plasma cell is of identical binding specificity to the antigen receptors on its parent B cell. Plasma cells with intracytoplasmic immunoglobulin accumulations (Russell bodies) are called Mott cells (Figure 11.9).

There are two distinct populations of plasma cells: a short-lived population that lives for 1–2 weeks and produces large amounts of antibodies shortly after antigen exposure, and a long-lived population that can survive for months or years.

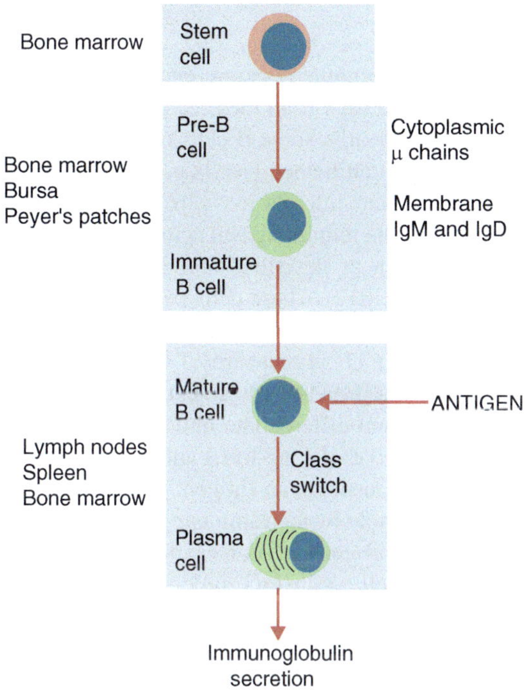

FIGURE 11.8

The progressive development of a B cell from stem cell to plasma cell.

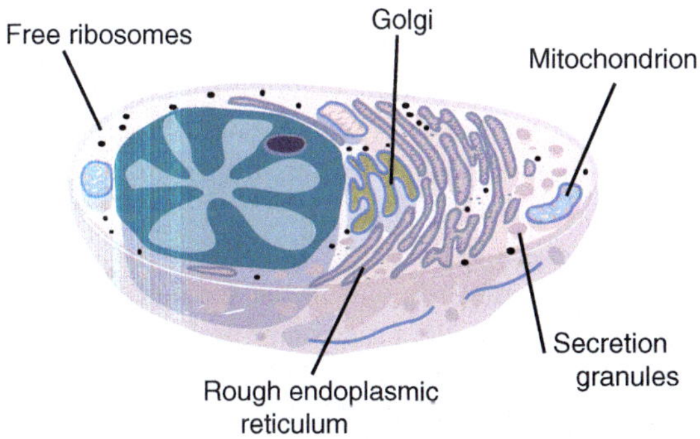

FIGURE 11.9

The structure of a typical plasma cell.

(In humans these plasma cells have a half-life of 8–15 years.) These antibodies provide immediate immunity to microbial pathogens. The short-lived cells are found in the spleen and lymph nodes soon after immunization. The long-lived plasma cells, in contrast, accumulate in the bone marrow.

Memory B cells

One reason why the primary immune response ends is that the responding B cells and plasma cells undergo apoptosis. If all these cells died, however, immunological memory could not develop. Clearly, some B cells must survive as memory cells. B cells are activated by antigen and helper T cells in the paracortex of lymph nodes. Most of these B cells differentiate into plasma cells and migrate to the bone marrow, spleen, and other organs, but the remaining cells proliferate, and form germinal centers. Asymmetric cell division as described above likely accounts for these two different fates (Barnett et al., 2012). These cells persist under the influence of programming and rescue signals. Thus, memory cells are first screened for their ability to bind antigens. This induces CD154 on nearby T cells, which in turn promotes the expression of bcl-2. Bcl-2 is a protein that protects them against apoptosis and so allows these cells to survive and differentiate into memory cells.

Memory cells form a reserve of long-lived antigen-sensitive cells to be called upon following subsequent exposure to an antigen. There are several subpopulations of memory B cells distinguishable by their immunoglobulin class, their location, and their passage through germinal centers. For example, one population consists of small, long-lived resting B cells with IgG antigen receptors. These cells, unlike plasma cells, look like generic lymphocytes. Their survival does not depend on antigen contact. On exposure to antigens, they proliferate and differentiate into plasma cells without undergoing further mutation. It has been calculated that in a secondary immune response, the clonal expansion of memory B cells results in 8- to 10-fold more plasma cells than does a primary immune response.

A second memory B cell population consists of large, dividing cells with IgM antigen receptors. These cells persist in germinal centers, where their continued survival depends on exposure to antigen by follicular dendritic cells. These long-lived plasma cells probably develop from a population of self-renewing, slowly dividing memory B cells (Ahuja et al., 2007). These memory B cells require a functional BCR to survive, suggesting that constant low-affinity antigen binding keeps them alive.

If a second dose of antigen is given to a primed animal, it will encounter large numbers of memory B cells that respond in the manner described previously for antigen-sensitive B cells. As a result, a secondary immune response is much greater than a primary immune response. The lag period is shorter since more antibodies are produced and they can be detected earlier. IgG subclasses are also produced in preference to the IgM characteristic of the primary response.

B cell subpopulations

B cells are heterogeneous and individual cells differ in both their phenotypes and functions. Thus, in mice, there are two subpopulations of B cells that develop from different precursor stem cells. These are called B1 and B2 cells. B1 cells originate from stem cells in the fetal liver or omentum rather than the bone marrow. They are innate-like cells that share some features with macrophages. They are, for example, phagocytic and microbicidal (they produce reactive oxygen species and can present antigens to $CD4^+$ T cells. B1 cells have a limited immunoglobulin V-region repertoire. They are potent producers of IL-10. They are commonly found in peripheral tissues but not in the bloodstream. 'B2 cells, in contrast, are the most common type of B cells and are found primarily in the bloodstream as well as the lymphoid follicles of the secondary lymphoid organs. They are responsible for producing the high-affinity antibodies during an infection. In species such as mice, humans, and cattle, these two B cell populations can be differentiated based on their expression of CD5. Thus, B1 cells are $CD5^+$ and B2 cells are $CD5^-$.

CD5 is expressed on a major subpopulation of equine B cells. These positive cells share some properties with B1 cells in humans. However, its expression on equine B cells is highly variable. Equine $CD5^{hi}$ and $CD5^{lo}$ B cells differentially express the B cell markers, CD2, CD21, and IgM (Prieto et al., 2017). The frequency of $CD5^{hi}$ cells varies with the animal's age and between horse tissues. Sequencing of light chain segments showed that $CD5^{hi}$ B cells generated diverse immunoglobulin repertoires.

Germinal centers

A key feature of the humoral immune response is the progressive increase in antigen-binding affinity over time. This process takes place as a result of somatic hypermutation occurring within B cells located in germinal centers (Figure 11.10).

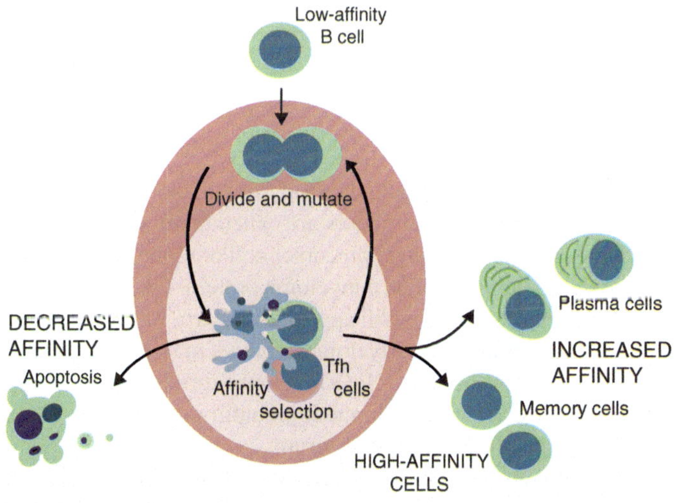

FIGURE 11.10 The functions of germinal centers.

These are sites where B cells increase their affinity for antigen as well as producing large numbers of memory cells.

Thus, germinal centers are sites where antigen-driven B cell proliferation, somatic hypermutation, and positive- and negative-selection of B cell populations occur (Berek, 1992). Germinal centers are divided into two zones based on their staining patterns: a light staining central zone containing dendritic cells, some B cells, and Tfh cells, and a darker staining peripheral zone that mainly consists of dividing B cells. In the early stages of the reaction, B cells stimulated by the antigen and Tfh cells migrate to the dark zone. There, they proliferate and as they do so, they mutate their antibody V genes. B cells divide every 6–8 h, so that within just a few days, a single B cell develops into a clone of several thousand cells. During this phase of rapid B cell division, the BCR V region genes mutate randomly, once per division (Dale et al., 2019). This repeated mutation generates populations of B cells whose BCRs differ slightly from the parent cell. Once these cells have been clonally expanded, a process that takes 10–20 days, they migrate to the light zone where they are presented with an antigen by the dendritic cells. Because of their altered V regions, some of these B cells have receptors that bind the antigen with greater affinity, while others bind it less strongly. A process of selection thus occurs. If a mutation has resulted in greater receptor binding affinity, this stimulates more B cell proliferation. Thus, cycles of rapid somatic hypermutation and selection lead to progressive improvement in antigen binding—a process called affinity maturation. These antigen-selected B cells eventually leave the germinal center to form either plasma cells or memory B cells.

In contrast, those B cells with BCRs that have reduced antigen-binding affinity undergo apoptosis. Thus, the B cell population that emerges from a germinal center is very different from the population of cells that entered it. In addition to somatic hypermutation of BCR V genes, BCRs also undergo class switching within germinal centers. Germinal centers eventually dissipate after the B cell response has peaked (Elsner & Shlomchik, 2020).

Myelomas

If a B cell turns cancerous, it may develop into a clone of immunoglobulin-producing plasma cells. Plasma cell tumors are called myelomas or plasmacytomas. Because myelomas arise from a single precursor cell or clone, they usually secrete a homogeneous immunoglobulin called a myeloma protein. On serum electrophoresis, this homogeneous myeloma protein will appear as a sharp, well-defined peak. This is called a monoclonal gammopathy. Myeloma proteins may belong to any immunoglobulin class, although in the horse, IgG myelomas predominate. The prevalence of myelomas expressing the various immunoglobulin classes in myeloma proteins correlates with their quantities in normal serum.

Plasma cell myelomas have been reported infrequently in horses, and most such reports describe individual cases. Quarter horses appear to be especially susceptible. Animals develop weight loss, anorexia, limb edema, anemia, lymphadenopathy, and bone pain. These malignant plasma cells can erode bone, so many equine cases present with lytic bone lesions. If located in the vertebrae, these may result in severe neurologic signs, including tetraparesis (Pelli et al., 2024). Monoclonal IgG antibodies can be detected in serum, while isolated light chains (Bence-Jones proteins) can be detected in the horse's urine (Edwards et al., 1993).

Serum immunoglobulins

Immunoglobulin G

IgG is the predominant serum immunoglobulin class in horses. It is also present in colostrum and on mucosal surfaces of the urinary tract and respiratory tract. It averages 1521 ± 29.6 mg/dL in aged horses 20 years and older, and slightly less (1447 ± 26.3 mg/dL in 5–12-year-old healthy animals (McFarlane et al., 2001). The horse is, however, unique in that it has seven different IgG isotypes, resulting from differences in their heavy chains and functionality (Lewis, Meehan, et al., 2008).

The most abundant isotype is IgG4/7 (IgGb), which accounts for about 68% of the immunoglobulins in an adult horse (Perkins & Wagner, 2015) (Fig. 11.11). This is followed by IgG3 plus IgG3/5 (IgG[T]), which account for about 14%. IgG1 (IgGa) accounts for 11.8% and IgG6 (IgGc) accounts for about 0.6%. The serum level of IgG2 is unclear since it is very low. All seven IgG subclasses are stabilized by interchain bonds composed of disulfide bridges. However, some IgG4 and IgG7 molecules are bound by non-covalent interchain bonds. All seven subclasses are N-glycosylated, with the glycosylation site located in their C_H2 domain. Additional glycosylation sites are present in the C_H1 domain of IgG3 and IgG5. In addition, IgG3 is has O glycosylated side chains attached to the heavy chain

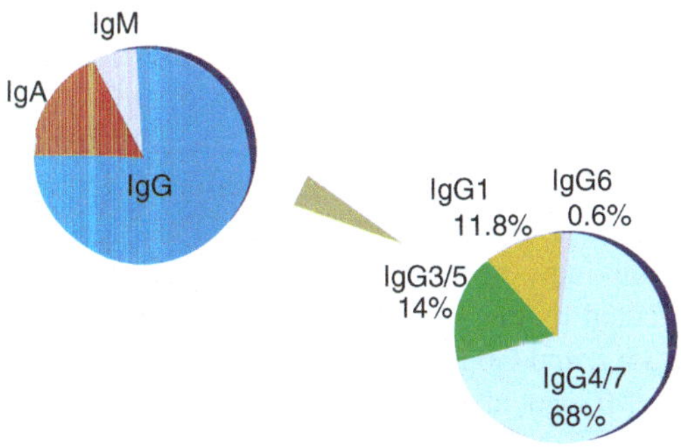

FIGURE 11.11

The relative concentrations of the major immunoglobulins as well as the major IgG subclasses in the horse. Remember however that they do vary greatly among horses of different breeds and ages. IgG2 levels are very low and difficult to measure.

- Data from Perkins, G. A., & Wagner, B. (2015). The development of equine immunity: Current knowledge on immunology in the young horse. Equine Veterinary Journal, 47, 267–274.

(Lewis, Wagner, & Woof, 2008). Staphylococcal protein A binds weakly to the equine IgGs. It binds most strongly to IgG1 and least strongly to IgG6. Protein G binds strongly to IgG4 and IgG7. Some subclasses, namely IgG1, IgG3, IgG4, IgG5, and IgG7, but not IgG2 or IgG6, can elicit a strong respiratory burst from equine blood lymphocytes. This reflects their ability to bind strongly to Fc receptors on effector cells. IgG1, IgG3, IgG4, and IgG7, but not IgG2, IgG5, or IgG6, can activate the classical complement pathway by binding to C1q.

Equine antibody responses are of two major types. In one, IgG3/5 predominates, while in the other IgG4/7 predominates. This appears to be determined, at least in part, by the activities of the two different helper T cell populations (These are described in Chapter 12). Thus, the production of IgG4/7 appears to be stimulated by a type 1 helper cell (Th1) response and is commonly directed at intracellular pathogens (Wagner, 2006). For example, the production of IgG4/7 is induced by viruses such as influenza, equine herpesvirus (EHV), and West Nile virus. In the case of EHV-1 infections, infected foals mount a Th1 response dominated by IgG1 and IgG4/7, while IgG3/5 and IgG6 responses are low (Larson & Wagner, 2021). In another study, a primary EHV-1 infection was shown to trigger a potent antibody response involving the production of IgG1, IgG4/7, and IgG3/5. (In effect, involving both Th1 and Th2 responses.) However, following prior sensitization with EHV-4. EHV-1-infected horses mounted a response dominated by IgG1 and IgG4/7 with no detectable IgG3/5 response (Bannai et al., 2011).

Likewise, both IgG4/7 and IgG3/5 predominate in the initial response of sick foals to the intracellular bacterium *Rhodococcus equi*. The presence of the IgG3/5 suggests that a Th2 response is occurring and is relatively unprotective in this case (Hooper-McGrevy et al., 2003). In another *R. equi* study, the Ig3/5:IgG4/7 ratio in the serum of non-surviving foals was significantly greater than in the survivors, reflecting its ineffectiveness against intracellular organisms (Mizuguchi et al., 2024).

Conversely, equine B cell responses to tetanus toxoid, to nematode parasites, to *Theileria equi*, or to Culicoides allergens consist of IgG3/5 antibodies predominantly. This suggests that these IgG3/5 responses are mediated through a Th2 helper cell (Th2) dependent pathway and are primarily directed against extracellular pathogens (Perkins & Wagner, 2015; Santos et al., 2021).

This interpretation may, however, be oversimplified since the IgG subclass response is also affected by the size of the challenge dose. Mild infections with *R equi* triggered G1, G4/7, and G6 responses, whereas high challenge doses promoted an IgG3/5 response (Mizuguchi et al., 2024). It is also unclear how Th1 cells influence B cell function.

Immunoglobulin M

IgM is produced by plasma cells in the secondary lymphoid organs. Its average concentration in horse serum is 191 ± 8.31 mg/dL in aged animals and less (75 ±

8.2 mg/dL) in younger animals (McFarlane et al., 2001). Other investigators have reported a range of 50–242 mg/dL (Perkins et al., 2003). When still attached to the B cell surface and acting as a BCR, IgM is a 180-kDa monomer. However, the secreted form of IgM consists of five 180-kDa units linked by disulfide bonds in a circular fashion. Its total molecular weight is then 900 kDa. A small J chain joins two of the units to complete the circle. IgM is the major immunoglobulin produced during primary immune responses. Smaller quantities are also produced in secondary responses. Although produced in small amounts, IgM is more efficient (on a molar basis) than IgG at complement activation, opsonization, virus neutralization, and agglutination. Because of their very large size, IgM molecules rarely enter tissue fluids, even at sites of acute inflammation.

Immunoglobulin A

IgA is found in the serum and mucosal secretions of horses. In serum, it averages 299 ± 13.4 mg/dL in aged and slightly less (261 ± 14.9 mg/dL in younger animals (McFarlane et al., 2001). IgA is the principal immunoglobulin in horse milk, tears, and nasal and bronchial secretions. IgA is mainly produced by plasma cells located under the body surfaces. Thus, they are located in the walls of the intestine, the respiratory tract, the urinary system, the skin, and the mammary glands. Although produced in large amounts, most of the IgA produced goes into the intestine and the respiratory tract. As a result, its serum concentration is usually lower than that of IgM (Lewis et al., 2010). It is a dimeric protein bound together by a J chain. The J chain is encoded by a gene on chromosome ECA3.

IgA produced in body surfaces is transported through epithelial cells into external secretions bound to the polymeric immunoglobulin receptor (pIgR) (also called secretory component) (Chapter 13). Secretory component is a 17 kDa peptide that binds to IgA dimers to form secretory IgA (SIgA). Equine PIgR is encoded by a gene located on chromosome ECA 5. It protects the IgA from digestion by microbial and intestinal proteases. IgA monomers have a molecular weight of 150 kDa, but they are normally secreted as dimers.

Immunoglobulin E

IgE, like IgA, is mainly made by plasma cells located beneath body surfaces. It is a typical Y-shaped, four-chain immunoglobulin with four constant domains in its ε heavy chains and a molecular weight of 190 kDa. Most IgE is bound to tissue mast cells and thus occurs in extremely low concentrations in serum. Interestingly, its physiological concentrations in horse serum are about a thousandfold higher than in human serum (Wagner, 2009). It is enriched in maternal colostrum and is therefore transferred to the suckling foal. In healthy normal horses, its concentration in serum averages 84.0 ± 90.9 mg/mL.

Immunoglobulin D

Horses possess what appears to be a fully functional gene locus encoding an IgD heavy chain (Wagner et al., 2004). It is expressed, at least at the mRNA level. IgD may be expressed in some equine B cells; however, this has yet to be demonstrated. Its functional significance is therefore unknown.

Antibody receptors

In addition to their antigen-binding abilities, the biological activity of immunoglobulins depends upon their ability to interact with cell surface receptors. These receptors bind to the Fc regions of the immunoglobulin heavy chains and hence are termed Fc receptors. Horses possess four of these receptors for IgG They include both activating and inhibitory receptors. The four IgG receptors are CD64 (FcγR1), CD32a (FcγRIIa), CD32b (FcγRIIb), and CD16 (FcγRIII) (Cacskovics, 2004).

CD64 (FcγRI) is a high-affinity receptor expressed on macrophages and dendritic cells. It is also expressed, to a limited extent, on neutrophils. Its binding affinity depends upon the IgG subclass involved. It consists of three extracellular immunoglobulin domains, a transmembrane domain, and a short cytoplasmic tail. To signal to a cell, CD64 must associate with the Fc receptor common gamma chain homodimer (FcRγ) which serves as a signal transducer.

CD32a and 32b (FcγRIIa and b) are low-affinity receptors expressed on macrophages. CD32a is an activating receptor, whereas CD32b is inhibitory. They have more than 90% sequence homology in their extracellular domains but differ in their cytoplasmic domains. Thus, horse CD32b lacks an immunotyrosine activating motif (ITAM) in its cytoplasmic tail.

CD16 (FcγRIII) is a 40-kDa type 1 transmembrane glycoprotein that binds IgG with low affinity. It is expressed on peripheral blood mononuclear cells. It is expressed on monocytes, macrophages, NK cells, neutrophils, and some DC subsets. It has two extracellular immunoglobulin domains, a transmembrane domain, and a cytoplasmic domain. It is usually complexed with the FcRγ chain. Antibody signaling through CD16 can trigger NK cell activation and consequent cell-mediated cytotoxicity (Chapter 10).

Horses possess a single IgA receptor, FcαR1 (EqCD89). FcαR1 is an activating receptor expressed on neutrophils, monocytes, macrophages, dendritic cells, and eosinophils. It is a protein of 271 amino acids. Signaling of IgA through this receptor can promote opsonization and phagocytosis, cytokine release, NETosis, a neutrophil respiratory burst, and macrophage antibody-dependent cell-mediated cytotoxicity. In addition to acting as an IgA receptor, CD89 also serves as a receptor for C-reactive protein and as a pattern recognition receptor for some bacteria (Morton, 2005). The CD89 gene (FCAR)is probably located within the horse lymphocyte receptor gene complex on ECA 10.

Horses have two IgE receptors. FcεRI is a high-affinity receptor expressed on mast cells. It can bind equine, bovine, and human IgE with very high affinity (Chapter 19). It plays a critical role in mast cell degranulation and the development of equine allergies. The second IgE receptor,CD23, or FcεRII, in contrast, is a low-affinity IgE receptor expressed on activated B cells, platelets, eosinophils, macrophages, NK cells, dendritic cells, and possibly even T cells. Both it and the neonatal Ig receptor (FcRn) are involved in immunoglobulin transport across epithelial surfaces such as the intestinal epithelium. They are described in Chapters 2 and 13. FcRn plays an important role in transporting colostral immunoglobulins into the mammary gland.

Donkey immunoglobulins

Donkeys possess the four major immunoglobulin classes, IgG, IgM, IgA, and IgE. Further analysis has demonstrated that the IGH locus is located on chromosome Eqas 7. The constant region genes in the donkey are arranged in order 5′-Cμ-Cδ-Cγ-Cε-Cα-3′, and this spans about 300 kb.

Analysis of the Cγ genes of the donkey has demonstrated that, like the horse, there are multiple donkey IgG subclasses. Those identified to date are IgG1, IgG2, IgG3, IgG5, IgG6 and IgG7. Their heavy chain constant regions contain glycans attached to a highly conserved glycosylation site (Marihonnaiah & Shivappa, 2024). Thus, among the mammals examined so far, the horse and donkey express the greatest number of IgG subclasses. As described previously, the different horse IgG subclasses have significant structural and functional differences. Similar differences may be expected in the donkey.

When the donkey IgG heavy chain gene sequences were compared to those of the horse, there was a match to 13 horse sequences. Thus, based on sequence similarity, it appears that donkeys possess heavy chains matching those found in horses (Marihonnaiah & Shivappa, 2024).

The donkey variable region within the IGH locus contains 117 V_H genes, of which 23 are functional, in addition to 44 D_H genes, and 8 J_H genes. The locus spans approximately 1189 kb. Certain gene segment combinations appear to be most common. These include, IGHV4-IGHD2-IGHJ6, IGHV4-IGHD4-IGHJ6, and IGHV4-IGHD2-IGHJ4. With respect to V(D)J recombination, onkeys and horses appear to differ in their N-nucleotide usage (Qiu et al., 2025).

References

Ahuja, A., Anderson, S. M., Khalil, A., & Siomchik, M. J. (2007). Maintenance of the plasma cell pool is independent of memory B cells. *Proceedings of the National Academy of Sciences, 105*, 4802–4807.

Bannai, H., Tsujimura, K., Kondo, T., Nemoto, M., et al. (2011). Induction of a Th1-biased IgG subclass response against equine herpesvirus type 1 in horses previously infected with type 4 virus. *Virology, 73*(4), 535–539.

Barnett, B. E., Ciocca, M. L., Goenka, R., Barnett, L. G., Wu, J., Laufer, T. M., et al. (2012). Asymmetric B cell division in the germinal center reaction. *Science, 335*(6066), 342–344.

Berek, C. (1992). The development of B cells and the B-cell repertoire in the microenvironment of the germinal center. *Immunological Reviews, 126*, 5–19.

Cacskovics, I. (2004). Fc receptors in livestock species. *Veterinary Immunology and Immunopathology, 102*(4), 351–362.

Cerutti, A., Qiao, X., & He, B. (2005). Plasmacytoid dendritic cells and the regulation of immunoglobulin heavy chain class switching. *Immunology & Cell Biology, 83*, 554–562.

Clark, M. R., Campbell, K. S., Kazlauskas, A., et al. (1992). The B cell antigen receptor complex: Association of Ig-α and Ig-β with distinct cytoplasmic effectors. *Science, 258*, 123–125.

Dale, G. A., Wilkins, D. J., & Bohannon. (2019). CD linkage consistent with templated mutagenesis. *Journal of Immunology, 203*, 1252–1264.

Durie, F. H., Foy, T. M., Masters, S. R., et al. (1994). The role of CD40 in the regulation of humoral and cell-mediated immunity. *Immunology Today, 15*, 406–411.

Edwards, D. F., Parker, J. W., Wilkinson, J. E., & Helman, R. G. (1993). Plasma cell myeloma in the horse: A case report and literature review. *Journal of Veterinary Internal Medicine, 7*, 169–176.

Elsner, R. A., & Shlomchik, M. J. (2020). Germinal center and extrafollicular B cell responses in vaccination, immunity and autoimmunity. *Immunity.* https://doi.org/10.1016/j.mmuni.2020.11.006

Faili, A., Aoufouchi, S., Flatter, E., et al. (2002). Induction of somatic hypermutation in immunoglobulin genes is dependent on DNA polymerase iota. *Nature, 419*, 944–946.

Gold, M. R. (2002). To make antibodies or not: Signaling by the B-cell antigen receptor. *Trends in Pharmacological Sciences, 23*, 316–324.

Hayashi, E. A., Akira, S., & Nobrega, A. (2005). Role of TLR in B cell development: Signaling through TLR4 promotes B cell maturation and is inhibited by TLR2. *Journal of Immunology, 174*, 6639–6647.

Hooper-McGrevy, K. E., Wilkie, B. N., & Prescott, J. F. (2003). Immunoglobulin G subisotype responses of pneumonic and healthy exposed foals and adult horses to *Rhodococcus equi* virulence-associated proteins. *Clinical and Diagnostic Laboratory Immunology, 10* (3), 345–351.

Kirkham, P. M., Mortari, F., Newton, J. A., & Schroeder, H. W. (1992). Immunoglobulin VH clan and family identity predicts variable domain structure and may influence antigen binding. *The EMBO Journal, 11*(2), 603–609.

Larson, E. M., & Wagner, B. (2021). Viral infection and allergy—What equine immune responses can tell us about disease severity and protection. *Molecular Immunology, 135*, 329–341.

Lazarevic, V., Glimcher, L. H., & Lord, G. M. (2013). T-bet: A bridge between innate and adaptive immunity. *Nature Reviews Immunology, 13*, 777–789.

Lewis, M. J., Meehan, M., Owen, P., & Woof, J. M. (2008). A common theme in interaction of bacterial immunoglobulin-binding proteins with immunoglobulins illustrated in the equine system. *Journal of Biological Chemistry, 283*(25), 17615–17623.

Lewis, M. J., Wagner, B., Irvine, R. M., & Woof, J. M. (2010). IgA in the horse: Cloning of equine polymeric Ig receptor and J chain and characterization of recombinant forms of equine IgA. *Mucosal Immunology*. https://doi.org/10.1038/mi.2010.38

Lewis, M. J., Wagner, B., & Woof, J. M. (2008). The different effector function capabilities of the seven equine IgG subclasses have implications for vaccine strategies. *Molecular Immunology, 45*, 818–827.

Manso, T. C., Groenner-Penna, M., Minozzo, J. C., Antunes, B. C., et al. (2018). Next generation sequencing reveals new insights about gene usage and CDR- H3 composition in the horse antibody repertoire. *Molecular Immunology*. https://doi.org/10.1016/j.molimm.2018.11.017

Marihonnaiah, S., & Shivappa, G. K. B. (2024). Site-specific N-glycoprofiling of immunoglobulin G subtypes from donkey milk. *Journal of Agricultural and Food Chemistry, 72*, 26547–26557.

McFarlane, D., Sellon, D. C., & Gibbs, S. A. (2001). Age-related quantitative alterations in lymphocyte subsets and immunoglobulin isotypes in healthy horses. *American Journal of Veterinary Research, 62*(9), 1413–1417.

Mizuguchi, Y., Tsuzuki, N., Ebana, M. D., Suzuki, Y., & Kakuda, T. (2024). IgG subtype response against virulence-associated protein A in foals naturally infected with *Rhodococcus equi*. *Veterinary Sciences*. https://doi.org/10.3390/vetsci11090422

Morton, H. C. (2005). IgA Fc receptors in cattle and horses. *Veterinary Immunology and Immunopathology, 108*, 139–143.

Morton, H. C., Pleass, R. J., Storset, A. K., Brandtzaeg, P., & Woof, J. M. (2005). Cloning and characterization of equine CD89 and identification of the CD89 gene in chimpanzees and rhesus macaques. *Immunology*. https://doi.org/10.1111/j.1365-2567.2005.02129.x

Navas, C., Manso, T., Martins, F., Minto, L., et al. (2022). The major role of junctional diversity in the horse antibody repertoire. *Molecular Immunology, 151*, 231–241.

Papavasiliou, F. N., & Schatz, D. G. (2002). Somatic hypermutation of immunoglobulin genes: Merging mechanisms for genetic diversity. *Cell, 109*, S35–S44.

Pasare, C., & Medzhitov, R. (2005). Control of B-cell responses by toll-like receptors. *Nature, 438*, 364–368.

Patel, R. S., Tomlinson, J. E., Divers, T. J., Van de Walle, G. R., & Rosenberg, B. R. (2021). Single-cell resolution landscape of equine peripheral blood mononuclear cells reveals diverse cell types including T-bet^{+} B cells. *BMC Biology*. https://doi.org/10.1186/s12915-020-00947-5

Pelli, A., Schiffbauer, V., Tommasa, S. D., Ulrich, R., et al. (2024). Paramedullary plasma cell myeloma originating from the first cervical vertebra (C1) in an 8-month-old Warmblood with tetraparesis: Clinical and pathological findings. *Equine Veterinary Education, 36*, e302–e307.

Perkins, G. A., Nydam, D. V., Flaminio, M. J. B. F., & Ainsworth, D. M. (2003). Serum IgM concentrations in normal, fit horses and horses with lymphoma or other medical conditions. *Journal of Veterinary Internal Medicine, 17*, 337–342.

Perkins, G. A., & Wagner, B. (2015). The development of equine immunity: Current knowledge on immunology in the young horse. *Equine Veterinary Journal, 47*, 267–274.

Prieto, J. M. B., Tallmadge, R. L., & Felippe, M. J. B. (2017). Developmental expression of B cell molecules in equine lymphoid tissues. *Veterinary Immunology and Immunopathology, 183*, 60–71.

Qiu, Y., Jiang, J., Yi, X., Wang, S., & Sun, X. (2025). Exploration of the differential expression patterns of immunoglobulin heavy chains in horses and donkeys. *Developmental & Comparative Immunology, 166*, Article 105360.

Santos, A. C., Nogueira, E. W., Moraes, B. S. S., Müller, V., et al. (2021). Immune responses of adult horses, pregnant mares and foals to an experimental vaccine with recombinant EMA-2 protein of Theileria equi. *Research in Veterinary Science, 239*, 186–192.

Schwab, U. E., Tallmadge, R. L., Matychak, M. B., & Felippe, J. B. (2017). Effects of autologous stromal cells and cytokines on the differentiation of equine bone marrow-derived progenitor cells. *American Journal of Veterinary Research, 78*, 1215–1228.

Sinkora, M., Stepanova, K., Butler, J. E., Sinkora, M., Jr., et al. (2022). Comparative aspects of immunoglobulin gene rearrangement arrays in different species. *Frontiers in Immunology.* https://doi.org/10.3389/fimmu.2022.823145

Sun, Y., Wang, C., Wang, Y., Zhang, T., Ren, L., et al. (2010). A comprehensive analysis of germline and expressed immunoglobulin repertoire in the horse. *Developmental & Comparative Immunology, 34*, 1009–1020.

Tallmadge, R. L., Tseng, C. T., King, R. A., & Felippe, M. J. B. (2013). Developmental progression of equine immunoglobulin heavy chain variable region diversity. *Developmental & Comparative Immunology, 41*(1), 33–43.

Tedder, T. F., Zhou, L.-J., & Engel, P. (1994). The CD19/CD21 signal transduction complex of B lymphocytes. *Immunology Today, 15*, 437–442.

Vadnais, M. L., Criscitiello, M. F., & Smider, V. V. (2017). In T. Protein, T. Vaughan, J. Osbourn, & B. Jallal (Eds.), *Antibodies in other species* (1Ed). Wiley Verlag.

Wagner, B. (2006). Immunoglobulins and immunoglobulin genes of the horse. *Developmental & Comparative Immunology, 30*, 155–164.

Wagner, B. (2009). IgE in horses: Occurrence in health and disease. *Veterinary Immunology and Immunopathology, 132*, 21–30.

Wagner, B. (2024). Monoclonal antibody development advances immunological research in horses. *Veterinary Immunology and Immunopathology.* https://doi.org/10.1016/j.vetimm.2024.110771

Wagner, B., Miller, D. C., Lear, T. L., & Antczak, D. F. (2004). The complete map of the Ig heavy chain constant gene region reveals evidence for seven IgG isotypes and for IgD in the horse. *Journal of Immunology, 173*, 3230–3242.

Walther, S., Rusitzka, T. V., Diesterbeck, U. S., & Czarny, C.-P. (2015). Equine immunoglobulins and organization of immunoglobulin genes. *Developmental & Comparative Immunology, 53*, 303–319.

Willis-Karp, M., & Finkelman, F. D. (2015). Untangling the complex web of IL-4- and IL-13-mediated signaling pathways. *Science Signaling.* https://doi.org/10.1126/scisignal.1.51.pe55

Wu, H., Bi, X., Cao, F., Zhu, C., et al. (2016). Molecular characterization of equine APRIL and its expression analysis during the adipogenic differentiation of equine adipose-derived stem cells in vitro. *Animal Biotechnology, 27*(4), 262–268.

Wu, H., Chen, S., Liu, M., Xu, X., et al. (2013). Molecular characterization and evolutionary analysis of horse BAFF-R, tumor necrosis factor receptor related to B cell survival. *International Immunopharmacology.* https://doi.org/10.1016/j.intimp.2013.11.019

CHAPTER

The central role of equine T cell systems

12

Antibodies bind to invading organisms in blood or tissue fluids, hastening their destruction. However, not all foreign invaders are found outside cells. All viruses and some bacteria grow inside cells at sites inaccessible to antibodies. Antibodies are therefore of limited use in defending horses against such invaders. Viruses and other intracellular organisms must be eliminated by other mechanisms. For this, the body uses two different cell-mediated processes. Either infected cells are killed rapidly by cytotoxic T cells so that the invader has no time to grow, or alternatively, activated macrophages develop the ability to destroy the intracellular organisms. In general, organisms such as viruses that enter the cell cytosol or nucleus are killed by cytotoxic T cells, whereas organisms such as bacteria or parasites that reside within endosomes are destroyed by activated macrophages. T cells mediate both processes. The antigens that trigger these immune responses are synthesized within the animal's own cells and are thus classified as endogenous antigens.

T cells

The T cells of the adaptive immune system must recognize and respond appropriately to diverse microbial pathogens. They must be able to assume different functional configurations depending on the nature of the microbial challenge. This is largely achieved by employing differentiated T-cell subpopulations. For example, horses mount a cell-mediated, type 1 immune response by activating Th1 cells, generating cytotoxic T cells, and destroying virus-infected cells, hence effectively combating viral invasion. Alternatively, they can trigger an antibody-mediated immune response by activating Th2 cells and B cells and so combat extracellular bacteria. In other situations, Th17 cells may be activated and promote local inflammation or generate antiviral interferons. If required, they can also act as regulatory (Treg) cells and prevent inappropriate immune responses. T cells can also change their phenotype rapidly if the situation demands it. This selection process involves the use of pattern recognition receptors, antigen-binding by MHC-encoded receptors, and the use of very specific antigen receptors. The responding T cells activate different transcription factors to generate different cytokine mixtures. These cytokine mixtures, in turn, trigger different forms of immune defense, ideally optimized to eliminate specific invaders.

The Immunology of Horses and Donkeys. https://doi.org/10.1016/B978-0-443-44863-8.00001-6

When newly generated T cells emerge from the foal's thymus, they migrate to sites throughout the body where they remain quiescent until they encounter an antigen that binds to their receptors. When they bind the appropriate antigen, signals are generated that cause these T cells to divide and differentiate into many different subpopulations based on the nature of the antigen, and their microenvironment. They include helper and regulatory T cells that regulate immune responses and effector or cytotoxic T cells that destroy abnormal cells. Each of these T cell types responds to antigens when they bind to their receptors, provided they receive appropriate costimulation. The nature of the costimulation determines their career pathway.

When dendritic cells (DCs) present their processed antigens to helper T cells, they generate three signals. The first signal is delivered when T cell antigen receptors bind antigen fragments attached to MHC class II molecules. The second signal amplifies this stimulation through other cell surface receptors, such as adhesion molecules. The third signal determines the direction in which naïve helper T cells will develop and is generated by multiple cytokines (Walsh & Mills, 2013). For example, some microbial antigens trigger DCs to secrete IL-12. These are called DC1 cells since their IL-12 activates Th1 pathways and triggers type 1 cell-mediated immune responses. Other microbial antigens can cause DCs to secrete IL-4 and IL-13. These cytokines stimulate Th2 cell differentiation and are produced by DC2 cells. Th2 cells activate B cells and trigger antibody-mediated type 2 responses. It may also be that the same dendritic cell can promote a type 1 or a type 2 response, depending on the dose and type of antigen encountered. The response may also depend on its location. For example, DCs in the intestine or airways preferentially secrete IL-4 and thus promote type 2 IgA-mediated antibody responses. T cell populations, therefore, differ in which antigen receptor chains they use, which costimulatory molecules they employ, and which cytokines they produce.

T cell antigen receptors

Each individual T cell expresses about 30,000 identical antigen receptors (TCRs) on its surface. Each TCR is constructed from two components: an antigen-binding component and a signal transduction component. The antigen-binding component consists of two peptide chains that form a heterodimer, with the antigen-binding site located between the two chains (Fig. 12.1). Based on their paired antigen-binding chains, there are two major classes of T cell antigen receptors. One class employs paired γ and δ (γ/δ) chains. The other employs α and β (α/β) chains. The data on this differentiation in equids is limited as a result of a lack of specific reagents. However, Tallmadge et al. (2018) examined the transcriptomes of immune genes in peripheral blood mononuclear cells in adult horses. They studied the cells expressing delta chain (TCRD) genes, presumably γ/δ cells, and the T cells expressing alpha chain (TCRA) genes, presumably α/β T cells, by flow cytometry. In the case of the delta gene, they detected 20 reads per million expressing TCRD and about 700 reads per million in cells expressing TCRA genes. This ratio suggests

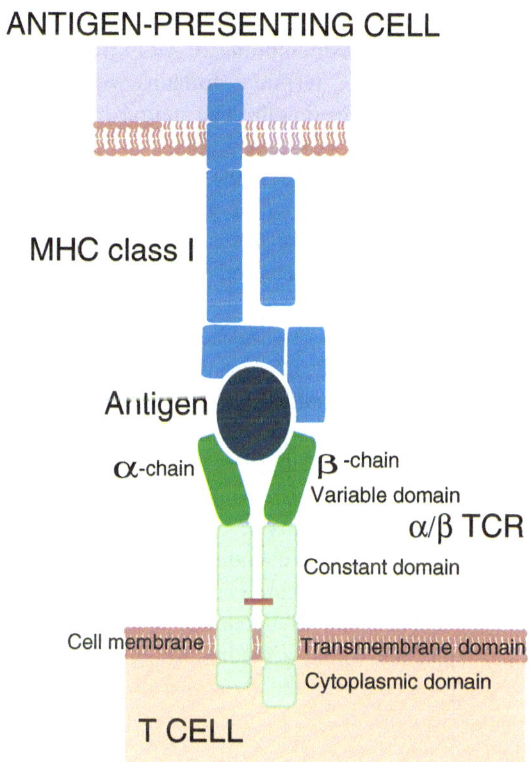

FIGURE 12.1 The structure of an α/β T cell antigen receptor and its ligand—antigen presented by an MHC class I molecule.

that γ/δ T cells account for about 2.7% of the circulating T cells (Tallmadge et al., 2018). In another study, Patel and colleagues examined equine peripheral blood mononuclear cells at the single-cell level in horses. They found that only 1.70% of perforin-positive T cells expressed γ/δ -receptors (Patel et al., 2021).

The four T cell antigen-binding chains (α, β, γ, and δ) are similar in overall structure, although they differ in size as a result of variations in glycosylation. The α/β receptors are 46–48 kDa heterodimers. The γ/δ receptors are more diverse. Examination of equine γ/δ T cells has revealed that they possess multiple different TCR structures. These share a similar 38 kDa δ chain but use many different γ chains.

Each antigen-binding chain is constructed from four domains. The paired N-terminal domains (α1 and β1) each contain about 100 amino acids, and their sequence varies greatly among T cells. These are the variable (V) domains, and their function is to bind peptides presented by MHC molecules. The second domains (α2 and β2) contain about 150 amino acids. These are constant (C) domains. A third, very small domain consists of about 20 hydrophobic amino acids, where the chains pass through the T cell membrane. This transmembrane domain contains a Conserved Antigen Receptor Transmembrane (CART) motif that plays a key role in TCR signal transduction. The C-terminal domains within the T cell cytoplasm are only five to 15 amino acids in length. The paired receptor chains are linked by a disulfide bond between their constant domains to form a stable heterodimer. As a result, a groove is present between the two V domains that serves as the antigen-binding site. The precise shape of the antigen-binding groove varies among different TCRs because of variations in the amino acid sequences of their V domains. The specificity of the binding between a TCR and an antigen is determined by the shape of this groove (Tizard, 2024).

As in immunoglobulin molecules, within each TCR V domain are regions where the amino acid sequences are very highly variable. These are the regions that actually come into contact with the antigen. For this reason, they are called the complementarity-determining regions (CDRs). The antigen-binding site of the TCR is formed by the paired CDRs from the two chains that constitute the walls of the groove. The rest of the V domain outside the CDRs has a relatively constant sequence and provides structural stability.

Each of these TCR peptide chains is encoded by a sequence of three or four genes called, variable (V), diversity (D), joining (J), and constant (C) genes. The V domains of the TCRs are encoded either by linked V, D, and J genes or by just V and J genes. For example, the α and γ chains are encoded by three genes: TRA (or TRG) V, J, and C. In contrast, the β, and δ chains also use an additional TRBD or TRDD gene. In general, γ/δ-expressing T cells have much less receptor diversity than α/β-expressing T cells (Su et al., 1999).

TCR genes

The four antigen-binding chains of equine TCRs are encoded by four gene complexes located in three loci on chromosome ECA4 (Schrenzel & Ferrick, 1995). The genes encoding the α and δ chains are combined in a single complex, the TRA/D locus. The genes encoding the beta and gamma chains are separate loci. Each complex contains one or more genes encoding the constant domains of these chains. These C genes are preceded by the V, D, and J genes encoding their variable antigen-binding sites (Fig. 12.2).

TRA/D genes

The equine TRA/D locus contains five unique TRAV genes (or gene segments) in five different subfamilies, five distinct TRAJ genes that have conserved 3′ residues but diverse residues at their 5′ ends, and a single TRAC gene. The TRAC gene has highly conserved transmembrane and cytoplasmic domains when compared to TRAC in other mammals. This conservation is almost certainly required to retain its ability to interact with the CD3 signaling peptides.

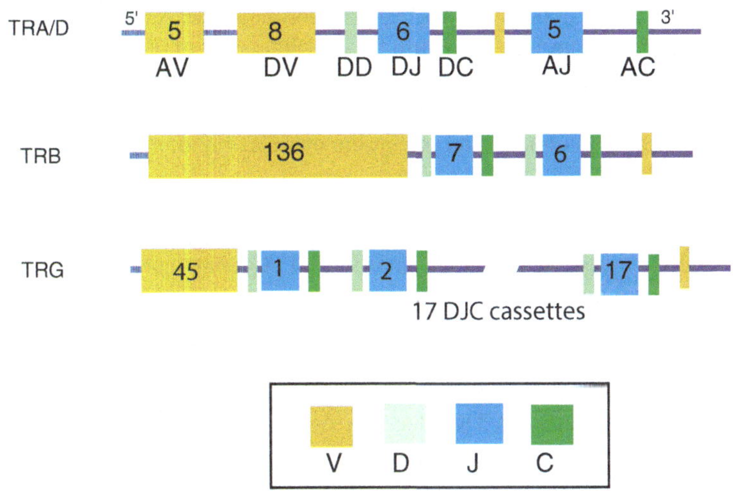

FIGURE 12.2 The organization of the three equine T cell antigen receptor gene loci.

The TRG locus may have up to 17 V-J-C cassettes. They are all located on chromosome ECA4.

The equine TRD locus contains eight unique TRDV genes from seven subfamilies. These result in significant junctional diversity in the V-J region. It is of interest to note that the equine TRDV genes most closely resemble those in the sheep. Given that both are grazers exposed to a similar spectrum of intestinal parasites, it may be speculated that these TRDV genes may have been selected by the same antigenic stimuli. Horses have six highly conserved TRDJ genes, of which three are functional. The locus also contains a single TRDC gene that is homologous to this gene in other mammals except for its connecting peptide region (Schrenzel & Ferrick, 1995).

TRB locus

The equine TRB gene locus is approximately 900 Kb in size so that it is the largest such locus yet recorded in mammals. It contains many more genes than other mammals. Thus it contains136 TRBV genes, 2 TRBD genes, 13 TRBJ, and two constant region (TRBC) genes (Antonacci et al., 2024).The TRBV genes are grouped into 29 subgroups based on 75% or greater similarities to the human sequences. Five of these subgroups consist of a single gene. The TRBV5 subgroup contains 20 genes while the TRBV7 subgroup contains 11 genes. CDR3 analysis suggests that theTRBJ2 cluster is preferentially used. The arrangement of the TRB locus is similar to the other TCR clusters with a cluster of 135 TRBV genes located upstream of two TRB(J)C clusters of 6.5 Kb each. and an inverted TRBV gene at the 3′ end of the last TRBC gene. Forty-seven of the TRBV genes appear to be functional. Eighty-four are pseudogenes and five are ORFs. There are also obvious TRBV polymorphisms among the five different horse breeds tested (Thoroughbred, Arabian, Standardbred, Quarter horse, and American miniature horse) (Schrenzel et al., 1994). Both of the constant region genes TRBC1 and TRBC2 encodes a peptide chain of 177 amino acids. These chains differ in nine amino acid residues, of which four are located in the transmembrane domain and one in the cytoplasmic domain.

TRG locus

The horse TRG locus located on chromosome ECA4 contains 45 variable (TRVG) genes that belong to seven mammalian subgroups as determined by nucleotide sequence identity and predicted functionality (Massari et al., 2023). The potential functional germline is limited to four out of the seven subgroups. TRFV1 and TRGV3 are the only multimember subgroups. It contains 25 TRGJ genes and 17 constant (TRGC) genes. The TRG locus is organized into 17 V-J-(J)-C cassettes. These occupy about 1100 kb. The number of gamma constant region genes is the largest yet reported in any mammal and is significantly higher than in the other domestic mammals. However, only nine of these TRGC genes appear to be functional. Three are classified as open reading frames (ORFs), and four appear to be pseudogenes. The TRGC1 cassette consists of TRGV genes from each subgroup. In addition to the multiple V-J rearrangements at this locus, there is a significant amount of trans-cassette recombination. As a result, the same V region gene can combine with a different TRJG gene in another cassette. Consequently, the TRG locus is highly polymorphic. It is speculated that these differences in their antigen receptors may determine the tissue distribution of equine γ/δ T cell populations (Schrenzel et al., 1994).

The TRG locus of the donkey (*E. asinus*) has also been sequenced. It is located on chromosome Eqas1 (Massari et al., 2023). The donkey TRG locus contains 34 TRGV, 21 TRGJ, and 14 TRGC genes. They are distributed in 14 VJC cassettes They occupy a region of approximately 860 kb. Each donkey VJC cassette matches a horse VJC cassette. This is the second-largest TRGC locus detected in mammals to date.

Gene rearrangement

TCR α and γ chains are constructed using only V, J, and C genes. TCR β and δ chains use V, D, J, and C genes, and they may also insert more than one D gene into the complete chain assembly. As a result, V-D-D-J-or longer constructs can be formed. This amount of gene recombination also means that the reading frame of the D genes may change and also yield productive rearrangements. Looping-out and deletion account for more than 75% of these TCR rearrangements. The remaining rearrangements result from either unequal sister chromatid exchange or gene inversion. That is, moving an inverted segment of one gene into a position beside a segment in the opposite orientation. These genes are separate in the germline but are first brought together by DNA rearrangement and are subsequently modified by base insertion or deletion as the T cells mature and differentiate (Olivieri et al., 2015).

Base insertion and deletion

Although in general, TCRs are constructed from a smaller V-, D-, and J-gene pool than immunoglobulins, their antigen-binding diversity tends to be similar as a result of junctional diversity. Random N-nucleotides may be inserted at the V, D, and J junctions using the enzyme terminal deoxynucleotidyl transferase (TdT). Up to five nucleotides may be added between V and D, and four between D and J genes. Likewise, random nucleotides may be removed by nucleases. This insertion of N-nucleotides and base deletion is probably the most significant contributor to TCR junctional diversity.

Receptor-antigen binding

T-cell receptors cannot bind free antigens. The antigen must first be processed within an antigen-processing cell, such as a dendritic cell or a virus-infected cell (Walsh & Mills, 2013). The processed antigen fragments are then bound to the antigen-binding groove of an MHC molecule. The antigen-MHC complex is then presented to a T cell. When an antigen-MHC complex and its T cell receptor bind, they interact through the side chains on the antigen and the MHC molecule and the CDRs of the TCR. There are three CDRs within each TCR V region. The first two have probably arisen through selection in the germline. The third CDR is by far the most variable and is generated when the V, D, and J genes recombine.

Signal transduction

CD3 complex

The ability of the immune system to mount a rapid and appropriate response to a specific invader depends on the responding T cells. Much of their decision-making depends upon the signals sent to the T cell by cell-bound antigen, together with multiple costimulatory signals from a mixture of cytokines. A key part of this pathway is the signal-transducing component of the TCR called the CD3 complex (Fig. 12.3). The genes that encode the proteins of the equine CD3 complex are clustered in chromosome ECA7. When an antigen binds to its TCR, a signal is generated by the CD3 complex that triggers the T cell response. The paired antigen-binding chains of each TCR are linked to the signal-transducing proteins of the CD3 complex. CD3 consists of five peptide chains with molecular weights ranging from 18 to 42 kDa (Blanchard-Channell et al., 1994). The five chains (γ, δ, ε, ζ, and η) are arranged in three dimers; γ-ε, γ-ε, and either ζ-ζ or ζ–η. The TCR β chain is linked to the γ-ε dimer, and the TCR α chain is linked to the γ-ε dimer to form two trimers (Nel, 2002). The complete hexamer interacts with CD3ζ to form the CD3 complex. The structure of CD3 also differs between the α/β and γ/δ TCRs (Göbel & Dangy, 2000).

CD4 and CD8

Two additional glycoproteins are closely associated with the TCR and the signals it generates. These are CD4 and CD8. Their expression tends to be mutually exclusive

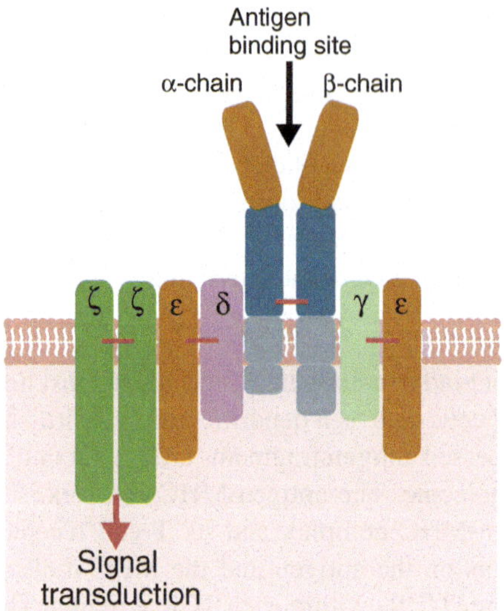

FIGURE 12.3 The structure of the equine CD3 complex.

Overall structure of the TCR/CD3 complex. The signal transduction proteins are collectively classified as CD3. About 80% of equine α/β TCRs use ζ-ζ dimers. The remaining 20% use ζ–η heterodimers.

but double-positive cells are found in the horse.There are four major subpopulations of α/β T cells in the peripheral blood of horses based on their expression of the costimulatory molecules, CD4 and CD8. $CD4^+$ T cells account for 44.8 ± 31.4% of total blood lymphocytes. $CD8^+$ cells account for 8.7 ± 1.3% (Tschetter et al., 1997). T cells in the thymus proceed from double negative through double positive stages to single positive $CD4^+$ or $CD8^+$ cells. A high proportion of $CD4^+$ cells also express a CD8α chain. CD8α is expressed on activated and memory $CD4^+$T cells (Holderness et al., 2013).

Absolute lymphocyte counts are decreased in horses over 20 years of age when compared to young animals under 12 years. This drop involves both $CD4^+$ and $CD8^+$ T cells as well as B cells (McFarlane et al., 2001). The decline in $CD8^+$ T cells is associated with an increase in the CD4:CD8 ratio in the aged population. Thus, the ratio is 4.07 ± 1.54 in old horses but only 3.30 ± 1.31 in young horses.

CD4

Equine CD4 is a single peptide glycoprotein of 60 kDa encoded by a gene located on chromosome ECA6. CD4 is noncovalently bound to the TCR. It recognizes and interacts with the invariant region of MHC class II on antigen-presenting cells. Its cytoplasmic domain is associated with the tyrosine kinase, $p56^{lck}$, and plays a key role in T cell activation. Thus, signals passing via CD4 and activating the tyrosine kinase are an essential part of T cell costimulation. Its expression can be modulated

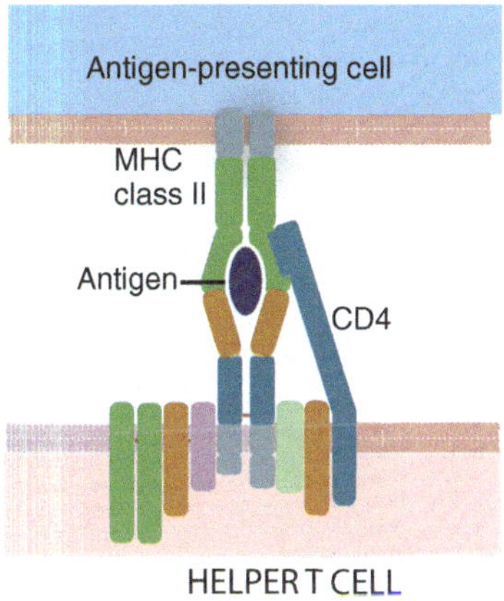

FIGURE 12.4 The function of CD4.

CD4 cross-links a T cell with the MHC class II molecule on an antigen-presenting cell, thus binding them together and triggering its helper cell functions.

by antigens or by phorbol esters. These activate protein kinase C, which results in CD4 internalization (Zhang et al., 1994) (Fig. 12.4).

CD8

Equine CD8 is a heterodimer consisting of alpha and beta chains. CD8α is a 39 kDa protein, while CD8β is a 32 kDa protein, and the dimer is 68 kDa in size. Both the alpha and beta chains of the CD8 heterodimer are expressed on T cells from blood, thymus, spleen, mesenteric lymph node, and ileal intraepithelial lymphocytes (Tschetter et al., 1997). However, in each of these tissues, there is also a T cell population that expresses a CD8α chain homodimer (Tschetter et al., 1997). The highest percentage of CD8αα cells is 37.7%, found among the intestinal intraepithelial lymphocytes. This compares to 23.9% in the blood, 18.8% in the spleen, 6.1% in the thymus, and 14.2% in the mesenteric lymph node (Fig. 12.5).

CD4 and CD8 determine the class of antigen-presenting MHC molecule that can be recognized by the T cell. For example, CD4, found only on helper T cells, binds MHC class II molecules on antigen-presenting cells. CD8, in contrast, is found only on cytotoxic T cells and binds MHC class I molecules on virus-infected or other abnormal cells. This CD4 and CD8 binding enhances TCR signal transduction by holding the T cell in contact with an antigen-presenting cell through the MHC for up to several hours while activating signals are exchanged.

During a primary antiviral response, $CD8^+$ cytotoxic T cells cannot respond to every virus-infected cell. There are about 10^{13} nucleated cells in a human-sized body, and possibly several hundred naïve T cells with receptors for each individual viral antigen. Clearly, these T cells can't find and kill all the virus-infected cells without help. In practice, dendritic cells link processed antigens to MHC class I molecules and carry them to lymphoid organs, where they are presented to $CD8^+$ T

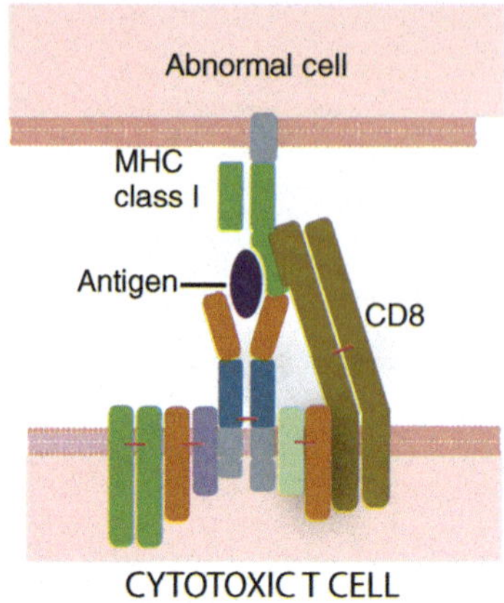

FIGURE 12.5 The binding role of CD8.

The CD8 heterodimer cross-links a cytotoxic T cell with a virus-infected target cell, thus binding them together and triggering a cytotoxic response.

cells. In order to respond fully, the $CD8^+$ cells must also be co-stimulated by $CD4^+$ helper cells. Co-stimulation is only effective when both $CD8^+$ and $CD4^+$ T cells recognize the antigen on the same presenting cell. Thus, a helper T cell first interacts with an antigen-presenting dendritic cell through CD40 and its ligand CD154. The helper T cells then activate the dendritic cells, upregulate their expression of MHC class I, and stimulate their production of IL-12. Once activated, dendritic cell MHC class I-linked peptides bind to $CD8^+$ T cells. However, only when correctly stimulated can the $CD8^+$ T cells respond fully and appropriately.

Different levels of stimulation can trigger different activation responses in $CD8^+$ T cells. As with helper cells, the duration of the stimulus is important. Although activated cytotoxic T cells can be triggered by brief exposure to an antigen, naïve T cells may have to be stimulated for several hours before responding. The required stimulation time may be shortened by increasing TCR occupancy or by providing additional co-stimulation. Once activated, naïve $CD8^+$ T cells divide. They undergo multiple rounds of division to generate large numbers of cytotoxic effector cells. Some calculations have suggested that they undergo as many as 19 cell divisions in the week following antigen exposure, and they probably divide every 4–6 hours (in rodents) (Nolz & Richer., 2020). All this is regulated by extracellular signals from the TCR, co-stimulatory molecules, and cytokines such as IL-2, IL-12, IL-21, and IL-27. These activated T cells migrate to peripheral sites and differentiate into effector and memory cells. Short-lived effector cells form the bulk of the population, and these mostly die once the foreign invades are eliminated.

As noted above, one critical trigger of T cell activation involves the binding of CD40 on an antigen-presenting cell to its ligand, CD154, on the responding T cell. CD154 is transiently expressed on $CD4^+$ T cells after TCR stimulation, but it is immediately internalized after binding to CD40. CD154 expression identifies antigen-reactive $CD4^+$ T cells. These $CD4^+$ $CD154^+$ cells are derived from both naive and activated/memory T cells. These activated cells produce IFN-γ and TNF-α.

Helper T cell subpopulations

As pointed out at the beginning of this chapter the immune system has to be flexible if it is to respond to a multitude of diverse invaders. Much of this flexibility comes from T cells. As naïve $CD4^+$ T cells develop and differentiate, four major subpopulations emerge. They are classified into helper 1 (Th1), helper 2 (Th2), helper 17 (Th17), and regulatory (Treg) cells. Each subpopulation is distinguished by the mixture of cytokines that they secrete. As always, many of the details of their function have been investigated in mice and humans, and it must not be assumed that they function in a completely identical manner in equids. Cell-mediated immune responses mediated through Th1 cells are classified as type 1 immune responses. Likewise, antibody responses mediated by Th2 cells are classified as type 2 responses. Inflammatory type 3 immune responses are mediated by Th17 cells (Annunziato & Romagnani, 2015) (Fig. 12.6).

Helper 1 T cells (Th1)

As in other mammals, horses utilize multiple populations of helper T cells. The most important of these are helper-1 (Th1) and helper-2 (Th2) cells. Th1 cells mediate cell-mediated immune responses, whereas Th2 cells mediate antibody mediated immune responses. Both of these helper cell populations have been identified in the horse (Aggarwal & Holmes, 1999). The production of Th1 cells is driven by IL-12 produced by antigen-presenting dendritic cells (cDC1), macrophages (M1), and B cells, plus co-stimulation by CD80. Complete Th1 cell activation, proliferation, and IFN-γ production is achieved by additional stimulation from IL-18. IL-18 and IFN-γ thus reinforce each other's activities. These cytokines activate the transcription factor T-bet. T-bet is the master regulator of Th1 cell differentiation. Once activated, Th1 cells produce IL-2, IFN-γ, TNF-α, and lymphotoxin (TNF-β). Th1 cells, therefore, promote cell-mediated immune responses such as macrophage activation. They mediate immunity to intracellular organisms such as Mycobacteria, Rhodococcus, and viruses. These "type-1"-associated cytokines may also inhibit type-2 immune responses (See below) (Fig. 12.7).

Interferon-γ has some antiviral activity, but its major function is the mediation of Th1 cell responses. IFN-γ is mainly produced by Th1 cells, $CD8^+$ cytotoxic T cells, and natural killer (NK) cells, with lesser amounts from antigen-presenting cells, B cells, and natural killer (NKT) T cells. It activates cells through the JAK-STAT pathway. It promotes macrophage activation, suppresses Th2 cells, and enhances NK cell activities.

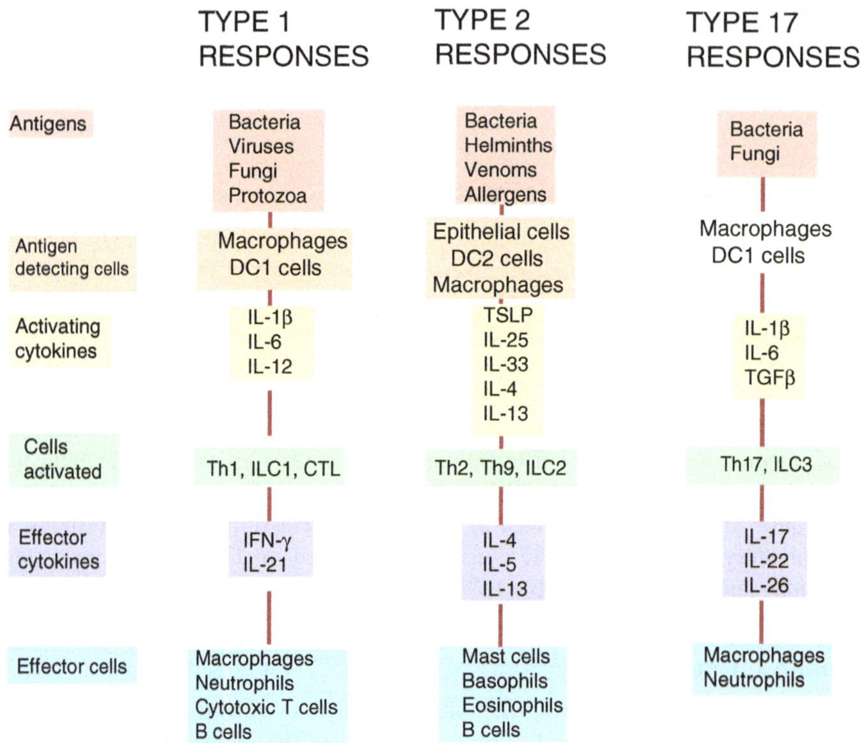

FIGURE 12.6 A summary diagram showing the diversity of T cell responses and the cytokines that control these responses.

IL-2 is produced by activated $CD4^+$ Th1 cells. Some is also produced by $CD8^+$ cells, NKT cells, dendritic cells, and mast cells. Its targets are T, B, and NK cells as well as macrophages. IL-2 is a potent stimulator of T cell proliferation, IFN-γ production, and antibody production by B cells. It enhances the cytotoxicity of $CD8^+$ T and NK cells. It promotes T cell differentiation into Th1 and Th2 subsets while also inhibiting Th17 differentiation. IL-2 is essential for the survival of regulatory T cells as well as for activation-induced cell death. Thus, it has a broad range of essential functions.

Given their importance in stimulating helper T cell functions, reports that foals produce smaller quantities of cytokines than adult horses may indicate defects in their helper cell functions. It has been confirmed that the amount of IFN-γ, IL-4, and IL-10 produced is quantitatively reduced in foals. compared to adult horses. However, the IFN-γ/IL-4 ratio shows a clear Th1 bias in the response in foals aged 6 and 12 weeks. Thus, by 5 days after birth, IFN-γ production by foal $CD4^+$ and $CD8^+$ T cells is similar to that in adults. However, IL-4 production remains low. This suggests that young foals have impaired Th2 responses while their Th1

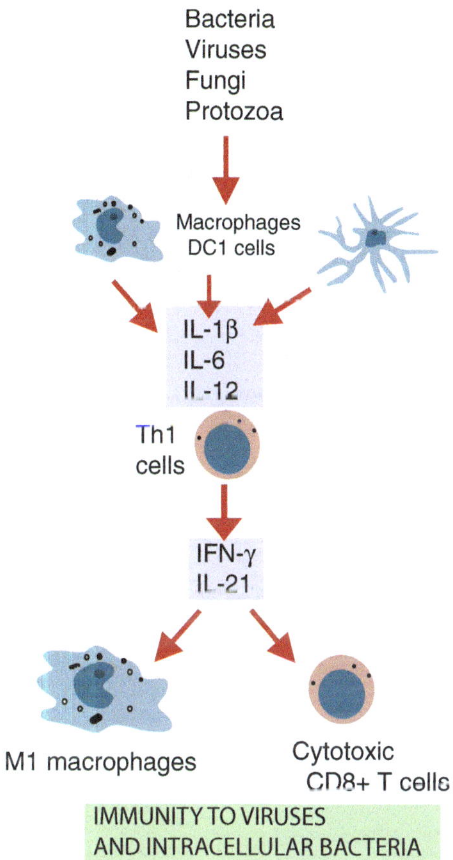

FIGURE 12.7 The generation and functions of Th1 cells.

responses are similar to those in adults. IL-10 production in young foals is also similar to that seen in adult horses (Wagner et al., 2010).

In the horse, Th1 cells appear to preferentially stimulate B cell production of the IgG subclass, IgG4/7. This differentiation is probably influenced by interferon-γ and interleukin-2 as well as by other B-cell maturation factors, although these have yet to be characterized in the horse (Isakov & Morrow, 1989; Sidman et al., 1984).

Helper 2 T cells (Th2)

Th2 cells are responsible for protective type 2 immune responses, including resistance to parasitic helminths, allergic diseases, and tissue repair. They are regulated, in turn, by dendritic cells. Conventional type 2 dendritic cells (cDC2) preferentially promote Th2 cell differentiation. The major Th2 stimulators are IL-33, IL-25, and

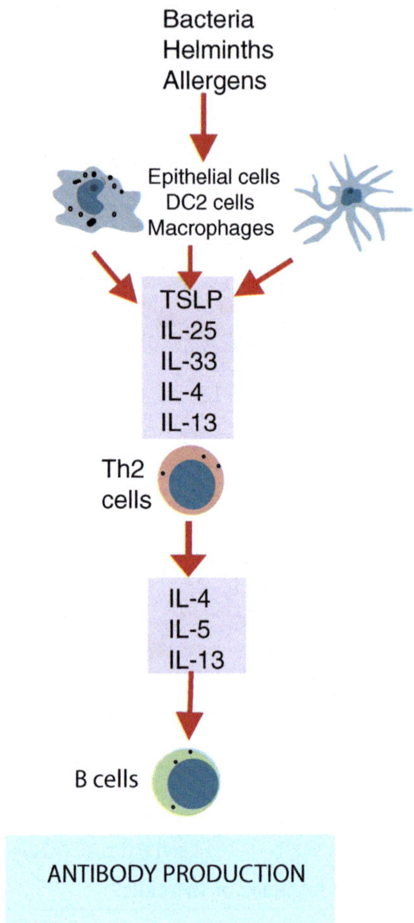

FIGURE 12.8 The generation and functions of Th2 cells.

TSLP. These Th2 cells respond optimally to antigens presented by cDC2 cells and macrophages and less well to antigens presented by B cells. The cDC2 cells provide additional co-stimulation through CD86. Th2 cells may also require co-stimulation by IL-1β from macrophages or dendritic cells (Walker & McKenzie, 2018) (Fig. 12.8).

Activated Th2 cells secrete IL-4, IL-5, IL-9, and IL-13 and so mediate "type 2" immune responses. These cytokines stimulate B cell proliferation and immunoglobulin secretion but tend to suppress cell-mediated responses. The cytokines from Th2 cells enhance B cell production of IgG, especially IgG3/5, and IgA up to 20-fold and production of IgE up to 1000-fold. Type 2 responses are not only associated with enhanced immunity to parasitic worms but also decreased resistance to mycobacteria and other intracellular organisms. They neutralize toxins and regulate wound and tissue repair following infection and injury. If not carefully regulated, type 2 responses can also trigger damaging allergic responses (Chapter 19).

Th17 cells

The third major population of $CD4^+$ T cells in horses produces the pro-inflammatory cytokine IL-17 and hence are called Th17 cells (Crome et al., 2010). Th17 cells are conventional lymphocytes that are abundant in mucosal surfaces. Their presence in these surface tissues is promoted by the gut microbiota (Bettelli et al., 2008). As a result, their frequency increases with age. They are also found in the bloodstream, spleen, and mesenteric lymph nodes. Conversely, γ/δ Th cells producing IL-17 did not show a similar increase in the blood and spleen. Th17 cells mediate type 3 immune responses (Schnell et al., 2023) (Fig. 12.9).

The development of Th17 cells is promoted by IL-23. IL-23 triggers the production of a unique transcription factor called ROR-γt. Th17 growth is then promoted by IL-1β, IL-6, and IL-21. These molecules induce the Th17 cells to produce a mixture of cytokines, namely IL-17A, IL-17F, IL-21, and IL-22 (Parrish-Novak et al., 2002). Th17 cells have two major functions: they mediate inflammation, and they are potent B-cell helpers. Cytokines of the IL-17 family play a key role in protective type 1 responses to extracellular bacteria and assist in the clearance of fungi. Under some circumstances, Th17 cells may convert into IFN-γ-producing Th1 cells. Likewise, they can differentiate into regulatory T cells (Tregs) when inflammation is resolved (Annunziato and Romagnani, 2015; Gagliani et al., 2015). The balance between Th17 and Treg cells is critical to maintaining homeostasis during immune and inflammatory responses.

Type 3 responses mediated by IL-17 play a key role in immunity to extracellular bacteria and fungi since they recruit neutrophils through their actions on stem cells. IL-17 also stimulates the production of GM-CSF, leading to a neutrophilia. It also promotes the recruitment and survival of macrophages, and it stimulates the production of pro-inflammatory cytokines and antibacterial peptides from many cell types. It attracts neutrophils and macrophages (but not eosinophils) to inflammatory sites. Th17 cell population growth is normally controlled by Treg cells as well as by the suppressive cytokines, IL-10, TGF-β and IL-35. Dysregulated IL-17 production contributes significantly to inflammatory diseases (McGeachy et al., 2019; Mills, 2023).

Follicular helper cells

Follicular helper T cells (Tfh cells) are a subpopulation of $CD4^+$ T cells that is specialized for providing help to B cells within germinal centers. Their production is tightly regulated to ensure a sufficient supply of functional B cells (Belanger & Crotty, 2016). Unlike the other helper T cell populations that are defined by the cytokines they produce, Tfh cells express the chemokine receptor CXCR5. As a result, they localize in the B-cell-rich areas of follicles and germinal centers. Tfh cells must

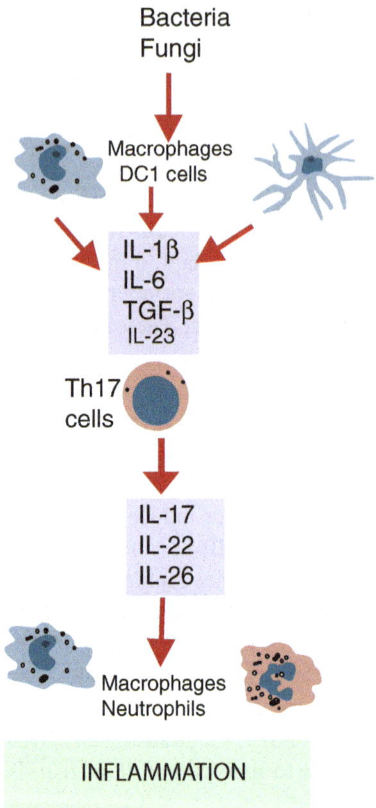

FIGURE 12.9 The generation and functions of Th17 cells.

be activated twice. They are initially activated by dendritic cells and subsequently activated by B cells. They promote B-cell survival, proliferation, and differentiation. They drive B-cell affinity maturation through IL-21 and CD154. Several different Tfh subsets have been identified in other mammalian species.

Cytotoxic T cells

$CD8\alpha^+$ $CD2^+$ T cells express cytotoxic surface receptors such as CD16 and NKp46, as well as perforins. Transcriptome analysis has shown that they express higher levels of mRNA encoding CD16, granulysin, NKG2D, granzyme A, and granzyme B. The largest populations of these cells are found in the lungs and the nasal mucosa. They kill target cells through contact and subsequent degranulation.

Granzymes are serine proteases found in T and NK cells, where they account for about 90% of their total granule contents. Horses possess at least two granzymes, A and B. Granzyme A is most abundant and triggers apoptosis of target cells. It destroys histones and releases a nuclear DNase. It is this enzyme that causes the DNA damage. Equine granzyme A has a molecular weight of 28.2 kDa. Granzyme B enters the target cell either by injection through the central pore of the perforin complex or by endocytosis. Equine granzyme B has been isolated and characterized (Piuko et al., 2007). It activates bcl-2 proteins, triggering the release of mitochondrial cytochrome C. The cytochrome C generates an apoptosome that, in turn, activates caspase 9 and the effector caspase cascade. The effector caspases activate endonucleases that trigger DNA fragmentation and so induce target cell death.

NK-lysin is a 33 kDa antibacterial lipid-disrupting basic peptide found in the granules of both cytotoxic T cells and NK cells in horses. It has broad-spectrum antibacterial activity against both Gram-positive and Gram-negative bacteria. Interestingly, it also has anti-inflammatory properties and downregulates the expression of IL-6 and TNF-α. Its highest concentrations are found in the intestinal tract, where it presumably suppresses inflammation.

Regulatory T cells

Regulatory T cells (Tregs) play a master role in regulating immune responses and maintaining the balance between peripheral tolerance and immunity. In addition to suppressing autoimmunity, they are implicated in tissue repair, maintenance, and regeneration (Fig. 12.10).

There are many Treg subpopulations, and they employ multiple suppressive mechanisms (Dikiy & Rudensky, 2023). Natural Treg cells originate in the thymus, whereas peripheral Treg cells are produced in secondary lymphoid organs, especially the intestine. The intestine is a major site of Treg development, and specialized intestinal dendritic cells promote this development through pathways that use a combination of transforming growth factor-β (TGF-β) and retinoic acid, a metabolite of vitamin A. The retinoic acid is generated by the bacterial microbiota in the gut and is required for normal T cell function. Changes in the microbiota may, therefore, reduce the Treg population while increasing the Th17 cell population. Intestinal Treg cells develop from naïve T cells in response to antigen and co-stimulation by IL-2 and TGF-β. These signals induce the transcription of FoxP3. FoxP3, in turn, induces transcription of the genes for CTLA-4, TGF-β, and IL-10. Equine Treg cells exert their suppressive functions by both cell-cell contact and cytokine-dependent pathways. The cytokines they employ are primarily IL-10 and TGF-β1 (Hamza et al., 2011).

Equine Treg cells are $CD4^+$, $CD25^+$ $FoxP3^+$. CD25 may also be transiently expressed on $CD4^+$ and $CD8^+$ cells (Wagner et al., 2024). They require IL-2 for activation, but excessive IL-2 may reduce their suppressive activity.

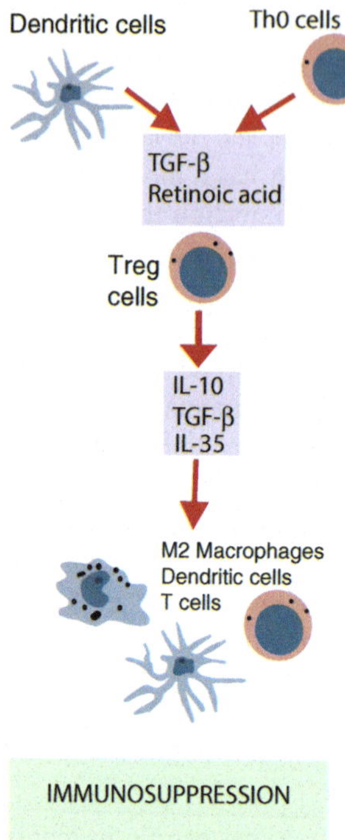

FIGURE 12.10 The generation and functions of Treg cells.

All activated T cells express CD25, but Treg cells are the only ones that express it when naïve. Their most characteristic feature, however, is their use of FoxP3. In a study of adult horses, Robbin et al. determined that a mean of 2.2% of $CD4^+$, and 0.5% of $CD8^+$ T cells expressed FoxP3. Interestingly, the proportion of $CD4^+$ $FoxP3^+$ cells was significantly reduced in horses over 15 years of age (1.5%). In horses 6 years of age and under, their frequency was 2.7%. There were no gender differences detected (Robbin et al., 2011). Thirty-five percent of activated $CD4^+$ $FoxP3^+$ T cells produced IFN-γ while 9% produced IL-10. It appears that $CD4^+$ $FoxP3^+$ T cells likely represent natural Tregs, while $CD4^+FoxP3^+$ $IL\text{-}10^+$ T cells may represent either activated natural Tregs or inducible Tregs. $CD4^+$, $FoxP3^+$ $IFN\text{-}\gamma^-$ cells are probably activated Th1 cells (Robbin et al., 2011).

The proportion of $FoxP3^+$ T cells is much higher in foals than in their mothers. Not only that, but they are functionally more suppressive. This presumably facilitates the development of neonatal tolerance (Hamza et al., 2015).

The importance of FoxP3 is readily seen in equine sarcoidosis caused by bovine papillomavirus (BPV) (Chapter 21). Equine sarcoids are infiltrated by large numbers of $CD4^+$ $CD8^+$ double-positive T cells that express FoxP3. Interestingly, FoxP3 is also expressed within the BPV-infected fibroblasts. As a result, sarcoid cells show increased transcription of TGF-β, resulting in an immunosuppressive tissue environment that permits viral growth (Wilson & Hicks, 2016).

Tregs suppress immune responses through multiple pathways (Dikiy & Rudensky, 2023). Thus, they can inhibit immune responses through direct cell-to-cell contact. This may be mediated by the delivery of suppressive molecules through gap junctions, by binding membrane-bound suppressive cytokines such as TGF-β, by producing cytotoxic granzymes and perforins, or by CTLA-4-mediated reverse signaling through CD80. CD25 on Treg cells may bind and hence reduce the availability of IL-2. Galectin-1 on Tregs can bind receptors on effector T cells, resulting in their cell cycle arrest. CTLA-4^+ cells can induce apoptosis of effector T cells by releasing granzymes or tumor necrosis factor-related apoptosis-inducing ligand (TRAIL). A second mechanism—inhibition by producing suppressive cytokines-is used predominantly by natural Treg cells. These cytokines include IL-10, TGF-β, and IL-35, as well as competitors for cytokine receptors. IL-10 is the most important of these suppressive cytokines.

As a result of all these mechanisms, Treg cells suppress the response of helper T cells to antigens and prevent inappropriate T cell activation in the absence of an antigen. Treg cells can also suppress $CD4^+$ and $CD8^+$ T cell responses by pathways independent of IL-10 and TGF-β. For example, they appear to shorten the interaction time between T cells and antigen-presenting cells and thus prevent activation. Treg cells may also suppress immune responses indirectly by promoting dendritic cell indoleamine dioxygenase expression (Chapter 2).

Treg cells are not the only way in which cellular control of immune responses is exercised. Many of the regulatory activities of T cells reflect the antagonistic functions of Th1 and Th2 cells. For example, IFN-γ from Th1 cells can suppress IgE production, whereas IL-10 from Th2 cells is suppressive for dendritic cell IL-12 production and thus for the production of Th1 cytokines.

Memory T cells

Horses possess memory T cells, as demonstrated by their anamnestic responses to vaccine boosting. When naïve T cells encounter antigens with appropriate co-stimulation, they differentiate into multiple effector T cell populations. These effector cells are usually short-lived because they are eliminated by apoptosis. However, some of these cells resist apoptosis and develop into long-lived memory cells. These can be thought of as "antigen-experienced" stem cells. Memory T cells can be the most abundant T cell population in the body, especially in older animals, since they accumulate throughout life. Compared to naïve T cells, memory cells are easier to activate, live longer, and have enhanced effector activity. As a result, they mount a strong, rapid cytokine response the next time they encounter the antigen. The differences in behavior between naïve and memory T cells likely result from epigenetic modifications that alter gene transcription (mainly histone methylation) and, hence, cell functions (Weng et al., 2012).

This development of effector and memory T cell populations results from asymmetric T cell division (Ciocca et al., 2012). Naïve T cells interact with antigen-presenting cells for several hours through a surface structure termed an immunological synapse (Padhan & Varma, 2020). Once it receives sufficient antigenic stimulation, the T cell begins to divide even before it separates from the presenting cell. The dividing T cell is polarized since one pole of the cell contains the antigen receptors within the immunological synapse. The other pole contains the molecules excluded from the synapse. Thus, when the cell divides, it forms two distinctly different daughter cells. The daughter cell adjacent to the synapse is the precursor of the effector T cells. The daughter cell formed at the opposite pole is the precursor of the memory T cells.

Three types of memory T cells have been characterized. These are central memory cells, tissue-resident memory T cells, and effector memory T cells (Schenkel & Masopust, 2014). Central memory T cells circulate through secondary lymphoid tissues, such as lymph nodes, awaiting the arrival of invaders. They lack immediate effector function but have very rapid recall responses. Effector memory T cells, in contrast, have receptors enabling them to home to inflamed tissues, where they immediately attack invaders without the need to differentiate further. Tissue-resident memory T cells provide a first response to pathogens invading through the body surfaces. They rapidly produce cytokines after infection. They do not circulate in peripheral blood. All memory T cell populations express either CD4 or CD8 and persist in the absence of antigen. $CD8^+$ memory cells tend to accumulate under epithelial surfaces, while $CD4^+$ memory cells are scattered through the tissues in memory lymphocyte clusters (Vezys et al., 2009). Effector memory T cells are $CD62^{lo}$ while central memory T cells are $CD62^{hi}$.

Memory cells slowly divide and replenish their numbers. The cytokines, IL-7 and IL-15 are required for the survival of memory $CD8^+$ T cells, whereas only IL-7 is needed for the survival of $CD4^+$ T cells. These cytokines maintain the cells in a state of slow proliferation. The size of the immune system is fixed somewhat, but the effector memory $CD8^+$ T cell pool can double without loss of preexisting memory cells. Bacterial PAMPs, such as lipopeptides, may also promote the long-term survival of memory T cells even in the absence of persistent antigens.

NKT cells

Horses have an established NKT cell-CD1d system (van Beeck et al., 2009). These natural killer T (NKT) cells are thymus-derived T cells that share a phenotype with NK cells. They are a subset of innate-like $CD3\varepsilon^+$ T cells found in some mammals. Unlike conventional α/β T cells that bind peptide antigens presented by classical MHC molecules, NKT cells can respond to endogenous glycolipid antigens presented by nonpolymorphic CD1d proteins expressed on some antigen-presenting cells and hematopoietic cells. This results in the rapid production of multiple effector cytokines, such as IFN-γ, and the mediation of a range of innate responses.

The NKT cells interact with the CD1d-bound antigens through a conserved invariant TCR (Chapter 10).

Unique T cell antigens

EqWC1 and EqWC2

When cell surface proteins characterized by binding to a specific monoclonal antibody cannot be assigned a specific cluster of differentiation (CD), they are provisionally given a "workshop cluster" (WC) designation. Horse lymphocytes express two of these unassigned, species-specific proteins (Lunn et al., 1998).

EqWC1 is present on a major T cell subset as well as on granulocytes and dendritic cells. It is found on 70% of equine T cells, 30% of B cells, and 50% of granulocytes. It may be an equine ortholog of the T cell surface antigen Thy1 or human CD90 (Chen et al., 2012).

A second unassigned protein, EqWC2, is expressed on granulocytes and most T cells. It is a protein of 160–180 kDa. It may be a low molecular weight isoform of CD45 or a member of the integrin family. It is also expressed on equine dendritic cells (Siedek et al., 1997).

Two other provisionally designated horse leukocyte WC antigens have now been identified and assigned their CD designation. EqWC3 is now considered to be CD2, a T cell marker, while EqWC4 is the equine ortholog of CD28.

References

Aggarwal, N., & Holmes, M. A. (1999). Characterization of equine T helper cells: Demonstration of Th1- and Th2-like cells in long-term equine T-cell cultures. *Research in Veterinary Science, 66*, 277–279.

Annunziato, F., & Romagnani, S. (2015). The 3 major types of innate and adaptive cell-mediated effector immunity. *The Journal of Allergy and Clinical Immunology, 135*, 626–635.

Antonacci, R., Giannico, F., Moschetti, R., Pala, A., et al. (2024). Comprehensive analysis of the genomic and expressed repertoire of the T-cell receptor beta chain in *Equus caballus*. *Animals*. https://doi.org/10.3390/ani14193817

Belanger, S., & Crotty, S. (2016). Dances with cytokines, featuring Tfh cells, IL-21, IL-4 and B cells. *Nature immunol, 17*(10), 1135–1136.

Bettelli, E., Korn, T., Oukka, M., & Kuchroo, V. K. (2008). Induction and effector functions of T(H)17 cells. *Nature, 453*, 1051–1057.

Blanchard-Channell, M., Moore, P. F., & Stott, J. L. (1994). Characterization of monoclonal antibodies specific for equine homologues of CD3 and CD5. *Immunology, 82*, 548–554.

Chen, C., Herzig, C. T. A., Alexander, L. J., Keele, J. W., et al. (2012). Gene number determination and genetic polymorphism of the gamma delta T cell co-receptor WC1 genes. *BMC Genetics, 13*, 86.

Ciocca, M. L., Barnett, B. E., Burkhardt, J. K., Chang, J. T., & Reiner, S. L. (2012). Cutting edge: Asymmetric memory T cell division in response to rechallenge. *Journal of Immunology, 188*(9), 4145–4148.

Crome, S. Q., Wang, A. Y., & Levings, M. K. (2010). Translational mini-review series on Th17 cells: Function and regulation of human T helper 17 cells in health and disease. *Clinical and Experimental Immunology, 159*, 109–119.

Dikiy, S., & Rudensky, A. Y. (2023). Principles of regulatory T cell function. *Immunity, 56*, 240–255.

Göbel, T. W. F., & Dangy, J.-P. (2000). Evidence for a stepwise evolution of the CD3 family. *Journal of Immunology, 164*, 879–883.

Gagliani, N., Amezcua Vesely, M. C., Iseppon, A., Brockmann, L., et al. (2015). Th17 cells transdifferentiate into regulatory T cells during resolution of inflammation. *Nature, 523* (7559), 221–225.

Hamza, E., Gerber, V., Steinbach, F., & Marti, E. (2011). Equine CD4+ CD25 high T cells exhivit regulatory activity by close contact and cytokine-dependent mechanisms in vitro. *Immunology, 134*, 292–304.

Hamza, E., Mirkovitch, J., & Steinbach, M. (2015). Regulatory T cells in early life: Comparative study of CD4+ CD25 high T cells from foals and adult horses. *PLoS One*. https://doi.org/10.1371/journal.pone.0120661

Holderness, J., Hedges, J. F., Ramstead, A., & Jutila, M. A. (2013). Comparative biology of γδ T cell function in humans, mice, and domestic animals. *Annual Review of Animal Biosciences, 1*, 99–124.

Isakov, N., & Morrow, P. R. (1989). Interleukin 2 regulates antigen-specific immunoglobulin response of naive murine B cells. *Cellular Immunology, 120*(2), 366–374.

Lunn, D. P., Holmes, M. A., Antczak, D. F., Agerwal, N., et al. (1998). Report of the second leukocyte antigen workshop, Squaw Valley, California, July 1995. *Veterinary Immunology and Immunopathology, 62*, 101–143.

Massari, S., Giannico, F., Paolillo, N. V., Pala, A., et al. (2023). Genomic and comparative analysis of the T cell receptor gamma locus in two Equus species. *Frontiers in Immunology*. https://doi.org/10.3389/fimmu.2023.1264949

McFarlane, D., Sellon, D. C., & Gibbs, S. A. (2001). Age-related quantitative alterations in lymphocyte subsets and immunoglobulin isotypes in healthy horses. *American Journal of Veterinary Research, 62*, 1413–1417.

McGeachy, M. S., Cua, D. J., & Gaffen, S. L. (2019). The IL-17 family of cytokines in health and disease. *Immunity, 50*, 892–906.

Mills, K. H. G. (2023). IL-17 and IL-17-producing cells in protection versus pathology. *Nature Reviews Immunology, 23*, 38–54.

Nel, A. E. (2002). T-cell activation through the antigen receptor. 1: Signaling components, signaling pathways, and signal integration at the T-cell antigen receptor synapse. *The Journal of Allergy and Clinical Immunology, 109*, 758–770.

Nolz, J. C., & Richer, M. J. (2020). Control of memory CD8+ T cell longevity and effector functions by IL-15. *Molecular Immunology, 117*, 180–188.

Olivieri, D. N., Gambon-Cerda, S., & Gambon-Deza, F. (2015). Evolution of V genes from the TRV loci of mammals. *Immunogenetics, 67*(7), 371–384.

Padhan, K., & Varma, R. (2010). Immunological synapse: A multi-protein signaling cellular apparatus for controlling gene expression. *Immunology, 129*, 322–328.

Parrish-Novak, J., Foster, D. C., Holly, R. D., & Clegg, C. H. (2002). Interleukin-21 and the IL-21 receptor: Novel effectors of NK and T cell responses. *Journal of Leukocyte Biology, 72*, 856–863.

Patel, R. S., Tomlinson, J. E., Divers, T. J., Van der Walle, G. R., & Rosenberg, B. R. (2021). Single-cell resolution landscape of equine peripheral blood mononuclear cells reveals diverse cell types including T-bet+ B cells. *BMC Biology*. https://doi.org/10.1186/s12915-020-00947-5

Piuko, K., Bravo, I. G., & Muller, M. (2007). Identification and characterization of equine granzyme B. *Veterinary Immunology and Immunopathology, 118*, 239–251.

Robbin, M. G., Wagner, B., Noronha, L. E., Antczak, D. F., & de Mestre, A. M. (2011). Subpopulations of equine blood lymphocytes expressing regulatory T cell markers. *Veterinary Immunology and Immunopathology, 140*, 90–101.

Schenkel, J. M., & Masopust, D. (2014). Tissue-resident memory T cells. *Immunity, 41*(6), 886–897.

Schnell, A., Littmann, D. R., & Kuchroo, V. K. (2023). T_H17 cell heterogeneity and its role in tissue inflammation. *Nature Immunology, 24*, 19–29.

Schrenzel, M. D., & Ferrick, D. A. (1995). Horse (*Equus caballus*) T-cell receptor alpha, gamma, and delta chain genes: Nucleotide sequences and tissue-specific gene expression. *Immunogenetics, 42*, 112–122.

Schrenzel, M. D., Watson, J. L., & Ferrick, D. A. (1994). Characterization of horse (*Equus caballus*) T-cell receptor beta chain genes. *Immunogenetics, 40*, 135–144.

Sidman, C. L., Marshall, J. D., Schultz, L. D., Gray, P. W., & Johnson, H. M. (1984). Gamma-interferon is one of several distinct B cell-maturing lymphokines. *Nature, 309*(5971), 801–804.

Siedek, E., Little, S., Mayall, S., Edington, N., & Hamblin, A. (1997). Isolation and characterization of equine dendritic cells. *Veterinary Immunology and Immunopathology, 60*, 15–31.

Su, C., Jakobsen, I., Gu, X., & Nei, M. (1999). Diversity and evolution of T-cell receptor variable region genes in mammals and birds. *Immunogenetics, 50*, 301–308.

Tallmadge, R. L., Wang, M., Sun, Q., & Felippe, M. J. B. (2018). Transcriptome analysis of immune genes in peripheral blood mononuclear cells of young foals and adult horses. *PLoS One*. https://doi.org/10.1371/journal.pone.0202646

Tizard, I. R. (2024). *Veterinary immunology* (11 ed.). St. Louis: Elsevier.

Tschetter, J. R., Davis, W. C., Perryman, L. E., & McGuire, T. C. (1997). CD8 dimer usage on αβ and γδ T lymphocytes from equine lymphoid tissues. *Immunobiology, 198*, 424–438, 98.

Van Beeck, F. A. L., Reinink, P., Hermsen, R., Zajonc, D., et al. (2009). Functional CD1d and/or NKT invariant chain transcript in horse, pig, African elephant, and Guinea pig, but not in ruminants. *Molecular Immunology, 46*, 1424–1431.

Vezys, V., Yates, A., Casey, K. A., et al. (2009). Memory CD8 T-cell compartment grows in size with immunological experience. *Nature, 457*, 196–200.

Wagner, B., Babasyan, S., Wilford, S., Robbin, M. G., et al. (2024). Monoclonal antibodies for equine CD25 improve detection of regulatory T cells in horses. *Veterinary Immunology and Immunopathology, 274*, Article 110790.

Wagner, B., Burton, A., & Ainsworth, D. (2010). Interferon-gamma, interleukin-4 and inteleukin-10 production by T helper cells reveals intact Th1 and regulatory Tr1 cell activation and a delay in the Th2 cell responses in equine neonates and foals. *Veterinary Research*. https://doi.org/10.1051/vetres/2010019

Walker, J. A., & McKenzie, N. J. (2018). T_H2 cell development and function. *Nature Reviews Immunology, 18*, 121–134.

Walsh, K. P., & Mills, K. H. (2013). Dendritic cells and other innate determinants of T helper cell polarisation. *Trends in Immunology, 34*(11), 521–530.

Weng, N. P., Araki, Y., & Subedi, K. (2012). The molecular basis of the memory T cell response: Differential gene expression and its epigenetic regulation. *Nature Reviews Immunology, 12*(4), 306–315.

Wilson, A. D., & Hicks, C. (2016). Both tumour cells and infiltrating T-cells in equine sarcoids express FOXP3 associated with an immune-suppressed cytokine microenvironment. *Veterinary Research*. https://doi.org/10.1186/s13567-016-0339-8

Zhang, C. H., Grunig, G., Davis, W., & Antczak, D. F. (1994). Downregulation followed by re-expression of equine CD4 molecules in response to phorbol myristate acetate. *Veterinary Immunology and Immunopathology, 42*, 71–82.

Immunity on equine body surfaces 13

Although horses and donkeys possess an extensive array of innate and adaptive defense mechanisms within their tissues and organs, it is at their surfaces that invading microorganisms are first encountered and largely repelled or destroyed. The skin is the most obvious of these surfaces, but it represents only a small fraction of the area of the body exposed to the exterior. The surface areas of the mucous membranes of the intestinal and respiratory tracts are at least 200 times larger. The majority of pathogens enter the body through these mucosal surfaces, and respiratory and enteric infections are the most significant causes of death in foals. While the immune systems ensure that the interior of the body remains largely free of microbial invaders, it is not possible to keep the surfaces of the body sterile. As a result, by far the greatest numbers of immune cells are found associated with these surfaces. The physical barriers to microbial invasion are also considerable and contribute significantly to host defenses (Fig. 13.1).

The skin

Equine skin carries out its barrier function effectively, and few bacteria can penetrate intact skin unaided. The skin forms a tough physical barrier supplemented by continuous desquamation, desiccation, and a low pH because of fatty acids in sebum. In

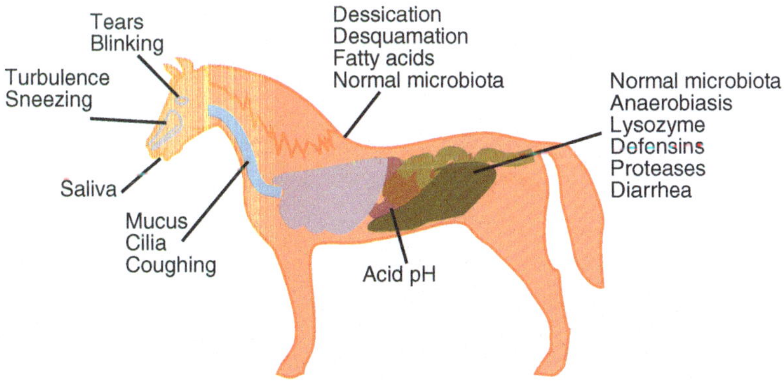

FIGURE 13.1

The wide diversity of physical and innate surface protection mechanisms in the horse.

The Immunology of Horses and Donkeys. https://doi.org/10.1016/B978-0-443-44863-8.00027-2

addition, the skin carries a resident microbiota that outcompetes, and excludes pathogenic bacteria and fungi. If the skin microbiota is disturbed, its protective properties are reduced, and microbial invasion may result. Thus, skin infections tend to occur in areas such as the axilla or groin, where both pH and humidity are high. Hair itself prevents desiccation and may protect against some fungal infections (Fig. 13.2).

Each layer of the skin has its own defensive mechanisms. For example, equine keratinocytes express multiple pattern recognition molecules (PRMs) such as TLR4 and TLR5, mannose receptors, and C-type lectins, so they can recognize molecular patterns associated with microbial invasion. As a result, when stimulated by these invaders, keratinocytes respond by producing a complex mixture of interleukins, interferons, chemokines, and growth factors, all of which assist in excluding microbes. Keratinocytes are also the main source of cathelicidins and β-defensins (Wingate et al., 2009). Equine keratinocytes produce significant quantities of IL-1β, IL-6, and CXCL8 in response to bacterial lipopolysaccharides (Leise et al., 2010). Stimulation of sensitized equine keratinocytes with Culicoides midge salivary allergens results in upregulation of the genes encoding the chemokines CCL5, CCL11, and CCL20, as well as IL-31. Stimulation by TLR1/2 ligands results in upregulation of the TLR and NOD receptor signaling pathways as well as the NF-κB pathway (Cvitas et al., 2022).

Mast cells and skin secretory cells, such as those within the apocrine and sebaceous glands, also add antimicrobial peptides and lipids to the protective barriers.

Under normal conditions, keratinocytes continually renew the epidermis in a coordinated manner. If the skin is wounded or inflamed, alterations in adhesion molecules, surface receptors, and the cytokine environment change the behavior of

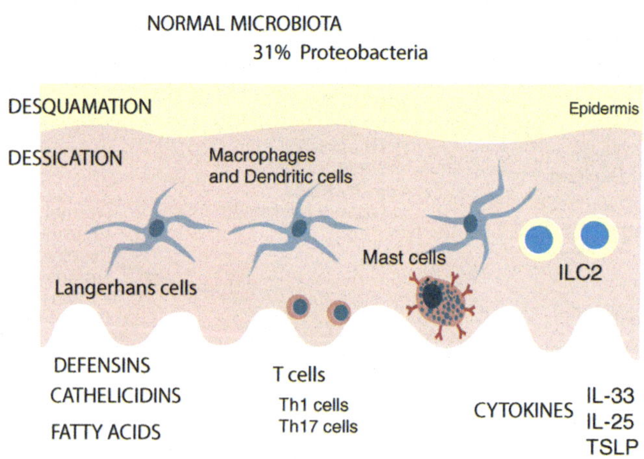

FIGURE 13.2 The innate and adaptive immune defenses of the skin.

These include antibacterial molecules in addition to competition from the normal microbiota, T cells, mast cells, Langerhans cells, and inflammatory cytokines.

the keratinocytes. Keratinocytes also express MHC class II molecules and may act as antigen-presenting cells (Coates et al., 2018).

Once they penetrate the skin, microbes encounter dendritic cells in large numbers. The best-known of these are Langerhans cells (Chapter 7). Langerhans cells bind microbial antigens and present them to nearby helper T cells. The dermis also contains resident DCs, as does the subcutaneous adipose tissue layer.

T cells are mainly located in the basal layer of healthy skin associated with Langerhans cells. $CD4^+$ and $CD8^+$ T cells are present in equal numbers. In other domestic mammals, a subset of circulating T cells that home to the skin and produce IL-22 (Th22 cells) has also been identified (Sonnenberg et al., 2011). Interleukin 22 is a 34 kDa member of the IL-10 family produced by activated Th17 cells, NK cells, and mast cells. It suppresses IL-4 production by Th2 cells and induces acute-phase protein production in the liver. It appears to be especially important in maintaining barrier function on exposed body surfaces. It promotes antimicrobial immunity, inflammation, and tissue repair and regeneration. Skin also contains resident memory T cells that can provide global skin immunity and thus protect non-involved skin. Treg cells facilitate cutaneous wound healing by enhancing local expression of the epithelial growth factor receptor. While not yet demonstrated in horse skin, it is clear that horses do produce IL-22, at least in the trophoblast of the equine chorionic girdle (Chapter 2). (Brosnahan et al., 2012)

Failure of the skin permeability barrier predisposes to secondary infections, while pathogen colonization aggravates the permeability defect. The antimicrobial barrier is also defective in cases of atopic dermatitis. Both defensins and cathelicidins are downregulated as a result of defective lamellar body functions. Lamellar bodies are secretory organelles found in keratinocytes. They fuse with the cell membrane and release the lipids that seal the gaps between keratinocytes and thus serve a skin barrier function. They also regulate the proteasess that cause skin desquamation (Leprince & Simon, 2025),). Reduced levels of free fatty acids and sphingosine reduce antimicrobial activity in the skin, and as a result, secondary infections will increase. Fungi such as Malassezia yeasts are important members of the equine skin microbiota (Shokri, 2015). As commensals, they interact with their host's immune system and play an important role in regulating host immune responses. They are regarded as a major predisposing factor in some forms of dermatitis, but it must be remembered that other factors, such as host immunity, epithelial barrier dysfunction, and environmental factors, also play a role.

The respiratory tract

The mammalian respiratory tract differs from other surfaces in that it is in intimate connection with the interior of the body yet is required by its very nature to allow unhindered access of air to the alveoli. This is especially important in equids that rely on rapid flight for protection against predators. Particles suspended in inhaled air are largely removed by turbulence that directs them onto its mucus-covered surfaces where they adhere. The turbulence is caused by the conformation of the turbinate bones, the trachea, and the bronchi. This turbulence filter serves to remove particles as small as 5 μm before they reach the alveoli (Iwasaki et al., 2016).

The respiratory mucus layer lining the airways is in continuous flow, being carried from the bronchioles up the bronchi and trachea by ciliary action or backward through the nasal cavity to the pharynx. Here, the "dirty" mucus is swallowed and digested in the intestinal tract. Particles that bypass this mucociliary escalator and reach the alveoli are phagocytosed by alveolar macrophages. Once these cells have successfully ingested particles, they migrate to the mucus escalator and are also carried to the pharynx (Fig. 13.3).

A blanket of mucus gel produced by goblet cells lines the upper respiratory tract. This mucus contains soluble host defense molecules such as lysozyme, lactoferrin, surfactant proteins, and cationic peptides such as the defensins and cathelicidins. Most microorganisms that enter the mucus layer are likely to be killed rapidly. The surfactant proteins SP-A and SP-D are also produced in the lungs of horses. They are synthesized by pulmonary intravascular macrophages located in the alveolar septa. They are present in both bronchiolar epithelial cells and type II alveolar epithelial cells, as well as in intravascular macrophages and neutrophils (Bocking & Singh., 2021) (Chapter 3). These surfactant proteins reduce surface tension at the alveolar surface so that a thin film of fluid forms on the surface and prevents lung collapse. SP-A and D, are C-type lectins that also bind to microbial carbohydrates and act as opsonins. SP-A and -D also activate macrophages, promote chemotaxis, and enhance the respiratory burst, as well as the production of inflammatory cytokines. These surfactant proteins also enhance the clearance of apoptotic cells from the lung. This is especially important in the resolution of inflammation since apoptotic neutrophils and their toxic contents must be removed from the alveoli by macrophages as promptly as possible. Surfactant proteins can also modulate

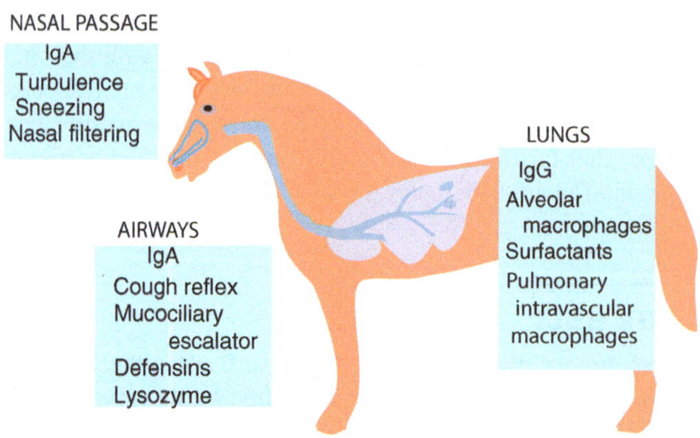

FIGURE 13.3

The physical and innate defenses of the equine respiratory tract.

the functions of dendritic cells and T cells. SP-A inhibits the maturation of dendritic cells, whereas SP-D enhances their uptake and presentation of antigens. Both SP-A and SP-D inhibit T cell proliferation. Pulmonary intravascular macrophages in 30-day-old foals contain both SP-A and SP-D (Bocking et al., 2021).

Equine pentraxin 3 (PTX3) is a 32 or 42 kDa protein produced by many different cell types within the lungs, especially neutrophils and macrophages. It has a major antibacterial role. Like other acute-phase proteins, PTX3 is produced in response to TNF-α, IL-1β, and some microbial components. PTX3 can bind to diverse bacteria, fungi, and viruses and promote their phagocytosis, as well as activating the terminal complement pathway and causing their lysis. It is present in significant amounts in bronchial epithelial cells and vascular endothelium of normal horse lungs. It is also present within equine bronchoalveolar macrophages, and pulmonary intravascular macrophages, as well as neutrophils, and epithelial cells. PTX3 acts on alveolar macrophages to enhance their phagocytic abilities (Townsend et al., 2023). Its production can be induced in vitro by exposing bronchiolar lavage fluid cells to dust particles (Ramery et al., 2010).

The respiratory tract of the horse contains bronchial lymphoid nodules as well as lymphocytes distributed diffusely throughout the lung and airways. The mucosa of the larynx contains many immunologically active cells, including large numbers of T cells. Antigen-sampling M cells may be associated with these lymphoid nodules, and are also abundant within the nasal mucosa. The nasal mucosa is also rich in IgA-producing plasma cells. These tissues mainly produce secretory IgA, especially in the upper regions of the respiratory tract. This IgA mixes with mucus molecules and so enhances the clearance of adherent bacteria. The polymeric immunoglobulin receptor (pIgR) is expressed at low levels on bronchial epithelial cells. In the bronchioles and alveoli, however, the secretions also contain a large proportion of IgG that binds to the mucus gel—"muco-trapping," and hence carries bound microorganisms up the mucus escalator to the pharynx (Schaefer & Lai, 2022). IgE is also synthesized in significant amounts in the lymphoid tissues of the upper respiratory tract.

Bronchoalveolar lavage fluid

Many cells may be washed out of the airways of equine lungs by flushing with saline. This bronchoalveolar lavage fluid (BALF) is a useful material to explore the defenses of the lungs. In healthy horses, about 50%–65% of the cells flushed out in bronchoalveolar washes are macrophages, 30%–44% are lymphocytes, and 3%–6% are neutrophils. 0%–1% are eosinophils, while 1%–2% are mast cells. Overall cell counts in BALF range from 150 to 510 × 10^6/L. These numbers change significantly in asthmatic horses with a relative increase in eosinophil numbers (Riihimaki et al., 2023). Lung T cells can produce cytokines, and alveolar macrophages are activated following infection with intracellular bacteria. Cell-mediated immune responses are therefore readily provoked among the cells within the lower respiratory tract (Pickles et al., 2002).

As expected, the numbers of leukocytes present in the bronchoalveolar fluid from newborn foals are relatively low. Initially, these are almost exclusively macrophages. Lymphocytes are essentially absent from the lungs at birth but climb slowly between two and 4 months (Flaminio et al., 2000) (Fig. 13.4).

The cellular populations in BALF from normal healthy donkeys are similar to those in horses but contain slightly higher percentages of macrophages (Mendoza et al., 2018).

The nasal mucosa is rich in MHC II- and CD1-positive dendritic cells, and all types of T cells, as well as IgA-producing plasma cells. It is also rich in mast cells located just under the epithelial surface. In nasal secretions from horses and foals over 28 days of age, IgA is the predominant immunoglobulin isotype. In animals less than 14 days of age, IgG is the predominant isotype in these secretions (Sheoran et al., 2000). The nasal IgA is largely responsible for immunity to upper respiratory

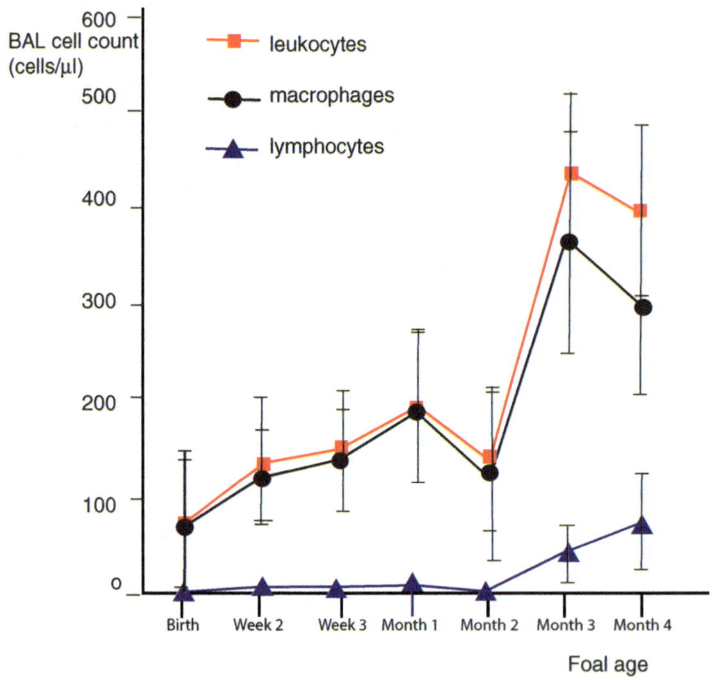

FIGURE 13.4 Bronchoalveolar lavage differential leukocyte counts in healthy foals from birth to 4 months of age.

Note that the population largely consists of macrophages. The results represent the mean and standard deviation of samples from 10 foals.

- From Flaminio, J. B. F., Rush, B. R., Davis, E. G., Hennessey, K., et al. (2000). Characterization of peripheral blood and pulmonary leukocyte function in healthy foals. Veterinary Immunology and Immunopathology, 73, 267–285, with permission.

tract infections such as those caused by *Streptococcus equi* (Galan & Timoney, 1985).

Two of the most vulnerable sites to infection in the horse are the guttural pouches. These are large diverticula that extend from the auditory tube. They play a role in cooling the blood supply to the brain. They are, however, susceptible to infections by organisms such as *Strep equi*, the cause of strangles. They appear to resist infections through the use of a layer of mucus containing diverse glycoproteins with high amounts of sulfated carbohydrates and sialic acids to cover their mucosal surfaces. These block access to cell surface proteins and potentially interfere with bacterial and viral adherence (Parillo et al., 2009). Interestingly, the walls of the urinary bladder use a similar heavily glycosylated mucus layer for protection.

The urogenital tract

The reproductive tract of the mare can be divided into a lower (vagina and cervix) and an upper part (uterus and fallopian tubes). The lower part is covered by stratified squamous epithelium, the upper by columnar epithelium. All are covered by microbicidal mucus. Within the lower part, the keratinocytes express pattern recognition molecules (PRMs) and produce cytokines and antimicrobial peptides. The upper part contains large numbers of macrophages, dendritic cells, and innate lymphoid cells.Healthy mares with normal reproductive tracts are usually resistant to chronic uterine infections (Fig. 13.5).

Plasma cells containing IgG, IgA, or IgM can be identified at all levels of the reproductive tract. Secretory component is present in the uterine epithelium but not in the oviduct, cervix, or vagina. The number of IgG and IgA-positive cells is roughly equal in both parts. The number of IgG-producing cells declines from the uterus to the vagina (Widders et al., 1985). While IgA accounts for about 5% of equine serum immunoglobulins, it accounts for 50% of the endometrial immunoglobulins. Conversely, while IgG accounts for 66% of serum immunoglobulins, it

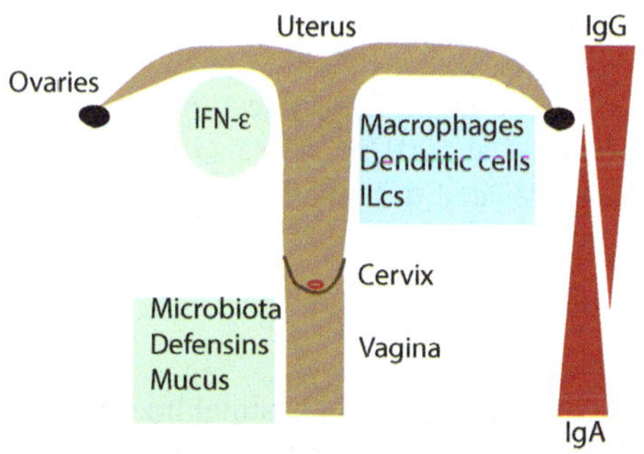

FIGURE 13.5

The innate and adaptive defenses of the mare's genital tract.

only accounts for 31% of the endometrial immunoglobulins (Liu, 1988). Uterine concentrations of IgG are significantly higher during the luteal phase of the mare's estrus cycle than during periods of estrus. The relative ratios of IgM, IgA, or IgG do not change over the cycle.

The predominant immunoglobulin in equine cervicovaginal mucus is IgA, whereas within the uterus, it is IgG. IgG also reaches the uterine lumen and the vagina by active transport mediated by FcRn. This receptor is pH-dependent. It binds IgG in the tissues where the pH is high and releases it in the vagina, where the pH is very low (Guenther et al., 2024) (Fig. 2.7).

A type I interferon, designated interferon-ε, is expressed in the epithelial cells of the female reproductive tract. IFN-ε induces typical IFN-regulated genes (Fung et al., 2013). It is not, however, induced by the conventional pattern recognition pathways involving receptors such as the TLRs. Instead, it is constitutively expressed and hormonally regulated. IFN-ε has been characterized in mares (Fischer et al., 2018).

The urogenital tract of stallions is also defended against microbial invasion. Antimicrobial peptides are found in the testes, seminal vesicles, and prostate. Epithelial cells lining the urethra express PRMs, and macrophages and dendritic cells are abundant. IgG is the predominant immunoglobulin in seminal plasma, and IgA is also present. The B cells that produce these immunoglobulins are mainly found in the penile urethra and prostate. T cells are also abundant in the urethra, testes, and prepuce. IgA is present in small amounts in normal urine, produced presumably, by B cells in the walls of the urinary tract.

The gastrointestinal tract

Oral cavity

A critical role in the immune defense of the oral cavity is played by salivary secretory IgA. The level of sIgA in equine saliva averages 7.4 mg/dL. There is also a limited quantity of IgG in equine saliva. It is about one-fifth of the concentration of IgA. Analysis of the IgG isotypes in saliva indicated that the saliva/serum ratio of IgG4/7 is about four times higher than that of IgG3/5. There is, however, great individual variability in these quantities, reflecting the significant contribution of local IgA synthesis (Palm et al., 2016). It is also interesting to note that salivary levels of IgA are greatly elevated in horses suffering from gastric ulcer syndrome (Botia et al., 2024).

Small intestine

The layer of enterocytes lining the gastrointestinal tract forms an enormous surface between the body and the external environment. Thus, the entire gastrointestinal tract, from mouth to anus is a potential route of microbial invasion. It must exclude not only potential pathogens but also the commensals of the normal microbiota. Thus, a mucosal "firewall" must be established to discourage invasion (Fig. 13.6).

The first cellular barrier to microbial invasion is the intestinal epithelium. This consists of a continuous layer of enterocytes and goblet cells. Collectively, these cells form an effective physical barrier by having tight junctions between cells and a glycocalyx on their luminal surface. In addition to the goblet cells that produce the mucus, enterocytes also produce a diverse mixture of antimicrobial peptides that limit microbial exposure. Enteric defensins accumulate within intestinal crypts and achieve very high concentrations in the mucus layer closest to the epithelium. They serve a barrier function since they prevent commensals from entering the crypt space and so reduce direct microbial contact with enterocytes. The defensin mixture selectively kills some bacterial species and, as a result, also regulates the composition of the microbiota.

Enterocytes possess a complete set of PRMs and can sense signals coming from the microbiota. They can then transmit these signals to the immune cells in the lamina propria. They are actively involved in shaping the intestinal immune environment since they help maintain balance between anti- and pro-inflammatory signals. They also block access of intact antigens to the lamina propria. Tight junctions between enterocytes help maintain this barrier. (Molecules larger than about 2 kDa are excluded.) Thus, they keep the normal intestinal microbiota away from the intestinal immune system. Enterocytes secrete or respond to regulatory cytokines. For example, they produce thymic stromal lymphopoietin (TSLP) that is required for the generation of Tregs. They also produce TGF-β and the B cell-stimulating cytokines, BAFF and APRIL. If an enterocyte becomes infected, it can respond by producing antimicrobial peptides and increasing mucin and cytokine production. It may also respond by undergoing inflammasome-mediated cell death.

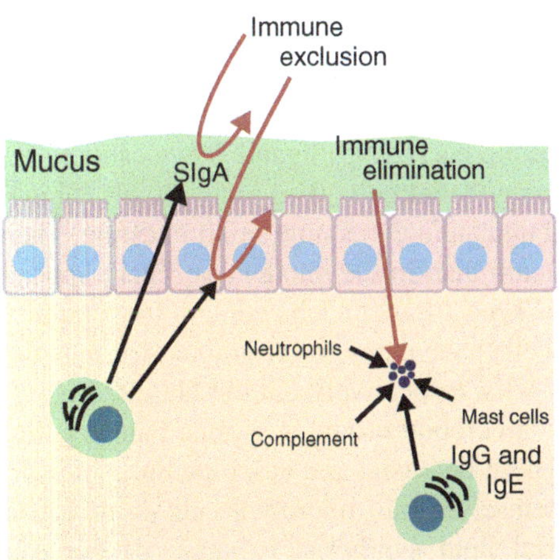

FIGURE 13.6 The major immune defenses of the equine gastrointestinal tract.

Invading organisms are either excluded or eliminated.

The gastrointestinal mucus layer is also critical to the exclusion of both commensals and pathogens. It consists of a gel containing mucins, glycoproteins, and lipids that prevents bacteria from contacting the epithelium (Johansson & Hansson, 2016). This mucus acts as a lubricant, blocks chemical insults, and can capture and then expel pathogens. The mucus forms two layers. The inner layer next to the enterocytes consists of firm mucus rich in defensins and lysozyme and contains few bacteria. The fluid mucus in the intestinal lumen is composed primarily of mucins produced by intestinal goblet cells. Many bacteria are embedded in this mucus, which prevents their washout. Its thickness and composition vary, but it tends to be thickest where the microbiota is most abundant. Both the inflammasome and autophagy pathways control the production of this mucus by goblet cells.

The enterocyte brush border is also covered by a glycocalyx, a layer of acidic polysaccharides and glycoproteins that binds to the apical surface of the cells and serves as a protective barrier while still permitting the absorption of nutrients. The glycocalyx also serves as a protective barrier on the endothelial surface of healthy blood vessels. Among the key components of the glycocalyx are syndecan-1, heparan sulfate, and hyaluronan. If the glycocalyx is damaged, it may result in the development of small intestinal colic in horses. Thus, serum and peritoneal fluid concentrations of syndecan-1 are elevated in horses suffering from inflammatory and strangulating lesions in the small intestine. Hyaluronan levels are also higher in diseased horses when compared to healthy control animals. There is also a greater number of heparan sulfate positive cells in diseased intestinal tissue (Hobbs et al., 2025).

Paneth cells

Among the epithelial cells that line the equine gastrointestinal tract are a population of granule-rich cells located at the bottom of the enteric crypts. These are Paneth cells. They are specialized secretory epithelial cells with an extensive endoplasmic reticulum, a large Golgi apparatus, and abundant large granules in their apical cytoplasm. These granules contain antimicrobial peptides, especially α-defensins. In addition, they also secrete fas (CD95) ligand. They can also act as phagocytic cells and remove apoptotic epithelial cells (Cui et al., 2023) (Fig. 13.7).

Paneth cells are abundant in the equine small intestine. Their numbers are higher in the jejunum and ileum than in the duodenum. There appear to be two structural subtypes in the horse. Type 1 Paneth cells contain large numbers of secretory granules, whereas type 2 cells have many fewer granules. It may well be that they represent young and aged cells, respectively (Cui et al., 2023).

When triggered by microbial products, equine Paneth cells secrete large quantities of α-defensins. These defensins are amphipathic molecules that act like detergents. They insert themselves into microbial cell walls, cause bacterial lysis, and interfere with bacterial lipid synthesis. IChapter 3) For example, equine alpha defensin-1 is lethal for *Rhodococcus equi*. Equine Paneth cells also produce large quantities of the antibacterial enzyme lysozyme.

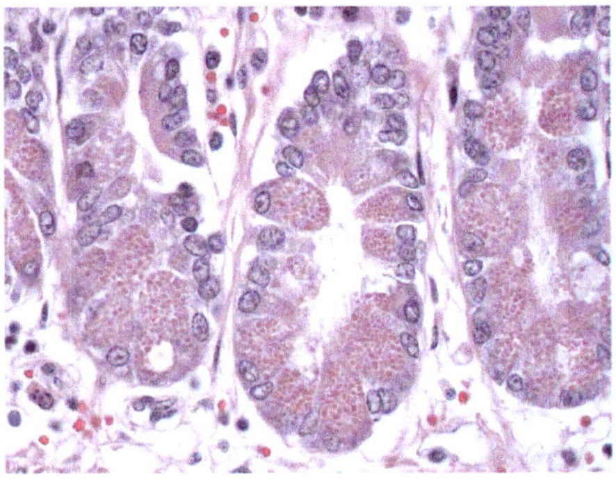

FIGURE 13.7 Paneth cells from the intestine of a horse.

The cells located at the base of the crypts are filled with large eosinophilic granules and are the major source of intestinal defensins and lysozyme Original magnification '60.

- Courtesy Dr. Brian Porter.

Mucosal lymphoid tissues

Because of the importance of preventing microbial invasion through the gastrointestinal mucosa, these surfaces contain large amounts of lymphoid tissue. Mucosal lymphoid tissues can be classified as sites where antigens are processed and immune responses are initiated (inductive sites) and sites where antibodies and cell-mediated defensive immune responses are generated (effector sites).

Inductive sites

The mucosa-associated lymphoid tissues (MALTs) contain all three cell types required to initiate adaptive immune responses: T cells, B cells, and dendritic cells. These tissues include lymphoid tissues in the eyelids, nasal mucosa, tonsils, pharynx, tongue and palate, Peyer's patches; solitary lymphoid nodules, and numerous lymphoid nodules in the lung. These lymphoid tissues are known by their acronyms. Thus, GALT (Gut-Associated Lymphoid Tissue) is the collective term for all the lymphoid nodules, Peyer's patches, and individual lymphocytes found in the intestinal walls. Similarly, BALT is the acronym used for the Bronchus-Associated Lymphoid Tissue in the lungs. These organized lymphoid tissues, unlike lymph nodes, do not react to foreign antigens delivered through afferent lymph but rather sample them directly from the mucosal surface. The tonsils are especially important in inducing immunity on mucosal surfaces in the oral cavity and pharyngeal region (Chapter 8).

Peyer's patches are the largest and most obvious of the mucosal lymphoid tissues. Peyer's patches consist of masses of lymphocytes clustered together in follicles and covered with an epithelium that contains M cells (Chapter 8). M cells are specialized epithelial cells involved in antigen transportation from the intestinal lumen to mucosal lymphoid tissues (Corr et al., 2008). They have microfolds (M) rather than microvilli on their surface. They are found in the dome epithelium overlying Peyer's patches. While scattered over the domes of duodenal and jejunal PP, they are the major cell type in the epithelium overlying the ileal PPs. The mucus layer tends to thin out over Peyer's patches (there are fewer goblet cells, so that the M cells protrude into the intestinal lumen. However, there are also deep intrafollicular invaginations in the duodenal dome epithelium that contain few M cells. M cells endocytose the proteins and microbes they encounter, but rather than destroying them, they transport the antigens to the underlying lymphoid tissue. M cells may also transport soluble macromolecules such as IgA, small particles, and even whole organisms.

Effector sites

Although Peyer's patches are full of lymphocytes, most intestinal IgA is produced in diffuse lymphoid nodules and by isolated plasma cells scattered throughout the submucosa of the intestine, in bronchi, and in salivary glands.

B cells

B cells respond to antigens that penetrate the enterocyte barrier. Some of these responding B cells migrate to regional lymph nodes and into intestinal lymphatics, from which they reach the thoracic duct and enter the bloodstream. These circulating IgA-positive B cells have an affinity for all body surfaces. As a result, they colonize not only the intestinal tract but also the respiratory tract, urogenital tract, and mammary glands. Thus, antigen priming at one location will permit antibodies to be synthesized and secondary responses to occur at locations remote from the priming site, reflecting the existence of a common mucosal immune system. The movement of IgA-positive B cells from the intestine to the mammary glands is especially important since it provides a route by which antibodies directed against intestinal pathogens in the mare can be transferred to the newborn foal through her colostrum and milk. Oral administration of an antigen to a pregnant mare will thus result in the appearance of antigen-specific IgA antibodies in her milk. In this way, antibodies directed against intestinal pathogens can flood the intestine of the newborn foal. T cells originating within the Peyer's patches also home specifically to the intestinal mucosa by using specialized vascular adhesive molecules. For example, mucosal addressin cell-adhesion molecule-1 (MAdCAM-1) is an adhesion molecule expressed on the high endothelial venules of Peyer's patches and on venules in intestinal lamina propria and the mammary gland. Its ligand is the lymphocyte integrin $\alpha4/\beta7$. B and T cells that express this integrin migrate preferentially to the intestine and the mammary glands.

T cells

T cells are found in the equine intestinal wall. They are mainly scattered throughout the lamina propria and in Peyer's patches. Some T cells are also situated between enterocytes immediately below the mucosal surface, where they are known as intraepithelial lymphocytes (IELs). Their location suggests that they play an important role in the defense of the mucosa. IELs regulate host-microbial interactions at the intestinal mucosal surface and are critical components in preventing invasion by the commensal microbiota. Intraepithelial lymphocyte function is, in turn, regulated by many different cytokines, including IL-2, IL-7, IL-15, and TGF-β.

T cells originate in the bone marrow, undergo thymic selection, and mature within the lamina propria just under the enterocytes. Wedged between epithelial cells, IELs can recognize antigens directly, possibly through the TLR-MyD88 pathway as well as their antigen receptors and secrete cytokines such as IFN-γ in response. The interferon, in turn, stimulates macrophages and nearby enterocytes to secrete protective nitric oxide (Van Kaer & Olivares-Villagomez, 2018).

In horses, IELs are MHC class II positive cells and may act as antigen-presenting cells. They regulate B-cell IgA responses. Some have NK cell activity, whereas others are cytotoxic T cells that may attack parasites within the intestinal lumen. They also play a role in the repair of damaged epithelia. Likewise, lamina propria cells and enterocytes, especially in the jejunum and ileum located close to Peyer's patches, are also MHC II positive. There are two different groups of intestinal lymphocytes that produce IL-17. One group consists of mucosal ILC3s that produce IL-17 spontaneously. The second group consists of Th17 cells that produce IL-17 following antigen processing and exposure to IL-23, driven by dendritic cells.

Adaptive immunity

Both antibody- and cell-mediated immune responses protect body surfaces. Some of these antibodies, most notably IgA and possibly IgM, act by immune exclusion—they keep the antigens out. The others, especially IgE and IgG, destroy any antigens that penetrate the surface tissues by immune elimination.

Immunoglobulin A

IgA is present in equine blood serum, colostrum, milk, and other body secretions such as saliva and tears. It is the predominant immunoglobulin in tears and saliva. In serum, IgA averages 299 ± 13.4 mg/dL in aged and slightly less (261 ± 14.9 mg/dL in younger animals (McFarlane et al., 2001). However, there are enormous breed differences. For example, in Shetland ponies, the mean serum IgA level is 153 mg/dL. This is slightly higher than IgM. In their tears, IgA levels range from 80 to 150 mg/dL. However, in milk it is 80–130 mg/dL and in colostrum 20–28 mg/dL (Rouse & Ingram, 1970). The predominant form of IgA found in the pony serum has an apparent molecular weight of about 350 kDa, suggesting that it is dimeric (McGuire & Crawford, 1972) (Fig. 13.8).

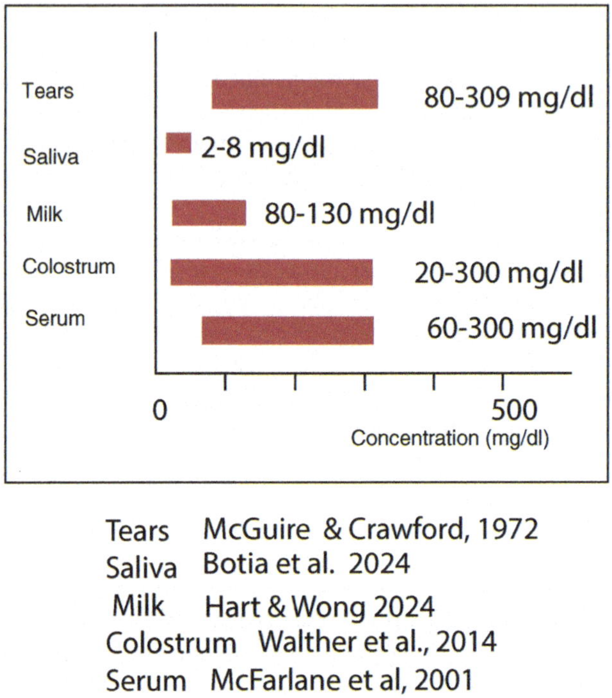

FIGURE 13.8

IgA levels in body fluids.

- Data from the references cited on the figure.

In another study, it was found that the mean IgA concentration in equine tears was higher in females than in males. This study found a mean level of 309 $\pm$ 30.7 mg/dL. This difference could be caused by many factors, including not only sample size, but also the breed of the horse and degree of antigenic challenge as well as the severity of the eye irritation caused by environmental dusts (Martin et al., 1997).

Structure

As in most other mammals, there is a single IGHA heavy chain gene within the horse IGH locus that occurs in four allelic forms. These differ in the length of their hinge region. The distribution of these alleles differs between breeds (Snoeck et al., 2006). IgA monomers are about 160 kDa in size and are typical four-chain, Y-shaped molecules. They are usually secreted as dimers or larger polymers linked by a 15 kDa J-chain. IgA has several extra cysteine residues in its heavy chains. As a result, these form multiple short interchain disulfide bonds that compact the chains and shield vulnerable sites from intestinal proteases. As a result, IgA is not readily destroyed by intestinal enzymes. When coexpressed with equine IgA, the J chain results in its effective dimerization (Lewis et al., 2010). The gene for the J chain is located on chromosome ECA 3 and consists of 4 exons.

Tissue distribution

IgA is present in equine serum and mucosal secretions. IgA predominates in equine surface secretions. At least 80% of all equine plasma cells are found in the intestinal lamina propria, and collectively they produce more immunoglobulin A than all other immunoglobulin isotypes combined. IgA is excreted in enormous amounts in saliva, intestinal fluid, mesenteric lymph, nasal and tracheal secretions, tears, milk, colostrum, urine, and the secretions of the urogenital tract. Because IgA is transported through enterocytes, it can also act inside these cells. Thus, IgA can bind to newly synthesized viral proteins inside these cells and interrupt viral replication. In this way, the IgA can prevent viral growth before the integrity of the epithelium is damaged. This is a unique example of antibodies acting in an intracellular location. The second unique function of intracellular IgA is to excrete foreign antigens. Thus, IgA can bind to antigens that have penetrated to the submucosa. Once bound, the IgA-antigen complexes bind to the pIgR and are then actively transported back across the enterocytes into the intestinal lumen. IgA can therefore act at three different levels to exclude foreign antigens: within the submucosa, within enterocytes, and within the intestinal lumen.

Production

IgA is synthesized and secreted by plasma cells located in the intestinal submucosa, especially in the crypt region. This dimeric IgA binds to the receptor for polymeric immunoglobulins (pIgR) on the basolateral surface of enterocytes. The receptor binds covalently to the Cα2 domain of one of the IgA monomers. The membrane-bound IgA-pIgR complex is then endocytosed and actively transported across the enterocyte. When it reaches the exterior surface, this endocytic vesicle fuses with the apical plasma membrane and exposes the complex to the intestinal lumen. The extracellular domains of the pIgR are then cleaved by proteases so that the IgA, with the receptor peptide still attached (secretory IgA), is released into the lumen. The receptor peptide is called secretory component. The production, transport, and secretion of secretory component occur even in the absence of IgA, so that free secretory component is found in high concentrations in intestinal contents. Equine pIgR has been cloned and sequenced. Its gene is located on chromosome ECA 5, and it contains 11 exons (Lewis et al., 2010) (Fig. 13.9).

To undergo a class switch and thus produce IgA, mucosal B cells must also receive signals from other cells, as well as the microbiota and retinoic acid from dietary vitamin A. Some IgA production is T cell independent and just requires costimulation by cytokines from dendritic cells and epithelial cells. Other B cells require help from Th2 cells to make the switch to IgA production.

T-dependent IgA production mainly occurs in Peyer's patches. Dendritic cells take the antigen from M cells and use it to generate Tfh cells. CD40-ligand

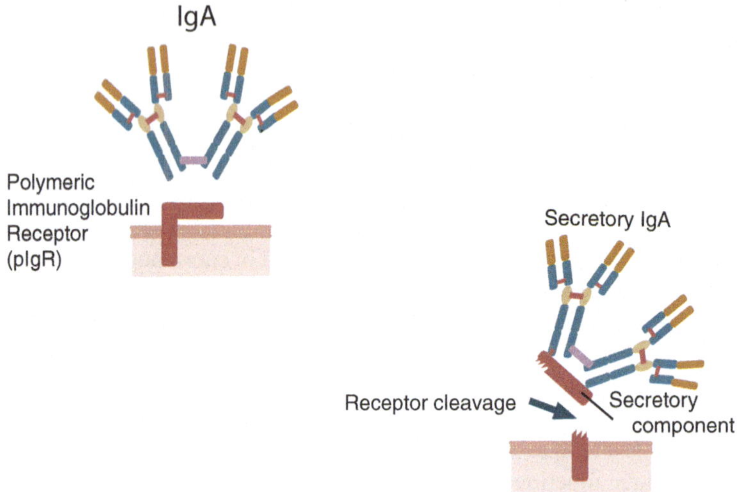

FIGURE 13.9

The role of secretory component in transporting IgA across intestinal epithelial cells.

(CD154) and IL-21 from these Tfh cells induce expression of activation-induced cytidine deaminase (AID) in the B cells. This promotes IgA class switch recombination. This pathway is stimulated by segmented filamentous bacteria attached to the enterocytes (Chapter 14). The B cells generated by this pathway are persistent. They can re-enter germinal centers and undergo somatic mutation. Thus, this IgA may be of very high affinity.

T-independent IgA production mainly occurs in B cells located in the lamina propria and isolated lymphoid follicles under the influence of BAFF and APRIL. ILC3 cells also contribute to this process. The IgA produced by this pathway is usually of low affinity and is directed primarily at antigens from the microbiota (Bunker & Bendelac, 2018).

Follicular dendritic cells secrete soluble B–cell–stimulating cytokines, including BAFF and APRIL (Chapter 6). The dendritic cells themselves are activated by intestinal neuropeptides, such as vasoactive intestinal peptide. Eosinophils are required for the maintenance of plasma cells in the lamina propria. They are also a major source of APRIL. As a result, they directly support the B cell class switch and are required for both T-independent, and T-dependent generation of IgA. These signals, together with CD40–CD154 interactions, trigger B cell IgA production in the absence of antigen. Enterocytes and intraepithelial lymphocytes also produce APRIL and promote B cell differentiation. B cells that require both antigen and Th2 cells to make the switch to IgA are stimulated by TGF-β. Other Th2 cytokines that promote this switch include IL-4, IL-5, IL-6, and even IL-10. The IgA response is relatively slow to develop and has a very high threshold for induction (10^9 bacteria). When boosted, the IgA response does not increase exponentially but grows progressively in an additive manner.

Functions/receptors

IgA is not bactericidal and does not activate the complement system. It can, however, neutralize viruses and some viral and bacterial enzymes. IgA-antigen complexes bind to monocytes and macrophages, neutrophils, and eosinophils through a low-affinity receptor, FcαR1 (CD89). In fact, much of the biological activities of IgA act through this receptor (Morton et al., 2005). When IgA-opsonized particles bind to CD89, they trigger superoxide production, opsonization, antibody-dependent cell-mediated cytotoxicity, as well as the release of inflammatory mediators. The most important function of IgA is to coat infectious agents and so prevent their adherence to epithelial surfaces resulting in immune exclusion. If bacteria or viruses cannot adhere to enterocytes, they are trapped in the mucus layer and simply pass along with the intestinal contents and are expelled without doing any harm.

CD89 has been characterized in the horse. Its sequence is highly homologous to that in humans and bovines. It contains 271 amino acids. It consists of a 204 amino acid extracellular region consisting of two immunoglobulin domains, a transmembrane region of 19 amino acids, and a 27 amino acid cytoplasmic tail. It can bind both serum IgA as well as secretory IgA. The IgA binding site is located at the domain furthest away from the cell membrane (Morton, 2005).

The presence of the gut microbiota also drives IgA production. Different commensals differ in their ability to induce an sIgA response. The gut microbiota is constantly being sampled at the inductive sites, and this triggers the generation of new IgA-secreting plasma cells. Thus, the IgA system is constantly responding to the microbiota. Conversely, most, but not all, commensals are coated with IgA, and this IgA affects their population composition. It is likely that the IgA-coated organisms are potential mucosal pathogens and are therefore excluded. For example, IgA preferentially coats the Enterobacteriaceae while ignoring the Bacteroides and Lactobacilli. Segmented filamentous bacteria are especially potent at triggering IgA responses (Yang et al., 2022).

IgA is released into the intestinal lumen, where it can bind to many but not all the members of the intestinal microbiota (Chapter 14). It is also produced in response to microbial invasion, and specific antibodies are present in the feces of infected horses. As a result, fecal IgA levels can be employed as a marker of mucosal immune dysfunction in horses with colic. Fecal IgA levels are significantly higher in horses with colic than in horses with normal intestinal function implying that they are undergoing microbial invasion (Zak-Bochenek et al., 2025).

Liver excretion

In rodents, polymeric immunoglobulin A is transferred from the bloodstream across hepatocytes into the bile through the use of the pIgR. In humans, the pIgR is expressed on biliary epithelial cells so IgA is transferred directly from serum to into the bile. Unfortunately, I have been unable to find any references indicating that IgA is present in equine bile.

Selective IgA deficiencies

Low levels of IgA tend to be correlated with the development of gastrointestinal and respiratory diseases. While inherited IgA deficiencies have not yet been identified in horses, they may result from stressful situations. For example, hospitalization in unfamiliar surroundings may be sufficiently stressful in horses to result in clinically significant IgA deficiencies. Likewise, surgical procedures may result in an IgA deficiency (Normal fecal IgA levels average 1.26 mg/g). Following general anesthesia, IgA concentrations in horses decrease significantly, independent of its duration or the type of surgery performed (May et al., 2024). High plasma cortisol levels are weakly correlated with low fecal IgA levels on the day of surgery. In addition to surgery, low fecal IgA levels are associated with transportation and hospitalization in general. Physical and psychological stress adversely affects local immune function.

Management practices may also influence equine IgA levels. For example, horses kept under intensive sanitary management—individually housed in concrete stalls, with fresh straw daily, manure removed as necessary were compared to horses housed in loose groups in a large paddock. The horses housed individually had lower immunoglobulin levels of all classes, but only the IgA decline was statistically significant. The intensively housed group had a mean serum IgA level of 246.3 mg/dL. The loose group had a mean IgA level of 332.6 mg/dL. Presumably, the intensively housed horses were exposed to fewer and less diverse environmental antigens. It is also clear that the intensively housed animals got considerably less exercise than those in the loose group (Souza et al., 2010).

Other immunoglobulins

Among the earliest immunoglobulins found in the intestine of the newborn foal are those of the IgM class (Chapter 2). IgM will also bind to pIgR and is carried through the enterocyte to the lumen. Because of its structure, however, secretory IgM is much more susceptible to digestion by intestinal proteases than secretory IgA.

Immunoglobulin E

Because IgA does not activate complement, it functions by immune exclusion. There is a second line of mucosal defense, however, that destroys antigens that penetrate the mucosal barrier (immune elimination). This is mediated by IgE. B cells producing IgE are mainly found under epithelial surfaces rather than in the lymph nodes or spleen. This IgE binds to mast cells in the mucosa of the intestine, respiratory tract, and skin. If invading organisms evade capture by IgA and gain access to the tissues, these mast cells will degranulate and IgE-mediated inflammation will be triggered. These responses involve rapid degranulation of mast cells and the release of their inflammatory mediators into the surrounding tissues. The mast cell contents such as histamine cause acute inflammation, increase the permeability of small blood vessels, and promote fluid leakage between enterocytes, leading to the outflow of mucus containing large quantities of IgG (Fig. 13.10).

This process occurs, for example, when parasitic worms invade the intestinal mucosa. IgA has little effect on these invaders, so they have no difficulty in burrowing

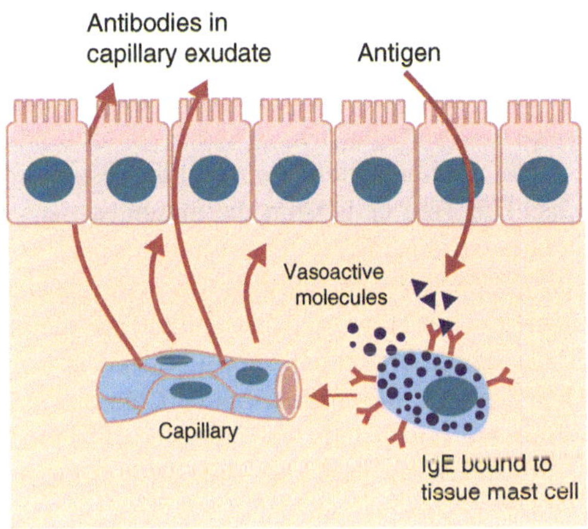

FIGURE 13.10

The defense of mucus membranes by local allergic responses.

into the superficial layers of the mucosa. When sensitized mast cells encounter parasite antigens, however, the release of vasoactive molecules, together with the intense local inflammation, changes in blood flow, and intestinal motility, may be sufficient to force the parasite to disengage—a phenomenon called "self-cure" (Chapter 18).

Thus, IgA and IgE work in concert. IgA normally is the first line of defense, and IgE serves as a backup system. If IgA production is defective, the IgE response may be triggered in excess. As a result, low levels of IgA can result in increased IgE production and predispose horses to the development of allergic responses to food and inhaled antigens.

Food tolerance

Normal horses are immunologically tolerant to the protein antigens they ingest in foods and, as a result, are normally unresponsive to ingested proteins. Dietary proteins are not normally antigenic for two reasons. First, the ingested proteins are degraded by the gut proteases into small, non-immunogenic peptides. Second, any dietary proteins absorbed intact normally generate a strong intestinal Treg cell response, resulting in oral tolerance. Tregs are abundant in the intestinal mucosa, where they mediate tolerance to food antigens as well as to much of the microbiota. These specialized Treg cells suppress Th2 cells, decrease B cell IgE production, suppress effector T cell emigration into tissues, induce IL-10 production by DCs, and inhibit the activation of mast cells, eosinophils, and basophils.

Antigenic food components that enter the gut lumen may leak into the body by passing between cells (paracytosis) or even through cells (transcytosis). Intestinal M cells may bind these food proteins and deliver them to DCs. Other food proteins may penetrate the gut barrier by transcytosis through goblet cells. Intestinal DCs can also extend their dendrites between the epithelial cells and capture proteins within the gut lumen. Once these proteins are captured, they are carried by the DCs to draining mesenteric lymph nodes or Peyer's patches. Specialized intestinal DCs produce molecules such as TGF-β and retinoic acid that instruct the responding T cells to differentiate into Treg cells. The Treg cells from the mesenteric lymph nodes of orally tolerant animals, in turn, secrete the suppressive cytokines TGF-β and IL-10. A specialized subpopulation of ROR-γt^+ intestinal dendritic cells, called Thetis cells, stimulates food antigen-specific Treg production and hence maintains oral tolerance (Akagbosu et al., 2022). These Thetis cells are produced in large numbers around weaning at a time when oral tolerance is developing (Cabric et al., 2025). As a result, secretory IgA responses are not usually generated against food antigens. A third mechanism by which oral tolerance may be induced is through the production of "tolerosomes." These are exosomes produced by enterocytes. They carry MHC class II molecules on their surface, and this binds antigenic peptides sampled from the gut lumen. Purified tolerosomes fed to animals induce tolerance. It is suggested that presentation of food antigens by tolerosomes to Thetis cells induces Treg formation (Ostman et al., 2005).

Food allergies have been reported in horse but are uncommon and not well documented. Wild oats, white clover, and alfalfa have been recognized as allergens in this species. Simultaneous hypersensitivities to multiple unrelated food allergens do occur (Chapter 19).

Donkey IgA

Like the horse, donkeys possess a single *IGHA* gene within their IGH locus. Their serum IgA levels of 0.5–2.4 mg/mL are comparable to those in the horse. Jenny's milk contains 0.9–2 mg of IgA/mL (Veronesi et al., 2014). However, it has also been demonstrated that in donkeys, total fecal IgA levels correlated with their strongyle fecal egg count, especially in donkeys in good physical condition. They did not, however, correlate in donkeys in poor condition (Tombak et al., 2020).

References

Akagbosu, B., Tayyebi, Z., Shibu, G., et al. (2022). Novel antigen presenting cell imparts Treg-dependent tolerance to gut microbiota. *Nature, 610*, 752–760.

Bocking, T., Johnson, L., Singh, A., Desai, A., et al. (2021). Expression of surfactant protein-A and D, and CD9 in lungs of 1 and 30 day old foals. *BMC Veterinary Research*. https://doi.org/10.1186/s12917-021-02943-5

Bocking, T., & Singh, B. (2021). Light and electron-microscopic localization of CD9 and surfactant protein A and D in normal lungs of the horse. *Canadian Journal of Veterinary Research, 85*, 170–176.

Botia, M., Martin-Cuervo, M., Martinez-Subiela, S., Ceron, J. J., et al. (2024). Changes in immunoglobulins G and A in saliva and serum of horses with equine gastric ulcer syndrome (EGUS) and their relationship with other immune and redox status biomarkers. *Biology*. https://doi.org/10.3390/biology13110891

Brosnahan, M. M., Miller, D. C., Adams, M., & Antczac, D. F. (2012). IL-22 is expressed by the invasive trophoblast of the equine (*Equus caballus*) chorionic girdle. *The Journal of Immunology, 188*, 4181–4187.

Bunker, J. J., & Bendelac, A. (2018). IgA responses to microbiota. *Immunity, 49*, 211–224.

Cabric, V., Parisotto, Y. F., Park, T., Akagbosu, B., et al. (2025). A wave of thetis cells imparts tolerance to food antigens early in life. *Science*. https://doi.org/10.1126/science.adp0535

Coates, M., Blanchard, S., & MacLeod, A. S. (2018). Innate antimicrobial immunity in the skin: A protective barrier against bacteria, viruses, and fungi. *PLoS Pathogens*. https://doi.org/10.1371/journal.ppat.1007353

Corr, S. C., Gahan, C. C. G. M., & Hill, C. (2008). M-cells: Origin, morphology and role in mucosal immunity and microbial pathogenesis. *FEMS Immunology and Medical Microbiology, 52*, 2–12.

Cui, C., Li, L., & Peng, J. (2023). Paneth cells in farm animals: Current status and future direction. *Journal of Animal Science and Biotechnology*. https://doi.org/10.1186/s40104-023-00905-5

Cvitas, I., Oberhaensli, S., Leeb, T., & Marti, E. (2022). Equine keratinocytes in the pathogenesis of insect bite hypersensitivity: Just another brick in the wall? *PLoS One*. https://doi.org/10.1371/journal.pone.o266263

Fischer, C. D., Wachoski-Dark, G. L., Grant, D. M., Bramer, S. A., & Klein, C. (2018). Interferon epsilon is constitutively expressed in equine endometrium and up-regulated during the luteal phase. *Animal Reproduction Science, 195*, 38–43.

Flaminio, J. B. F., Rush, B. R., Davis, E. G., Hennessey, K., et al. (2000). Characterization of peripheral blood and pulmonary leukocyte function in healthy foals. *Veterinary Immunology and Immunopathology, 73*, 267–285.

Fung, K. Y., Mangan, N. E., Cumming, H., et al. (2013). Interferon-ε protects the female reproductive tract from viral and bacterial infection. *Science, 339*, 1088–1090.

Galan, J. E., & Timoney, J. F. (1985). Mucosal nasopharyngeal immune responses of horses to protein antigens of *Streptococcus equi*. *Infection and Immunity, 47*(3), 623–628.

Guenther, M. C., Borowicz, P. P., Hirchert, M. R., Semanchil, P. L., et al. (2024). Identifying the immunoglobulin G transporter in equine tissues: A look at the neonatal Fc receptor. *Journal of Equine Veterinary Science, 139*, Article 105131.

Hobbs, K. J., Ludwig, E. K., Martin, E. M., Bayless, R., et al. (2025). Endothelial glycocalyx damage is associated with small intestinal disease in horses. *Journal of the American Veterinary Medical Association*. https://doi.org/10.2460/ajvr.25.07.0251

Iwasaki, A., Foxman, E. F., & Molony, R. D. (2016). Early local immune defenses in the respiratory tract. *Nature Reviews Immunology*. https://doi.org/10.1038/nri.2016.117

Johansson, M. E., & Hansson, G. C. (2016). Immunological aspects of intestinal mucus and mucins. *Nature Reviews Immunology, 16*, 639–649.

Leise, B. S., Yin, C., Pettigrew, A., & Belknap, J. K. (2010). Proinflammatory cytokine responses of cultured equine keratinocytes to bacterial-associated molecular pattern motifs. *Equine Veterinary Journal, 42*(4), 294–303.

Leprince, C., & Simon, M. (2025). Epidermal lamellar bodies, essential organelles for skin barrier function. *Frontiers in Cell and Developmental Biology*. https://doi.org/10.3389/fcell.2025.1597884

Lewis, M. J., Wagner, B., Irvine, R. M., & Woof, J. M. (2010). IgA in the horse: Cloning of equine polymeric Ig receptor and J chain and characterization of recombinant forms of equine IgA. *Mucosal Immunology.* https://doi.org/10.1038/mi.2010.38

Liu, I. K. M. (1988). Uterine defense mechanisms in the mare. *Veterinary Clinics of North America: Equine Practice, 4*(2), 221–228.

Martin, E., Molleda, J. M., Ginel, P. J., Novales, M., et al. (1997). Total protein and immunoglobulin concentrations in equine tears. *Journal of Veterinary Medicine A, 44*, 461–465.

May, A., Gerhards, H., & Wollanke, B. (2024). Effect of hospitalization on equine local intestinal immunoglobulin A (IgA) concentration measured in feces. *Journal of Equine Veterinary Science, 137*, Article 105078.

McFarlane, D., Sellon, D. C., & Gibbs, S. A. (2001). Age-related quantitative alterations in lymphocyte subsets and immunoglobulin isotypes in healthy horses. *American Journal of Veterinary Research, 62*(9), 1413–1417.

McGuire, T. C., & Crawford, T. B. (1972). Identification and quantitation of equine serum and secretory immunoglobulin A. *Infection and Immunity, 6*(4), 610–615.

Mendoza, F. J., Toribio, R. E., & Perez-Ecija, A. (2018). Donkey internal medicine—Part II: Cardiovascular, respiratory, neurologic, urinary. opthalmic, dermatology and musculoskeletal disorders. *Journal of Equine Veterinary Science, 65*, 86–97.

Morton, H. C. (2005). IgA Fc receptors in cattle and horses. *Veterinary Immunology and Immunopathology, 108*, 139–143.

Morton, H. C., Pleass, R. J., Storset, A. K., Brandtzaeg, P., & Woof, J. M. (2005). Cloning and characterization of equine CD89 and identification of the CD89 gene in chimpanzees and rhesus macaques. *Immunology.* https://doi.org/10.1111/j.1365-2567.2005.02129.x

Ostman, S., Taube, M., & Telemo, E. (2005). Tolerosome-induced oral tolerance is MKC dependent. *Immunology, 116*, 464–476.

Palm, A.-K., Wattle, O., Lundstrom, T., & Wattrang, E. (2016). Secretory immunoglobulin A and immunoglobulin G in horse saliva. *Veterinary Immunology and Immunopathology, 180*, 59–65.

Parillo, F., Arias, M. P., & Supplizi, A. V. (2009). Glycoprofile of the different cell types present in the mucosa of the horse guttural pouches. *Tissue and Cell, 41*, 257–265.

Pickles, K., Pirie, R. S., Rhind, S., et al. (2002). Cytological analysis of equine bronchoalveolar fluid. Part 2: Comparison of smear and cytocentrifuged preparations. *Equine Veterinary Journal, 34*, 292–296.

Ramery, E., Fievez, L., Fraipont, A., Bureau, F., & Lekeux, P. (2010). Characterization of pentraxin 3 in the horse and its expression in airways. *Veterinary Research.* https://doi.org/10.1051/vetres/2009066

Riihimaki, M., Fegraeus, K., Nordlund, J., Waern, I., et al. (2023). Single cell transcriptomics delineates the immune cell landscape in equine lower airways and reveals upregulation of FKBP5 in horses with asthma. *Scientific Reports.* https://doi.org/10.1038/s41598-023-43368-4

Rouse, B. T., & Ingram, D. G. (1970). The total protein and immunoglobulin profile of equine colostrum and milk. *Immunology, 19*, 901–907.

Schaefer, A., & Lai, S. K. (2022). The biophysical principles underpinning muco-trapping functions of antibodies. *Human Vaccines & Immunotherapeutics.* https://doi.org/10.1080/21645515.2021.1939605

Sheoran, A. S., Timoney, J. F., Holmes, M. A., Karzenski, S. S., & Crisman, M. V. (2000). Immunoglobulin isotypes in sera and nasal mucosal secretions and their neonatal transfer and distribution in horses. *American Journal of Veterinary Research, 61*(9), 1099–1105.

Shokri, H. (2015). Occurrence and distribution of Malassezia species on skin and external ear canal of horses. *Mycoses*. https://doi.org/10.1111/myc.12430

Snoeck, V., Peters, I. R., & Cox, E. (2006). The IgA system: A comparison of structure and function in different species. *Veterinary Research, 37*, 455–467.

Sonnenberg, G. F., Fouser, L. A., & Artis, D. (2011). Border patrol: Regulation of immunity, inflammation and tissue homeostasis at barrier surfaces by IL-22. *Nature Immunology, 12* (5), 383–390.

Souza, C. M., Miotto, B. A., Bonin, C. P., & Camargo, M. M. (2010). Lower serum IgA levels in horses kept under intensive sanitary management and physical training. *Animal*. https://doi.org/10.1017/s175173111000131X

Tombak, K. J., Budischak, S. A., Hauck, S., Martinez, L. A., & Rubenstein, D. I. (2020). The non-invasive measurement of faecal immunoglobulin in African equids. *IJP: Parasites and Wildlife, 12*, 105–112.

Townsend, M., Fowler, B., Aulakh, G. K., & Singh, B. (2023). Expression of pentraxin 3 in equine lungs and neutrophils. *Canadian Journal of Veterinary Research, 87*(1), 9–16.

Van Kaer, L., & Olivares-Villagomez, D. (2018). Development, homeostasis and functions of intestinal intraepithelial lymphocytes. *Journal of Immunology, 200*, 2235–2244.

Veronesi, M. C., Dall'Ara, P., Gloria, A., Servida, F., et al. (2014). IgG, IgA and lysozyme in Martina Franca donkey jennies and their foals. *Theriogenology, 81*, 825–831.

Widders, P. R., Stokes, C. R., David, J. S., & Bourne, F. J. (1985). Immunohistochemical studies of the local immune system in the reproductive tract of the mare. *Research in Veterinary Science, 38*(1), 88–95.

Wingate, K. V., Torres, S. M., Silverstein, K. A. T., Hendrickson, J. A., & Rutherford, M. S. (2009). Expression of endogenous antimicrobial peptides in normal canine skin. *Veterinary Dermatology, 20*, 19–26.

Yang, C., Chen-Liaw, A., Spindler, M. P., Tortorella, D., et al. (2022). Immunoglobulin A antibody composition is sculpted to bind the self-gut microbiome. *Science Immunology, 7* (73). https://doi.org/10.1126/sciimmunol.abg3208

Zak-Bochenek, A., Drabkova, Z., Sergedaite, V., Swinska, N., et al. (2025). Fecal secretory IgA and lactate level as a biomarker of mucosal immune dysfunction in horses with colic. *Journal of Veterinary Internal Medicine*. https://doi.org/10.1111/jvim.70073

CHAPTER

The microbiota and the equine immune system

14

The external body surfaces of horses and donkeys consist of multiple nutrient-rich ecosystems where millions of microbes thrive. Each external surface is populated by enormous numbers of bacteria, archaea, fungi, and viruses, collectively termed the microbiota. The bacteria are the best studied of these. Thus, bacteria live on the skin, in the respiratory tract, in parts of the genitourinary tract, and sometimes within the body, but mainly within the gastrointestinal tract, especially the large intestine. It has been estimated that in the human body, at least half of all its cells are microbial. In hindgut fermenters such as horses and donkeys, the proportion of microbial cells is probably much greater. As a result of their lifelong, intimate association with body surfaces, the microbiota can be considered to be an integral part of the body—"a virtual organ." As such, they profoundly influence both innate and adaptive immunity, and conversely, they are influenced by signals generated by their host. Microbial metabolites, immune cells, and neurons interact in a coordinated manner that influences both health and disease susceptibility. Microbial metabolites influence immune modulation, epithelial integrity, oral tolerance, and inflammation. This has given rise to the concept that animals and their microbiota together form "superorganisms" (or holobionts) that share nutrition and exchange energy and metabolites, and whose complex interactions are largely regulated by immune mechanisms (Rodrigues-Hoffmann et al., 2017). The net result is that the microbiota of the horse and the donkey have a significant influence on their immunity, health, and performance. This is especially significant in neonatal life when the developing microbiota influences a foal's immune system development and thus disease susceptibility.

The normal equine microbiota

It is now well accepted that the body's surface microbiota both contribute to local host defenses and also have effects on the immune system and metabolism that extend throughout the body (Fig. 14.1). Nutrients and microbial metabolites are continually released into the body, where they influence both innate and adaptive immune functions. The immunological defenses on body surfaces are therefore faced with the task of coexisting with the "good" microbiota, while at the same time preventing microbial invasion through breaks in the epithelial barriers (Belkaid & Hand, 2014).

The Immunology of Horses and Donkeys. https://doi.org/10.1016/B978-0-443-44863-8.00019-3

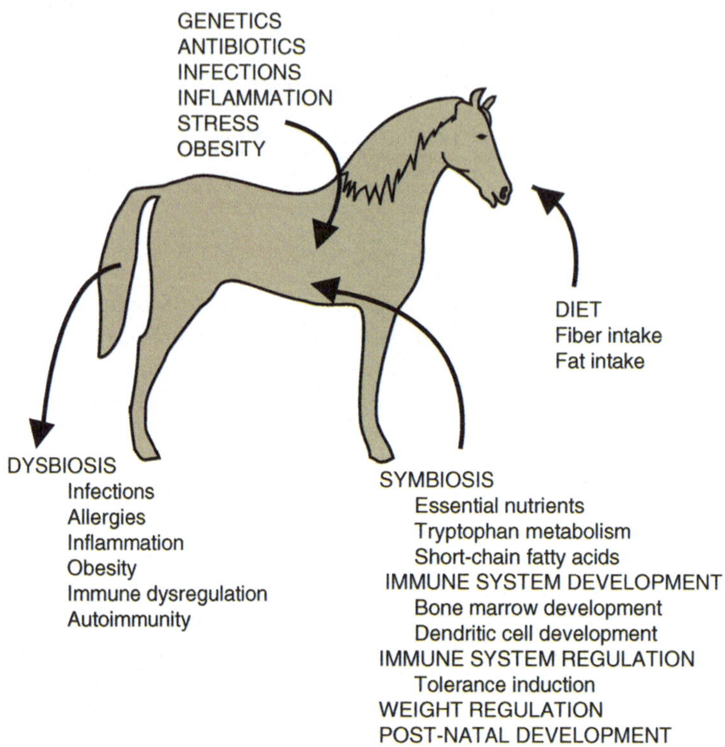

FIGURE 14.1

The factors that influence the composition of the microbiota and the diverse effects of the microbiota on equine body surfaces.

Each horse's microbiota is unique, and its composition is determined by management, diet, gender, genetics, breed, age, and environmental factors. The composition of the microbiota also changes along the intestinal tract under the influence of nutrient availability and the local microenvironment.

Four bacterial phyla dominate body surface populations. They are the Firmicutes (also called the Bacillota), the Actinobacteria (Actinomycetota), the Bacteroidetes (Bacteroidota), and the Proteobacteria (Pseudomonadota). The Firmicutes consist of Gram-positive bacteria with a low G + C content in their DNA. Many are spore-forming. Important members include the Clostridia, which may be beneficial or pathogenic. They also include potentially pathogenic Streptococci and Staphylococci. The Actinobacteria are also Gram-positive bacteria, but they have a higher G + C content than the Firmicutes. Important members include the Mycobacteria. The phylum Bacteroidetes consists of Gram-negative bacilli that can degrade otherwise indigestible plant carbohydrates to produce short-chain fatty acids (SCFAs). The Proteobacteria are also a major phylum of Gram-negative enterobacteria. They include pathogens such as *Escherichia coli* and *Klebsiella*.

The skin microbiota

Horse skin, as in other mammals, is home to trillions of microorganisms. These are found on the surface of keratinocytes and extend into sebaceous glands and hair follicles. The skin is not, however, a hospitable environment (Ross et al., 2019). The outer cell layers are constantly shed and replaced by new cells from below. It is cool in some areas and hot in others. Some areas of skin may be very dry, and may have a high salt content, as well as being hydrophobic, acidic, or nutrient-poor. Other areas may be moist but bathed in a complex mixture of proteases, enzymes, and antimicrobial peptides such as β-defensins and cathelicidins. The skin microbiota can be divided into a resident population that is relatively stable and consistent—a true commensal population, and a population of transient bacteria that may only survive on the skin for hours or days. Both populations contain a mixture of commensals and potential pathogens, yet invasion and disease are relatively uncommon (Mulder et al., 2009) (Fig. 14.2).

An analysis of samples taken from four skin sites on clinically healthy horses (dorsum, ventral abdomen, pastern, and groin) identified bacteria from 38 phyla and 1665 genera. The most common phyla identified in all samples were Proteobacteria, Firmicutes, Actinobacteria, and Bacteroidetes. The Proteobacteria were the predominant phylum on the abdomen, groin, and pastern skin, accounting for a mean relative abundance (MRA) of 60%, 41%, and 58% of the gene sequences, respectively. These were followed by Firmicutes (27%, 34%, and 31%, respectively). The Firmicutes were the dominant phylum on the dorsum, accounting for an MRA of 38% of sequences, followed by the Proteobacteria at 36%. The Actinobacteria and Bacteroidetes were present in the lowest numbers at all four sites. There were no significant differences in species richness or diversity between the four sites or between individual horses. The alpha diversity was higher in winter and summer

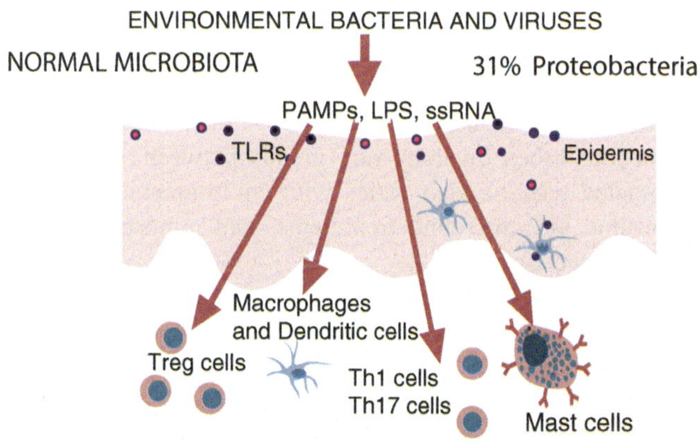

FIGURE 14.2

The mechanisms by which the body surface microbiota assist in protecting surfaces from pathogen colonization.

than in spring or autumn (in Canada). The Proteobacteria were most abundant in the autumn and spring, accounting for 83% and 72% of sequences, respectively. Conversely, Firmicutes were most abundant in summer and winter with a mean relative abundance of 51% and 49%, respectively (O'Shaughnessy-Hunter et al., 2021).

In a similar study in Shetland ponies, Strompfova and Stempelova detected the presence of 18 phyla and 119 families on the pony skin (Strompfova & Stempelova, 2024). They found that the most abundant phyla were Proteobacteria (30.8%), Actinobacteria (20.4%), Firmicutes (19.5%), Bacteroidetes (8.5%), and Deinococcota (7.2%). Among the bacteria, Corynebacteria were the most abundant genus (7.4%).

Investigations into the role of the skin microbiota in equine wound healing have also been undertaken. This was performed on full-thickness wounds on both the body and limbs (Kamus et al., 2018). The anatomical location significantly affected the microbial population of the healing wounds. Fusobacterium and Actinobacillus were associated with the limb wounds during the initial healing stages. Bandaging also significantly affected the skin microbiota during the healing process. The microbiota rapidly returned to normal once wound healing was complete.

Because of their prominence and relatively weak eye defenses, horses appear to be especially prone to developing corneal infections. If their tear film is insufficient, horses may develop fungal infections of the conjunctiva and cornea. Fungi are considered part of the conjunctival microbiota, but their prevalence is relatively high compared to other species. They are especially high in horses housed indoors and exposed to dust from hay and straw, as well as in hot, humid tropical regions (Mo et al., 2023).

The respiratory tract microbiota

Like all body surfaces exposed to the external environment, the respiratory tract houses a dense, dynamic, and complex microbiota. It has been calculated that a human inhales 10^5 bacteria/day just breathing normally. A horse will inhale considerably more, especially if living in a dusty stable!! As a result, the respiratory tract houses a diverse microbiota consisting of at least 94 different taxa. As at other sites, the number of taxa and their diversity vary greatly between individual horses. The nature of the inhaled bacteria also varies with environmental conditions such as the type of housing, any microbial treatments, and atmospheric dust levels, as well as the animal's feed.

The colonization of the respiratory tract begins with the first breaths taken by the newborn foal. The initial population of inhaled bacteria comes from the mare's vagina and teat skin. Weaning has significant effects on the gastrointestinal and, thus, the respiratory microbiota. Overall, the predominant equine respiratory phyla are the Firmicutes, Proteobacteria, and Actinobacteria. The respiratory microbiota also changes with the age of the foal and only tends to stabilize around the time of weaning. The details of this process are influenced by both maternal and environmental factors. Suckling will result in the inhalation of maternal udder and skin microbes.

The stress of weaning, plus management issues such as crowding and transportation, will affect the process. Stress and abrupt dietary changes may result in dysbiosis.

The respiratory tract presents diverse environments, but, for convenience, it can be divided into two distinct ecosystems: the upper and lower respiratory tracts. In the upper tract (nasopharynx and larynx), many nasal bacteria are also present on the skin, while others are common environmental bacteria. Deeper in the airways, in the lower respiratory tract (trachea and lungs), there is also a diverse bacterial population (O'Dwyer et al., 2016). There are also significant differences in the microbiota between the nasal and oral cavities. Thus, in one study, there was a greater proportion of Firmicutes in transtracheal aspirates, while bronchoalveolar lavage samples contained increased numbers of Actinobacteria and fewer Firmicutes. Gemellaceae and Streptococcaceae had a greater abundance in nasopharyngeal and tracheal samples, while Bacilli and Propionibacteria were more abundant in bronchoalveolar lavage samples (Bishop, Migliorisi, et al., 2024) (Fig. 14.3). The upper respiratory tract microbiota also shows great individual variability and is relatively unstable. Given the conditions under which many horses are housed,

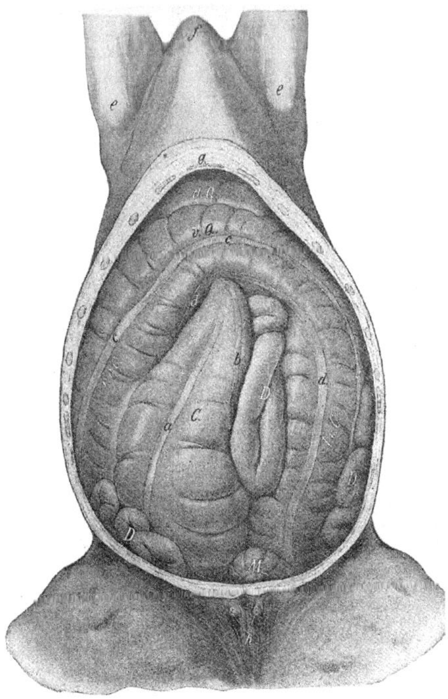

FIGURE 14.3

A ventral view of the abdominal cavity of the horse showing the extremely large size of its cecum and colon, the sites of hindgut fermentation.

- From Sisson, S., & Grossman, J.D. (1953). The large intestine. In Anatomy of the domestic animals *(4th ed., p. 429). Philadelphia, PA: W.B. Saunders Company.*

especially in dusty environments, it is unsurprising that the nasal microbiota is highly complex. Compared to the lower tract, the prevalence of Moraxella is increased, whereas Cupriavidus is increased in the lower tract.

Healthy horse lungs also harbor a complex microbiota, related to, but much less dense and complex than that found in the upper respiratory tract. As described in Chapter 20, the lung microbiota is also altered in horses suffering from inflammatory airway disease (Bond et al., 2017). Commensal organisms generally persist within the mucus layer of the airways and include not only bacteria, but also fungi (yeasts), and viruses such as bacteriophages. In the absence of this microbiota, the airways are prone to mount exaggerated Th2 responses. The presence of the microbiota induces Treg activity that suppresses these responses. It is also clear that microbes on one mucosal surface can affect immunity at distant surfaces. Thus, the intestinal microbiota can shape immunity in the airways as well as the development of equine asthma (Leduc et al., 2024) (Chapter 20). The intestinal microbiota also regulates pulmonary adaptive responses (Dang & Marsland, 2019). For example, segmented filamentous bacteria (SFB) in the intestine regulate pulmonary immunity to bacteria and fungi. The gut microbiota stimulates type 2 innate lymphoid cells to migrate from the gut to the lungs, where they promote IL-33 production (Pu et al., 2021). Conversely, influenza infection in the lungs generates type I interferons. These, in turn, induce changes in the gut microbiota, such as depletion of obligate anaerobic bacteria and an increase in Proteobacteria, resulting in intestinal dysbiosis. Thus, the outcome of infectious diseases is affected by the collective influence of both local and distant microbial communities (Christodoulou & Clarke, 2024).

The blood microbiota

Venous blood is not always sterile in healthy horses (Simms et al., 2025). Blood collected from the jugular vein of healthy horses revealed the presence of 55–70 bacterial genera in samples from individual horses. Collectively, 293 different bacterial genera were isolated from the blood of 20 horses. The most dominant taxa were *Gardnerella*, *Sporomusaceae*, *Kapabacteriales*, *Beijerinckiaceae*, and *Phascolarcticobacterium*. There were great differences between individual horses. Some of the genera isolated included potential pathogens, such as *Bacteroides*, *Clostridium*, *Peptostreptococcus*, and *Staphylococcus*. The significance of these results is debatable. Some of the organisms found in blood may simply be transient contaminants. It is also possible that they have escaped from body surfaces such as the gastrointestinal tract.

The reproductive tract microbiota

Like all organs that communicate directly with the external environment, the reproductive tract of mares houses a dense and complex microbiota. If this microbiota is disrupted and dysbiosis results, then this predisposes to diseases such as endometritis, a common cause of fertility problems in mares (Gil-Miranda, Macnicol, et al., 2024). As with the respiratory tract, the microbiota changes progressively the deeper it penetrates into the animal's body. For many years, it was believed that the interior of the uterus was sterile. That is not the case. The cervix itself has its own diverse microbiota. The microbiota of the vagina and uterus are similar to each other but differ from that in the clitoral area and on the skin (Fig. 14.4).

As with other populations, Firmicutes, Actinobacteria, Proteobacteria, and Bacteroidetes are the predominant phyla in both the vagina and uterus of healthy maiden mares. There is no dominant species at the genus level. There is a higher proportion of Proteobacteria in the vaginal samples compared to the uterine samples. Streptococci and staphylococci are present in abundance in both vaginal and uterine samples. Lactobacilli account for less than 10% (Gil-Miranda, Caddey, et al., 2024). Populations change during estrus, and *Lactobacillus*, *Escherichia*, *Streptococcus*, *Blautia*, *Staphylococcus*, *Klebsiella*, *Acinetobacter*, and *Peptoanaerobobacter* may be detected at variable levels of abundance during estrus (Poole et al., 2023). It is also important to point out that the composition of the equine reproductive

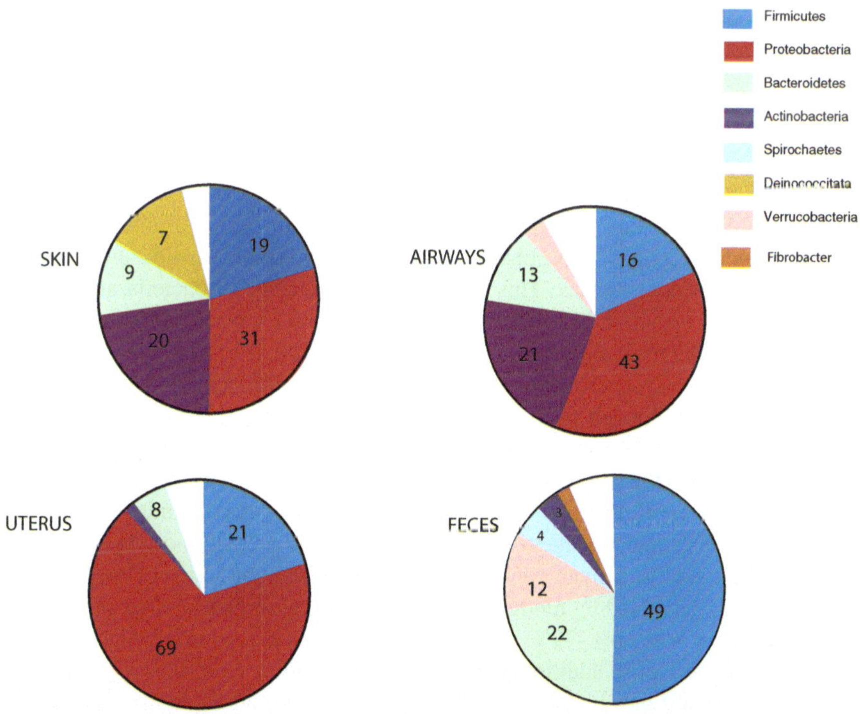

FIGURE 14.4 The distribution of the normal microbiota in the skin, lungs, and uterus of horses as well as in their feces.

Note that the composition of the fecal microbiota is very different from that on other body surfaces.

microbiome may also differ significantly between different geographical and climatic regions (Holyoak et al., 2022).

The gastrointestinal microbiota

The horse with its enormous cecum and colon requires its microbiota in order to utilize its cellulose-rich diet. As a result, the horse's gut may contain up to 10^{15} bacterial cells. The anterior digestive tract contains many environmental bacteria, such as the Proteobacteria, consumed with the forage. In the hindgut, the predominant resident bacteria include Firmicutes, Bacteroidetes, and Verrucomicrobia. Firmicutes constitute 40%–90% of this microbiota and include Clostridia and Bacilli. The horse cecum also contains a dense population of methanogenic archaea. These organisms are potent sources of SCFAs such as butyrate. As in other species, diets influence the composition of the microbiota. Thus, a high starch diet in horses may result in the proliferation of Lactobacilli, resulting in lactic acidosis and the development of laminitis.

When sampled 20 min after birth, foal fecal meconium contains small amounts of bacterial DNA with a profile related to the composition of the mare's feces. The intestine is rapidly colonized. By 24 h after birth, the foal's rectum is colonized by Firmicutes and Proteobacteria. By 7 days of age, the foal fecal microbiota is still different from that of adults. The mare's vaginal microbiota contributes significantly to both the 24-hour and the 7-day neonatal fecal populations (Husso et al., 2020).

Equids are grazing herbivores adapted to living in open grasslands. They ingest their diet of grasses and high-fiber plants in small amounts. It passes rapidly through the stomach before being exposed to the enzymes within the small intestine. Adult horses do not undertake coprophagy. However, they cannot avoid some contact with the feces of other horses. This facilitates the exchange of bacteria and viruses as well as intestinal parasites. Sports and leisure horses housed indoors generally have two or three meals daily of forages plus concentrate. The digesta subsequently passes into the two compartments of the large intestine, the cecum and colon, where it is subjected to prolonged microbial fermentation and degradation. The availability of food substrates to the large intestinal microbiota is greatly affected by the digestibility of the food in the small intestine. Thus, by the time the digesta reaches the large intestine, the plant cellulose cell walls remain undigested. Indeed, hindgut fermenters have a shorter intestinal passage time than ruminants. As a result, their digestive tract is less efficient, and they must compensate with a higher food intake. However, volatile fatty acids generated by hindgut fermentation and absorbed by the colon appear to provide as much as 60%–79% of the energy available to the horse. Microbial proteins also provide some additional nutrition. The hindgut microbial population is therefore essential if the animal is to extract any energy remaining in the digesta after the stomach and small intestine have done their work. This fermentation within the cecum–colon ecosystem serves to maximize the effectiveness of the digestive tract.

Oral cavity and tonsils

The oral cavity of horses has its own complex microbiota. The tonsils appear to function as a reservoir site for numerous bacteria and viruses. The oral cavity is dominated by the genera *Gemella* and *Actinobacillus*. In horses with periodontitis, there is a higher microbial diversity, and the dominant phyla are *Prevotella* and *Veillonella*. The periodontitis oral samples also have a higher relative abundance of *Methanobacteriaceae* and *Thermoplasmatales*. Potential oral pathogens such as *Treponema*, *Tannerella*, and *Porphyromonas* are present at low levels in all the samples (Kennedy et al., 2016). In a separate study focusing on Gram-negative bacteria within the equine oral cavity, it was found that 55 Gram-negative isolates were identified, of which 89% were potentially zoonotic (Pimenta et al., 2023)!

The ingested food is held for a limited period in the equine stomach. The stomach is not, however, sterile. It contains a high concentration of anaerobes as well as Lactobacilli and Streptococci. The microbiota of the stomach, as with the oral cavity, reflects, in large part, the most recent meal of the horse.

The small intestine

Digesta passes rapidly through the equine small intestine. As a result, this is where the most accessible carbohydrates and proteins are digested and absorbed. The equine small intestinal microbiota is a complex community containing bacteria, archaea, fungi, and viruses. The most obvious of these are trillions of bacteria belonging to hundreds of different species. It is dominated by Firmicutes and Proteobacteria. The proportion of Bacteroidetes drops while Proteobacteria increase steadily from the stomach to the colon. There are significant differences between the microbial communities in the small and large intestines. These differences appear to be associated with changes in oxygen tension as well as nutrient availability. As a result, the colon microbiota is very much richer in species than in the small intestine and more similar between individual horses. There are also differences between the luminal microbiota and the mucosal-associated microbiota. A large proportion of available carbohydrates and proteins are digested and absorbed in the ileum (85%–95% and 10%–70%, respectively) (Santos et al., 2011).

Hindgut fermentation

The colon and cecum of the horse are very large chambers that occupy much of its peritoneal cavity (Fig. 14.3). They must be large since, like the rumen, they provide for much of the animal's energy needs. It has been estimated that the digesta may reach the cecum and ventral colon 30–45 min after leaving a horse's stomach (Santos et al., 2011). Hindgut fermenters such as the horse and donkey are monogastric herbivores that digest fibrous plant carbohydrates by anaerobic fermentation in the cecum and colon (Costa et al., 2015). The SCFAs produced are absorbed through the mucosa. (The equine colonic microbiota is estimated to generate about 20% of the methane generated by the bovine rumen.) (Haspel, 2025). Fatty acids reach their greatest concentration 5–8 h after a meal and include acetic acid, propionic acid, butyric acid, and lactic acid. The relative concentration of each acid varies with the horse's diet. Once within the large intestine, the digesta is subjected to further microbial digestion for 48–72 h. It is subsequently pushed into the rectum, where some water is removed to form the feces (Fig. 14.3).

The cecal bacteria can be classified into cellulolytic, proteolytic, and glycolytic species. The proportion of cellulolytic bacteria is especially high in the cecum. Organisms such as *Ruminococcus flavefaciens, Ruminococcus albus*, and *Fibrobacter succinogenes* appear to be the dominant species. (These are different from the isolates found in the bovine rumen.) The strains appear to be equine-specific. Firmicutes are the main bacterial phylum (especially Clostridia), but the predominant organism is a member of the Verrucomicrobia. Other phyla found in the equine large intestine include Spirochetes, and Bacteroidetes. The large intestinal microbiota is also vulnerable to severe stresses, and as a result, changes in the colonic microbiota can cause other problems. For example, under certain conditions, such as carbohydrate overload, the microbiota of the large gut changes drastically, as a result of which their pH drops and bacterial PAMPs escape into the bloodstream. This can result in the development of acute laminitis (Chapter 5) (Fig. 14.4).

The fecal microbiota of the horse is dominated by Firmicutes (15%–85%). The next common phyla are Bacteroidetes and Verrucomicrobia (Chaucheyras-Durand et al., 2022). The fecal microbiota probably reflects the composition of the colonic microbiota.

Nutritional efficiency

The composition and metabolism of the gut microbiota are critically dependent on diet. Thus, the microbiota in horses fed a low-fat, high-plant polysaccharide diet is very different from that in animals on a high-fat, high-sugar, and low-plant polysaccharide diet. Variations in meal size and frequency can also have an effect. Fluctuations in the intestinal microbiota may require an animal to adjust its metabolic and immunologic performance in response to nutritional and environmental changes (Venable et al., 2017).

To obtain nutrition from plant-based foods, a horse must be able to extract energy from plant polysaccharides. This is largely the function of the anaerobes within the large intestine that convert the complex carbohydrates to SCFAs. The most important of these are species of Clostridium, Eubacterium, and Butyrivibrio. SCFAs such as acetate, propionate, and butyrate are the major products of colonic fermentation. SCFAs derived from a fiber-rich diet act not only as energy sources but also function as protective molecules. They can enter cells by passive diffusion or by binding to transporter molecules.

SCFAs are not only a key energy source, but they also regulate both innate and adaptive immune responses. Depending upon their concentration, they may be either pro- or anti-inflammatory. For example, butyrate inhibits neutrophil expression of some chemotactic factor receptors such as CXCR2. It, therefore, slows their immigration into inflammatory sites. It also inhibits neutrophil NET formation (Yao et al.,

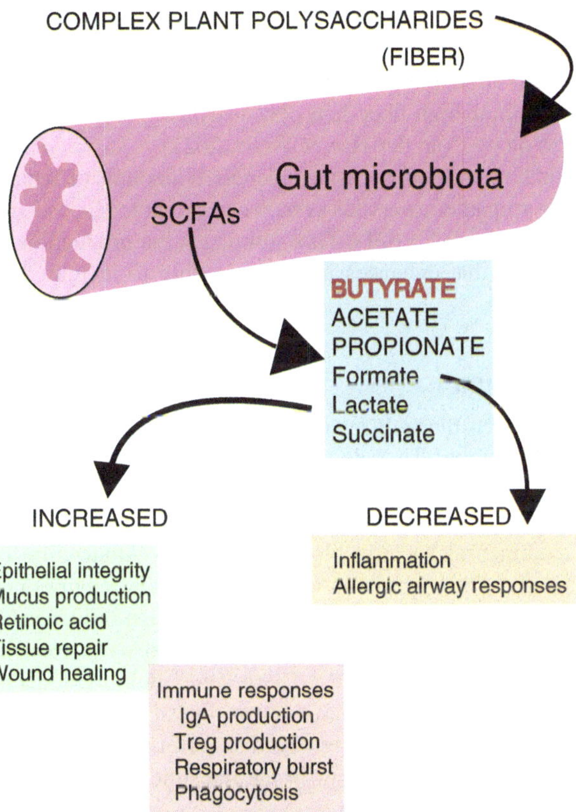

FIGURE 14.5 The importance of short-chain fatty acids, especially butyrate, in promoting immunity.

These fatty acids are generated by the digestion of complex carbohydrates and are also a major source of energy in herbivores. They are produced in large quantities by the microbial digestion of plant cellulose fibers.

2022). Butyric acid has anti-inflammatory effects since it acts on macrophages to enhance their antibacterial peptide production and prevents epigenetic changes by inhibiting histone deacetylases (Schulthess et al., 2019). Butyrate also increases barrier functions by stimulating enterocytes and increasing goblet cell differentiation and mucus production (Fig. 14.5).

SCFAs inhibit the development of monocytes into macrophages and DCs by inhibiting histone deacetylation. SCFAs also act on DCs to inhibit lipopolysaccharide-induced maturation and reduce their production of IL-12. They can also inhibit the production of some chemokines, such as monocyte chemoattractant protein-1. SCFAs promote the differentiation of ILC1 and ILC3 cells but suppress ILC2 cell production. They can promote the differentiation of B cells into plasma cells and so promote intestinal IgA responses. Butyrate can inhibit the proliferation of $CD4^+$ T cells but does not affect the proliferation of FoxP3$^+$ Treg cells. SCFAs also inhibit the differentiation of intestinal T cells and inhibit the production of Th1 cytokines. Butyrate induces intestinal Treg cell differentiation and stimulates IL-10 secretion (Mann et al., 2024). As a result, SCFAs from high-fiber diets play a key role in regulating intestinal inflammation and physiology (Van der Hee & Wells, 2021).

If the intestinal microbiota generates increased amounts of acetate, then this will activate the parasympathetic nervous system and promote glucose-stimulated insulin production (Takeuchi et al., 2021). This stimulates the production of a hunger hormone called ghrelin that enhances appetite, leading to increased food intake and obesity.

Intestinal protection

The microbiota protects the body against colonization by pathogens and prevents the overgrowth of pathobionts. They do this by competing for essential metabolites and nutrients and by inducing intestinal immune responses (Kamada, Chen, et al., 2013; Kamada, Seo, et al., 2013). By fully occupying and exploiting the intestinal microenvironment, commensal bacteria block subsequent colonization by less adapted pathogenic bacteria. The microbiota also modifies local environmental conditions by keeping the pH and oxygen tension low. This is also influenced by the diet; for example, the intestine of milk-fed animals contains many lactobacilli that produce bacteriostatic lactic and butyric acids. These acids inhibit colonization by *E. coli*, so foals suckled naturally tend to have fewer digestive disturbances than animals weaned early in life. There is a strong negative correlation between the level of lactobacilli and the number of pathogens in the intestine (Blander et al., 2017).

Microbiota signals

Bacteria, be they on the skin, respiratory tract, genital tract, oral cavity, or intestine, communicate directly and effectively with their host's immune system through the release of soluble metabolites. Indeed, this interaction is essential to the proper functioning of innate and adaptive immune responses. Alterations or imbalances in the microbiota, therefore, can have profound effects on the functions of the immune system (Ennamorati et al., 2020). The proper interaction between the immune system and the microbiota is required for optimal equine health (Arpaia & Rudensky, 2014).

Responses to the microbiota

For many years, it was believed that the role of the immune system was simply to ensure the complete exclusion of all invading microbes by distinguishing between self and not-self and eliminating foreign antigens. We now know, however, that decision alone is insufficient to ensure health. The immune system also determines the degree of threat posed by the microbes it encounters and adjusts its response accordingly. It must maintain tolerance to the microbiota or food antigens while, at the same time, being highly responsive to invading pathogens. This discrimination is determined in part by the way in which enteric microbial antigens are processed and the behavior of enterocytes. It is also determined by intestinal T and B cells as well as by the gut microenvironment. The members of the intestinal microbiota must either be tolerated or ignored if an animal is to remain healthy. An animal cannot afford to act aggressively toward its own microbiota. The presence of all these bacterial products has the potential to trigger massive acute inflammation, but this inflammation must not happen unless essential for the defense of the body.

Enterocytes

The intestinal epithelium is not simply a barrier. It is a highly responsive tissue that employs innate and adaptive immune cells to restrain the microbiota without triggering unnecessary inflammation, but is always ready to activate more potent defensive responses should the need arise. Enterocytes interact with the intestinal microbiota. They produce many peptides that kill specific bacteria and, as a result, shape the composition of the population. Enterocytes block access of intact antigens to the lamina propria. They ensure that a balance exists between inflammation and tolerance. They secrete and respond to regulatory cytokines. They present antigens to dendritic cells. Within the epithelium and the underlying lamina propria are intraepithelial T lymphocytes (IELs) that, upon appropriate stimulation by microbiota-induced IL-1β or IL-23, can regulate their differentiation into effector or regulatory cells (Schachtschneider et al., 2013).

Enterocytes express pattern recognition molecules (PRMs) for many microbial-associated molecular patterns (MAMPs), including TLRs-1, -2, -3, -5, and -9 as well as NOD-2. As a result, when exposed to MAMPs, recruitment of MyD88 and TRIF results in NF-κB and MAP kinase activation and cytokine synthesis. In practice, bacterial signals trigger the production of some antimicrobial peptides and cytokines but not inflammation. This is because the PRMs are not expressed on the luminal side of enterocytes, where they would normally come into contact with commensals. They are located at the base of the cells and in intracellular locations. Thus, they are activated only when bacteria penetrate the epithelial barrier. By excluding microbes, enterocytes also prevent the development of inflammation within the intestinal wall. Some of the cytokines produced by enterocytes also influence the regulatory activities of antigen-processing cells, such as macrophages and dendritic cells. IL-10 inhibits the TLR-MyD88 pathway, whereas IL-2 inhibits TLR-independent pathways.

The antimicrobial peptides within the inner mucus layer a well as the enterocyte glycocalyx keep most of the microbiota from contacting the enterocytes and thus ensure that the microbiota remains safely within the intestinal lumen. Thus, they not only protect the host from microbial invasion but also from the potentially harmful inflammatory response that would occur if MAMPs are absorbed into the body.

ILC3 cells

Type 3 innate lymphoid cells also regulate the interactions between the microbiota and its host (Chapter 10). They are found in the mucosa of the gastrointestinal tract (lamina propria, tonsils, and Peyer's patches) as well as in the lungs and skin. They respond to IL-23, IL-1β, and TSLP from dendritic cells by producing IL-17 and IL-22. These attract neutrophils and promote the production of antimicrobial peptides, especially the defensins in the small intestine. These defensins interact with the mucus layer to maintain a relatively bacteria-free zone adjacent to the mucosal surface. ILC3 cells also activate B cells and stimulate IgA production. They can promote tolerance to food antigens by producing IL-22, which in turn promotes Treg production. ILC3 cell production is regulated by the aryl hydrocarbon receptor as well as by butyrate generated by the intestinal microbiota (Kim et al., 2017).

B cells

The intestinal lymphoid tissues such as the Peyer's patches in conventional animals are in intimate contact with the billions of bacteria that make up the gut microbiota. As a result, developing B cells are exposed to a diverse universe of products generated by these commensal organisms. It is believed that this complex mixture promotes B-cell diversification and enhances the development of the pre-immune repertoire. Products derived from the microbiota are required for proper development not only of the gut-associated lymphoid tissue (GALT) but also of the antibody system itself. Products from the intestinal bacteria, acting through pattern recognition receptors, activate the developing B cells and promote immunoglobulin V region diversification. This diversification may also depend upon the presence of selected bacterial species such as *Bacillus subtilis*, *Bacteroides fragilis,* and certain Clostridia. Bacterial structural components such as lipoarabinomannans, lipopolysaccharides, some superantigens such as Staphylococcal protein A, or even metabolites such as fatty acids and retinoic acid, may also influence the B-cell diversification process. Likewise, endogenous stimulatory molecules from helper cells such as IL-4, IL-13, or IL-33 may also be required. Two very obvious cytokines that promote B-cell development are BAFF (B-cell-activating factor) and APRIL (a proliferation-inducing ligand), are upregulated by bacterial products and promote B-cell proliferation in an autocrine fashion (Maynard et al., 2012) (Chapter 11).

Although the microbiota is separated by the inner mucus layer and glycocalyx from direct contact with enterocytes, intestinal dendritic cells can extend their processes into the intestinal lumen and sample the microbiota. These bacteria may persist within the dendritic cells for several days while the cells carry them into the mucosa and mesenteric lymph nodes, process them, and present them to B cells. In addition, some bacteria are taken up by specialized antigen-capturing M cells, penetrate the

Peyer's patches, and become resident within the tissues. Although most of these invading bacteria are killed by macrophages, some are also presented to B cells. The B cells produce IgA in response, which may also modify the composition of the microbiota and can block further mucosal penetration. Bacteria are also prevented from breaching the mucosal barrier by the ongoing IgG response, while the complex of mesenteric lymph nodes of the horse form an additional barrier that prevents the commensals from reaching the systemic immune system (Fig. 8.4) (Mu et al., 2021).

T cells

The key to successful accommodation with the intestinal microbiota depends on the body's ability to control inflammation in the gut wall. This is achieved by maintaining a balance between pro-inflammatory Th17 cells and anti-inflammatory Treg cells. Intestinal helper T-cell phenotypes are "plastic" and precursor cells can differentiate into either Treg or Th17 cells, while Th17 cells may further differentiate into Th1 cells. This differentiation is regulated by signals from the microbiota. In effect, the microbiota programs the T-cell system to optimize its function (Ennamorati et al., 2020). Additionally, helper T-cell differentiation is determined by cytokines. For example, the development of both Tregs and Th17 cells is promoted by TGF-β. Treg cells require TGF-β plus retinoic acid and IL-2, whereas Th17 cells require TGF-β plus IL-6 and IL-23. The major transcription factors used by Tregs and Th17 are Foxp3 and ROR-γt, respectively, and these are coexpressed in naïve and effector $CD4^+$ cells (Gensollen et al., 2016).

Treg cells

Intestinal Treg cells are required to maintain the body's commensal relationship with its microbiota. Treg cells produce IL-10 as well as express high levels of CTLA-4 (cytotoxic T lymphocyte antigen 4), the inhibitory ligand for CD80. Treg production occurs in response to signals from both the microbiota and enterocytes. These Treg cells, when acted on by pro-inflammatory cytokines, can convert to IL-17 or IFN-γ-expressing effectors and so "break" tolerance. Under some circumstances, Th17 cells can also give rise to IFN-producers that functionally resemble Th1 cells, and many intestinal Th1 cells likely develop through this pathway. Under other circumstances, the Treg cells may be converted to helper cells and promote the B cell switch to IgA production. Indeed, about 75% of the IgA reactive to the microbiota is produced through a pathway controlled by Treg cells.

Mucosal inflammation is actively suppressed by the production of large numbers of IL-10-producing $Foxp3^+$ Tregs. Under stable, healthy conditions, the production of Treg cells is favored while that of Th17 cells is suppressed. It is also clear, however, that this tolerance can only go so far. Should a potential pathogen seek to invade the body from the intestine, then the immune system must be prepared to respond aggressively. This is mediated by pro-inflammatory Th17 cells.

Th17 cells

As described in Chapter 12, Th17 cells are a subset of $CD4^+$ T cells that regulate inflammation and maintain the intestinal epithelial barrier. Under the influence of IL-23, they produce the proinflammatory cytokines IL-17A, IL-17F, and IL-22. Like Treg cells, the development of Th17 cells is regulated by signals from both the microbiota and enterocytes. Th17 cell development is specifically stimulated by the attachment of SFBs to enterocytes. Enterocytes can sense this tight attachment (Ivanov et al., 2009). The mechanism by which these bacteria affect enterocytes is unclear, but they cause the enterocytes to produce serum amyloid A (SAA). The SAA acts as a cytokine and stimulates IL-23 production by macrophages, leading to ILC3 secretion of IL-22 and IL-17. This, in turn, triggers the development of Th17 cells. Lamina propria macrophages and dendritic cells can also detect SFB-derived molecules through their TLRs and produce IL-23 and TGF-β, so promoting further Th17 cell differentiation. As a result, the T cells differentiate into ROR-γt-expressing Th17 cells. Th17 cells regulate the abundance of

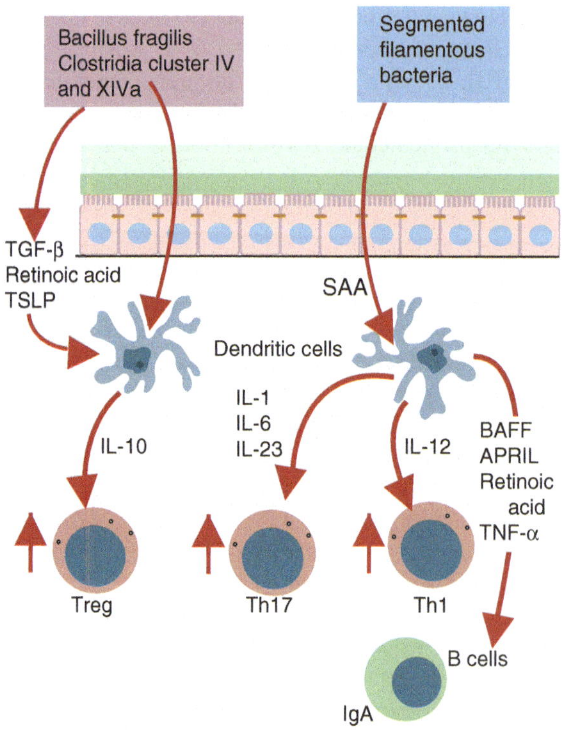

FIGURE 14.6

The role of segmented filamentous bacteria and Clostridial clusters in regulating T-cell subset formation and thus suppressing unwanted intestinal inflammation.

SFBs by promoting the production of antibacterial peptides such as β-defensins, lipocalins, and calprotectin by enterocytes (Fig. 14.6).

Retinoic acid

Commensal bacteria can provide the horse with a direct source of retinoic acid, the active metabolite of vitamin A. Retinoic acid is a critical regulator of mucosal immunity. It is produced by SFB (Woo et al., 2021). SFB are unique spore-forming, long filamentous Gram-positive anaerobic commensals found in the ileum of horses (Lowden & Heath, 1995). (Their scientific name is "*Candidatus savagella*"—the provisional name given to unculturable bacteria.) They bind tightly to the upper third of the intestinal villi. They have a unique ability to stimulate the maturation of T and B cells and especially to stimulate Th17 responses and IgA production. They can also upregulate host innate defense genes, inflammatory cytokines, and lymphokines (Wu et al., 2010). SFBs attach very strongly to the epithelial cells overlying Peyer's patches, where they are in a good position to be sampled by dendritic cells. (Most other bacteria remain within the mucus layer.) SFBs induce the development of germinal centers in Peyer's patches and other intestinal lymphoid organs and also increase the production of IgA and Th17 cells (Gaboriau-Routhiau et al., 2009). Thus, in addition to activating the T-cell population, the microbiota also ensures that the entire intestinal tract contains functional cells and that there are no gaps in the defenses.

Interleukin-22

IL-22, a member of the IL-10 family, plays an important role in maintaining intestinal mucosal barrier integrity. While it has been identified in the horse, its properties and functions in this species have not been closely examined. In other mammals, it is produced by Th17 cells, activated T cells, and ILC3s in response to IL-23. IL-22-producing ILC3s are present in normal intestinal tissues, especially in cryptopatches. In other herbivores, the IL-22 acts on nearby Paneth cells to release their granules rich in antimicrobial peptides (defensins and lysozymes) and hence influences the composition of the microbiota. IL-22 acts on cells of the skin and the digestive and respiratory systems to increase the expression of several β-defensins and thus promotes innate immunity and repair in these tissues. It promotes enterocyte growth and survival. On exposure to IL-22, enterocytes produce defensins that protect the intestinal epithelium. ILC3-derived IL-22 also inhibits T-cell-mediated intestinal inflammation by suppressing those cells that respond to antigens from commensal bacteria. IL-22 from ILC3s also inhibits the growth of SFB (Valle-Noguera et al., 2021).

Calprotectin

Calprotectin consists of two S100 proteins, S100A8 and S100A9 that normally form a heterotetramer. The complex has significant antimicrobial properties because it is a metal chelator that restricts the availability of the essential trace elements Zn and Mn to bacteria. Calprotectin is found in neutrophils, monocytes, macrophages, and epidermal cells. It forms about 60% of neutrophil cytosolic protein and is released in large amounts into blood and tissue fluid in inflammation. Fecal calprotectin is used as a marker for intestinal inflammation, such as inflammatory bowel disease (IBD) and other diseases of the gastrointestinal tract in horses. For example, in the healthy horse, the normal level of fecal calprotectin is 0.056–0.278 mg/mL. Horses suffering from colitis have calprotectin levels well above this value (Bishop, Shanthappa, et al., 2024). It is also significantly elevated in the saliva of horses with equine gastric ulcer syndrome (Munoz-Prieto et al., 2023). In both these cases, the calprotectin assays do not differentiate between gastrointestinal and other inflammatory diseases.

Juglone, the toxin that causes black walnut poisoning, induces a systemic inflammatory response as a result of increased inflammatory cytokine production in the lungs, liver, colon, and laminae of the hoof. The result is that horses develop severe laminitis. Investigations have revealed that calprotectin levels are increased in the laminar epidermis as a result of a neutrophil infiltration. It is suggested, therefore, that calprotectin may play a critical role in the development of this form of laminitis (Faleiros et al., 2009).

Dysbiosis

Because of its size and complexity, the equine gastrointestinal microbiota is readily disturbed by stress originating outside or inside the body. Thus, it is sensitive to changes in diet, age, and especially levels of starch, fiber, and fat (Raspa et al., 2024). Other stresses, such as transportation, estrus, and excessive work or exercise, also influence its composition (Li et al., 2024; Perry et al., 2018). It is clear from the above discussion that the gut microbiota exerts a significant influence on the systemic immune response. If this microbiota becomes unstable or imbalanced, dysbiosis occurs. One common cause is abrupt changes in the diet. Thus, weaning may cause a severe dysbiosis that results in postweaning diarrhea. At weaning, foals are suddenly fed with a carbohydrate-rich diet from diverse cereals as well as crude proteins. This in turn results in a decrease in enteric lactobacilli and microbial diversity, accompanied by an increase in the numbers of Clostridia, Prevotella, and facultative anaerobes. such as the Proteobacteria. The precise changes depend upon the sources of the fibers and proteins fed. Dysbiosis may also result from allergic diseases that themselves do not directly affect the gastrointestinal tract, such as asthma (Boucher et al., 2024).

Equine inflammatory bowel disease

Several different forms of IBD occur in horses. There are diverse innate and adaptive immune mechanisms involved, but in general, they cause malabsorption and a failure to receive sufficient nutrients. Thus, IBD results in weight loss, colic, and chronic diarrhea. The different forms are classified based on the predominant infiltrating cell population. The intestinal cellular infiltrates may be eosinophilic, lymphoplasmacytic, or granulomatous. There are several different forms of the eosinophilic disease. These diseases may well be caused by immune responses to components of the intestinal microbiota or the mycobiota. They may also result from allergic reactions to foods and intestinal parasites as well. These diseases primarily involve the small intestine, but in severe cases, the lesions may also extend to the cecum and colon (Timko, 2024).

Clinical signs in affected horses range from mild digestive disturbances to severe unremitting colic and chronic diarrhea. They usually reflect malabsorption problems, as evidenced by inappetence, weight loss with edema, and hypoalbuminemia. Standardbred and Thoroughbred horses appear predisposed to these diseases.

The pathogenesis of IBDs is complex and multifactorial. It has been suggested that they result, in part, from a dysbiosis resulting in an imbalance between Treg cells and Th17 cells. Rectal biopsies of horses suffering from chronic IBD show an increase in the expression of IL-17 mRNA. TLR4 expression is also elevated in horses with chronic active disease. Thus, it is clear that Th17 cells are actively engaged in the inflammatory process while Tregs appear to be unable to suppress it (Olofsson et al., 2015).

Limited attempts have been made to determine the etiology of equine IBD. One study, however, investigated whether affected horses have antibodies directed against the gluten-derived protein, gliadin and the autoantigen transglutaminase 2. It was found that some horses did indeed possess antibodies directed against transglutaminase 2. These antibody-positive horses included both IBD horses as well as horses on a high-gluten diet. There was, however, no significant difference in antibody titers between the IBD horses and the gluten-fed control animals. Interestingly, a single IBD horse had high levels of autoantibodies against not only transglutaminase two but also against deamidated gluten peptides and equine endomysium. After 6 months on a gluten-free diet, this horse recovered clinically and had significantly improved duodenal histopathology (Van der Kolk et al., 2012).

Eosinophilic diseases may affect many locations along the gastrointestinal tract. There are three recognized forms of eosinophilic enteritis in the horse: Focal, diffuse, and multisystemic. They all probably reflect an aberrant type 2 immune response in the intestinal tract. Some are attributed to parasites such as the protozoan *Balantidium coli* (Headley et al., 2008).

A multisystemic eosinophilic epitheliotrophic disease (MEED) has been reported in young Standardbreds. Affected horses develop an eosinophilic infiltration of multiple organs, including the skin, oral cavity, esophagus, salivary glands, liver, lung, and mesenteric lymph nodes, in addition to the intestinal tract. The lesions may also contain lymphocytes and macrophages. Affected horses may also suffer from exudative dermatitis affecting the face, limbs, and ventral abdomen that resembles the autoimmune disease, pemphigus foliaceus (Chapter 22). The hepatobiliary system may also be affected. Diagnosis is by biopsy of affected organs.

Some horses may develop a diffuse eosinophilic enterocolitis. This involves massive infiltration of the mucosa with eosinophils plus lymphocytes, and macrophages. Depending on the mucosal layer involved, it can result in recurrent colic rather than diarrhea. The infiltrates may be diffuse or segmental. Circumferential mural bands may also develop and result in intestinal blockage. The lesions in these cases are usually restricted to the gastrointestinal tract and affected animals do not necessarily develop an eosinophilia.

Granulomatous enteritis may be focal or systemic. It may preferentially occur in young Standardbreds. In some cases, it reflects chronic infections with bacteria such as Mycobacteria, Listeria, or Salmonella. Animals usually have diffuse lesions in the small intestine. They suffer from villous atrophy, and the lesions consist of macrophages, lymphocytes, and epithelioid cell aggregates. Occasional giant cells may be present. (In many respects, this resembles Johne's disease in cattle!) The granulomatous lesions may spread to other nearby organs such as the liver, spleen, and kidneys (Schumacher et al., 2000).

Lymphoplasmacytic enteritis is a rare disease characterized by a lymphocyte and plasma cell infiltrate in the lamina propria of the intestine. It results in a chronic enterocolitis and segmental or diffuse thickening of the small intestine. Villous atrophy is usually present. There is no apparent breed or sex predisposition, and horses of all ages appear susceptible. Affected horses are thin, lethargic, depressed, and suffer from chronic diarrhea. They are commonly hypoproteinemic and hypoalbuminemic. Diagnosis requires a biopsy, but it is difficult to diagnose antemortem. It has been suggested that this disease may, in fact, be the early premalignant stage of an intestinal lymphosarcoma (Kemper et al., 2000).

It must be emphasized, however, that bacterial infections remain the major cause of equine diarrhea. *Salmonella enterica*, serotypes Agona, Anatum, and Typhimurium are pathobionts that can adapt to the colon microenvironment, and are a common cause of equine enteritis. Studies have shown that about 3% of horses are carriers that can transmit Salmonellosis to others. They may shed the organisms intermittently, especially when stressed. Clinical disease and the resulting diarrhea vary greatly in severity. It may result in bacteremia and sepsis (Smith et al., 1978).

Diagnosis of equine IBD is one of exclusion. It, therefore, requires hematology, fecal egg counts, and bacterial cultures, looking especially for Salmonella. Hypoproteinemia is a common finding. Rectal palpation may be useful in detecting a thickened bowel wall. Likewise, transabdominal ultrasound may identify thickened walls or lymphadenopathy. A rectal biopsy is diagnostic in about a third of patients.

Diverse drugs have been used to treat these diseases, although this is often unrewarding. These include steroids (dexamethasone or prednisolone), antibiotics, hydroxychloroquine, metronidazole, and sulfasalazine. Prolonged treatment is required. Anthelmintics may be used if the eosinophilic disease is attributed to parasites.

Some horses may respond positively to dietary changes. Under some circumstances, it may prove possible to make permanent changes in the intestinal microbiota in such a way that a horse's health and productivity may benefit significantly. This is generally done through the use of probiotics. Probiotics are bacterial cultures administered in sufficient numbers and for a sufficient time to make these changes.

The horse virome

In addition to the bacteria, the normal equine microbiota also contains Archaea, fungi, and numerous viruses. The viral component of the microbiota is called the virome—the collection of all viruses found within an animal. It is estimated that the horse intestine may contain more than 2000 viral genotypes (Babenko et al., 2020). This virome differs between individual horses and may be even more diverse than the bacterial microbiota. The equine virome, as in other mammals, is dominated by bacteriophages that prey on the dense bacterial population. The horse fecal virome is richer than that of humans and has a greater diversity of phages. None of the phage species appears to dominate (Babenko et al., 2020). Nevertheless, they play an important role in determining the composition of the intestinal microbial community. In addition to the bacteriophages, the horse intestinal virome may contain potential pathogens. These can include parvoviruses, herpesviruses, and hepaciviruses (Li et al., 2015). These may also include endogenous viruses that are integrated into and form a significant component of equine genomes.

The donkey microbiota

Donkeys, like horses, possess complex microbial populations on all their external surfaces. Their oral microbiota complexity increases significantly after weaning, with significant increases in the Firmicutes and Myxococcota. As in the horse, the donkey's gastrointestinal tract contains the largest and most complex of these populations. The donkey cecum contains numerous bacterial genera such as Prevotella, Desulfovibrio, Alistipes, and Treponema (Kahn et al., 2025). *Clostridiales*, *Ruminococcaceae*, and *Strep equinus* predominate in the dorsal colon. *Prevotella* and *Treponema* are most abundant in the cecum (Li et al., 2022). Overall, Firmicutes and Bacteroidetes dominate in the donkey hindgut, while Firmicutes dominate in the foregut. *Lactobacilli* are the predominant genus in the anterior intestinal tract. As in the horse, there is greater microbial diversity in the adherent bacterial population than in the liquid intestinal contents. Likewise, high-energy diets increase the Firmicutes-to-Bacteroidetes ratio and increase the prevalence of *Prevotellaceae* while reducing the prevalence of *Ruminococcaceae*. As in horses, stresses such as transportation significantly alter the donkey intestinal microbiota (Kahn et al., 2025). Li et al. (2022) have found that genes related to the immune system such as IL-17R, IL-1R, IL-33, C1QA, and MMP3 are upregulated in the donkey colon reflecting the presence of functional immune defenses in this organ.

References

Arpaia, N., & Rudensky, A. Y. (2014). Microbial metabolites control gut inflammatory responses. *Proceedings of the National Academy of Sciences of the United States of America, 111*, 2058–2059.

Babenko, V. V., Millard, A., Kulikov, E. E., Spasskaya, N. N., et al. (2020). The ecogenomics of dsDNA bacteriophages in feces of stabled and feral horses. *Computational and Structural Biotechnology Journal, 18*, 3457–3467.

Belkaid, Y., & Hand, T. W. (2014). Role of the microbiota in immunity and inflammation. *Cell, 157*, 121–141.

Bishop, R. C., Migliorisi, A., Holmes, J. R., Kemper, A. M., et al. (2024). Microbial populations vary between the upper and lower respiratory tract, but not within biogeographic regions of the lung of healthy horses. *Journal of Equine Veterinary Science*. https://doi.org/10.1016/j.jevs.2024.105141

Bishop, R. C., Shanthappa, N., Connolly, S. L., Wilkins, P. A., & McCoy, A. M. (2024). Reference intervals for equine fecal calprotectin and calprotectin:protein ratio in horses with colic and colitis. *American Journal of Veterinary Research*. https://doi.org/10.2460/ajvr.24.09.0271

Blander, J. M., Longman, R. S., Iliev, I. D., Sonnenberg, G. F., & Artis, D. (2017). Regulation of inflammation by microbiota interactions with the host. *Nature Immunology, 18*, 851–860.

Bond, S. L., Timsit, E., Workentine, M., Alexander, T., & Leguillette, R. (2017). Upper and lower respiratory tract microbiota in horses: Bacterial communities associated with health and mild asthma (inflammatory airway disease) and effects of dexamethasone. *BMC Microbiology*. https://doi.org/10.1186/s12866-017-1092-5

Boucher, L., Leduc, L., Leclere, M., & Costa, M. C. (2024). Current understanding of equine gut dysbiosis and microbiota manipulation techniques: Comparison with current knowledge in other species. *Animals*. https://doi.org/10.3390/ani14050758

Chaucheyras-Durand, F., Sacy, A., Karges, K., & Apper, E. (2022). Gastrointestinal microbiota in equines and its role in health and disease: The black box opens. *Microorganisms*. https://doi.org/10.3390/microorganisms10122517

Christodoulou, C., & Clarke, T. B. (2024). Gut microbes coordinate pulmonary immunology. *Proceedings of the National Academy of Sciences*. https://doi.org/10.1073/pnas.2408800121

Costa, M. C., Silva, G., Ramos, R. V., Staempfli, H. R., et al. (2015). Characterization and comparison of the bacterial microbiota in different gastrointestinal tract compartments in horses. *The Veterinary Journal, 205*, 74–80.

Dang, A. T., & Marsland, B. J. (2019). Microbes, metabolites, and the gut-lung axis. *Mucosal Immunology, 12*, 843–850.

Ennamorati, M., Vasudevan, C., Clerkin, K., et al. (2020). Intestinal microbes influence development of thymic lymphocytes in early life. *Proceedings of the National Academy of Sciences of the United States of America, 117*, 2570–2578.

Faleiros, R. R., Nuovo, G. J., & Belknap, J. K. (2009). Calprotectin in myeloid and epithelial cells of laminae from horses with black walnut extract-induced laminitis. *Journal of Veterinary Internal Medicine, 23*, 174–181.

Gaboriau-Routhiau, V., Rakotobe, S., Lecuyer, E., Mulder, I., et al. (2009). The key role of segmented filamentous bacteria in the coordinated maturation of gut helper T cell responses. *Immunity, 31*, 677–689.

Gensollen, T., Iyer, S. S., Kasper, D. L., & Blumberg, R. S. (2016). How colonization by microbiota in early life shapes the immune system. *Science, 352*, 539–544.

Gil-Miranda, A., Caddey, B., Orellana-Gurrero, D., Smith, H., et al. (2024). Vaginal and uteine microbiota of healthy maiden mares during estrus. *Veterinary Sciences*. https://doi.org/10.3390/vetsci11070323

Gil-Miranda, A., Macnicol, J., Orellana-Gurrero, D., Samper, J. C., & Gomez, D. E. (2024). Reproductive tract microbiota of mares. *Veterinary Sciences*. https://doi.org/10.3390/vetsci11070324

Haspel, T. (2025). *The case for eating wild horses out west*. https://www.washingtonpoast.com.food/2025/08/01/wild-horses-overpopulation-food-eating/.

Headley, S. A., Kummala, E., & Sukura, A. (2008). *Balantidium coli* infection in a Finnish horse. *Veterinary Parasitology, 158*(1–2), 129–132.

Holyoak, G. R., Premathilake, H. U., Lyman, C. C., Sones, J. L., et al. (2022). The healthy equine uterus harbors a distinct core microbiome that varies with geographical location. *Scientific Reports*. https://doi.org/10.1038/s41598-022-18971-6

Husso, A., Jalanka, J., Alipour, M. J., Huhti, P., et al. (2020). The composition of the perinatal intestinal microbiota in the horse. *Scientific Reports*. https://doi.org/10.1038/s41598-019-57003-8

Ivanov, I. I., Atarashi, K., Manel, N., et al. (2009). Induction of intestinal Th17 cells by segmented filamentous bacteria. *Cell, 139*, 485–498.

Kahn, M. Z., Li, Y., Zhu, M., Li, M., et al. (2025). Advances in donkey disease surveillance and microbiome characterization in China. *Microorganisms*. https://doi.org/10.3390/microorganisms13040749

Kamada, N., Chen, G. Y., Inohara, N., & Nunez, G. (2013). Control of pathogens and pathobionts by the gut microbiota. *Nature Immunology, 14*, 685–690.

Kamada, N., Seo, S.-U., Chen, G. Y., & Nunez, G. (2013). Role of the gut microbiota in immunity and inflammatory disease. *Nature Reviews Immunology, 13*, 321–333.

Kamus, L. J., Theoret, C., & Costa, M. C. (2018). Use of next generation sequencing to investigate the microbiota of experimentally induced wounds and the effect of bandaging in horses. *PLoS One*. https://doi.org/10.1371/journal.pone.0206989

Kemper, D. L., Perkins, G. A., Schumacher, J., Edwards, J. F., et al. (2000). Equine lymphocytic plasmacytic enterocolitis: A retrospective study of 14 cases. *Equine Veterinary Journal, 32*, 108–112.

Kennedy, R., Lappin, D. F., Dixon, P. M., Buijs, M. J., et al. (2016). The microbiome associated with equine periodontitis and oral health. *Veterinary Research*. https://doi.org/10.1186/s13567-016-0333-1

Kim, S.-H., Cho, B.-H., Kiyono, H., & Jang, Y.-S. (2017). Microbiota-derived butyrate suppresses group 3 innate lymphoid cells in terminal ileal Peyer's patches. *Scientific Reports*. https://doi.org/10.1038/s41598-017-02729-6

Leduc, L., Costa, M., & Leclere, M. (2024). The microbiota and equine asthma: An integrative view of the gut-lung axis. *Animals*. https://doi.org/10.3390/ani14020253

Li, L., Giannitti, F., Low, J., Keyes, C., et al. (2015). Exploring the virome of diseased horses. *Journal of General Virology, 96*, 2721–2733.

Li, Y., Ma, Q., Shi, X., Liu, G., & Wang, C. (2022). Integrated multi-omics reveals novel microbe-host lipid metabolism and immune interactions in the donkey hindgut. *Frontiers in Immunology*. https://doi.org/10.3389/fimmu.2022.1003247

Li, J., Toyama, H., Matsumoto, T., Qasimi, M. I., et al. (2024). Changes in fecal microbiota during estrus cycle in healthy thoroughbred mares. *Journal of Equine Veterinary Science*. https://doi.org/10.1016/j.jevs.2024.105434

Lowden, S., & Heath. (1995). Segmented filamentous bacteria associated with lymphoid tissues in the ileum of horses. *Research in Veterinary Science, 59*, 272–274.

Mann, E. R., Lam, Y. K., & Uhlig, H. H. (2024). Short-chain fatty acids: Linking diet, the microbiota and immunity. *Nature Reviews Immunology, 24*, 577–595.

Maynard, C. L., Elson, C. O., Hatton, R. D., & Weaver, C. T. (2012). Reciprocal interactions of the intestinal microbiota and immune system. *Nature, 489*, 231–241.

Mo, P. M., Picard, J., & Gummow, B. (2023). The conjunctival fungal microbiota of horses in a North Queensland tropical environment and their in vitro susceptibilities to antifungal agents. *Veterinary Research Communications, 47*, 1641–1651.

Mu, Q., Swartwout, B. K., Edwards, M., Zhu, J., et al. (2021). Regulation of neonatal IgA production by the maternal microbiota. *Proceedings of the National Academy of Sciences of the United States of America, 118*(9), Article e2015691118.

Mulder, I. E., Schmidt, B., Stokes, C. R., Lewis, M., et al. (2009). Environmentally-acquired bacteria influence microbial diversity and natural innate immune responses at gut surfaces. *BMC Biology, 7*, 79. https://doi.org/10.1186/1741-7007-7-79

Munoz-Prieto, A., Contreras-Aguilar, M. D., Ceron, J. J., Ayala de la Pena, I., et al. (2023). Changes in calprotectin (S100A8-A9) and aldolase in the saliva of horses with equine gastric ulcer syndrome. *Animals*. https://doi.org/10.3390/ani13081367

O'Dwyer, D. N., Dickson, R. P., & Moore, B. B. (2016). The lung microbiome, immunity, and the pathogenesis of chronic lung disease. *Journal of Immunology, 196*, 4839–4847.

O'Shaughnessy-Hunter, L. C., Yu, A., Rousseau, J. D., Foster, R. A., & Weese, J. S. (2021). Longitudinal study of the cutaneous microbiota of healthy horses. *Veterinary Dermatology, 32*, Article 467-e128.

Olofsson, K., Hjertner, B., Fossum, C., Press, C. M., & Lindberg, R. (2015). Expression of T helper type 17 (Th17)-associated cytokines and toll-like receptor 4 and their correlation with Foxp3 positive cells in rectal biopsies of horses with clinical signs of inflammatory bowel disease. *The Veterinary Journal, 206*, 97–104.

Perry, E., Cross, T.-W. L., Francis, J. M., Hilscher, H. D., et al. (2018). Effect of road transport on the equine cecal microbiota. *Journal of Equine Veterinary Science, 68*, 12–20.

Pimenta, J., Pinto, A. R., Saavedra, M. J., & Cotovio, M. (2023). Equine Gram-negative oral microbiota: An antimicrobial resistance watcher? *Antibiotics*. https://doi.org/10.3390/antibiotics12040792

Poole, R. K., Soffa, D. R., McAnally, B. E., Smith, M. S., et al. (2023). Reproductive microbiomes of domestic livestock: Insights using 16SRNA gene amplicon community sequencing. *Animals, 13*, 484.

Pu, Q., Lin, P., Gao, P., Wang, Z., et al. (2021). Gut microbiota regulate gut-lung axis inflammatory responses by mediating ILC2 compartmental immigration. *Journal of Immunology, 207*, 1–11.

Raspa, F., Chessa, S., Bergero, D., Sacchi, P., et al. (2024). Microbiota characterization throughout the digestive tract of horses fed a high-fiber vs. a high-starch diet. *Frontiers in Veterinary Science*. https://doi.org/10.3389/fvets.2024.1386135

Rodrigues-Hoffmann, A. (2017). The cutaneous ecosystem: The roles of the skin microbiome in health and its association with inflammatory skin conditions in humans and animals. *Veterinary Dermatology, 28*, Article 60-e15.

Ross, A. A., Rodrigues-Hoffmann, A., & Neufeld, J. D. (2019). The skin microbiome of vertebrates. *BMC Microbiome*. https://doi.org/10.1186/s40168-019-0694-6

Santos, A. S., Rodrigues, M. A. M., Bessa, R. J. B., Ferreira, L. M., & Martin-Rosset, W. (2011). Understanding the equine cecum-colon ecosystem: Current knowledge and future perspectives. *Animals*. https://doi.org/10.1017/s1751731110001588

Schachtschneider, K. M., Yeoman, C. J., Isaacson, R. E., White, B. A., et al. (2013). Modulation of systemic immune responses through commensal gastrointestinal microbiota. *PLoS One, 8*(1). doi:10.1371/journal.pone.0053969.

Schulthess, J., Pandey, S., Capitani, M., Rue-Albrecht, K. C., et al. (2019). The short-chain fatty acid butyrate imprints an antimicrobial program in macrophages. *Immunity, 50*, 432–445.

Schumacher, J., Edwards, J. F., & Cohen, N. D. (2000). Chronic idiopathic inflammatory bowel disease of the horse. *Journal of Veterinary Internal Medicine, 14*, 258–265.

Simms, N., Bertone, J. J., Melgarejo, T., O'Shea, C., & Linde, A. (2025). Equine blood microbiome in a cohort of clinically healthy trail riding horses. *Journal of Veterinary Internal Medicine*. https://doi.org/10.1111/jvim.70082

Sisson, S., & Grossman, J. D. (1953). The large intestine. In *Anatomy of the domestic animals* (4th ed., p. 429). Philadelphia, PA: W.B. Saunders Company.

Smith, B. P., Riena Guerra, M., & Hardy, A. J. (1978). Prevalence and epizootiology of equine salmonellosis. *Journal of the American Veterinary Medical Association, 172*(3), 353–356.

Strompfova, V., & Stempelova, L. (2024). Composition and diversity of the 16S RNA based skin bacterial microbiome in healthy horses. *Veterinary Research Communications, 48*, 2847–2855.

Takeuchi, T., Miyauchi, E., Kanaya, T., Kato, T., et al. (2021). Acetate differentially regulates IgA reactivity to commensal bacteria. *Nature, 595*, 560–564.

Timko, K. (2024). Approach to inflammatory bowel disease. *Vet Clin Equine, 40*, 287–306.

Valle-Noguera, A., Ochoa-Ramos, A., Gomez-Sanchez, M. J., & Cruz-Adalia, A. (2021). Type 3 innate lymphoid cells as regulators of the host-pathogen interaction. *Frontiers in Immunology*. https://doi.org/10.3389/fimmu.2021.748851

Van der Hee, B., & Wells, J. M. (2021). Microbial regulation of host physiology by short-chain fatty acids. *Trends in Microbiology, 29*. https://doi.org/10.1016/j.tim.2021.02.001

van der Kolk, J. H., van Putten, L. A., Mulder, C. J., Grinwis, G. C. M., et al. (2012). Gluten-dependent antibodies in horses with inflammatory small bowel disease (ISBD). *Veterinary Quarterly, 32*, 3–11.

Venable, E. B., Fenton, K. A., Braner, V. M., Reddington, C. E., et al. (2017). Effects of feeding management on the equine fecal microbiota. *Journal of Equine Veterinary Science, 49*, 113–121.

Woo, V., Eshleman, E. M., Hashimoto-Hill, S., Whitt, J., et al. (2021). Commensal segmented filamentous bacteria-derived retinoic acid primes host defense to intestinal infection. *Cell Host & Microbe, 29*, 1744–1756.

Wu, H.-J., Ivaniv, I., Darce, J., Hattori, K., et al. (2010). Gut-residing segmented filamentous bacteria drive autoimmune arthritis via T helper 17 cells. *Immunity*. https://doi.org/10.1016/j.immumi.2010.06.001

Yao, Y., Cai, X., Fei, W., Ye, Y., et al. (2022). The role of short-chain fatty acids in immunity, inflammation and metabolism. *Critical Reviews in Food Science and Nutrition, 62*(1), 1–12.

CHAPTER

Horse and donkey vaccines

15

There are more than 3.6 million horses in the United States, 2.5 million in Argentina, and up to 1.2 million in the UK, Germany, and France. Infectious diseases are of significant concern in all these animals, although the specific threats they face differ according to their use and location. As with other species, travel and intermingling of animals from multiple sources greatly increases their risk of acquiring infectious diseases. These diseases can result not only in health issues and even death, but can also adversely affect their performance. Unlike other species, horses travel internationally on many occasions, especially in the racing and show-jumping industries. Well-considered vaccination is, by far, the most effective method of preventing disease spread. Owners should be reminded that vaccination is cheap compared to the value of a horse. It should, however, also be pointed out that while mild exercise will promote immune responses, especially in older horses, extreme stressful exercise and overtraining as well as long confinement and transportation can be significantly immunosuppressive (Edwards & Booy, 2013) (Chapter 24)

As with other animal vaccines, equine vaccines can be divided into "core" vaccines and optional or risk-based vaccines. Core vaccines are those directed against endemic diseases that a horse may be unable to avoid, diseases of public health significance, and very severe, life-threatening diseases. In North America, these include the vaccines directed against rabies, tetanus, and the viral encephalitides, Eastern, Western, and West Nile (Desanti-Consoli et al., 2022).

Optional vaccine use is based upon a veterinarian's professional experience and perception of risk, as well as the specific circumstances of each individual horse. They include vaccination against bacterial diseases such as Potomac horse fever, Strangles, Leptospirosis, and Botulism, as well as against viral diseases such as Equine influenza, Equine herpesviruses, and Equine viral arteritis.

Core vaccines

Tetanus

Clostridium tetani is a member of the microbiota in the intestinal tract of horses and is therefore abundant in the soil on many horse farms. Its spores persist in the environment for many years. *Cl. tetani* grows in the anaerobic environment of deep puncture wounds, surgical incisions, umbilical wounds in foals, and the uterus associated with retained placenta or other trauma. It should be noted that the size or severity of the

The Immunology of Horses and Donkeys. https://doi.org/10.1016/B978-0-443-44863-8.00008-9

wound is not always predictive of tetanus development. As the organism grows, it secretes a neurotoxin called tetanospasmin that is responsible for the clinical disease.

Tetanus vaccines consist of purified, formalin-inactivated toxoids. Tetanus toxoid is a potent antigen, especially when adjuvanted, and it stimulates a strong, protective antibody response. Circulating antibodies alone can neutralize tetanus toxin. Thus, all horses are at risk of tetanus, and tetanus toxoid is a core vaccine for all horses. The duration of immunity is at least 1 year, so annual revaccination is required. It takes about 2 weeks for immunity to develop after primary vaccination. It is also essential to vaccinate pregnant mares 4–8 weeks before foaling. This not only protects their foals through colostral antibodies but also protects the mares against foaling-related tetanus. Tetanus immune globulin should also be administered to any unvaccinated horse that requires immediate immunity as a result of a potentially contaminated wound.

Rabies

While not a common disease in horses, equine rabies is invariably lethal and is of Public Health significance in many countries. Rabies vaccine should therefore be considered a core requirement. There are five licensed rabies vaccines currently approved for use in horses in the United States. All are inactivated and tissue culture-derived. They are injected intramuscularly and are highly effective in young healthy horses.

Some veterinarians prefer that mares be vaccinated prior to breeding. Given the potency of these rabies vaccines, the mare's antibody levels will remain high throughout the pregnancy and still provide sufficient colostral antibodies to assure protection of their foals.

If confronted with foals from mares with an unknown rabies vaccination history, one may assume that they have been vaccinated and boost accordingly. An alternative approach is to test their serum for antibodies against rabies about 24 hours after birth, at a time when they would be predicted to have received colostral antibodies. If negative, they should be treated as if the mares were unvaccinated, whereas if positive, one must assume that the mares had been vaccinated.

If a vaccinated horse has been bitten by a rabid animal, then it should be immediately revaccinated by a veterinarian and then placed under observation for 45 days as directed by the regulatory authorities. If an unvaccinated horse is exposed to a rabid animal, it may be euthanized immediately. If this is an unacceptable procedure, then the horse should be monitored for 6 months under veterinary supervision and with the approval of the appropriate authorities. This may also include isolation and immediate vaccination.

Eastern and Western equine encephalitis (EEE and WEE)

Both EEE and WEE are caused by alphaviruses in the family Togaviridae. These viruses are maintained in the environment by circulating through birds and transmitted by mosquitoes. They are not common diseases but do occur sporadically in midsummer and fall across the United States. Outbreaks may be especially common in very wet years when pools of stagnant water form and mosquitoes thrive. Clinical EEE cases are primarily restricted to the Eastern coastal plains and the Gulf coast. Conversely, WEE primarily occurs in Western and Midwestern states and the Southeast. A variant of EEE virus (Madariaga virus) occurs in South America. Thus, both of these diseases can be considered endemic across both North and South America. Both diseases present with fever, anorexia, and depression. Severe cases can result in blindness, ataxia, behavioral changes, convulsions, and death within 2–3 days. EEE is nearly always fatal in horses (75%–80% mortality) while WEE causes about 30%–40% mortality. Recovered horses likely have lifelong immunity. Combined vaccines against EEE and WEE are core vaccines that should be boosted annually. In areas with a prolonged mosquito season, it may be appropriate to give two doses annually, one in the spring and one in the fall. Likewise, horses that were not vaccinated in the previous year should receive two doses 3–6 weeks apart.

All currently available EEE/WEE vaccines are formalin-inactivated whole viral products. It has not yet been possible to produce effective modified live vaccines. These vaccines may be combined with vaccines containing antigens from tetanus, influenza, and West Nile Virus. Current research activities are focused on the production of effective cross-reactive vaccines where a single dose can protect against all three encephalitis viruses (Stromberg et al., 2020).

As in humans, there is a growing tendency to employ vaccines that contain multiple antigens in a single dose. This is much less stressful for the animal and equally protective. For example, there is a 7-component vaccine available that contains West Nile virus, three encephalitis viruses, influenza, and rhinopneumonitis virus, in addition to tetanus toxoid. The three encephalitis vaccines are Eastern, Western, and Venezuelan. The rhinopneumonitis component includes both equine herpesviruses, EHV-1 and EHV-4. It is administered to horses over 4 months of age with two priming doses and annual revaccination.

West Nile virus

West Nile virus (WNV) is currently the most significant insect-borne encephalitis virus in North America. It is classified as a Flavivirus. WNV is now found across the entire United States and most of Canada, and Mexico. WNV affects birds, humans, and horses, but horses are by far the most susceptible species, representing over 95% of clinically affected mammals. Affected horses develop ataxia and motor deficits ranging from mild to an inability to walk. Fever is not a consistent feature. About 30% of infected horses die, and the survivors may show residual damage, including altered gait and abnormal behavior. Because of its distribution and significance, WNV vaccination is considered essential. At the present time in the USA, there are two licensed inactivated tissue culture adjuvanted whole virion vaccines, a canary pox recombinant vectored vaccine, and an inactivated yellow fever chimera vaccine.

The two inactivated vaccines may not prevent infection, but they do reduce disease severity and prevent the development of a viremia (Cendejas & Goodman, 2024). A recombinant canarypox vectored WNV vaccine is available that will not replicate in vaccinated horses but persists for a sufficient period to stimulate a protective response (Siger et al., 2006).

The chimeric vaccine consists of a genetically engineered vaccine strain (17D) of yellow fever virus as a vector with inserted West Nile pre-membrane (PreM) and envelope (E) proteins to generate a chimeric virus-like particle. The remaining nucleocapsid proteins, as well as the nonstructural proteins and untranslated gene termini, are those of the yellow fever virus.

Antibodies to WNV are detectable by 21 days post-vaccination and reach maximal titers by about 4 weeks. WNV antibody titers may be somewhat lower in response to combined vaccines when compared to single antigen vaccines. Recovered horses probably develop lifelong immunity. However, antibody titers do decline over time, even in convalescent horses. Thus, regular serological testing and, if necessary, revaccination should be undertaken in WNV endemic areas (Tolnai et al., 2025). Box 15.1.

Risk-based vaccines

Anti-bacterial vaccines

There are many diverse antibacterial vaccines available for use in horses. These primarily consist of killed whole organisms—bacterins, toxoids, or attenuated live organisms. Fig. 15.1.

Botulism

Botulism results from ingestion of the neurotoxins of *Clostridium botulinum*. These toxins cause a flaccid paralysis by inhibiting the release of acetylcholine from motor neurons. *Cl. botulinum* can produce seven different neurotoxins. Types A, B, and C are associated with botulism outbreaks in horses, but type B accounts for more than 85% of equine botulism cases in the USA. This organism is found in soil, so it can contaminate wounds. *Cl. botulinum* can also cause a rapidly fatal shaker foal syndrome (toxicoinfectious botulism) as a result of ingestion of spores on contaminated

Box 15.1 Equine vaccination Guidelines

Comprehensive guidelines for vaccinating horses in North America have been produced by the American Association of Equine Practitioners (AAEP). They are available at https://aaep.org/guidelines-resources/vaccination-guidelines/resource-library/

These guidelines are neither regulations nor directives. It is left to the discretion of the attending veterinarian to use vaccines in an appropriate manner to ensure the optimal health care programs for their clients.

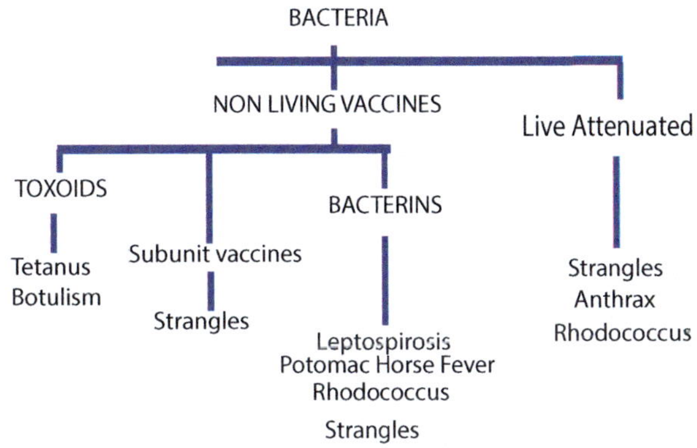

FIGURE 15.1

The diversity of equine antibacterial vaccines.

vegetation. Likewise, forage poisoning occurs when preformed toxin is ingested with improperly baled hay or contaminated feed.

A formalin-inactivated toxoid against botulinum toxin type B is licensed for use in horses in the United States. There are no toxoids available for types A or C. Vaccination is warranted for all horses since they may move into recognized endemic areas. It is especially recommended for horses that reside in the endemic areas in Kentucky and the Mid-Atlantic states. The horses at greatest risk are those fed baled hay, haylage, and silage, as well as foals born to unvaccinated mares. Shaker foal syndrome is a significant problem in endemic areas in foals 2 weeks to 8 months of age.

Strangles

Streptococcus equi subspecies *equi* causes strangles in horses, donkeys, and mules. Clinical disease includes abrupt pyrexia, pharyngitis, and dysphagia, so that horses have difficulty swallowing and anorexia. Lymphadenopathy then develops, leading to abscess formation in the submandibular and retropharyngeal lymph nodes. When these abscesses burst, their contents contribute to a copious, purulent, and highly infectious nasal discharge. Metastatic strangles is characterized by abscesses in other lymph nodes, especially in the abdomen and thorax. While most severe in weanlings and yearlings, horses of any age can develop the disease. As of 2017, strangles has been a reportable disease in the United States. Recovery from clinical disease results in prolonged immunity that lasts for at least 5 years. This immunity is associated with the production of antibodies against *S. equi* M protein. Strains of *S. equi* show little genomic diversity, and strangles vaccines should offer cross-protection against most circulating strains of the bacteria. Vaccination is recommended where strangles is a persistent endemic problem or for horses at a high risk of exposure. Several different strangles vaccines are available. They use diverse technologies. For example, killed vaccines are available in some countries. Inactivated injectable *S. equi* bacterins are associated with a relatively high prevalence of injection site reactions (soreness or abscesses at the injection site and occasional cases of purpura hemorrhagica). In addition, any protection conferred by these vaccines is short-lasting. *Strep. equi* bacterins give immunity for less than 1 year, even though recovery from a natural case of strangles may confer lifelong immunity in horses. A vaccine containing purified Streptococcal M-protein given intramuscularly is available in the United States. This vaccine may not prevent the disease. It will, however, reduce the severity of clinical disease and reduce disease prevalence by about 50% (Boyle et al., 2018).

A subunit strangles vaccine that contains a mixture of eight soluble recombinant streptococcal fusion proteins is also available. The proteins were identified by analysis of the bacterial genome and studies in mice. They consist of a combination of surface and secreted proteins. The cloned proteins are generated in *E. coli*, purified, and then combined. A saponin-based adjuvant is subsequently added. This vaccine is administered intramuscularly and requires a primary course of two injections. It also has an excellent safety profile (Rendle et al., 2024). This vaccine has DIVA capability (Vaccinated animals can be differentiated from infected animals) since none of the antigens are included in diagnostic ELISA tests (SEQ_2190—antigen A, and SeM—Antigen B) are present in the vaccine. It is commercially available in Europe (Robinson et al., 2018, 2020).

Several attenuated live strangles vaccines are available globally. For example, a live intranasal vaccine containing a non-encapsulated strain of *Strep. equi* is available in the USA and New Zealand. After administration, the attenuated bacteria should ideally reach the lingual and pharyngeal tonsils, where they stimulate local immunity. It may be anministered to horses aged 9 months or older. The vaccine organisms can be isolated from vaccinated horses up to 46 days after vaccination. In some cases, the attenuated bacteria may cause the slow development of mandibular or retropharyngeal abscesses, a nasal discharge, and occasional cases of purpura hemorrhagica (Cursons et al., 2015). These may be severe in young foals. Because this attenuated organism retains the ability to infect wounds, no other vaccines should be delivered concurrently, and no invasive procedures performed at the same visit. This vaccine was generated by treating a wild-type isolate with a mutagen. It differs from the original strain of *Strep equi* by about 68 mutations, but it is not known which of these are responsible for its attenuation. Its activity depends on the production of nasopharyngeal mucosal IgG and IgA responses directed against the bacterial M protein.

Another modified live Strangles vaccine is also available in Europe. This contains a live attenuated *aroA* deletion mutant (Strain TW928) that lacks 932 base pairs of the *aroA* gene. This vaccine is administered by submucosal injection into the inside of the upper lip but painful reactions at the injection sites may occur. Immunity to experimental challenge persists for about 3 months. This vaccine is not DIVA-compatible. Because of the risk of purpura, horses known to have had strangles within the previous year and horses with high antibody levels (titers>1:3200) should not be vaccinated (Robinson et al., 2015, 2018).

Anthrax

Anthrax is a fatal septicemia caused by *Bacillus anthracis*. The infection can be acquired by ingestion, inhalation, or wound contamination. It is restricted to certain regions in North America associated with alkaline soils. Vaccination is not required outside these endemic areas. The anthrax vaccine, the Sterne 34F strain, is an attenuated non-encapsulated spore vaccine. It may cause temporary injection site swelling in young foals and should not be used in pregnant mares. Since this is a live bacterial vaccine, it is important to ensure that antibiotics are not given to the horse at the same time. A live anthrax vaccine containing spores has been reported to cause an immune-mediated necrotizing vasculitis in miniature horses. The lesions contained significant quantities of IgM. However, the mechanisms involved are unknown (Wobeser, 2015).

Leptospirosis

Leptospirosis is a sporadic disease of horses. The leptospires cause equine recurrent uveitis, abortions, and renal disease (Chapter 22). The bacteria are spread via the body fluids of infected horses, especially their urine. The commonest serovars in horses in the United States are *L. interrogans*, serovar Pomona type kennewicki, and *L. kirchneri* serovar Grippotyphosa. A killed whole-cell monovalent bacterin against serovar Pomona has been approved for use in horses (Correia et al., 2017).

Potomac horse fever

Equine neorickettsiosis, (Potomac Horse Fever) is caused by an obligate intracellular bacterium, *Neorickettsia risticii*. It is transmitted by the accidental ingestion of aquatic insects harboring the metacercaria of an infected trematode. The infection results in abortion in mares as well as depression, fever, leukopenia, enterocolitis with profuse diarrhea, and laminitis. A killed, adjuvanted whole-cell vaccine is available. It may be beneficial in endemic areas, but *N. risticii* is genetically very heterogeneous, and as a result, the vaccine does not protect against all strains. The vaccine should be administered the spring in advance of the trematode/insect season in summer and fall. Studies have investigated the effectiveness of using monovalent or multivalent vaccines (incorporating rabies vaccine), and have confirmed its poor immunogenicity. Only a third of the horses in this study demonstrated seroconversion at any time point after vaccination (McKenzie et al., 2019).

Inactivated vaccines are widely used to control Potomac horse fever. However, inactivated vaccines are generally unable to stimulate a strong cell-mediated response. As a result, the existing vaccines are relatively ineffective. and Potomac horse fever occurs despite widespread vaccination. The vaccines induce relatively low antibody titers and insignificant neutralizing activity (Dutta et al., 1998). Thus, a combination of poor immunogenicity and perhaps an inappropriate adaptive immune response results in horses remaining vulnerable to this infection.

Rhodococcus equi

Rhodococcus equi is a facultative intracellular bacterium that causes lethal bronchopneumonia and pyogranulomatous lung lesions in foals 3 weeks to 6 months of age. The organism elicits both antibody and cell-mediated immune responses in foals. Protection is attributed to a type 1 immune response mediated by IgG1 antibodies. Traditional live, killed, and attenuated vaccines have proved to be ineffective. Encouraging results have however, been obtained when pregnant mares are vaccinated against poly-N-acetyl glucosamine, a highly conserved capsular polysaccharide. It is assumed that this immunity results from the transfer of maternal antibodies in colostrum (Giles et al., 2015). Passive immunization with hyperimmune serum against whole bacteria or against poly-N-acetyl glucosamine may also be of significant benefit when treating infected foals (Cywes-Bentley et al., 2018).

It has also been shown that enteral immunization of newborn foals with live virulent *R. equi* on days 1 and 3 results in the foals developing enhanced innate and adaptive immune responses by 28 days. These foals were protected against intrabronchal challenge with *R. equi* (Petri da Silviera et al., 2025). This appears to be a form of trained immunity.

Lyme disease

Lyme disease caused by *Borrelia burgdorferi* can occur in horses. Most infected animals show minimal clinical signs. In others it causes stiffness and lameness as well as neurologic signs such as ataxia and paresis. There are currently no USDA-licensed equine Lyme disease vaccines available in the United States. Experimental studies using a commercial German vaccine containing outer surface proteins (Osp) A and C have been shown to induce strong antibody responses in horses (Knödlseder et al., 2019). For example, ponies were completely protected against experimental infection by vaccination using an aluminum adjuvanted recombinant OspA antigen vaccine. This followed exposure to Borrelia-infected ticks 92 days after receiving a third vaccine dose (Chang et al., 1999).

Anti-viral vaccines

Horses are susceptible to many viruses that can cause serious, life-threatening infections. As a result, many diverse and innovative vaccines have been developed to prevent these diseases. They include inactivated, modified-live, and subunit vaccines. Fig. 15.2.

Venezuelan equine encephalitis (VEE)

VEE, as its name implies, is endemic in tropical wet forest areas of South and Central America. It is caused by an Alphavirus, in the Togaviridae family, and is maintained in a rodent reservoir and transmitted by mosquitoes. It can cause debilitating and potentially lethal encephalitis in horses and humans. VEE has not been diagnosed in the United States since 1971. It is therefore a reportable foreign animal

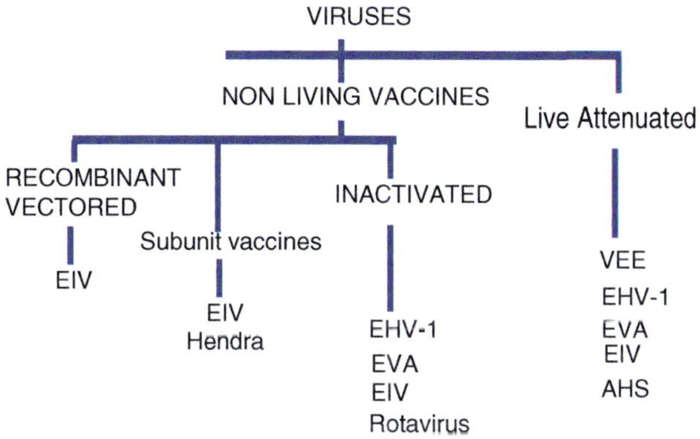

FIGURE 15.2 The diversity of equine antiviral vaccines

Note that equine influenza (EIV) vaccine has a greater diversity of available vacines than other equine virus. This presumably reflects its importance as a potentially zoonotic disease.

disease. Should VEE recur, an inactivated vaccine may be given to horses in a two-dose primary series, 3–4 weeks apart, with annual revaccination. Vaccination against EEE and WEE will induce antibodies that cross-react with VEE and may provide partial protection.

A modified live vaccine strain of VEE, C-84, is also used in horses. The vaccine must be kept cold, reconstituted, and used immediately, and given as a single dose to horses over 3 months of age. Horses should be revaccinated annually. This vaccine has been conditionally approved in the United States. Obviously, it cannot be used in the USA at the present time but would be released should a VEE outbreak occur (Paessler & Weaver, 2009).

Equine rhinopneumonitis

Equid herpesvirus type 1 (EHV-1) and type 4 (EHV-4) cause respiratory and neurologic disease and abortion. They are endemic in horse populations worldwide. Many foals become infected in the first weeks or months of life, but infections also occur when horses from different locations are mingled. Both viruse types cause rhinopneumonitis with fever, lethargy, anorexia, nasal discharge, cough, and mandibular lymphadenopathy. Both EHV-1 and EHV-4 can also cause abortion in naïve mares, weak nonviable foals, or a relatively infrequent paralytic neurologic disease (equine herpesvirus myeloencephalopathy, EHM). EHV-4 causes especially severe abortion outbreaks.

Like other herpesviruses, these viruses readily establish a latent infection in horses, which then become asymptomatic carriers. Most horses are therefore re-infected multiple times during their lifetime, usually sub-clinically. Viral reactivation occurs when horses are stressed, resulting in a viremia and short-term viral shedding. If this reactivation occurs in pregnant mares, they may abort.

Routine vaccination is required for the prevention of abortion and to reduce the severity of rhinopneumonitis in young or other at-risk horses. Although horses develop serum antibodies after infection, these antibodies are not correlated with protection. However, an intranasal antibody response consisting of virus-neutralizing IgG4/7 antibodies correlates well with prevention of shedding and viremia as well as protection (Perkins et al., 2019). Current vaccines are not effective in preventing the development of neurologic disease.

Many different inactivated vaccines are available for the control of EHV-1 and -4. These include some licensed for protection against respiratory disease alone, and others that are used for protection against both rhinopneumonitis and abortion. One inactivated vaccine is given intramuscularly for two doses, but the third dose may be given intranasally! Not all these vaccines are equally protective, and immunity is generally short-lasting.

A modified live EHV-1 vaccine is also available. It is used for protection against rhinopneumonitis in horses over three months-of-age. Like other live herpesvirus vaccines, it causes a rapid onset of protection as a result of interferon production. Because the duration of immunity is relatively short, multiple doses may be administered annually. Even infected, recovered horses probably only remain immune for up to 6 months. Horses less than 5 years of age, horses in contact with pregnant mares, horses that come into extensive contact with frequently moved horses, and show horses in high-risk environments should receive EHV-1 vaccines. Equestrian organizations may require such vaccination (Bannai et al., 2018). An experimental vaccine containing multiple deletion mutants of EHV-1 is, as expected, highly attenuated and appears to be effective in horses (Balena et al., 2022).

Equine viral arteritis

Equine viral arteritis is caused by an enveloped, positive-stranded RNA virus (EAV) in the genus Arterivirus. It occurs in horses worldwide. EAV can cause abortion in pregnant mares and establish a long-term carrier state in breeding stallions. Foals infected during the first few months of life may develop edema, conjunctivitis, urticaria, and rarely, a severe pneumonia, enteritis, or pneumoenteritis. The majority of primary EAV infections are, however, subclinical or asymptomatic. Persistent carrier stallions are the natural reservoir of EAV. All horses should be serologically tested, and a negative antibody titer should be documented by a licensed laboratory before vaccinating.

Protective, virus-neutralizing antibodies are directed against a viral envelope glycoprotein G_L (Castillo-Olivares et al., 2003). An inactivated adjuvanted vaccine is licensed for use in certain European countries. This vaccine is used in breeding and non-breeding horses. Interestingly, another inactivated vaccine has been developed in Japan. It is stored in anticipation of an outbreak of EVA occurring in Japan. It is not commercially available.

A modified live EAV vaccine is licensed for use in the USA and Canada. It contains a virus attenuated by multiple serial passages in primary equine and rabbit kidney cells and in equine dermal cells. It is safe and effective in stallions and non-pregnant mares. It should not be given to pregnant mares. Mild febrile reactions and transient lymphopenia do occur. In first-time vaccinates, the frequency, duration, and amount of vaccine virus that is shed via the respiratory tract is less than that observed with natural infection. Vaccination in the face of an EVA outbreak has been successful in controlling disease spread. When considering vaccinating against EVA, it is important to consult with state and/or federal animal health officials ahead of time to ensure that the vaccine complies with any official control program.

Breeding stallions should receive annual revaccination against EVA no later than 4 weeks prior to each breeding season. Before initial vaccination, all stallions must undergo serologic testing and be confirmed negative for antibodies to EAV. All first-time vaccinated stallions should then be isolated for 3 weeks after vaccination before being used for breeding. Some countries prohibit entry of any horse that is serologically positive for antibodies to EAV, regardless of its vaccination history. Countries that do accept EVA-vaccinated horses typically require stallions or colts to have a certified vaccination history and confirmation of pre-vaccination negative serological status. To resolve some of these issues, studies on inactivated marker vaccines are ongoing (Castillo-Olivares et al., 2003).

Equine influenza

Equine influenza virus (EIV) causes an acute respiratory disease in horses, donkeys, and mules worldwide. This disease, caused by the orthomyxovirus equine influenza A type 2 (A/equine 2), is one of the most common and important infectious diseases of horses. It is highly contagious and spreads rapidly between animals by the respiratory route. It is endemic in many countries and causes major outbreaks once sufficient antigenic drift occurs and the horse population is no longer immune. It causes high morbidity with significant economic consequences. Mortality is uncommon, but the virus may kill donkeys and colostrum-deprived foals (Paillot, 2014).

EIV, like other influenza viruses, undergoes continuous antigenic drift as a result of mutations in its RNA genome that result in amino acid substitutions in its hemagglutinin and consequent alterations in its structure and antigenicity. Continuous virus surveillance and characterization are essential for its control. Influenza vaccines only work when they match the circulating strains, and they must be updated periodically if failures are to be avoided. This update is based on a formal review of circulating strains by an expert committee of the OIE (The World Organization of Animal Health).

Influenza viruses have two major surface proteins, the hemagglutinin (H) and the neuraminidase (N). The hemagglutinin is the major target of neutralizing antibodies and an essential antigen in influenza vaccines. Equine influenza viruses are classified by their subtype, as well as the location and year they were first isolated. For example, H7N7 was first isolated in Prague in 1956, while H3N8 was first isolated in Miami, Florida, in 1963. H7N7 strains have not been detected since the late 1970s (Branda et al., 2025).

The original H3N8 equine influenza virus strain changed very little between 1963 and 1988. In 1989, however, it subsequently diverged into two antigenically and genetically distinct lineages, one Eurasian and one American. The Eurasian lineage has not been isolated for many years and is believed extinct. The American lineage subsequently evolved into Kentucky, Argentinian, and Florida lineages. The Kentucky and Argentinian lineages have not been isolated recently. Sometime after 2000, the Florida lineage in turn diverged into two sub-lineages, clades 1 and 2. These are now the dominant H3N8 EIV lineages circulating internationally. Florida clade 2 viruses have predominated in Europe and Asia, while clade 1 viruses predominate in North America. (However, in October 2018, clade 1 was introduced into Europe from North America and triggered a large outbreak. Florida clade 1 includes A/eq/Ohio/03, A/eq/Wisconsin/03, and A/eq/South Africa/03 viruses. Florida clade 2 includes A/eq/Italy/99, A/eq/Newmarket/03, and A/Richmond/07 viruses. H3N8 viruses from these two sub-lineages are sufficiently antigenically different as to require the presence of both in vaccines. Vaccination against one clade may not fully protect against the disease caused by the other. Currently, it is recommended that horses traveling internationally should receive vaccines containing both Florida clade 1 and clade 2 viruses. Antigenic drift continues to occur however, and recent isolates are diverging from both clades. Newly emerged strains of clade 2 may be responsible for outbreaks of influenza in vaccinated horses in the UK and France (Ryan et al., 2015). The disease is currently most prevalent in the UK based on the number of reported outbreaks between 2019 and 2024 (Branda et al., 2025). Fig. 15.3.

Influenza outbreaks generally follow the introduction of an infected horse into a stable, where the virus spreads rapidly through susceptible animals. Thus, quarantine of newly arriving horses and timely vaccination are required for disease control. All horses should be vaccinated regularly against influenza with the currently

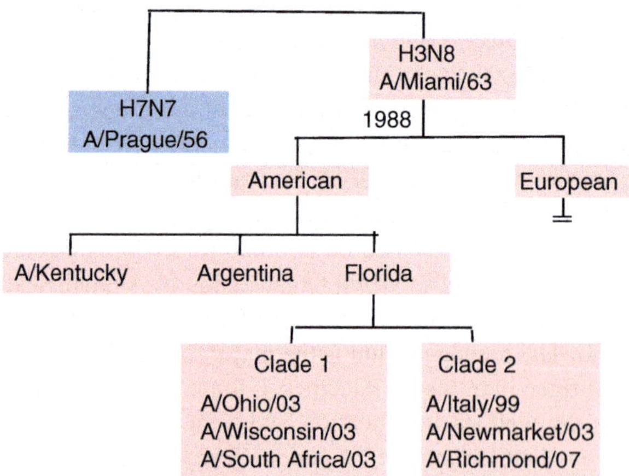

FIGURE 15.3 Recent equine influenza strains

The original split from the H7N7 virus to the H3N8 virus occurred around 1963. Since then the virus has diversified considerably.

recommended strains (Reemers et al., 2020). Vaccination reduces both clinical signs and viral shedding, although vaccinated infected horses may, however, still shed some virus (Pouwels et al., 2014).

Should an outbreak of influenza occur, it may be necessary to establish a buffer zone surrounding that area. In the 2007–08 Australian outbreak caused by the Florida clade 1 strain A/eq/Sydney/07, the disease was compartmentalized by ring vaccination that blocked viral spread.

In some countries, influenza vaccination is mandatory for horses participating in equestrian activities under the rules of International Equestrian Organizations. Some require that horses be vaccinated vetween 6 months and 21 days prior to competing. Some of these organizations require biannual rather than annual revaccination since antibody levels appear to drop after 4–6 months. It is absolutely critical that equine influenza vaccines contain epidemiologically relevant strains since there is minimal cross-strain protection (Horspool LJ. & King, 2013). Studies on different vaccine formulations have suggested that there are minimal differences in their antigenicity. However, many vaccinated horses, while protected against clinical disease, may remain infected with the influenza virus (Entenfellner et al., 2020).

There are four types of EIV vaccine currently available: whole inactivated and subunit vaccines, an intranasal modified-live cold-adapted vaccine, and a recombinant canarypox vectored vaccine.

The earliest flu vaccines consisted of whole, inactivated products. Inactivated influenza vaccines may contain many different antigens from multiple strains of influenza A clade 2. They contain whole viruses combined with adjuvants such as carbomer, aluminum hydroxide, or ISCOM-matrix. The viruses are first grown in embryonated chicken eggs or tissue culture, concentrated, and purified before they are inactivated with formaldehyde or beta-propiolactone. They induce antibodies against the viral hemagglutinin, neuraminidase, and other conserved viral antigens. However, immunity is often short-lived. Thus, most of these vaccines require two injections for priming, although three are better. They are most suitable for vaccination of pregnant mares in order to boost colostral antibodies. They may be combined with other viral antigens such as the equine herpesviruses, the encephalitis viruses, and tetanus.

A subunit influenza vaccine is also available. It contains the purified HA and NA subunits from A/equine-2/South Africa/4/03 and A/equine-2/Newmarket/2/93. It is adjuvanted with ISCOM/ISCOM-matrix. It is currently available in the European Union (Paillot & Prowse, 2012).

A modified-live cold-adapted intranasal vaccine against H3N8 is also available. A/Equine 2/Kentucky/91 was attenuated by cold adaptation in embryonated eggs. As a temperature-sensitive agent, it can replicate in the upper respiratory tract but not deeper within the body. It is approved for vaccination of non-pregnant horses over 11 months of age, followed by revaccination every 6 months. As with other live intranasal vaccines, horses can shed the vaccine virus. However, this shedding generally lasts for less than a week. The onset of protective immunity occurs by 7 days post-vaccination. It is best not to use this vaccine in pregnant mares. In addition to safety concerns, this vaccine does not elicit high serum antibody levels, so colostral antibodies may not be elevated. This is not entirely surprising since the intranasal immune response is primarily restricted to the nasal mucosa. This vaccine is only available in the USA. (Heldens et al., 2004)

A canarypox-vectored vaccine encoding the hemagglutinin genes from A/eq/Ohio/03 and A/eq/Richmond/1/07 is available in North America and Europe. It contains an adjuvant and is administered intramuscularly. During the 2007 Australian outbreak, it was shown to significantly reduce the severity and duration of disease and viral shedding (Paillot & El-Hage, 2016). An accelerated vaccination schedule with only 14 days between vaccination and boosting was applied in emergencies. Ideally, it should be administered at least 4 weeks before an event. This vaccine induces high anti-hemagglutinin levels, so it should induce colostral antibodies in pregnant mares. The advantage of this vaccine is that it has DIVA capability. Vaccinated horses only have antibodies against the hemagglutinin, whereas infected horses develop antibodies against multiple other viral antigens, such as the neuraminidase.

In general, horses receive two priming doses of vaccine 4–6 weeks apart, followed by revaccination 5–6 months later. Foals should be vaccinated at 6–7 months and annually or biannually thereafter. If necessary, vaccination of foals at 3 months may be effective. Antibody levels appear to wane rapidly between the second and third vaccination, and if the interval between these boosters is too long, there may be an "immunity gap" lasting several weeks. Horses infected during this time may develop subclinical infection and shed significant amounts of live infectious virus, posing a risk to naïve contacts. Interestingly, there also appears to be a negative correlation between the number of doses of vaccine received by a horse and its antibody titers. The reasons for this are unclear, but it has been suggested that newly formed plasma cells displace older memory plasma cells resulting in a loss of pre-existing antibodies. Mares have significantly higher antibody levels than stallions for reasons unknown.

DNA- and mRNA-based equine influenza vaccines are currently under development (Ault et al., 2012). Likewise, an equine influenza vaccine containing neuraminidases and hemagglutinins derived by reverse genetics has shown very encouraging results (Ohta et al., 2022). Virus-like particle-based vaccines are also under development.

Strategic vaccination may be appropriate, such as timing revaccination to correspond to periods of exposure to other horses. Vaccination in the face of an outbreak may be effective if the outbreak is detected sufficiently early. In unvaccinated horses, the rapid onset of immunity that occurs after the use of the intranasal product suggests that this would be the logical vaccine to use.

Rotaviruses

Group A rotaviruses, non-enveloped RNA viruses, are a major cause of foal diarrhea. Morbidity is often high while mortality is low. Rotavirus vaccination of pregnant mares results in a decrease in the prevalence and severity of foal diarrhea on infected farms, probably as a result of rotavirus antibodies in mares' colostrum. An inactivated vaccine that contains rotavirus Group A is specifically licensed for intramuscular use in pregnant mares in order to induce colostral antibodies (Nemoto & Matsumura, 2020).

Other equine vaccines

African Horse Sickness

African Horse Sickness (AHS) is an insect-borne disease affecting all equidae and caused by an unenveloped double-stranded RNA Orbivirus related to ruminant bbluetongue virus. It is transmitted by *Culicoides* midges and is endemic in sub-Saharan Africa. Nine antigenically distinct viral serotypes of AHSV have been identified. Both monovalent and polyvalent modified live vaccines are commercially available. These contain virus attenuated by growth in Vero cells, and most provide good protection, although they have the potential to revert to virulence, undergo reassortment, and possibly be transmitted by their vectors. Some are more reactive than others, and protection may be incomplete. Additionally, the currently available vaccines may cause fetal abnormalities when given to pregnant mares. Annual revaccination is required. Encouraging results have been obtained using baculovirus recombinant vaccines incorporating the major neutralizing epitope, VP2 (Aksular et al., 2018). The use of live AHS vaccines is prohibited in many unaffected countries.

Inactivated AHS vaccines are also available. However, immunity is slow to develop, and the duration of immunity is short. Horses require revaccination every 6 months (Rodriguez et al., 2020). As a result, studies are ongoing on the use of effective adjuvants with these vaccines (van Rijn et al., 2020).

Hendra virus

Hendra virus is a *Henipavivirus* in the subfamily Paramyxovirinae. It occurs in horses in Australia, where it causes a high fever and severe respiratory disease with pulmonary edema. It causes 58% mortality in humans and 75% mortality in horses. A vaccine containing the viral G protein (required for cell attachment) is available for use by licensed veterinarians in Australia. It should be given to foals over 4 months with two boosters at 3-week intervals, followed by annual revaccination (Middleton et al., 2014).

Immune contraception

Healthy feral horse populations can double their numbers every four or 5 years. Under these circumstances, it is desirable to control the size of these horse populations without killing individuals. This may be accomplished by fertility control. Contraceptive vaccination is one technique that can do this. It is easily administered, cost-effective, and efficacious in multiple species. Killing is irreversible, while vaccination is not. However, this method of contraception relies on inducing an autoimmune response in a recipient animal. It also involves rounding up large numbers of widely dispersed feral animals. Not an easy task!

Gonadotropin-releasing hormone (GnRH)

A successful contraceptive vaccine immunizes animals against gonadotropin-releasing hormone (GnRH) (Stout & Colenbrander, 2004). GnRH produced by the hypothalamus controls the pituitary release of follicle-stimulating hormone and luteinizing hormone. As a result, it controls gamete production and fertility. It also regulates male and female sexual activity. Thus, vaccination against GnRH can be used to control inappropriate sexual behavior in both stallions and mares. In mares, the reduction in GnRH leads to a decline in estrogen levels so that behavioral estrus ceases. Blocking of GnRH production can be accomplished by vaccination (Janett et al., 2009). GnRH is a small, poorly immunogenic peptide. To make the vaccine work, multiple GnRH peptides are therefore chemically conjugated to a large immunogenic carrier protein such as hemocyanin. The GnRH-hemocyanin conjugate is adjuvanted with a water-in-mineral oil emulsion. Several commercial GnRH vaccines are available for use in horses.

One such vaccine, named GonaCon has been developed as a reproduction inhibitor by the National Wildlife Disease Center of the USDA. GonaCon induces antibodies that bind and neutralize GnRH and effectively block the release of follicle stimulating hormone and luteinizing hotmone from the pituitary. This, in turn, inhibits breeding and its behaviors in both males and females. Antibodies peak about 2 weeks after the second vaccine dose. Cyclical estrus behavior will start to decline within 2 weeks after the second dose as the ovaries shrink.

GonaCon has induced contraception with a single dose for up to 5 years in wild horses. It is currently registered by the Environmental Protection Agency as a contraceptive for white-tailed deer and wild horses, thus effectively managing overabundant wildlife populations. (The vaccine is classified as a "restricted use pesticide")! It has also been employed to control population size in donkey sanctuaries.

In some regions of the world, overpopulation by donkeys is also of significant concern. Studies on donkeys vaccinated using an experimental zona pellucida contraceptive vaccine adjuvanted with Freund's complete adjuvant have found that they cause severe stress to female animals. Acute stress with increased cortisol levels occurred with the first dose, and chronic stress, as measured by decreased cortisol, followed the second injection, especially in those donkeys that developed injection site lesions (Peterson et al., 2022).

Adverse events

As with other vaccines, the commonest side-effects are associated with in horses and donkeys are directly associated with the injection site. In descending order, these are swelling (edema), pain, stiffness, infection, and inflammation. The vaccine itself may induce a temporary state of lethargy and anorexia, perhaps accompanied by a fever and malaise (Fig. 15.4).

Allergic reactions, while uncommon, may occur in horses in response to vaccine antigens. In severe anaphylaxis, the major shock organs of horses are the lungs and the intestines (Chapter 19). Bronchial and bronchiolar constriction leads to coughing, dyspnea, and eventually apnea. The major mediatorsof anaphylaxis in horses are histamine and kinins. Anaphylaxis requires prompt epinephrine treatment administered intramuscularly or intravenously.

Local injection site reactions may occur, especially in response to strangles vaccines and some polyvalent vaccines, especially those containing adjuvants (Horohov et al., 2015). However, ongoing studies are resulting in significant improvements in adjuvant safety and efficacy (Carnet et al., 2023). While usually transient, these reactions may be treated with non-steroidal anti-inflammatory drugs as well as the use of warm compresses. Some adjuvants can also cause severe local lesions, including skin ulceration (Peterson et al., 2022).

Following exposure to *Strep. equi* antigens, some horses may develop purpura hemorrhagica, an acute, immune-complex-mediated, vasculitis. Other triggers of purpura hemorrhagica include infections with *Corynebacterium pseudotuberculosis*, *R. equi*, equine influenza virus, and equine herpesvirus type 1. In some cases, it develops in the absence of any obvious prior infection. Clinical signs develop within 2–4 weeks following natural or vaccinal exposure to streptococcal antigens (Chapter 20). There are great variations in disease severity and the clinical course ranges from a mild transient reaction to fatal disease.

Adverse reactions are inherent risks of vaccination and unpredictable. Some horses may develop transient systemic signs of innate immunity, including fever, anorexia, colic, diarrhea, and tachycardia. Intranasal vaccines may trigger a slight nasal discharge. Therefore, it is recommended that horses not be vaccinated in the 2 weeks prior to shows, performance events, sales, or domestic transport. Some veterinarians may elect not to vaccinate horses within 3 weeks of international transport (Barquero et al., 2007).

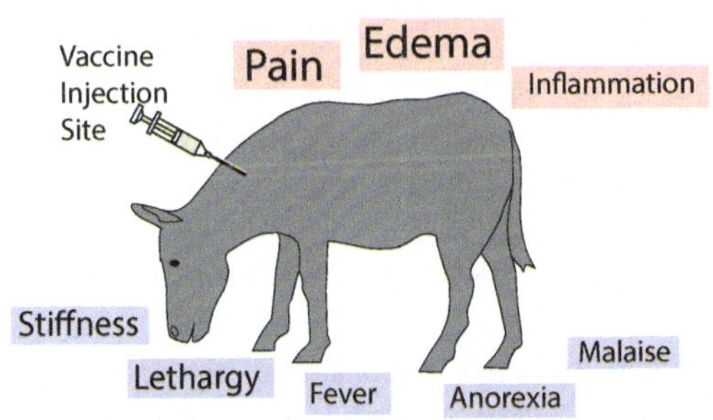

FIGURE 15.4 The local and systemic adverse events commonly observed in horses and donkeys following vaccination

Text size indicates their prevalence.

International vaccine requirements

The International Federation for Equestrian Sports (FEI) has a mandatory biosecurity policy that requires that horses competing in international horse show events must be vaccinated every 6 months against both clade 1 and clade 2 Florida sublineage equine influenza viruses (Horspool & King, 2013). Horses are issued with a "Passport" that records every vaccine they receive. These passports are checked to ensure that participating horses have indeed been vaccinated. Horses may also require other vaccines depending on their environment; for example, tetanus, equine herpesvirus, and West Nile virus infections or GnRH vaccination. These vaccines must also be recorded in the horse's passport. These include details of the vaccine, serial/batch number, date, and route of administration. All entries must be signed by the veterinarian and stamped with the veterinarian's clinic stamp. Competing horses must have been vaccinated against influenza between 6 months and 21 days of the previous booster vaccination. However, they cannot compete if they have been vaccinated within 7 days of arrival. In the United States, the United States Equestrian Federation (USEF) issues the passports for FEI competition. The passport must be renewed every 4 years and updated when ownership changes (Paillot et al., 2017).

Antiserum production

Diphtheria toxin was first identified in 1888. Subsequently, Emil Behring and his colleague Kitasato Shibasaburo in Berlin, and Emile Roux and Andre Yersin in Paris, showed that the serum from immune animals could neutralize its toxic effects. In late 1891, two seriously ill diphtheritic children were saved by the administration of serum from an immunized sheep produced by Emil Behring. Sheep are small and do not produce a lot of serum. Emile Roux therefore switched to horses that produced a lot more serum than the sheep and at a higher antibody titer. By 1894, both groups of investigators had treated hundreds of children and shown that equine antitoxin treatment had more than halved diphtheria mortality rates (Mortimer, 2011). This was the first specific cure for any infectious disease,—ever! Behring won the first Nobel Prize for Medicine for this discovery in 1901. Equine antiserum production is still widely employed for passive immunization because of low costs, relative simplicity, and short production time.

Equine immune serum is used to treat multiple infectious diseases, such as tetanus, rabies, and botulism, as well as for the treatment of envenomation by snakes, spiders, and scorpions. After receiving multiple doses of antigen (the number is related to the individual animal's response and the level of antibodies desired) and producing the desired level of antibodies, the horse is bled, and antibodies (immune globulins) are purified from the plasma.

Horses used for antiserum production receive multiple repeated doses of vaccine in order to produce very high levels of specific antibodies. This prolonged and intense stimulation of their immune system results in several health issues, especially amyloidosis. Thus, a single dose of a vaccine such as influenza or West Nile vaccine causes a transient acute phase response reflected in an increase in serum SAA levels that peak on day two post-vaccination but return to normal by day nine (Baumgarten et al., 2024). Horses that are employed for antiserum production for several years, and are thus repeatedly immunized, can develop progressive systemic inflammation and prolonged elevated SAA levels. Even horses that have been retired from antiserum production for 2 years may have persistently high levels of fibrinogen and globulins as well as amyloid deposits in their liver and kidneys (Arifianto et al., 2024).

Donkey vaccines

There is remarkably little information available on the vaccination of donkeys. There do not appear to be any commercially available vaccines specifically formulated for use in donkeys. Studies have confirmed that they respond to tetanus and influenza vaccination in essentially the same manner as horses. They mount a strong T cell response to these vaccines (Perzyna et al., 2025). Consequently, they should receive the same core vaccines as horses, but revaccination will depend on their specific circumstances and geographic location, as well as a careful risk assessment. They should be vaccinated from 3 months of age. The core vaccines for donkeys in North America include rabies, tetanus, Eastern and Western equine encephalomyelitis, and West Nile virus. Influenza/rhinopneumonitis vaccine is also recommended. The use of other risk-based vaccines will, in part, depend upon their degree of contact with other equids. There is no evidence to support the use of lower doses of horse vaccines in donkeys. After all, miniature horses and foals still get the same vaccine dose (Perzyna et al., 2025).

References

Aksular, M., Calvo-Pinilla, E., Marin-Lopez, A., Ortego, J., et al. (2018). A single dose of African horse sickness virus (AHSV) VP2 based vaccines provides complete clinical protection in a mouse model. *Vaccine*. https://doi.org/10.1016/j.vaccine.2018.09.065

Arifianto, D., Esfandiari, A., Wilbawan, I. W. T., Amrozi, A., et al. (2024). Assessment of health impacts in retired antisera-producing horses: Blood biochemistry and serum amyloid A analysis. *Veterinary World, 17*(9), 2136–2143.

Ault, A., Zajac, A. M., Kong, W. P., Gorres, J. P., et al. (2012). Immunogenicity and clinical protection against equine influenza by DNA vaccination of ponies. *Vaccine, 30*, 3965–3974.

Balena, V., Pradhan, S. S., Bera, B. C., Anand, T., et al. (2022). Double and quadruple deletion mutant of EHV-1 is highly attenuated and induces optimal immune response. *Vaccine*. https://doi.org/10.1016/j.vaccine.2022.12.044

Bannai, H., Nemoto, M., Tsujimura, K., Yamanaka, T., et al. (2018). Comparison of protective efficacies between intranasal and intramuscular vaccination of horses with a modified live equine herpesvirus type-1 vaccine. *Veterinary Microbiology, 222*, 18–24.

Barquero, N., Daly, J. M., & Newton, J. R. (2007). Risk factors for influenza infection in vaccinated racehorses: Lessons from an outbreak in Newmarket, UK in 2003. *Vaccine, 25*, 7520–7529.

Baumgarten, C. M., Delph Miller, K. M., Davis, E. G., Beard, L. A., et al. (2024). Serum amyloid A increases following routine vaccination of healthy adult horses. *Journal of the American Veterinary Medical Association, 262*(9), 1181–1187.

Boyle, A. G., Timoney, J. F., Newton, J. R., Hines, M. T., et al. (2018). *Streptococcus equi* infections in horses: Guidelines for treatment, control, and prevention of strangles-revised consensus statement. *Journal of Veterinary Internal Medicine, 32*, 633–647.

Branda, F., Yon, D. K., Albanese, M., Binetti, E., et al. (2025). Equine influenza: Epidemiology, pathogenesis, and strategies for prevention and control. *Viruses*. https://doi.org/10.3390/v17030302

Carnet, F., Perrin-Cocon, L., Paillot, R., Lotteau, V., et al. (2023). An inventory of adjuvants used for vaccination in horses: The past, the present, and the future. *Veterinary Research*. https://doi.org/10.1186/s13567-023-01151-3

Castillo-Olivares, J., Wieringa, R., Bakonyi, T., de Vries, A. F., et al. (2003). Generation of a candidate live marker vaccine for equine arteritis virus by deletion of the major virus neutralization domain. *Journal of Virology, 77*(15), 8470–8480.

Cendejas, P. M., & Goodman, A. G. (2024). Vaccination and control methods of West Niler virus infection in equids and humans. *Vaccines*. https://doi.org/10.3390/vaccines2950485

Chang, Y., Novosol, V., McDonough, S. P., et al. (1999). Vaccination against Lyme disease with recombinant Borrelia burgdorferi outer-surface protein A (rOspA) in horses. *Vaccine, 18*, 540–548.

Correia, L., Martins, G., & Lilenbaum, W. (2017). Detection of anti-Leptospira inhibitory antibodies in horses after vaccination. *Microbial Pathogenesis, 110*, 494–496.

Cursons, R., Patty, O., Steward, K. F., & Waller, A. S. (2015). Strangles in horses can be caused by vaccination with Pinnacle I. N. *Vaccine, 33*, 3440–3443.

Cywes-Bentley, C., Rocha, J. N., Bordin, A. I., Vinacur, M., et al. (2018). Antibody against poly-N-acetyl glucosamine provides protection against intracellular pathogens: Mechanism of action and validadion in horse foals challenged with *Rhodococcus equi*. *PLoS Pathogens, 14*, Article e1007160. https://doi.org/10.1371/1/journal.ppat.1007160

Desanti-Consoli, H., Bouillon, J., & Chapuis, R. J. J. (2022). Equids' core vaccines guidelines in North America: Considerations and prospective. *Vaccines*. https://doi.org/10.3390/vaccines10030398

Dutta, S. K., Vemulapalli, R., & Biswas, B. (1998). Association of deficiency in antibody response to vaccine and heterogeneity of *Ehrlichia risticii* strains of Potomac Horse Fever vaccine failure in horses. *Jorunal of Clinical Microbiology, 36*(2), 506–512.

Edwards, K. M., & Booy, R. (2013). Effects of exercise on vaccine-induced immune responses. *Human Vaccines & Immunotherapeutics, 9*(4), 907–910.

Entenfellner, J., Gahan, J., Garvey, M., Walsh, C., et al. (2020). Response of sport horses to different formulations of equine influenza vaccine. *Vaccines*. https://doi.org/10.3390/vaccines8030372

Giles, C., Vanniasinkam, T., Ndi, S., & Barton, M. D. (2015). *Rhodococcus equi* (*Prescottella equi*) vaccines; the future of vaccine development. *Equine Veterinary Journal, 47*, 510–518.

Heldens, J. G., Pouwels, H. G., & van Loon, A. A. (2004). Efficacy and duration of immunity of a combined equine influenza and equine herpesvirus vaccine against challenge with an american-like equine influenza virus (A/equi-2/Kentucky/95). *The Veterinary Journal, 167*, 150–157.

Horohov, D. W., Dunham, J., Liu, C., Betancourt, A., et al. (2015). Characterization of the in situ immunological responses to vaccine adjuvants. *Veterinary Immunology and Immunopathology, 164*, 24–29.

Horspool, L. J., & King, A. (2013). Equine influenza vaccines in Europe: A view from the animal health industry. *Equine Veterinary Journal, 45*, 774–775.

Janett, F., Stump, R., Burger, D., & Thun, R. (2009). Suppression of testicular function and sexual behavior by vaccination against GnRH (Equity) in the adult stallion. *Animal Reproduction Science, 115*, 88–102.

Knödlseder, J. M., Fell, S. F., & Straubinger, R. K. (2019). A study with a commercial vaccine against Lyme borreliosis in horses using two different vaccination schedules: Characterization of the humoral immune response. *Vaccine, 37*(49), 7207–7212.

McKenzie, H. C., Funk, R. A., Trager, L., Werre, S. R., & Crisman, M. (2019). Immunogenicity of Potomac horse fever vaccine when simultaneously co-administered with rabies vaccine in a multivalent vaccine or as two monovalent vaccines at separate sites. *Equine Veterinary Journal, 51*, 774–778.

Middleton, D., Pallister, J., Klein, R., Feng, Y-R., et al. (2014). Hendra virus vaccine, a one health approach to protecting horse, human, and environmental health. *Emerging Infectious Diseases, 20*(3), 372–379.

Mortimer, P. P. (2011). The diphtheria vaccine debacle of 1940 that ushered in comprehensive childhood immunization in the United Kingdom. *Epidemiology and Infection, 139*, 487–493. https://doi.org/10.1017/s095026881000302X

Nemoto, M., & Matsumura, T. (2021). Equine rotavirus infection. *Journal of Equine Science, 32*(1), 1–9.

Ohta, M., Kambayashi, Y., Mita, H., Kuroda, T., et al. (2022). Protective efficacy of a reverse genetics-derived inactivated vaccine against equine influenza virus in horses. *Vaccine, 40*, 6362–6366.

Paessler, S., & Weaver, S. C. (2009). Vaccines for Venezuelan equine encephalitis. *Vaccine*. https://doi.org/10.1016/j.vaccine.2019.07.095

Paillot, R. (2014). A systematic review of recent advances in equine influenza vaccination. *Vaccines, 2*, 797–831.

Paillot, R., & El-Hage, C. M. (2016). The use of a recombinant canarypox-based equine influenza vaccine during the 2007 Australian outbreak: A systematic review and summary. *Pathogens, 5*.

Paillot, R., Marcillaud Pitel, C., D'Ablon, X., & Pronost, S. (2017. 5). Equine vaccines: How, when and why? Report of the Vaccinology Session, French Equine Veterinarians Association, 2016, Reims. *Vaccines (Basel)*.

Paillot, R., & Prowse, L. (2012). ISCOM-matrix-based equine influenza (EIV) vaccine stimulates cell-mediated immunity in the horse. *Veterinary Immunology and Immunopathology, 145*, 516–521.

Perkins, G., Babasyan, S., Stout, A. E., Freer, H., et al. (2019). Intranasal IgG4/7 antibody responses protect horses against equid herpesvirus 1 (EHV-1) infection including nasal virus shedding and cell-associated viremia. *Virology, 531*, 219–232.

Perzyna, M., Grzedzicka, J., Milczek-Haduch, D., Dabrowska, I., et al. (2025). Immunological responses to tetanus and influenza vaccination in donkeys. *Journal of Veterinary Internal Medicine, 39*(4). https://doi.org/10.1111/jvim.70137

Peterson, E. W., Segabinazzi, L. G. T. M., Gilbert, R. O., Bergfelt, D. R., & French, H. M. (2022). Evaluation of stress accompanying immunocontraceptive vaccination in donkeys. *Animals*. https://doi.org/10.3390/ani12040457

Petri da Silviera, B., Kahn, S. K., Legere, R. M., Bray, J. M., et al. (2025). Enteral immunization with live bacteria reprograms innate immune cells and protects neonatal foals from pneumonia. *Scientific Reports*. https://doi.org/10.1038/s41598-025-02060-5

Pouwels, H. G., et al. (2014). Efficacy of a non-updated, Matrix-C-based equine influenza subunit-tetanus vaccine following Florida sublineage clade 2 challenge. *The Veterinary Record, 174*, 633.

Reemers, S., Sonnemans, D., Horspool, L., van, B.s, et al. (2020). Determining equine influenza vaccine efficacy—The specific contribution of strain versus other vaccine attributes. *Vaccines*. https://doi.org/10.3390/vaccines8030501

Rendle, D., Bowen, M., Cavalleri, J., De Brauwere, N., et al. (2024). Strangles vaccination: A current European perspective. *Equine Veterinary Education, 37*(2), 90–97.

Robinson, C., Frykberg, L., Flock, M., Guss, B., Waller, A. S., & Flock, J. I. (2018). Strangvac: A recombinant fusion protein vaccine that protects against strangles, caused by *Streptococcus equi*. *Vaccine, 36*, 1484–1490.

Robinson, C., Heather, Z., Slater, J., Potts, N., et al. (2015). Vaccination with a live multi-gene deletion strain protects horses against virulent challenge with *Streptococcus equi*. *Vaccine, 33*, 1160–1167.

Robinson, C., Waller, A. S., Frykberg, L., Flock, M., et al. (2020). Intramuscular vaccination with Sreabgvac is safe and induces protection against equine strangles caused by Streptococcus equi. *Vaccine, 38*, 4861–4868.

Rodriguez, M., Joseph, S., Pfeffer, M., Raghavan, R., & Wernery, U. (2020). Immune response of horses to inactivated African horse sickness vaccines. *BMC Veterinary Research*. https://doi.org/10.1186/s12917-020-02540-y

Ryan, M., Gildea, S., Walsh, C., & Cullinane, A. (2015). The impact of different equine influenza vaccine products and other factors on equine influenza antibody levels in Thoroughbred racehorses. *Equine Veterinary Journal, 47*, 662–666.

Siger, L., Bowen, R., Karaca, K., Murray, M., et al. (2006). Evaluation of the efficacy provided by a recombinant canarypox-vectored Equine West Nile virus vaccine against an experimental West Nile virus intrathecal challenge in horses. *Veterinary Therapeutics, 7*(3), 249–256.

Stout, T. A., & Colenbrander, B. (2004). Suppressing reproductive activity in horses using GnRH vaccines, antagonists or agonists. *Animal Reproduction Science, 82*, 633–643.

Stromberg, Z. R., Fischer, W., Bradfute, S. B., Kubicek-Sutherland, J. Z., & Hraber, P. (2020). Vaccine advances against Venezuelan, Eastern, and Western encephalitis viruses. *Vaccines*. https://doi.org/10.3390/vaccines8020273

Tolnai, C. H., Forgach, P., Marosi, A., Feher, O., et al. (2025). Long-term humoral immune response after West Nile virus convalescence in horses in a geographic area of multiple orthoflavivirus circulation. *Journal of Veterinary Internal Medicine*. https://doi.org/10.1111/jvim.70176

van Rijn, P. A., Maris-Veldhuis, M. A., Grobler, M., Wright, I. M., et al. (2020). Safety and efficacy of inactivated African horse sickness (AHS) vaccine formulated with different adjuvants. *Vaccine*. https://doi.org/10.1016/l.vaccine.2020.08.072

Wobeser, B. K. (2015). Anthrax vaccine associated deaths in miniature horses. *Canadian Veterinary Journal, 56*, 359–360.

CHAPTER

16 Immunity to selected equine bacterial and fungal diseases

Horses and donkeys are subject to numerous infectious diseases caused by bacteria. Thus, a major function of their immune systems involves defense against such infections. Although horses live in a world densely populated with bacteria and house a dense and complex microbiota in their intestinal tract, most of these organisms neither invade their tissues nor cause disease. This is unsurprising for several reasons. First, the combined efforts of the innate and adaptive immune systems are sufficient to prevent invasion. Second, even organisms that successfully invade the animal body gain very little by harming their host. On the contrary, illness or death of the host animal reduces the survival of most bacteria and is, therefore, normally avoided. Indeed, as discussed in Chapter 14, the bacterial microbiota is essential for the animal's well-being since it protects against other invaders, provides energy by digesting foods such as cellulose, and optimizes the functioning of the immune system.

The ability of many bacteria to survive within an animal also depends on their virulence factors. Many of these virulence factors are encoded on mobile genetic elements that can be transmitted between species (e.g., plasmids). These virulence factors permit the bacteria to adapt to a specific environment and promote their transmission between hosts. Depending on their niche within the body, bacteria can use virulence factors to penetrate surface epithelia, bind to cell surfaces, acquire iron, evade immune responses, hide within cells, and promote transmission to another host (Collins, 2008). Some of these strategies result in damage to host tissues and must be prevented by the immune system. It should also be pointed out that many bacteria are unable to invade and cause disease in healthy, normal hosts, but will take the opportunity offered by immunosuppression or other weaknesses in host defenses to invade the body. Dead bodies have no defenses and decompose

Innate immunity

Antimicrobial immunity is mediated by an early innate response followed by a sustained adaptive response. Recognition of invading bacteria through toll-like receptors (TLRs) and other pattern recognition molecules induces cytokine release, complement activation, inflammation, and phagocytosis. If this is insufficient to eliminate the invaders, adaptive immune mechanisms take over. Thus, dendritic cells

The Immunology of Horses and Donkeys. https://doi.org/10.1016/B978-0-443-44863-8.00016-8

and macrophages capture invading bacteria and initiate adaptive immunity by secreting cytokines and triggering both T and B cell responses. TLRs are responsible in large part for the initial recognition of invading bacteria. The binding of microbial pathogen-associated molecular patterns (PAMPs) to TLRs triggers a signal cascade that activates genes encoding proteins that are critical in host defense (Fig. 16.1).

Type I interferons are also produced in response to bacterial PAMPS. IFN-α and IFN-β both boost macrophage cytotoxicity by enhancing their production of IFN-γ, nitric oxide, and TNF-α.

Natural killer (NK) cells also play a protective role in bacterial, protozoan, and fungal infections. For example, some bacteria may activate NK cells by upregulating the expression of NKG2D ligands on infected cells. Activated NK cells produce a large amount of IFN-γ which, in turn, activates both macrophages and dendritic cells (Mancuso et al., 2007).

Although many bacteria are destroyed by phagocytosis, others are killed when free in the circulation. Bacteria are destroyed by complement acting through the alternate or lectin pathways. Bacterial cell walls, lacking sialic acid, inactivate factor H and stabilize the alternate C3 convertase (C3bBbP). As a result, these bacteria are either opsonized or lysed. Activation also leads to the production of membrane attack complexes (MACs). These MACs alone may be unable to insert themselves

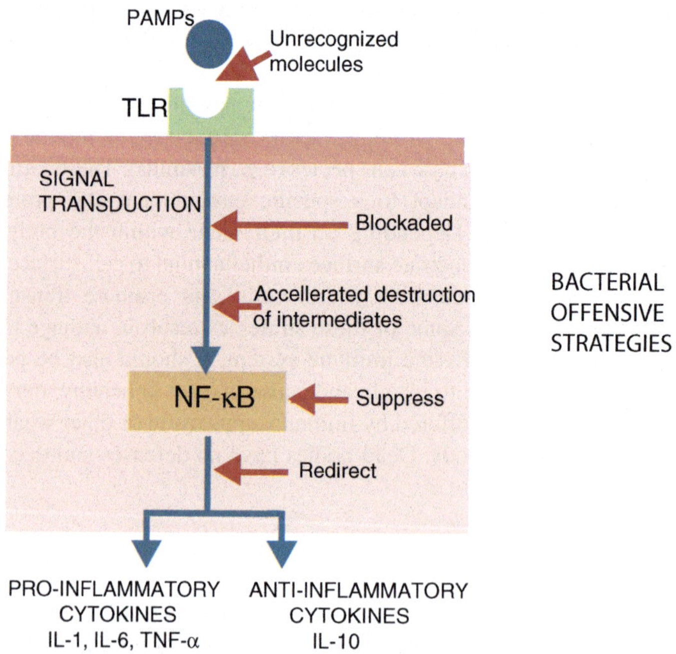

FIGURE 16.1 Innate immunity to bacterial pathogens and the offensive strategies employed by bacteria to overcome it.

into the carbohydrate layers of the microbial cell wall. However, lysozyme in the blood may partially digest the cell wall and so enable the MACs to insert themselves into the lipid bilayer of the inner bacterial membrane and lyse it. Horses produce multiple antimicrobial peptides that are also critical for defense against bacteria (Chapter 3). Once activated, platelets release many antibacterial peptides as well as reactive oxygen species (ROS). Platelets also bind to bacteria to form heterotypic aggregates that are readily phagocytosed by neutrophils or captured in NETs.

Antimicrobial peptides

A key component of equine innate immunity is the production of diverse bactericidal peptides. These include lysozyme, five cathelicidins, nine defensins, one psoriasin, one hepcidin, and five equinins (Bruhn et al., 2011). Neutrophils are the major source of these peptides. They also include the neutrophil antibacterial peptides NAP-1 and -2. Stem cells also secrete antimicrobial peptides that kill many bacteria involved in wound infections.

C-type lectins

Some equine glycoproteins bind strongly to carbohydrates expressed on microbial surfaces. They do so in a calcium-dependent manner and hence are classified as C-type lectins (CTLs). The most important of these in horses are mannose-binding lectin, dectin-1, histidine-rich glycoprotein, and the pulmonary surfactant proteins.

Mannose-binding lectin

One of the most important antibacterial lectins in horses binds to mannose-rich oligosaccharides on bacterial surfaces. This mannose-binding lectin (MBL) is synthesized in the liver. It is found in large amounts in equine blood. It is constructed from 32 kDa subunits, but it circulates as trimers or multimers (Podolsky et al., 2006). MBL is a member of the collectin family of proteins and is related to the pulmonary surfactant proteins (Chapter 3). Equine MBL has multiple sites that can bind microbial oligosaccharides, such as *N*-acetylglucosamine, mannose, glucose, galactose, and *N*-acetylgalactosamine. In addition to its mannose-binding abilities, equine MBL activates the complement system through the lectin pathway by activating an MBL-associated serine protease (MASP). MASP activates C4b2a, which acts as a C3 convertase. As a result, bacteria coated by MBL are either lysed by complement or opsonized and readily ingested by phagocytic cells. However, MBL levels are lower in sick horses than in healthy horses, although it is unclear whether this is a cause or effect of the infection.

Dectin-1

Some C-type lectins are pattern recognition receptors expressed on cell surfaces where they can bind bacteria, fungi, and some viruses. The most important of these are the dectins. The dectins bind β-glucans on fungal and bacterial cell walls. Dectin-1 is a 28 kDa protein that, like MBL, spontaneously forms dimers and tetramers. (It is classified as CD369.) Dectin-1 interacts with many different bacterial and fungal species. In association with TLR2, it activates macrophages. As a result, it plays an important role in immune defenses by triggering inflammatory responses and promoting intracellular destruction (Yadav & Schorey, 2006). Dectin-1 is expressed by neutrophils, macrophages, monocytes, and dendritic cells, including Langerhans cells. When it binds to bacterial and fungal carbohydrates, it triggers the production of IL-1β. Dectin-1 is present in the bronchoalveolar lavage fluid of horses housed indoors in stables, but its levels are considerably lower in horses at pasture. This presumably reflects the presence of suspended microbial particles such as fungal spores in dusty indoor air. It is also expressed in bronchial epithelial cells (Di Pietro et al., 2023).

Histidine-rich glycoprotein

Histidine-rich glycoprotein is an abundant protein of 70 kDa produced by liver cells smd found in horse serum. Its levels drop by about 50% in horses with a systemic inflammatory response. It appears to act on lipopolysaccharide-stimulated neutrophils to reduce their adherence to surfaces, and it reduces their chemotactic responsiveness to CXCL8 (IL-8). It reduces their oxidative response to ingested particles as detected by chemoluminescence. However, it also promotes neutrophil phagocytosis and lysosomal maturation. Thus, it appears to play a role as a dual regulator of equine neutrophils. It may play a role in minimizing neutrophil-induced tissue damage while still retaining their antimicrobial properties (Muko et al., 2021).

Adaptive immunity

There are five mechanisms by which the adaptive immune responses combat bacterial infections: (1) neutralization of toxins or enzymes by antibodies; (2) killing of bacteria by the classical complement pathway; (3) opsonization of bacteria by antibodies and complement, resulting in their phagocytosis and destruction; (4) destruction of intracellular bacteria by activated macrophages; and (5) direct killing of bacteria by cytotoxic T cells and NK cells. The relative importance of each of these processes depends upon the species of bacteria, their location, and their pathogenic mechanisms (Fig. 16.2).

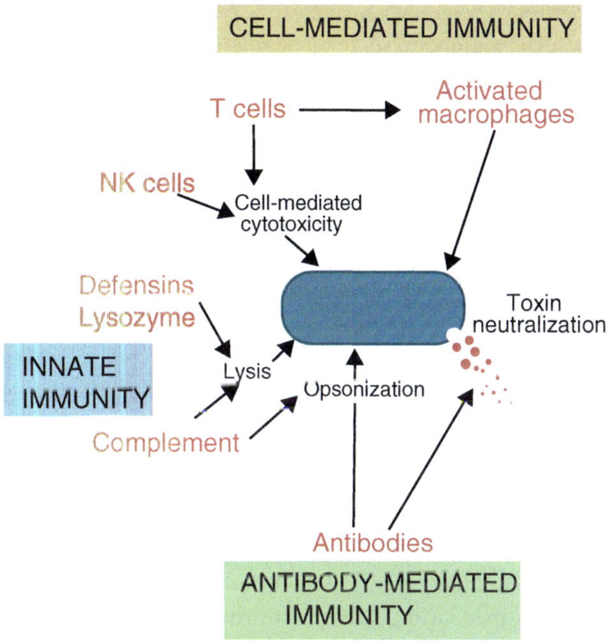

FIGURE 16.2 Adaptive immunity to bacterial pathogens.

Both cell-mediated and antibody-mediated defenses contribute to resistance.

Immunity to toxigenic bacteria

In diseases caused by toxigenic bacteria such as *Clostridium tetani* and *C. botulinum,* the immune response must not only eliminate the invading bacteria but also neutralize the lethal bacterial toxins. Destruction of the bacteria, however, may be difficult if they are embedded in a mass of necrotic tissue, and toxin neutralization is therefore a priority. Neutralization occurs when antibodies prevent the toxin from binding to its receptors on a target cell. The neutralization process, therefore, involves competition between receptors and antibodies for the toxin molecule.

Immunity to invasive bacteria

Protection against invasive bacteria is usually mediated by antibodies directed against their surface antigens. Efficient phagocytosis requires that the bacteria be coated with opsonins that can trigger attack by phagocytic cells. These opsonins include antibodies and C3b in addition to the innate opsonins such as mannose-binding lectin. Antibodies are not only effective opsonins in their own right but also increase the binding of C3b by activating the classical complement pathway. Antibodies directed against capsular (K) antigens may neutralize the antiphagocytic properties of bacterial capsules, thus permitting their destruction. In bacteria lacking capsules, antibodies directed against somatic (O) antigens act as opsonins. Some antibodies have direct antimicrobial activities. Antibodies against *E. coli* may be bacteriostatic since they interfere with the production of the iron-binding protein enterochelin and thus prevent bacterial iron scavenging. Some antibodies can generate oxidants and may kill bacteria directly.

When bacteria are stressed, they produce many new proteins. These stressors include heat, starvation, and exposure to oxidants; toxins such as heavy metals, protein synthesis inhibitors, and viral infections. The heat-shock proteins (HSPs) are the best understood of these new proteins. Low levels of HSPs are present in bacteria at normal temperatures. Mild stress, such as a low-grade fever, induces HSP production. For example, HSP levels climb from 1.5% to 15% of the total protein in stressed *E. coli*. There are three major bacterial HSPs: HSP 90, HSP 70, and HSP 60. (The number refers to their molecular weight in kDa.) When a bacterium is phagocytosed and exposed to the neutrophil respiratory burst, its stress triggers the production of bacterial HSPs. As a result, HSP 60 is the dominant bacterial antigen produced in infections caused by Mycobacteria and Borrelia species. These HSPs are highly antigenic for several reasons. First, they are produced in abundance within the infected host; second, they are readily processed by antigen-presenting cells; and third, the immune system may possess large numbers of B and T cells capable of responding to HSPs. Thus, anti-HSP responses may induce significant protection against many bacterial pathogens (Kaufmann & Dorhoi, 2016).

Immunity to intracellular bacteria

Autophagy is a key process in the destruction of intracellular bacteria. The cellular machinery used to destroy unwanted or damaged intracellular organelles, such as mitochondria, can also be employed to eliminate unwanted intracellular organisms. For example, phagocytosed bacteria that escape into the cytosol may be surrounded by an autophagosome-like structure and subsequently destroyed by lysosomal enzymes. Autophagy (or more correctly, xenophagy) may also play a key role in delivering processed microbial antigens to the MHC ELA molecules for presentation to helper T cells (Fig. 16.3).

Immunity to intracellular bacteria is mediated by cell-mediated mechanisms (Harris et al., 2009). Early in the immune response, activated M1 macrophages and cDC1 dendritic cells secreting IL-12 and TNF-α are most important (Benoit et al., 2008) (Chapter 7). Although macrophages from unimmunized animals cannot usually destroy these bacteria, this ability is acquired about 10 days after infection. Later in the response, IFN-γ from Th1 cells and the activities of cytotoxic $CD8^+$ T cells, become critical. IFN-γ, especially in association with TNF-α, greatly enhances the production of cytokines such as TNF-α, IL-6, IL-1β, IL-12, and IL-32, in addition to enzymes such as indoleamine 2,3-dioxygenase (IDO), and the release of reactive oxygen species. M1 macrophage

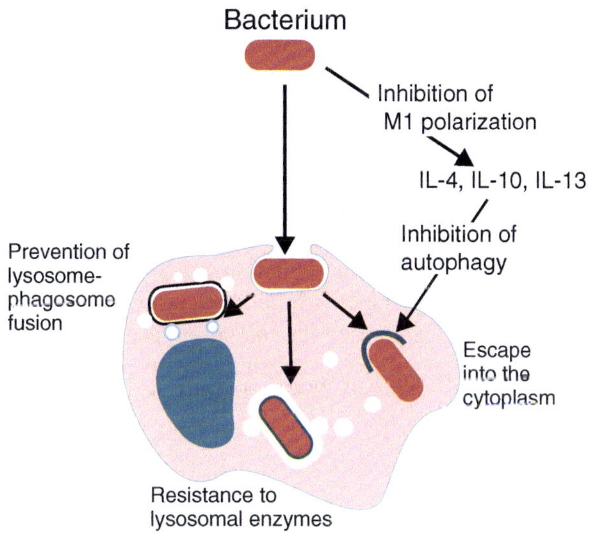

FIGURE 16.3 Immunity to intracellular bacteria.

activation has been shown to be important in resistance to *L. monocytogenes,S. enterica* Typhimurium, *Rhodococcus equi*, and *Mycobacteria*. For example, IFN-γ and TNF-α produced by primed T cells generate M1 macrophages, acidify their phagosomes, and kill mycobacteria. Uncontrolled M1 activation by bacteria such as Streptococci and *E. coli,* however, can contribute to disease pathology by inducing septic shock, tissue damage, and organ failure. The response of these activated macrophages tends to be nonspecific, and M1-activated macrophages can destroy many normally resistant bacteria. The development of M1 macrophages often coincides with the appearance of delayed (type IV) hypersensitivity responses to intradermally administered antigens (Chapter 20).

NK and cytotoxic T cells also participate in immunity to intracellular bacteria. These cytotoxic cells bind to target cells and use perforins to generate pores that allow the delivery of lytic granule contents into the infected cells. Granulysin B then penetrates the bacterial cell wall and so permits granzymes to enter the bacteria. These granzymes generate reactive oxygen species (ROS) that disrupt key enzyme pathways. Granzymes may also trigger apoptosis in the target cell, which may also limit bacterial survival.

NK cells can kill bacteria, and fungi, in addition to infected cells described above. This cytotoxicity is mediated by secreted perforins. The NK cells bind bacteria through NKp46 and NKG2D. Their perforins and granzymes can kill bacteria such as *Mycobacterium tuberculosis*, and *L. monocytogenes* (Mody et al., 2019). They are also cytotoxic for fungi such as Cryptococcus and Aspergillus.

Evasion of the immune response

The outcome of any infection depends upon the continuously evolving battle between the host and the microbe. To survive within an animal, bacteria must evade or inhibit the immune defenses. The complex interrelationships between bacteria and their animal hosts include the role of commensal bacteria on mucosal surfaces in regulating the growth and development of the immune system. These commensal bacteria generally do not aggressively seek to invade the body, so equilibrium can be achieved. Nevertheless, any invading microorganism may become a pathogen because it can invade a horse, evade its immune defenses, and survive at least for a time within its host. Pathogenic bacteria, like all organisms, try to avoid destruction. They have evolved many different mechanisms to overcome host innate and adaptive immune responses.

Evasion of innate immunity

The key to successful microbial invasion, at least initially, is evading innate immunity. Bacteria employ diverse mechanisms to prevent or at least delay an unpleasant fate. Only some selected examples can be mentioned here (Baxt et al., 2013; Reddick & Alto, 2014) (Fig. 16.4).

For example, some bacteria interfere with TLR signaling pathways and inflammasome activation. The methods used include the production of modified PAMPs that will not trigger TLRs, masking of PAMPs, blockage of TLR signaling pathways,

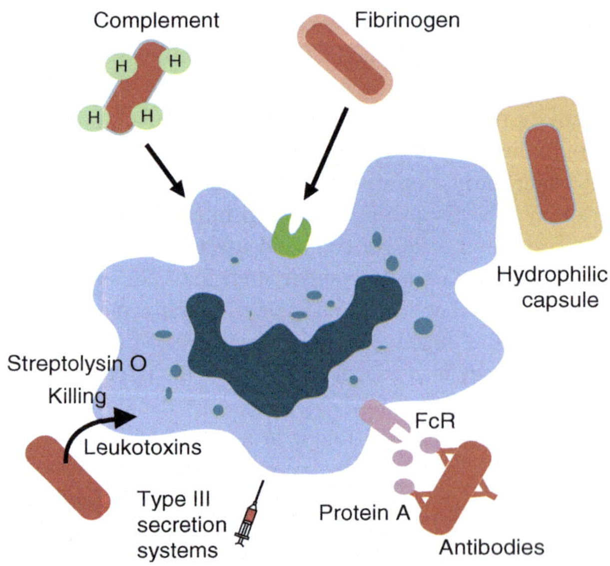

FIGURE 16.4 How bacteria evade immune destruction.

destruction of signaling molecules, destruction of NF-κB, and misdirection of signaling pathways toward anti-inflammatory pathways. Thus, *M. tuberculosis* uses a masking lipid to cover its PRRs. Leptospira have lipopolysaccharides that are recognized by TLR2 but not by TLR4. Bacteria also differ in the amount of CpG dinucleotides in their DNA and, so, differ in their ability to trigger TLR9 (Andersen-Nissen et al., 2005).

Many bacteria can block phagocytosis. For example, *S. aureus* expresses protein A. Protein A attaches to IgG Fc regions and so prevents antibodies from binding to its receptors on phagocytic cells or activating the classical complement pathway. Many bacteria can evade destructtion by complement. For example, the M protein of Streptococci binds fibrinogen and masks C3b-binding sites. It also binds factor H and so inactivates bound C3b. *S. aureus* produces a protein that blocks C3 convertases. Other bacteria produce proteases that can destroy complement components. *S. enterica* Typhimurium has a gene called *Rck* that confers resistance to complement-mediated lysis by preventing the insertion of the membrane attack complex into the bacterial outer membrane (Garcia et al., 2016).

Some strains of *Streptococcus* readily activate C3, leading to deposition of C3b on their surface and promoting their opsonization. This does not occur on Streptococci growing within biofilms, where the binding of C-reactive protein and C1q is reduced. Conversely, recruitment of factor H, the regulator of the alternative complement pathway, is enhanced in biofilms (Cerca et al., 2006). Thus, biofilm formation is an efficient method of evading both the classical and alternative complement pathways. *S. aureus* and *P. aeruginosa* can also evade phagocytosis by switching from planktonic growth to biofilm production (Domenech et al., 2013).

Bacteria can, of course, avoid being eaten simply by killing phagocytic cells. Leukotoxins are a relatively crude method of assassination (Narayanan et al., 2002). Nevertheless, it works for *Strep equi*. Some bacteria use more sophisticated methods, such as injecting toxins into their targets. Gram-negative bacteria such as *Salmonella*, *Pseudomonas*, and *E. coli* have developed an elaborate needle complex, a type III secretion system, to convey effector molecules directly into the cytosol of effector cells. These injection systems are turned on when a bacterium is ingested by a cell and exposed to a low pH within the phagosome. Once the needle complex penetrates the cytosol and detects its neutral pH, injection of effector molecules occurs. These molecules activate guanosine triphosphatases and disrupt intracellular signaling pathways. At high concentrations, they generate transmembrane pores and kill the cells.

Although killing leukocytes is an effective way to avoid phagocytosis, other bacteria are content to simply survive within phagocytic cells. Some generate a resistant cell wall to protect themselves against lysosomal enzymes. For example, *S. aureus* uses a cell wall peptidoglycan that is completely resistant to lysozyme. *Strep equi* uses an effective capsule containing hyaluronic acid. Some bacteria produce antioxidants that neutralize the products of the respiratory burst. For example, the carotenoid pigments responsible for the yellow color of *S. aureus* can quench singlet oxygen. *S. enterica* Typhimurium can prevent the production of nitric oxide (NO) and downregulate host NOS2 activity. *S. aureus* produces catalase that degrades hydrogen peroxide, and the free radicals produced during the respiratory burst. It also produces lactate dehydrogenase, which helps it to resist NO-mediated oxidation. *E. coli* can defend themselves against hypochlorite through the actions of a molecular chaperone called Hsp33. This protein unfolds on exposure to hypochloride and then binds and protects essential proteins against bleach-induced aggregation.

Bacteria such as enteropathogenic *E. coli*, secrete molecules that can protect them against neutrophils. For example, *E. coli* produces lysozyme inhibitors. Other bacteria ensure that they are never exposed to these enzymes by interfering with phagosomal maturation. Mycobacteria can establish themselves within vacuoles that exclude proteases and oxidants by blocking lysosome-phagosome fusion. In the case of *M. tuberculosis*, the bacterium enters the macrophage through cholesterol-enriched membrane microdomains that are coated on the cytosolic side with tryptophan-aspartate-containing coat protein that prevents phagosome maturation. Thus, lysosomes cannot fuse with the phagosome. They remain distributed within the cytosol, and the bacteria survive and grow (Pieters & Gatfield, 2002). Mycobacteria can also prevent the acidification of phagosomes by preventing the recruitment of the proton pump adenosine triphosphatase from the vacuolar membrane so that lysosomal cathepsins remain inactive. Another mechanism used by bacteria to avoid destruction is simply to escape from the phagosome by migrating into the cytosol, surrounded by a coat of polymerized actin. This method is employed by mycobacteria and by *L. monocytogenes*. Listeria secretes listeriolysin O that destroys cell membranes and so permits the organism to enter the macrophage cytosol (*L. monocytogenes* causes an uncommon meningoencephalitis in horses that is associated with macrophage pleocytosis (Phelps et al., 2023)).

Even extracellular killing can be inhibited by some bacteria. Neutrophils and macrophages can release intranuclear DNA and associated chromatin proteins, resulting in the formation of extracellular traps. This extracellular chromatin is coated with antimicrobial proteins, including granule components that can kill bacteria. However, bacteria such as the pneumococci and *S. aureus* can secrete endonucleases that degrade this chromatin net (Thammavongsa et al., 2013). Additionally, the released phosphonucleotides can be dephosphorylated by another Staphylococcal enzyme and generate deoxyadenosine, which then triggers apoptosis and eliminates any nearby macrophages!

Evasion of adaptive immunity

Bacteria may also avoid or modify adaptive immune responses—a more difficult task (Sansonetti & Di Santo, 2007). A horse will not respond effectively to organisms it cannot detect or to organisms that it encounters for the first time. Some bacteria secrete proteases that can destroy immunoglobulins or cytokines. These organisms can thus prevent opsonization and Fc receptor-mediated phagocytosis.

Bacteria may also interfere with macrophage polarization to promote their survival. Some Salmonella and Mycobacteria can neutralize M1-related effectors or inhibit M1 cytokine secretion or expression. Proteins from *M. tuberculosis* can inhibit activation of NF-κB. Responding Mycobacteria may induce the synthesis of IL-10, and TGF-β and hence prolong their survival. IL-10 is especially effective in inhibiting macrophage activation, suppressing oxidant production, and reducing MHC class II expression. The evolution of bacterial diseases into persistent chronic infections is associated with a tendency to M2 polarization mediated by IL-10. As described below, *R. equi* expresses a virulence associated protein, VapA, that interferes with endolysosome formation, thus enabling it to survive within macrophages (Rofe et al., 2016).

Once activated, platelets also release antibacterial peptides and reactive oxygen species (ROS). They also bind to bacteria to form heterotypic aggregates that are readily phagocytosed by neutrophils or captured in NETs. Horse platelets exposed to bacterial lipopolysaccharide from *E. coli* or lipotechoic acid from *Staph. aureus* can inhibit bacterial growth as a result of the release of reactive oxygen species (Aktan et al., 2013). Nevertheless, many commensal bacteria are also pathobionts. For example, *Clostridium tetani* and *Clostridium perfringens* are commonly found among the intestinal microbiota of horses. Bacterial disease is not, therefore, an inevitable consequence of the presence of pathogenic organisms on a body surface. The development of disease is related to many other factors, including the immunity of the host, the presence of damaged tissues, the location of the bacteria, and their virulence (Giguere & Prescott, 2000).

Selected horse bacterial diseases

Rhodococcus equi

Rhodococcus equi is a facultative, intracellular, Gram-positive coccobacillus and an opportunistic pathogen. (Its taxonomy is debated and is also classified as a species in the Genus *Prescottell*a, but this nomenclature has not been widely adopted by veterinarians (Sangal et al., 2022)). While it is a soil saprophyte, it is also a member of the normal equine intestinal microbiota. It is a common bacterium and up to 60% of foals may acquire the organism as a result of inhaling infected dust particles. It also causes serious infections in pigs as well as cattle, goats, dogs, cats and immunosuppressed humans.

R. equi is the most important cause of severe, pyogranulomatous pneumonia in foals under 6 months of age. The most severe infections occur in foals less than 1 month of age. It can also cause disease in immunodeficient older horses. *R. equi* can also invade the small and large intestines, especially the cecum, colon, and mesenteric lymph nodes (Uzal et al., 2022). Foals acquire Rhodococcus infection by inhaling or ingesting the dust from contaminated soil. Many develop subclinical infections. Up to 50% may develop pneumonia. The death rate is 2%–5%. Foals that survive develop lifelong immunity.

A genome-wide survey has been conducted to identify the horse genes associated with susceptibility to *R. equi* infection. A region located on chromosome ECA26 is associated with susceptibility. Within this region is the gene, *TRPM2,* that encodes a protein belonging to the transient receptor potential cation channel family. It plays a key role in the generation of neutrophil extracellular traps. It thus contributes to the development of antibacterial immunity (Tripathi et al., 2018). Another potentially important gene involved in *R. equi* resistance is Nramp 1 (*SLC11A1*). It is expressed in macrophages and plays a role in controlling intracellular iron concentrations. Some transferrin genes are also linked *to R. equi* susceptibility (Tallmadge et al., 2020).

Pathogenesis

Inhaled *R equi* is readily phagocytosed by foal alveolar macrophages. (For this purpose, it uses the type 3 complement receptor (Mac-1).) Virulent strains carry a large plasmid of 80–90 kb that contains a pathogenicity island of 21 kb that encodes multiple virulence-associated protein (VAP) genes. The most important of these appears to be the gene for virulence-associated protein A (VapA). VapA interferes with endolysosomal function by preventing their acidification and reducing cathepsin B activity. VapA thus allows *R equi* to survive within alveolar macrophages by inhibiting protein degradation within lysosomes (Rofe et al., 2016). The bacteria therefore persist and grow within the phagosomes that fail to develop into functional lysosomes, and as a result, the pH of their contents remains high. Strains of *R. equi* that lack VapA are avirulent (Vail et al., 2021).

Thus, Rhodococcus can persist within these macrophage vacuoles. It is interesting to note a recent finding that alveolar macrophages play two roles. They phagocytose and destroy invading microorganisms. They also act to minimize inflammation within the lungs. Controlling inflammation appears to be their first priority, and as a result, they may permit excessive bacterial growth by default (Better et al., 2025) (Fig. 16.5).

Immunity

The presence of *R. equi* within macrophages stimulates a type I interferon response and consequent expression of interferon-stimulated genes (Vail et al., 2021). This response is triggered by activation of the cGAS/STING pathway. This pathway is triggered when DNA escapes into the cell cytoplasm. The bacterial dsDNA activates cGAS that then binds and activates an adaptor molecule, known as stimulator of interferon genes (STING). STING then activates the IRF3 and NF-κB pathways. The activation of these pathways leads to the production of large quantities of type 1 interferons, especially IFN-β as well as the NF-κB-mediated expression of inflammatory cytokines (Motwani et al., 2019).

Some phagosomes containing *R equi* bind galectins-3, -8, and -9. However, even in this location, they can activate the foal's innate immune defenses. They act through the toll-like receptors to provoke the production of IFN-γ and TNF-α. If these are insufficient to activate the macrophages, then the Rhodococci will survive

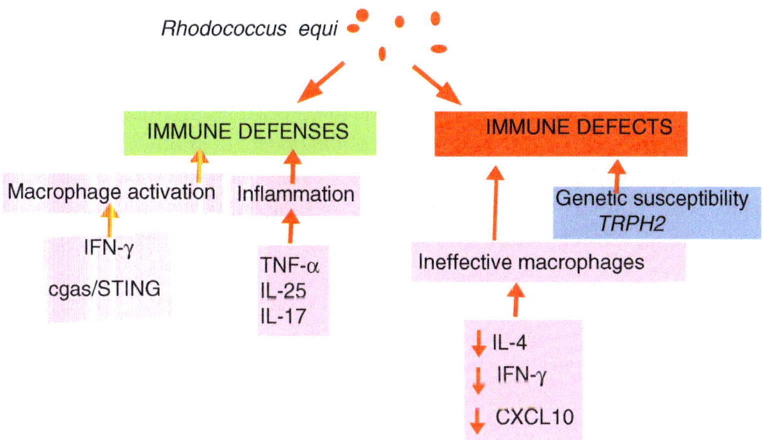

FIGURE 16.5 The immune factors affecting *R. equi* infections in foals.

and prosper. As described in Chapter 7, the IFN-γ activates the macrophages so that they develop an M1 phenotype, produce reactive oxygen species, and hence kill the invader. It should be pointed out, however, that *R equi* also produces a unique lipoglycan that may serve to enhance its survival within foal macrophages (Garton et al., 2002).

Given that *R. equi* is a normal member of the intestinal microbiota, it is unsurprising that healthy horses have antibodies to it. For example, naturally *R. equi*—infected foals mount IgM and IgA antibody responses irrespective of whether they develop clinical disease. IgM antibodies can be detected in healthy foals between 5 and 9 weeks of age. IgA antibody levels also peak around this time, but at much lower serum levels (Takai et al., 1986). Serum concentrations of VapA-specific IgA of 19 foals did not rise significantly during their first 28 days of age but increased nearly 10-fold by 56 days. Similarly, in the foal bronchoalveolar fluid, relative concentrations of IgA increased progressively with age (Aucoin et al., 2026).

Infected foals mount an antibody response to *R. equi* virulence-associated proteins (Hooper-McGrevy et al., 2003). Relative concentrations of serum VapA-specific IgG1, IgG3/5, and IgG4/7, of 19 healthy foals did not differ significantly during the first 28 days of age but increased nearly 10-fold by age 56 days.

In experimentally infected foals, following intratracheal or oral inoculation with *R. equi*, IgG antibodies were first detected, followed by IgM and IgA, reflecting foal B cell ontogeny. Significant levels of IgM and IgA antibodies developed only in a pneumatic foal infected intratracheally with *R. equi*. Anti-*R. equi* IgG and IgA antibodies appeared in lung washings of this intratracheally infected foal. The humoral immune responses to *R. equi* are clearly affected by the route and severity of *R. equi* exposure (Takai et al., 1987).

The antibody response to *R. equi* in sick foals. is characterized by a significant bias toward the production of IgG1, IgG4/7 and IgG3/5. The latter is the result of a Th2 based response and tends therefore to be somewhat ineffective against an intracellular pathogen such as *R, equi*. IgG1, in contrast, is produced by healthy immune foals and is induced by a Th1 helper cell response. In another *R. equi* study, the Ig3/5:IgG4/7 ratio in the serum of non-surviving foals was significantly greater than in the surviving animals thus confirming the lack of protection afforded by IgG3/5 (Mizuguchi et al., 2024). This interpretation may, however, be oversimplistic since the IgG subclass response to *R. equi* also changes with the challenge dose. Mild infections with *R equi* triggered IgG1, IgG4/7 and IgG6 responses, whereas high challenge doses promoted an IgG3/5 response (Mizuguchi et al., 2024).

Cytotoxic $CD3^+$ $CD8^+$ T cells can be obtained by bronchoalveolar lavage from the lungs of adult horses. These pulmonary T cells can lyse *R. equi*-infected alveolar macrophages and peripheral blood mononuclear cells, but not uninfected target cells. However, these cytotoxic T cells are not active in three-week-old foals. In some foals, they were active at 6 weeks of age and in all foals by 8 weeks. Interestingly, this cytotoxic effect is not ELA restricted (Patton et al., 2005).

Inflammation

After detecting *R. equi*, neutrophils express increased amounts of interleukin-23 (IL-23). This IL-23 promotes Th17 cell differentiation. Driven by transforming growth factor-β (TGF-β) and IL-6, the Th17 cells then promote inflammation. Not only do these Th17 cells produce IL-17, but also IL-6, GM-CSF, G-CSF, chemokines, and metalloproteases. They thus trigger local inflammation and coordinate early neutrophil recruitment to infection sites, especially on epithelial surfaces (Curis & Way, 2009). Unlike macrophages, foal neutrophils appear to be fully functional at birth. When stimulated by *Rhodococcus equi,* they increased their mRNA production of IL-6. CXCL8, IL-23p19, and TNF-α (Liu et al., 2009).

In a separate study on the cytokine responses of neonatal foals to *R. equi*. Liu et al. (2011) demonstrated significant upregulation of cytokines produced by all three helper cell populations: Th1, Th2, and Th17. IL-17 was detected in bronchoalveolar fluid. They produced a similar level of transcripts for IFN-γ throughout the first 3 weeks after birth, suggesting that there was no impairment of the Th1 response during this time. However, IL-4 production was significantly reduced at birth, while IL-17 was reduced during the first week but rapidly recovered thereafter (Liu et al., 2011).

Foal immune defects

The adult equine cell-mediated immune system is well capable of combating *R. equi* infection. However, this is not the case in newborn foals (da Silviera et al., 2025). Young foals mount an inadequate innate immune response. Their innate and adaptive immune systems are too immature. Their most significant deficit appears to be an inability to produce sufficient IFN-γ. As a result, their Th1, cell-mediated response is inadequate. In addition, they cannot fully activate their M1 alveolar macrophages nor their cytotoxic T cells They produce insufficient reactive oxygen species. Their alveolar macrophages thus fail to control the infection, and hence the bacteria can survive and multiply within them.

The production of cytokines by neonatal foals has been investigated (Liu et al., 2009). Newborn foals produce limited amounts of the chemokine, CXCL10, as well as interleukins 2, 4, and 17 (CXCL10 production is normally induced by IFN-γ). The CXCL10 deficiency means that T cells are not recruited to infection sites. The failure to produce IL-17 means that Th17 responses are impaired. Conversely, the Th2 cytokine IL-4 is largely undetectable during the first 3 months of life. This delayed onset of Th2 activity explains, in part, why young foals respond very poorly to vaccination. It is clear that the basal production of IFN-γ and IL-6 is also impaired in neonatal foals. Conversely, the basal production of CXCL8, IL-12p35/p40, and IL-23p19/p40 is either comparable to or greater than adult levels. These are probably absorbed from colostrum (Mariella et al., 2017). The immaturity of their antigen-presenting cells is reflected by a local deficiency of CD1, which is involved in innate cell-mediated. immune responses (da Silviera et al., 2025).

Given the defects in the innate immune system of newborn foals, it makes sense to seek to enhance their innate immune responses by "training" (Chapter 10). For example, foals treated orally with virulent *R. equi* at 1 and 3 days of age demonstrate significantly enhanced innate immune responses (Petri da Silviera et al., 2025). Foals treated in this way demonstrated changes in the epigenetic profile of their monocytes and over a 1000 differentially expressed genes in their neutrophils. Among the upregulated genes are IL-1α, IL-6, CXCL8, IL-15, IL-18, and IL-32. Their adaptive system also responds with elevated levels of IgG1 and IgG4/7 and increased T cell production of IFN γ. As a result, these foals are protected against subsequent intrabronchial challenge with *R. equi.*

While *R. equi*-affected foals are too young to mount a protective antibody-mediated immune response, some have been recorded as developing a severe immune-mediated hemolytic anemia. It is a very rare complication, and its pathogenesis has not been investigated (Johns et al., 2011).

There is currently no vaccine available against *R. equi.* Thus treatment is by passive immunization. The standard of care of *R. equi* pneumonia in foals involves transfusion with 1 or 2 liters hyperimmune plasma. The results are highly variable since they depend upon the source of the immune plasma. However, antibodies may also be delivered to foal lungs by aerosol. For example, encouraging results have been obtained by nebulizing foals with the mRNA encoding the light and heavy chains of a monoclonal IgG1 antibody directed against the virulence-associated protein A (VapA). The mRNA is incorporated into bronchoalveolar cells that then make protective antibodies (Legere et al., 2025).

Potomac horse fever (PHF)

This disease, technically called equine neorickettsiosis, is a lethal enterocolitis caused by *Neorickettsia risticii.* First identified in Maryland, it is now known to be much more widespread and is found in Europe and South America as well as across North America. It is caused by an intracellular bacterium that invades intestinal epithelial cells, monocytes, macrophages, and mast cells. It causes an enterocolitis, so that clinical signs include fever and depression associated with diarrhea, and colic, leading to dehydration and laminitis. Affected horses are severely neutropenic. Mortality may reach 25%. Infected horses mount an antibody response mediated primarily by IgG. These antibodies can readily neutralize the organism in vitro. Neutralizing antibody titers reach a maximum around 25 days postinfection. However, as an intracellular organism, the bacterium can easily evade the lethal effects of antibodies by residing within cells. Thus, it appears that a cell-mediated response involving activation of M1 macrophages is required to fully control the infection (Dutta et al., 1998).

Strangles

Strangles is caused by *Streptococcus equi* spp *equi.* It is highly contagious and is one of the commonest and most important bacterial diseases of horses. It also affects donkeys and mules. The bacteria penetrate the nasal and oral mucus membranes, enter the lymphatics and invade local lymph nodes. It is characterized by the development of a fever, a profuse nasal discharge, and the formation of abscesses within the retropharyngeal and submandibular lymph nodes. The bacteria multiply extracellularly within the nodes. They appear to activate the complement system and, as a result, generate the chemotactic peptides C3a and C5a. Neutrophils are therefore attracted in large numbers to the sites of invasion. Horses also develop a marked leukocytosis. Unfortunately, these neutrophils are relatively ineffective in phagocytosing and killing the Streptococci (Timoney, 1993). This is probably a consequence of the antihemolytic effects of its hyaluronic acid capsule, an antiphagocytic M protein, in addition to the production by the bacteria of a potent leukotoxin.

The M protein of *Streptococcus equi* subsp *equi* is a cell wall protein also called fibrinogen-binding protein. Studies have indicated that it also binds preferentially to IgG4/7. Its binding site is located at the immunoglobulin CH2–CH3 interface. At this location, the M protein blocks the binding of complement component C1q and, as a result, prevents activation of the classical complement pathway. This permits *Strep equi* to evade destruction by the complement system (Lewis et al., 2008). The fibrinogen also appears to inhibit the intracellular killing of the Streptococci. The M protein of *Strep equi* also binds the FH protein of the alternative complement pathway and so inhibits the production of the key complement enzyme, C3 convertase.

Strangles abscesses develop within the lymph nodes over a period of 4–22 days. As they enlarge, they restrict the airways and interfere with the horse's breathing. They block lymph flow that contributes to additional edema formation. This edema may affect the lungs and cause respiratory distress. Hence the name strangles. When the abscesses rupture, they release thick, purulent pus that can drain through the skin or the guttural pouch and out of the nostrils. Most horses recover rapidly after abscess rupture. The overall mortality rate of strangles is 1%–2%. However, if complications develop, mortality can rise as high as 40%. If the drainage of the abscesses is incomplete, then up to 10% of horses, although apparntly healthy, may be persistently infected and intermittently shed *Strep equi*.

Horses mount a mucosal immune response against *Strep equi*. Thus, the nasopharyngeal mucus of infected horses contains both IgA and IgG-specific antibodies. These nasopharyngeal antibodies are directed against two major bacterial antigens, proteins of 41 and 46 kDa. Infected horses also mount serum antibody responses against a protein of 62 kDa in addition to multiple other bacterial antigens (Galan & Timoney, 1985).

Streptococcal M protein appears to be the major protective antigen of *Strep equi*. It is a key component of commercial strangles vaccines. *Strep equi* also employs a virulence factor called S protein. This molecule facilitates bacterial invasion and cell adherence (Cohen et al., 2024). Investigations have revealed that naturally infected horses do not make antibodies to this S protein. The S protein is, however, strongly antigenic when employed as a vaccine. Most horses that recover from strangles are resistant to reinfection for at least 5 years. This resistance does not correlate with serum antibody levels but with the nasopharyngeal antibody levels. Thus, the serum antibodies are probably not significantly protective.

Strep equi subspecies *zooepidemicus* also causes respiratory disease and endometritis in horses. However, it does cross-react with ssp *equi* so that vaccines such as "Strangvac" can protect against both subspecies. A significant adverse consequence is the development of purpura hemorrhagica (Chapter 20).

Contagious equine metritis

Contagious equine metritis is a genital infection of horse and donkey mares caused by a Gram-negative coccobacillus called *Taylorella equigenitalis*. It causes a local vaginitis accompanied by a mucopurulent uterine discharge. As expected, infected horses mount both a systemic and local immune response against this organism. Nevertheless, mares that recover may carry the organism for extended periods. As with strangles, the invading organism is covered by an antiphagocytic capsule that inhibits ingestion by neutrophils. In addition, the organism binds IgG but not IgA to its surface. This binding appears to involve not the classical antibody binding site of the immunoglobulin but its hinge region (Widders et al., 1985). Presumably, this is a mechanism by which the organism reduces opsonization and blocks complement activation and hence phagocytosis. As a result of this mechanism, systemic antibody responses are not protective. Even animals with high circulating antibody titers are still susceptible to experimental challenge. Animals that recover spontaneously from the infection are not resistant to subsequent challenge (Fernie et al., 1980).

Glanders

Glanders is a fatal infection of horses and donkeys caused by *Burkholderia mallei,* a facultative intracellular bacterium. It is an ancient disease that has killed large numbers of horses. It was mentioned by the Greek physician, Hippocrates in 330 BCE. One notable disease outbreak, caused such losses of cavalry horses in the French Army that it resulted in their defeat at the Battle of Blenheim in 1704. As a result, the french king, Louis XV, established the first Veterinary school in Lyons in 1761, to study the problem! The last recorded outbreak in the United States occurred in 1942. However glanders is still present in parts of Africa, Asia and South America.

Infected horses develop a nasal discharge, abscessation of lymph nodes throughout the body, and disseminated nodular abscesses within organs such as the liver, lungs, and spleen, as well as the skin and limbs. The acute disease may be associated with septicemia and sudden death. ("Glanders" is the name given to the respiratory disease. "Farcy" is the name of the skin disease.) As expected, affected horses and donkeys mount a strong antibody response against the secretory proteins of the organism, such as Hcp1, TssA, and Tssb. They also mount a significant cellular immune response with elevated levels of IFN-γ, TNF-α, IL-12, IL-17, and IL-6 (Saini et al., 2022). Nevertheless there are currently no licensed vaccines available against glanders. Some experimental vaccines have shown promise in small-animal models yet fail to provide satisfactory protection in horses, specilly against the chronic disease (Torres, 2025).

B. mallei has the ability to suppress the host's innate immune pathways. Thus, the secretory bacterial proteins listed above interact with the equine ubiquination degradation system and so suppress antigen presentation; They interfere with signaling by the TNF receptor and the NF-κB pathway; this modulates macrophage cytokine secretion, for example, increasing their production of IL-6 and IL-10. *B. mallei* lipopolysaccharide has an unusual structure so that it is a weaker macrophage activator than enterobacterial LPS and generates much less, IL-6, TNF-α, or IL-1β compared to other equine bacterial pathogens (Saikh & Mott, 2017).

The persistence of *B. mallei* in an intracellular environment appears to result from its ability to exploit the host's immune signaling pathways. Thus, *B. mallei* can block the cellular autophagy pathways, the pathways that are normally employed to get rid of unwanted intracellular organisms and bacteria. Collectively, blockage of these pathways can prevent an infected horse from eliminating *B. mallei* from the body and account in large part for its lethality as well as the lack of an effective vaccine (Aschenbroich et al., 2016). Experimental studies of *B. mallei*-infected laboratory rodents have confirmed that the organism can persist within the animal's macrophages. As a result, experimental activation of macrophages to the M1 phenotype by exposure to IFN-γ appears to work well in these species. Interleukin 12 and IL-18 appear to be especially effective in mediating this activation step (Rowland et al., 2006).

Equine proliferative enteropathy

Equine proliferative enteropathy is caused by the obligate intracellular Gram-negative bacterium *Lawsonia intracellularis*. It occurs primarily in post-weaning foals during the fall and winter months. Infected foals develop a chronic disease with severe anorexia and malabsorption resulting in a fever, loss of body condition, ventral edema, lethargy, colic, and diarrhea (Uzal et al., 2022). The animals develop a severe hypoalbuminemia and leukocytosis. In some cases, the disease may be acute and fatal.

L. intracellularis is a microaerophilic organism that resides within the apical cytoplasm of enterocytes. The organism is endocytosed by the enterocytes, but the phagosomal membrane breaks down rapidly, releasing the bacteria into the cytoplasm, where they proliferate. As a result, multiple bacteria are found in crypt enterocytes. These enterocytes continue to proliferate in the absence of any obvious inflammatory response. Transcripts show that several gene pathways are upregulated, including those encoding matrix metalloprotease 7 (MMP7), transglutaminase 2 (TGM2) and oncostatin M (OSM) (Leite et al., 2019). It is also apparent that the bacteria stimulate the β-catenin/Wnt and Notch signaling pathways to promote cell proliferation and reduce apoptosis (Huan et al., 2017).

The disease gets its name from the proliferative lesions that develop in the terminal ileum in the chronic disease, proliferative intestinal adenomatosis. These lesions result in an increase in the thickness of the ileal wall. These proliferative lesions are located near the ileocecal junction. The lesions may be diffuse or present as distinct nodules or polyps. The proliferation involves the intestinal epithelium, and the villous architecture is lost. The infected crypt cells fail to mature and are not shed. As a result, the crypts elongate and are distorted. In addition, they fail to differentiate into goblet or absorptive cells. This disease also occurs in pigs, and equine strains show 98% homology to the 16S-rDNA gene of porcine strains (Pusteria & Gebhart, 2013).

An inflammatory response is associated with these lesions, and is characterized by infiltration with $CD8^+$, $CD25^+$ T cells that peak between 14- and 24-days post-infection at a time corresponding to peak bacterial infiltration. Blood TNF-α, IL-6, and IFN-γ levels are elevated for up to 40 days. IL-10 and TGF-β levels may also be high during the first 5–10 days. IgA also accumulates within the enterocytes. It is unclear whether this is directed against the intracellular bacteria or reflects a breakdown in the transport of IgA through the epithelial cells to the intestinal lumen. In the hemorrhagic disease, the inflammatory response is more severe with T cell infiltration, cell lysis, and shedding of enterocytes into the gut lumen. The number of $CD8^+$ T cells in the lesions declines within 14 days of infection (Macintyre et al., 2003).

Immunity to fungal infections

Fungi are ubiquitous. They are found in abundance in the equine environment and are significant members of the equine surface microbiota—the mycobiota. Under some circumstances, they can invade and cause serious illness in horses. The primary predisposing factor is that the animal be significantly immunosuppressed

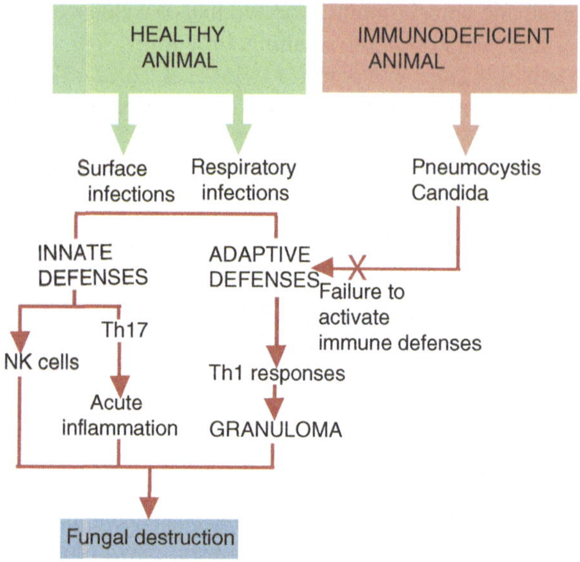

FIGURE 16.6 Mechanisms of immunity to fungal pathogens.

(Fig. 16.6). Thus, stresses including viral infections, neoplasia, or even malnutrition can predispose. Excessive and prolonged use of corticosteroids can be immunosuppressive, while excessive antibiotic use may result in dysbiosis (Rivera, 2014).

Equine fungal infections can be classified based on their degree of tissue penetration. These include, for example, the superficial mycoses, which are primary infections by fungi that can survive within the stratum corneum of the skin. The second type includes the cutaneous mycoses that can invade the skin and damage hair, hoofs, and skin. The other types are subcutaneous and deep mycoses that can invade organs such as the respiratory tracts, in addition to internal organs (Cafarchia et al., 2013).

Examples of fungi that cause a superficial mycosis in horses are the Malassezia yeasts. They cause a hyperplastic dermatitis accompanied by a mononuclear cell infiltration. Cutaneous infections can also affect keratinized tissue, including the skin and hoofs. The most important examples of these are the Dermatophytes that cause "ringworm." The most important of the subcutaneous mycoses is histoplasmosis. *Histoplasma capsulatum* causes localized infections of many tissues, including the lungs, gastrointestinal tract, bone marrow, and lymph nodes. It triggers a T cell-mediated defensive response. As a result, a histoplasmin skin test will yield a positive delayed hypersensitivity response (Chapter 20). This is, however, of limited usefulness since surveys have shown that up to 70% of healthy horses in endemic areas carry the organism and give a positive skin test result (Cafarchia et al., 2013). Disease dissemination depends in large part on the state of the horse's immune system. Epizootic lymphangitis, in horses, is caused by *Histoplasma capsulatum* var *farciminosum.* This is an endemic disease in horses, donkeys, and mules in North Africa and parts of Asia. It is a wound infection that is also spread by tick bites and biting flies. Affected animals show thickening of the lymphatics and lymphadenitis.

Deep mycoses are serious infections caused by organisms such as Aspergillus, Candida, Coccidioidomycosis, Cryptococcosis, and Pneumocystis. The primary risk factors include immunodeficiencies in addition to prolonged use of corticosteroids and antibiotics. Pneumocystis is well recognized as an opportunistic pathogen that causes serious pneumonia in immunosuppressed humans with AIDs or dogs with distemper. The commonest species recognized in horses is *P. carinii,* which mainly affects foals. One contributing factor to the development of Pneumocystis pneumonia in foals is a decrease in the numbers of $CD4^+$ and $CD8^+$ T cells in peripheral blood (Flaminio et al., 1988).

Like other infectious agents, fungi trigger both innate and adaptive immune responses. Fungal PAMPs acting either through TLRs or NLRs or through cell-surface C-type lectins such as the dectins, mannose-binding lectins, and scavenger receptors such as DC-SIGN (CD209) (Chapter 3) play a key role in early innate defenses (Plato et al., 2015). Thus, dectin-1 (CD369) binds to fungal β-glucans and triggers IL-22 and IL-23 production. Both contribute to anti-aspergillus resistance (Di Pietro et al., 2023). IL-23 activates Th17 cells. The IL-17 produced by these cells then activates both neutrophils and endothelial cells and promotes acute inflammation. It is of interest to note that culturing T cells and monocytes in the presence of *Candida* hyphae promotes the generation of Th17 cells. In contrast, culture in the presence of *Candida* yeast forms promotes production of IL-12 and a Th1 response (Sharma et al., 2022). Because of their size, neutrophils cannot totally ingest invading fungi. Nevertheless, by releasing enzymes and oxidants into the tissue fluid, neutrophils may severely damage fungal hyphae. Small fungal fragments or spores may be ingested and destroyed by macrophages or by NK cells.

Once established, fungal infections are mainly destroyed by Th1-mediated mechanisms. For example, some species of *Aspergillus* are facultative intracellular parasites, and chronic or progressive fungal diseases are commonly associated with defects in the T cell system. Th1 cells function in fungal infections by activating macrophages and by promoting epidermal growth and keratinization. Some T and NK cells can exert a direct cytotoxic effect on yeasts such as *Cryptococcus neoformans* and *Candida albicans* (Fig. 16.6).

Some donkey bacterial diseases

As expected, donkeys and mules suffer from the same infectious diseases that infect horses. However, donkeys and mules are not involved in racing or other athletic endeavors, and frequently live into old age, which may affect disease susceptibility. One of the most significant of these diseases is glanders. Donkeys are more susceptible to glanders than horses, whereas mules show an intermediate resistance and develop chronic disease (Barrandeguy & Carossino, 2018). Strangles is also a disease that affects donkeys and mules in addition to horses. Tetanus is, of course, a widespread disease associated with physical injuries. It is probably underreported in many populations. It is also clear that, given the use of donkeys in less developed communities, they are usually significantly under-vaccinated.

References

Aktan, I., Dunkel, B., & Cunningham, F. M. (2013). Equine platelets inhibit *E. coli* growth and can be activated by bacterial lipopolysaccharide and lipoteichoic acid although superoxide anion production does not occur, and platelet activation is not associated with enhanced production by neutrophils. *Veterinary Immunology and Immunopathology, 152*, 209–217.

Andersen-Nissen, E., Smith, K. D., Strobe, K. L., et al. (2005). Evasion of toll-like receptor 5 by flagellated bacteria. *Proceedings of the National Academy of Sciences of the United States of America, 102*, 9247–9252.

Aschenbroich, S. A., Lafontaine, E. R., & Hogan, R. J. (2016). Melioidosis and glanders modulation of the innate immune system: Barriers to current and future vaccine approaches. *Expert Review of Vaccines.* https://doi.org/10.1586/14760584.2016.1170598

Aucoin, A. A., Zhidkov, V., Legere, R. M., Borba, K. E. R., et al. (2026). The trajectories of relative concentrations of antirhodococcal immunoglobulin A differ from those of immunoglobulin G subisotypes in bronchoalveolar lavage fluid but not serum of foals. *Journal of the American Veterinary Medical Association.* https://doi.org/10.2460/ajvr.25.11.0402

Barrandeguy, N. E., & Carossino, M. (2018). Infectious diseases in donkeys and mules: An overview and update. *Journal of Equine Veterinary Science, 65*, 98–105.

Baxt, L. A., Garza-Mayers, A. C., & Goldberg, M. B. (2013). Bacterial subversion of host innate immune pathways. *Science, 340*, 697–701.

Benoit, M., Desnues, B., & Mege, J. L. (2008). Macrophage polarization in bacterial infections. *Journal of Immunology, 181*, 3733–3739.

Better, J., Estiri, M., Matt, et al. (2025). Cell type-specific efferocytosis determines the functional plasticity of alveolar macrophages. *Science Immunology.* https://doi.org/10.1126/sciimunol.ad13852

Bruhn, O., Grotzinger, J., Cascorbi, I., & Jung, S. (2011). Antimicrobial peptides and proteins of the horse—Insights into a well-armed organism. *BMC Veterinary Research.* https://doi.org/10.1186/1297-9716-42-98

Cafarchia, C., Figueredo, L. A., & Otranto, D. (2013). Fungal diseases of horses. *Veterinary Microbiology, 167*, 215–234.

Cerca, N., Jefferson, K. K., Oliviera, R., et al. (2006). Comparative antibody-mediated phagocytosis of *Staphylococcus epidermidis* cells grown in a biofilm or in the planktonic state. *Infection and Immunity, 74*, 4849–4855.

Cohen, N. D., Hughes, E. V., Bayne, C., Morris, E. R. A., et al. (2024). Immunization, but not natural infection of horses, results in antibody activity against the S protein of *Streptococcus equi* subsp *equi*. *American Journal of Veterinary Research.* https://doi.org/10.2460/ajvr.24.08.0228

Collins, H. L. (2008). Withholding iron as a cellular defense mechanism: Friend or foe? *European Journal of Immunology, 38*, 1803–1806.

Curis, M. M., & Way, S. S. (2009). Interleukin-17 in host defense against bacterial, mycobacterial and fungal pathogens. *Immunology, 126*, 177–185.

da Silviera, B. P., Cohen, N. D., Lawhon, S. D., Watson, R. O., & Bordin, A. I. (2025). Protective immune response against *Rhodococcus equi*: An innate immunity focused review. *Equine Veterinary Journal, 57*, 563–586.

Di Pietro, R., Dubuc, V., Manguin, E., Giroux-Lafond, R., et al. (2023). Characterization of fungal exposure and dectin-1 expression in healthy horses and horses with severe asthma. *American Journal of Veterinary Research*. https://doi.org/10.2460/ajvr.21.09.0143

Domenech, M., Ramos-Sevillano, E., Garcia, E., Moscoso, M., & Yuste, J. (2013). Biofilm formation avoids complement immunity and phagocytosis of *Streptococcus pneumonia*. *Infection and Immunity, 81*, 2606–2615.

Dutta, S. K., Vemulapalli, R., & Biswas, B. (1998). Association of deficiency in antibody response to vaccine and heterogeneity of *Ehrlichia risticii* strains of Potomac Horse Fever vaccine failure in horses. *Journal of Clinical Microbiology, 36*(2), 506–512.

Fernie, D. S., Batty, I., Walker, D., Platt, H., et al. (1980). Observations on vacine and post-infection immunity in contagious equine metritis. *Research in Veterinary Science, 28*, 362–367.

Flaminio, M. J. B. F., Rush, B. R., Cox, J. H., & Moore, W. E. (1988). CD4+ and CD8+ T-lymphopenia in a filly with *Pneumocystis carinii* pneumonia. *Australian Veterinary Journal, 76*, 399–402.

Galan, J. F., & Timoney, J. F. (1985). Mucosal nasopharyngeal immune responses of horses to protein antigens of *Streptococcus equi*. *Infection and Immunity, 47*(3), 623–628.

Garcia, B. L., Zwarthoff, S. A., Rooijakkers, S. H., & Geisbrecht, B. V. (2016). Novel evasion mechanisms of the classical complement pathway. *Journal of Immunology, 197*, 2051–2060.

Garton, N. J., Gilleron, M., Brando, T., Dan, H.-H., et al. (2002). A novel arabinomannan from the equine pathogen *Rhodococcus equi*. *Journal of Biological Chemistry, 277*(35), 31722–31733.

Giguere, S., & Prescott, J. F. (2000). Equine immunity to bacteria. *Veterinary Clinics of North America: Equine Practice, 16*(1), 29–47.

Harris, J., Master, S. S., DeHaro, S. A., et al. (2009). Th1-Th2 polarization and autophagy in the control of intracellular Mycobacteria by macrophages. *Veterinary Immunology and Immunopathology, 128*, 37–43.

Hooper-McGrevy, K. E., Wilkie, B. N., & Prescott, J. F. (2003). Immunoglobulin G subisotype responses of pneumonic and healthy exposed foals and adult horses to *Rhodococcus equi* virulence-associated proteins. *Clinical and Diagnostic Laboratory Immunology, 10* (3), 345–351.

Huan, Y. W., Bengtsson, R. J., MacIntyre, N., Guthrie, J., et al. (2017). *Lawsonia intracellularis* exploits b-catenin/Wnt and notch signaling pathways during infection of intestinal crypt to alter cell homeostasis and promote cell proliferation. *PLoS One*. https://doi.org/10.1371/journal.pone.0173782

Johns, I. C., Desrochers, A., Wotman, K. L., & Sweeney, R. W. (2011). Presumed immune-mediated hemolytic anemia in two foals with *Rhodococcus equi* infection. *Journal of Veterinary Emergency and Critical Care, 21*(3), 273–278.

Kaufmann, S. H., & Dorhoi, A. (2016). Molecular determinants in phagocyte-bacteria interactions. *Immunity, 44*, 476–491.

Legere, R. M., Ott, J. A., Poveda, C., Vanover, D., et al. (2025). Nebulization of an mRNA-encoded monoclonal antibody for passive immunization of foals against *Rhodococcus equi*. *Molecular Therapy*. https://doi.org/10.1016/j.ymthe.2025.06.025

Leite, F. L., Abrahante, J. E., Vasquez, E., Vannucci, F., et al. (2019). A cell proliferation and inflammatory signature is induced by *Lawsonia intracellularis* infection in swine. *mBio, 10*(1), e01605–01618.

Lewis, M. J., Meehan, M., Owen, P., & Woof, J. M. (2008). A common theme in interaction of bacterial immunoglobulin-binding proteins with immunoglobulins illustrated in the equine system. *Journal of Biological Chemistry, 283*(25), 17615–17623.

Liu, M., Bordin, A., Liu, T., Russell, K., & Cohen, N. (2011). The expression b of innate Th1-, Th2-, and Th17-type cytokines during early life of neonatal foals in response to *Rhodococcus equi*. *Cytokines, 56*, 356–364.

Liu, M., Liu, T., Bordin, A., Nerren, J., & Cohen, N. (2009). Activation of foal neutrophils at different ages by CpG deoxynucleotides and *Rhodococcus equi*. *Cytokine, 48*, 280–289.

MacIntyre, N., Smith, D. G. E., Shaw, D. J., Thomson, J. R., & Rhind, S. M. (2003). Immunopathogenesis of experimentally induced proliferative enteropathy in pigs. *Veterinary Pathology Online, 40*, 421–432.

Mancuso, G., Midiri, A., Biondo, C., et al. (2007). Type I IFN signaling is crucial for host resistance against different species of pathogenic bacteria. *Journal of Immunology, 178*, 3126–3133.

Mariella, J., Castagnetti, C., Prosperi, A., Scagliarini, A., & Peli, A. (2017). Cytokine levels in colostrum and in foals' serum pre- and post-suckling. *Veterinary Immunology and Immunopathology*, 34–37.

Mizuguchi, Y., Tsuzuki, N., Ebana, M. D., Suzuki, Y., & Kakuda, T. (2024). IgG subtype response against virulence-associated protein A in foals naturally infected with *Rhodococcus equi*. *Veterinary Sciences*. https://doi.org/10.3390/vetsci11090422

Mody, C. H., Ogbomo, H., Xiang, R. F., Kyei, S. K., et al. (2019). Microbial killing by NK cells. *Journal of Leukocyte Biology, 105*, 1285–1296.

Motwani, M., Pesiridis, S., & Fitzgerald, K. A. (2019). DNA sensing by the cGAS-STING pathway in health and disease. *Nature Reviews Genetics*. https://doi.org/10.1038/s41576-0151-1

Muko, R., Matsuda, H., Oikawa, M., Shin, T., et al. (2021). Histidine-rich glycoprotein functions as a dual regulator of neutrophil activity in horses. *Journal of Equine Veterinary Science*. https://doi.org/10.1016/j.jevs.2021.103620

Narayanan, S. K., Nagaraja, T. G., Chengappa, M. M., & Stewart, G. C. (2002). Leukotoxins of gram-negative bacteria. *Veterinary Microbiology, 84*, 337–356.

Patton, K. M., McGuire, T. C., Hines, M. T., Mealey, R. H., & Hines, S. A. (2005). *Rhodococcus equi* specific cytotoxic T lymphocytes in immune horses and development in asymptomatic foals. *Infection and Immunity, 73*(4), 2083–2093.

Petri da Silviera, B., Kahn, S. K., Legere, R. M., Bray, J. M., et al. (2025). Enteral immunization with live bacteria reprograms innate immune cells and protects neonatal foals from pneumonia. *Scientific Reports*. https://doi.org/10.1038/s41598-025-02060-5

Phelps, S., Chong, D., McKenzie, E., Kiupel, M., & Gorman, E. (2023). Mononuclear pleocytosis and meningoencephalitis caused by *Listeria monocytogenes* in an adult horse. *Canadian Veterinary Journal, 64*, 363–366.

Pieters, J., & Gatfield, J. (2002). Hijacking the host: Survival of pathogenic mycobacteria inside macrophages. *Trends in Microbiology, 3*, 142–146.

Plato, A., Hardison, S. E., & Brown, G. D. (2015). Pattern recognition receptors in antifungal immunity. *Seminars in Immunopathology, 37*, 97–106.

Podolsky, M. J., Lasker, A., Flaminio, M. J. B. F., Gowda, L. D., et al. (2006). Characterization of an equine mannose-binding lectin and its roles in disease. *Biochemical and Biophysical Research Communications, 343*, 928–936.

Pusteria, N., & Gebhart, C. (2013). *Lawsonia intracellularis* infection and proliferative enteropathy in foals. *Veterinary Microbiology, 167*, 34–41.

Reddick, L. E., & Alto, N. M. (2014). Bacteria fighting back: How pathogens target and subvert the host innate immune system. *Molecular Cell, 54*, 321–328.

Rivera, A. (2014). Protective immune responses to fungal infections. *Parasite Immunology, 36*, 453–462.

Rofe, A. P., Davis, L. J., Whittingham, J. L., Latimer-Bowman, E. C., et al. (2016). The *Rhodococcus equi* virulence protein VapA disrupts endolysosome function and stimulates lysosome biogenesis. *MicrobiologyOpen, 6*(2). https://doi.org/10.1002/mbo3.416

Rowland, C. A., Lertmemongkolchai, G., Bancroft, A., Haque, A., et al. (2006). Critical role of type I cytokines in controlling initial infection with *Burkholderia mallei*. *Infection and Immunity, 74*(9), 5333–5340.

Saikh, K. U., & Mott, T. M. (2017). Innate immune response to *Burkholderia mallei*. *Current Opinion in Infectious Diseases, 30*, 297–302.

Saini, S., Singha, H., Shanmugasundaram, K., & Tripathi, B. N. (2022). Characterization of immunoglobulin and cytokine responses in *Burkholderia mallei* infected equids. *Microbial Pathogenesis*. https://doi.org/10.1016/jmicpath.2021.105310

Sangal, V., Goodfellow, M., Jones, A. L., & Sutcliffe, I. (2022). A stable home for an equine pathogen: Valid publication of the binomial Prescottella equi gen. non./comb.nov., and reclassification of four rhodococcal species into the genus Prescottella. *International Journal of Systematic and Evolutionary Microbiology*. https://doi.org/10.1099/ijsem.0.005551

Sansonetti, P. J., & Di Santo, J. P. (2007). Debugging how bacteria manipulate the immune response. *Immunity, 26*, 149–161.

Sharma, J., Mudalagiriyappa, S., & Nangappa, S. G. (2022). T cell responses to control fungal infections in an immunological memory lens. *Frontiers in Immunology*. https://doi.org/10.3389/fimmu.2022.905867

Takai, R., Kawazu, S., & Tsubaki, S. (1986). Immunoglobulin and specific antibody responses to *Rhodococcus (Corynebacterium) equi* infection in foals as measured by enzyme-linked immunosorbent assay. *Journal of Clinical Microbiology, 23*(5), 943–947.

Takai, R., Kawazu, S., & Tsubaki, S. (1987). Humoral immune response of foals to experimental infection with *Rhodococcus equi*. *Veterinary Microbiology, 14*(3), 321–327.

Tallmadge, R. L., Antczak, D. F., & Felippe, M. J. B. (2020). Genetics of immune disease in the horse. *Veterinary Clinics of North America: Equine Practice, 36*, 273–288.

Thammavongsa, V., Missiakas, D. M., & Schneewind, O. (2013). *Staphylococcus aureus* degrades neutrophil extracellular traps to promote immune cell death. *Science, 342*, 863–865.

Timoney, J. F. (1993). Strangles. *Veterinary Clinics of North America: Equine Practice, 9*(2), 365–374.

Torres, A. G. (2025). Glanders: An ancient and emergent disease with no vaccine or treatment on site. *PLoS Neglected Tropical Diseases*. https://doi.org/10.1371/journal.pntd.0013160

Tripathi, J. K., Sharma, A., Sukumaran, P., et al. (2018). Oxidant sensor cation channel TRPM2 regulates neutrophil extracellular trap formation and protects against pneumoseptic bacterial infection. *The FASEB Journal, 32*, 6848–6859.

Uzal, F. A., Arroyo, L. G., Navarro, M. A., Gomez, D. E., et al. (2022). Bacterial and viral enterocolitis in horses: A review. *Journal of Veterinary Diagnostic Investigation, 34*(3), 354–375.

Vail, K. J., da Silveira, B. P., Bell, S. L., Cohen, N. D., et al. (2021). The opportunistic intracellular pathogen *Rhodococcus equi* elicits type 1 interferon by engaging cytosolic DNA sensing in macrophages. *PLoS Pathogens*. https://doi.org/10.13471/journal.ppat.1009888

Widders, P. R., Stokes, C. K., Newby, T. J., & Bourne, F. J. (1985). Nonimmune binding of equine immunoglobulin by the causative organism of contagious equine metritis, Taylorella equigenitalis. *Infection Immunity, 48*(2), 417–421.

Yadav, M., & Schorey, J. S. (2006). The β-glucan receptor dectin-1 functions together with TLR2 to mediate macrophage activation by mycobacteria. *Blood, 108*, 3168–3175.

CHAPTER

Immunity to selected equine viruses

17

Since viruses are obligate intracellular organisms, their very existence is threatened if they are destroyed by the immune system or by the death of their host. Because of this, both viruses and their hosts have been subjected to rigorous selection and adaptation. Viruses are selected for their ability to evade the host's immune responses, while at the same time, animals have been selected for survival despite virus-induced disease. Viruses that are eliminated before they replicate cannot spread. Hosts eliminated by viruses can no longer serve as hosts. An "oversuccessful" virus will reduce the availability of susceptible hosts, whereas a very successful host will be the largest target for the next generation of viruses. As a result, there can never be a "solution" to the problem of viruses.

For example, in infections where virus-host adaptation is poor, diseases tend to be lethal. Rabies is an excellent example of this. The virus is inevitably lethal in horses because they are unnatural hosts. On the other hand, in its "natural" hosts, such as bats and skunks, the rabies virus persists and may be shed in saliva for a long period without causing clinical disease. From the virus's "point of view," infection of horses is unprofitable since they almost never transmit rabies to skunks. Vaccination is relatively successful in this type of infection since the virus has not adapted to its host's defenses.

When the virus and its host are more adapted, although the disease may be severe, mortality may not be high, and the virus may be persistent. In this type of disease, further attacks may occur as a result of infection by variants of the same virus. An example of this type of virus infection is Equine influenza. Vaccination against influenza is complicated by the great diversity of influenza viruses. Even more adapted viruses can cause a persistent infection because the immune system is unable to eliminate them. An example is Equine Infectious Anemia. Vaccination against this disease is essentially unsuccessful. As their adaptation increases, viruses may cause latent infections and relatively mild, non-lethal disease. Equine herpesvirus infections also fall into this category. In studying the nature of the equine immune responses to viruses, it is well to recognize that this continuing selective pressure on both host and virus exists and profoundly influences the outcome of all viral infections.

The Immunology of Horses and Donkeys. https://doi.org/10.1016/B978-0-443-44863-8.00029-6

Virus structure and antigens

Virus particles, consist of a nucleic acid core surrounded by a layer of proteins. This protein layer, called the capsid, is made up of subcomponents called capsomeres. The virions may also be covered by a tegument and a lipid envelope. The complexity of viruses varies. Some, such as equine herpesviruses, are complex with a double-stranded DNA genome, a capsid, a tegument, and an envelope, whereas others, such as African Horse Sickness virus, are relatively simple. Antibodies can be induced against epitopes on all the proteins situated inside and on the surface of the virion.

Pathogenesis of virus infections

Adsorption, the first step in the invasion of a cell by a virus, occurs when a virus binds to cell surface receptors. These receptors are not there for the convenience of viruses but have some other physiological function. Thus, rabies virus binds to the receptor for acetylcholine, a neurotransmitter. The chemokine receptor CCR5 is the receptor used by West Nile virus. The nature, number, and distribution of their cell receptors determine the host range and tissue tropism of a virus. Once bound, the virion is taken into the cell through endocytosis or by fusion with the plasma membrane. Once inside a cell, the capsid is dismantled so that its nucleic acid is released into the cytoplasm, a process called uncoating. Once the virus genome is uncoated, replication begins. Host cell DNA transcription is inhibited so that only viral genetic information is processed. If the virus, for example, equine herpesvirus, contains DNA, this viral DNA is replicated. The new viral DNA is then transcribed into viral messenger RNA (mRNA), and this mRNA is translated into new capsid proteins. These new proteins are then assembled into virions. The host cell also replicates the viral nucleic acid so that large quantities of viral DNA are produced. The viral DNA is packaged inside the new capsids so that complete virions are formed. If the virus is not enveloped, the infected cells simply rupture, and multiple virions are released into the tissues. If the virions are enveloped, they leave the cell by budding through the cell surface. The cell membrane that encloses them serves as the new envelope. The released virions may then spread to nearby cells and invade them in turn.

Innate immunity

Rapid, powerful innate immune responses limit many viral infections. Interferons are especially important in this process. The enzyme lysozyme can also destroy viruses, as can many intestinal enzymes and bile. C-type lectins bind to viral glycoproteins and block virus interaction with host cells. For example, mannose binding lectin, and the surfactant proteins, SP-A, and SP-D can all bind and thus inactivate influenza viruses. Defensins from leukocytes and mucosal epithelial cells play a dual role in antiviral defenses since they can act both on the virus and on infected host cells. Thus, defensins can inactivate enveloped virions by disrupting their envelopes or by interacting with their glycoproteins. Some defensins can block intracellular signaling pathways in infected cells and interfere with transcription of viral RNA. Finally, cells invaded by viruses may undergo premature apoptosis, thus effectively preventing successful viral invasion and replication (Klotman & Chang, 2006).

Pattern-recognition molecules

Viruses, unlike bacteria and fungi, do not contain easily recognizable microbe-specific structures since they are constructed from host-derived components. For this reason, animal cells have evolved the ability to recognize the predominant virus-specific components, namely their nucleic acids (Ranjan et al., 2009). Three pattern recognition receptor (PRR) systems recognize viral nucleic acids. One system consists of two classes of nucleic acid receptors found within the cytosol of all nucleated cells. These are retinoic acid inducible gene -1 receptors (RIG-1) and melanoma differentiation-associated protein 5 receptors (MDA5). Both receptor classes can bind viral dsRNA and then signal through several adaptor proteins to activate the interferon-β (IFN-β) gene. The second system is mediated by toll-like receptors. TLR3 recognizes dsRNA. TLR7 and TLR8 recognize single-stranded RNA viruses such as the influenza viruses (Lund et al., 2005). TLR9 detects unmethylated CpG motifs in DNA. These motifs are common in both DNA viruses and bacteria. The third pattern recognition receptor system uses receptors with nucleotide-binding oligomerization (NOD) -like domains.

Interferons

The most important innate defense system against viral invasion is the interferon system. Interferons are antiviral cytokines. There are three types of interferons: type I, which includes, most importantly, IFN-α and IFN-β in addition to six others; type II IFNs, which include IFN-γ; and type III IFNs, which include the IFN-λs. The most important sources of type I interferons are plasmacytoid dendritic cells. Activated PRRs signal through specific signaling pathways such as MyD88 and TRIF to activate IRF-3 and IRF-7, as well as NF-κB. These are then translocated into the nucleus where they initiate the synthesis of multiple cytokines and type I interferons (Lazear et al., 2019) Fig. 17.1.

Viruses are not the only organisms that can trigger type I interferon production. For example, the opportunistic intracellular bacterium, *Rhodococcus equi*, triggers type I interferon production when it is phagocytosed by equine alveolar macrophages. It also activates the macrophage DNA-sensing pathways (Vail et al., 2021).

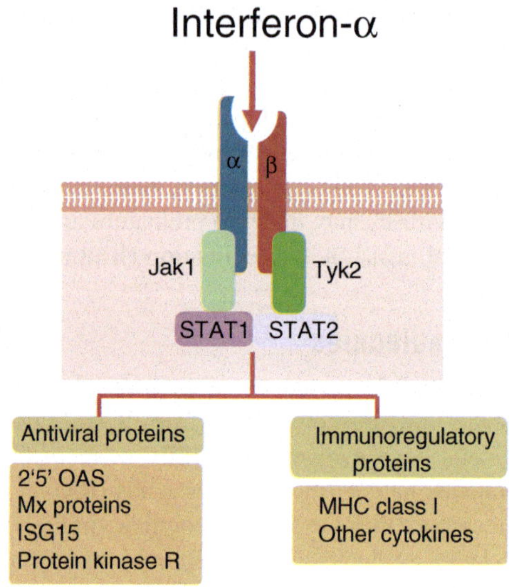

FIGURE 17.1

IFNAR—the receptor for the type I interferons

Ligand binding triggers the JAK-STAT transduction pathway and eventually activates both antiviral and immunoregulatory pathways.

Once released, interferons bind to cell surface receptors, heterodimers of IFNAR1 and IFNAR2. The receptors, in turn, activate a signal transduction cascade to eventually form a complex called interferon-stimulated gene factor 3 (ISGF3). This, in turn, binds to the promoter region of specific target genes. When interferons act on cellular targets, they upregulate the expression of hundreds of interferon-stimulated genes (ISGs)—the interferome.

Type I interferons

Twenty-six functional IFN genes have been identified on equine chromosome ECA23. These encode multiple type 1 interferons (Detournay et al., 2013). Thus, there appear to be six different IFN-α genes, four IFN-β genes, 12 IFN-ω genes of which four are pseudogenes, four IFN-δ genes (one pseudogene), one IFN-κ gene, and one IFN-ε gene. There are also three loci encoding interferons, classified as IFN-μ. (When first described, IFN-μ was classified as IFN-αω. However, subsequent studies demonstrated that in the horse, it is distinctly different from IFN-αω in other species.) (Detournay et al., 2013) Equine leukocytes exposed to live Sendai virus in vitro, readily express the mRNA for IFN-α, IFN-β, IFN-δ, IFN-μ and IFN-ω. However, fibroblasts only express IFN-β (Stetson & Medzhitov, 2006).

The equine type I interferons therefore include multiple forms of IFN-α and IFN-β, as well as multiple single gene products such as IFN- δ, IFN-ε, and IFN-κ. All are involved in the regulation of immune responses in addition to having antiviral activities. It is unclear if and how the different IFN-α gene products differ in their biological activities. The presence of only six in the horse is relatively few compared to the other domestic mammals. IFN-α is produced in large quantities by plasmacytoid dendritic cells (pDCs) and in much smaller amounts by lymphocytes, monocytes, and macrophages. IFN-β can be produced by almost any virus-infected cell. IFN-κ is produced by keratinocytes.

IFN-ε is a member of the type I family whose expression is limited to reproductive and brain tissues (Fischer et al., 2018). It has potent antiviral activity on both homologous and heterologous cells. It acts through the JAK/STAT pathway. It plays an important role in protecting the female reproductive tract, where it is expressed constitutively in the endometrium. In most cases, these molecules act on virus-infected cells to inhibit viral growth. The trophoblast interferons also regulate the maternal immune response to the fetus. Other interferons also play a role in equine pregnancy. For example, IFN-α, IFN-δ, and IFN-ω are all expressed by the embryonic trophoblast (de Amorin et al., 2023).

Type III interferons

Two equine type III interferons have been characterized, IFN-λ1 (CD28A) and IFN-λ3. They are both proteins of 191–195 amino acids (~21.5 kDa). The lambda-1 gene is located on chromosome ECA 22, whereas the lambda-3 gene is on ECA 10. These type III interferons are mainly produced by epithelial cells on mucosal surfaces. They signal through a unique receptor complex consisting of IL-10Rβ and IL-28Rα. While structurally unrelated to the type I interferons, they share signaling pathways and induce a similar gene response profile (Ichihashi et al., 2013). Their effects are most apparent at the intestinal and respiratory epithelia and the blood-brain barrier. They thus serve as a first line of defense against viral invasion.

Antiviral activities

The two major type I interferons (IFN-α and IFN-β) are produced within a few hours of viral invasion, and high concentrations are achieved long before adaptive immunity develops. IFN-α and IFN-β are produced when cells are triggered by viral nucleic acids binding to TLR-7 and TLR-9 or to RIG-1. Both bind to heterodimeric receptors (IFNAR) on nearby cells and activate JAK/STAT signaling pathways. These pathways activate at least 300 genes, many of which encode antiviral proteins. The result is the development of an "antiviral state" within a few minutes that peaks by 5–8 hours.

IFN-stimulated gene products act through many different pathways and have diverse effects on viruses. Some inhibit viral growth while others target specific viruses. They may target different stages of viral replication, such as viral entry, envelope uncoating, genome replication, protein assembly, or viral release. The existence of six IFN-α isoforms, even though they signal through a common receptor, suggests that they may have different functional roles. Interferons also target cells to promote viral clearance or induce apoptosis. These include increased neutrophil survival, activation of macrophages and regulation of NK cells, DCs, B cells, $CD8^{+}$T cells, and Th1 cells. They are, in effect, broad-spectrum antivirals.

One of the most important interferon-induced pathways is the 2′5′ A pathway, which upregulates transcription of the genes encoding 2′ 5′-oligoadenylate synthetases (2′ 5′-OAS). These enzymes are activated by exposure to long dsRNA from viruses in the cytoplasm. They act on adenosine triphosphate (ATP) to form 2′ 5′ adenylate oligomers. These oligomers bind and activate a ribonuclease called RNAase L. RNAase L degrades viral RNA and so inhibits viral growth. Fig. 17.2.

Another important interferon-mediated pathway is the Mx guanosine triphosphatase (GTPase) pathway. Mx proteins are large interferon-induced GTPases that accumulate as oligomers on intracellular membranes. Following viral infection, Mx monomers

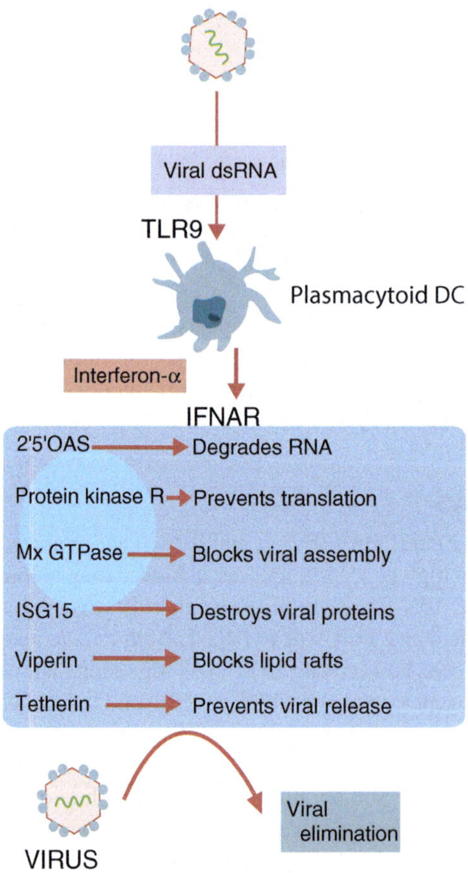

FIGURE 17.2

Some of the mechanisms by which the interferons can exert their antiviral activities.

are released. These bind and trap viral nucleocapsids and other essential viral components, and so block the assembly of new viruses. Mx proteins are expressed in many different cell types, such as hepatocytes, endothelial cells, and immune cells. They inhibit a wide range of RNA viruses, including the equine influenza viruses (Verhelst et al., 2013).

Protein kinase R (PKR) is induced by type I interferons. The kinase accumulates in the cell nucleus and cytoplasm. PKR regulates several cell signaling pathways and phosphorylates an initiation factor called eIF2α, which then prevents translation initiation by viral mRNA. Viperin is a protein that has direct antiviral activity and is induced by all three classes of interferon, double-stranded DNA and RNA, and by many different viruses. It appears to act on cellular lipids and interferes with lipid raft formation at different stages in the viral life cycle (Helbig & Beard, 2014). Tetherin is a small membrane protein that physically crosslinks (tethers!) virions to the plasma membrane and thus inhibits the release of enveloped viruses such as influenza from the cell surface. Tetherins from both horses and donkeys have similar antiviral abilities. They can both induce NF-κB signaling (Yin et al., 2014). However, equine infectious anemia virus encodes an accessory protein that antagonizes equine tetherin and therefore promotes the release of viral particles from infected cells (Bai et al., 2025).

The ability of cells to produce interferons varies. Virus-infected leukocytes, especially pDCs, directly interact with virus-infected cells to produce large amounts of IFN-α; almost any virus-infected cell can produce IFN-β; while antigen-stimulated T cells are the major source of IFN-γ (Assil et al., 2019).

Natural killer (NK) cells can kill virus-infected cells. NK cell cytotoxicity is stimulated by type I interferons and, as a result, is important early in a virus infection. Indeed, activated NK cells provide the first line of defense against many viruses. NK cells also produce large amounts of IFN-γ and perforins, and these, too, have direct antiviral effects. NK cells may therefore reduce the severity of viral infections long before the development of adaptive immunity and the appearance of specific cytotoxic T cells (Scalzo, 2002).

IFN-α not only activates NK cells but also most other immune cell populations. Thus, it stimulates the differentiation of monocytes into dendritic cells, as well as the maturation and activity of dendritic cells. IFN-α stimulates memory T cell proliferation, activates naïve T cells in chronic viral diseases, and enhances antigen-specific T cell priming. It promotes B cell functions such as IgG production and MHC expression (Shekhar & Yang, 2015).

RNA interference

RNA interference (RNAi) is an innate antiviral pathway that is employed in mammals including horses (Sagan & Sarnow, 2013). Viral double-stranded RNA (dsRNA) is broken up by an intracellular endonuclease called DICER into fragments of 21–23 nucleotides. Equine DICER is a protein of 218 kDa encoded by a gene on chromosome ECA2. The fragments produced act as amall interfering RNAs (siRNAs) These siRNAs are loaded into an RNA-induced silencing complex (RISC) that then binds to the viral RNA and destroys it, thus preventing viral growth. These siRNAs have been detected in a mouse germ cell line. Conversely, they are absent from somatic cells of adult mice. Embryonic cell lines cannot produce type 1 interferons, but adult somatic cells can. It has been suggested, therefore, that germ cell lines rely on RNA interference, but as they develop, they lose this pathway and replace it with the interferon response (Maillard et al., 2013). Fig. 17.3.

RNA interference is effective in protecting cultured horse skin cells from infection with equine arteritis virus (EAV). Thus, when target cells were transfected with siRNA and then challenged with EAV, virus titers were significantly reduced. Likewise, when siRNAs were used to treat cells already infected with EAV, it resulted in significantly improved cell survival rates (Heinrich et al., 2009).

Adaptive immunity

Antibodies prevent viral invasion of cells by blocking the adsorption of virions to target cells, by stimulating virus phagocytosis, by triggering complement-mediated virolysis, or by causing viral clumping and thus reducing the number of infectious units available for cell invasion. The binding of antibodies alone does not destroy viruses since splitting of virus-antibody complexes will release infectious virions.

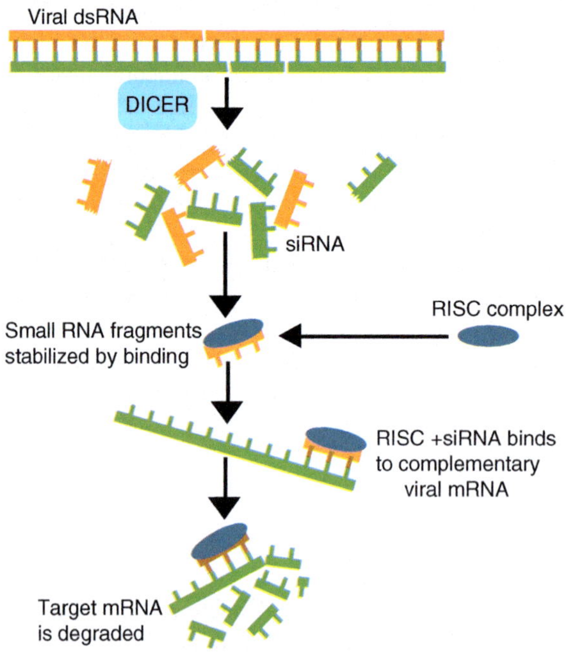

FIGURE 17.3

How viral interference inhibits viral replication.

Antibodies are not only directed against virion proteins but are also directed against new viral encoded proteins expressed by infected cells. As a result, these infected cells may also be destroyed. Antibodies may kill infected cells using complement or antibody-dependent cell-mediated cytotoxicity (ADCC). The cytotoxic cells include T cells, macrophages, and NK cells, using their Fc receptors, CD16, to bind to antibody-coated target cells.

Virus-neutralizing antibodies include IgG and IgM in serum and IgA in secretions. As in antibacterial immunity, IgG is quantitatively the most significant immunoglobulin, whereas IgM is qualitatively superior. Fig. 17.4.

Cell-mediated immunity

Although antibodies and complement can neutralize free virions and destroy virus infected cells, cell-mediated immune responses are much more important in controlling viral infections. Viral antigens may be expressed on infected cells long before progeny viruses are produced. When this endogenous antigen is presented by MHC class I molecules to cytotoxic $CD8^+$ T cells, the infected cells are recognized as foreign and killed. Viruses require host cells in which to replicate. Elimination of infected cells thus prevents viral spread. Although antibodies and complement or ADCC can assist, T cell-mediated cytotoxicity is the major protective mechanism. Cytotoxic T cells recognize peptide-MHC complexes and kill the presenting cells. Type I interferons

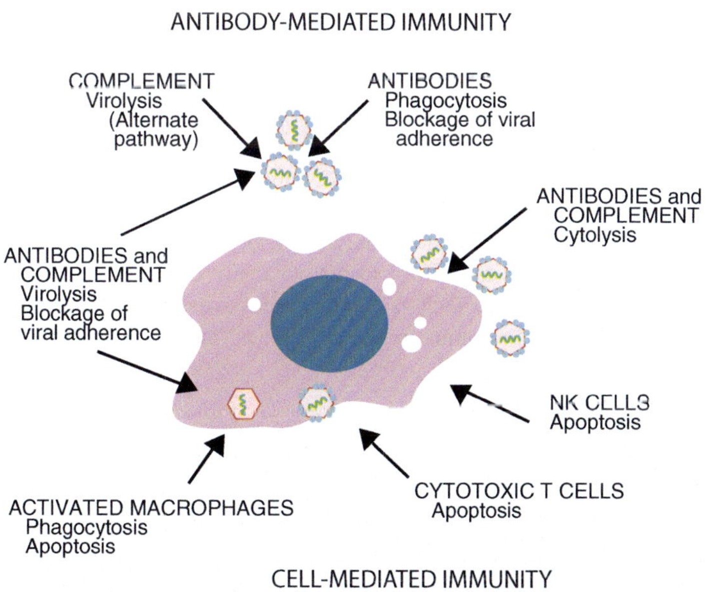

FIGURE 17.4

The diverse ways in which the adaptive immune system can protect a horse cell against viral invasion.

can sensitize virus-infected cells to this cytotoxic effect. Under some circumstances, cytotoxic T cells may kill intracellular viruses without killing the infected cells. This effect is mediated by T cell-derived IFN-γ and TNF-α. These cytokines activate two virucidal pathways. One pathway eliminates viral nucleocapsid particles, including their contained genomes. The second pathway destabilizes viral RNA.

Some viral antigens may act as superantigens by binding directly to TCR Vβ chains. For example, the rabies virus nucleocapsid binds to mouse $V\beta8^{+}$ T cells. By stimulating helper T cell activity in this way, rabies viruses can switch on Th2 cells. This, in turn, can result in an enhanced immune response to rabies viruses, as well as a polyclonal B cell response.

Macrophages develop antiviral activity following M1 activation. Viruses are readily endocytosed by macrophages and are then usually destroyed. If the viruses are noncytopathic and can grow inside macrophages, a persistent infection may result. Under these circumstances, the macrophages must be activated to eliminate the virus. Thus, M1 macrophage activation mediated by IFN-γ is a feature of equine infectious anemia (Cardeti et al., 2024).

The duration of immunological memory to viruses is highly variable. Antiviral antibodies may persist for many years in the absence of the virus. On the other hand, cytotoxic T cells die soon after virus elimination, while memory T cells can persist for many years (Chapter 12).

Evasion of the immune responses

As discussed above, during the millions of years they have coexisted with mammals, viruses have evolved numerous methods of evading host immune responses (Alcami & Koszinowski, 2000). RNA viruses have a very small genome with little room to spare for genes dedicated to suppressing immunity. As a result, RNA viruses tend to rely on genetic instsbility resulting in antigenic variation as their principal mechanism of immune evasion (Iannello et al., 2006). On the other hand, DNA viruses have a larger genome and can afford to devote many different genes to immune evasion. In large DNA viruses such as equine herpesvirus, as much as half the total genome may be devoted to immunoregulatory genes (Haig, 2001). Fig. 17.5.

Negative cytokine regulation

Viruses can block interferon activities. Methods range from blocking interferon receptor signal transduction to synthesizing soluble interferon receptors. Some viruses inhibit IFN-γ production by blocking the activities of IL-18 and IL-12, both of which are required for its production. Equine herpesvirus-1 (EHV-1) suppresses IFN-β production, and as a result, the expression of viperin is also suppressed. IFN-α production is also suppressed when EHV-1 invades mucosal surfaces such as the nasopharynx (Holmes et al., 2024). Some viruses make their own versions of cytokines and

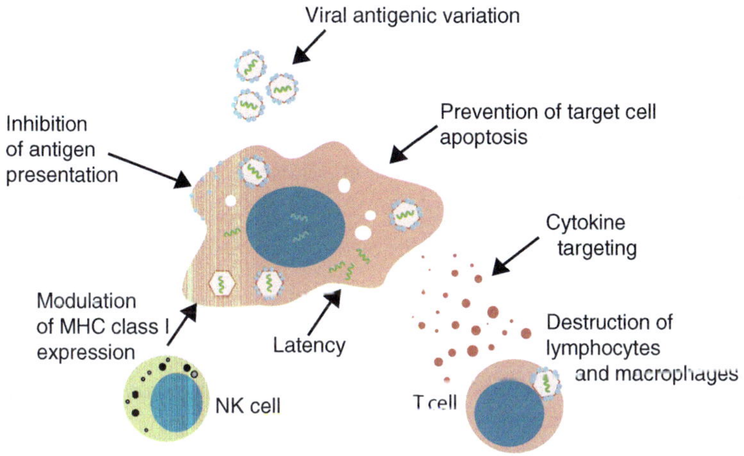

FIGURE 17.5

Some of the ways by which viruses evade destruction by the horse's immune system.

chemokines, and their receptors. For example, equine herpesvirus makes soluble CCR3, the receptor for CCL11. This effectively prevents it binding to the virions.

Interference with antigen processing

Many viruses interfere with the expression of MHC class I molecules and so inhibit antigen presentation (Rigden et al., 2002). They use many different suppressive techniques, including reducing transcription of MHC genes; blocking transporter protein function and thus the transport of peptides into the endoplasmic reticulum; inhibiting proteasomal degradation of viral proteins; inhibiting the intracellular transport of MHC class I α chains; preventing delivery of the loaded MHC to the cell surface; and ubiquinating and hence destroying MHC molecules. For example, equine herpesvirus-1 suppresses the expression of MHC class I molecules by interfering with transporter protein functions and down-regulating the expression of mRNA for MHC class I molecules. Other viruses may cause MHC class I molecules to be retained within a cell; they may prevent peptide binding to transporter proteins, prevent proteasomal degradation, redirect MHC molecules to lysosomes for degradation, or even encode inhibitors that block caspase activity. Influenza A viruses can stimulate the production of glucocorticosteroids, resulting in profound immunosuppression and secondary infections (Jamieson et al., 2010). They can also block macrophage differentiation into dendritic cells.

Evasion of natural killer cells

NK cells kill virus-infected cells at an early stage of infection before T and B cells are fully activated. Cytotoxic T cells kill targets that express foreign antigens on

MHC class I molecules. NK cells kill targets that fail to express these MHC class I molecules. For a virus to survive, it must induce the selective down-regulation of some MHC class I molecules, enabling the virus-infected cells to evade destruction by T cells while at the same time preventing NK cell activation (Lanier, 2008). This appears to be a strategy employed by equine herpesvirus-1 to ensure its persistence within infected horses (van der Meulen et al., 2006).

Alterations in the B cell system

One of the simplest mechanisms of viral immune evasion involves antigenic variation of RNA viruses. Multiple point mutations accompanied by poor editing functions of RNA polymerases permit the generation of many closely related but structurally, and antigenically, distinct viruses. The most significant examples of this occur among the influenza A viruses.

As influenza viruses spread through a population, they mutate and gradually change the structure of their hemagglutinins and neuraminidases. These changes alter the antigenicity of the virus. This gradual change is called antigenic "drift," and it permits the virus to persist in a population for many years. In addition, influenza viruses sporadically undergo a sudden, major genetic change in which a new strain develops whose hemagglutinins show no apparent relationship to the hemagglutinins of prior strains. Such a major change, called an antigenic "shift," is not due to mutation but results from recombination between two different virus strains. This occurs readily since the influenza virus has a segmented genome. It is the development of these naturally recombinant influenza viruses with a completely new antigenic structure that accounts for the periodic panzootics of influenza in horses.

Viral evasion through latency

In contrast to the short-lived immune response against bacteria, antiviral immunity is, in many cases, very long-lasting. One reason for this is related to virus persistence within cells, perhaps in a slowly replicating or a non-replicating form, as typified by equine herpesviruses. It is usually difficult to isolate viruses from an animal that has recovered from a herpesvirus infection. Sometime later, however, especially when the animal is stressed, the herpesvirus may reemerge and may even cause disease. During the latent period, when it is present in the host but cannot be reisolated, the virus nucleic acid persists in host cells, but its transcription is blocked, and no viral proteins are made. The persistent virus may periodically boost the immune response of the infected animal and, in this way, generate long-lasting immunity to superinfection. The immune responses in these cases, although unable to eliminate the virus, may prevent the development of clinical disease and therefore serve a protective role. Immunosuppression may permit clinical disease to recur in persistently infected animals. The association between stress and the development of some viral diseases is well recognized. It is likely that the increased steroid production in stressful situations may be sufficiently immunosuppressive to permit activation of latent viruses or infection by exogenous ones. For example, the stresses of transportation may result in horses redeveloping herpesvirus respiratory disease (Muscat et al., 2018).

Inhibition of apoptosis

Apoptosis may be considered a protective response since viruses also die when an infected cell dies. This is especially significant if a cell dies before virions are released. It is therefore to a virus's advantage to delay apoptosis until progeny viruses can be released. Thus, some herpesviruses, including equine herpesvirus-2, encode apoptosis inhibitors in their genomes.

Antibody-dependent enhancement

There are examples of virus infections in which the presence of antibodies results in increased susceptibility or severity of infection. Several mechanisms are involved in this, and many are poorly understood. This can involve antibody coating of virions so that their entry into cells through Fc receptors is facilitated. This FcR-mediated entry may be less effective than other routes in triggering interferon production. Virus-bound complement may similarly enhance virus infections. Equine infectious anemia viruses (EIAV) may increase their survival chances within an animal by similar mechanisms.

Some selected equine viral diseases

RNA viruses

RNA viruses have a relatively small genome. As a result, RNA viruses tend to rely on antigenic variation as their principal mechanism of immune evasion. Among the most important RNA viruses that affect horses are equine infectious anemia virus, the equine encephalitis viruses, equine arteritis virus, and equine influenza virus. Because of their antigenic variability, RNA viruses tend to cause more diverse disease problems than DNA viruses.

Equine infectious anemia

Equine infectious anemia is caused by a retrovirus within the lentivirus family,—EIAV. It is spread by biting flies such as Tabanids. The resulting disease may be acute, chronic, or inapparent (McGuire et al., 2002). Affected horses develop disease beginning about 7–15 days post-infection. They develop weight loss, ventral edema, and petechial hemorrhages. Following recovery from the first attack of disease characterized by anemia, fever, thrombocytopenia, and depression. Infected horses may remain healthy for weeks or months. However, three or four relapses and recurrent febrile episodes at 2- to 8-week intervals may occur before the horse either develops a chronic wasting disease or becomes clinically normal. Each episode of the disease tends to be milder than the previous one. The fevers are lower, and the anemia is less severe. All seropositive horses are considered infectious for life although they usually have a normal lifespan.

Antibody responses

Infected horses mount both antibody- and cell-mediated immune responses to EIAV, but despite this they remain infected for life. The detection of these antibodies by an immunoprecipitation assay (The Coggins Test) forms the basis of EIA control programs. However, cytotoxic $CD8^+$ T cells can be detected concurrently with viral clearance while neutralizing antibodies develop later, Horses infected with EIAV have unusually low levels of IgG3/5, although their circulating lymphocytes appear to be unaffected and respond normally to mitogens such as phytohemagglutinin.

Horses mount a significant antibody response aginst several different EIA viral core and envelope glycoproteins resulting in a hypergammaglobulinemia. This is especially marked in horses that suffer from repeated febrile episodes (Sellon, 1993).

Cell-mediated responses

it appears that cytotoxic T cells are primarily responsible for the control of the primary EIA viremia. These are MHC class I-restricted T cells. They are directed primarily against viral group specific (*gag*) epitopes. However, there is also evidence that envelope (*env*) epitopes are also the target of protective immunity (Hammond et al., 1997).

Another form of cell-mediated immunity to EIAV involves its destruction by activated macrophages. EIAV infects cells of the monocyte/macrophage lineage. It primarily replicates in organs containing large populations of macrophages, such as the liver, spleen, lungs, and lymph nodes. EIAV grows especially well in blood monocytes rather than tissue macrophages (Raabe et al., 1998). Thus, infected horses generate M1 macrophages that express metalloprotease 13 as well as interleukin-6 (Cardeti et al., 2024). These cells can then kill the virus.

Antigenic variation

The waves of viremia in EIA cases result from sequential antigenic variation in the viral envelope glycoproteins. EIAV, like other lentiviruses, undergoes random mutation, and new, antigenically different variants are produced at intervals. The elimination of each variant is determined by both $CD4^+$ and $CD8^+$ MHC-restricted cytotoxic T cells. Later, as new variants are produced, infected horses make neutralizing antibodies to that variant, and as a result, the viremia ends. Variants of EIAV, however, appear rapidly and randomly (Carpenter et al., 1987). The appearance of a new non-neutralizable variant leads to a viremic wave and clinical relapse. After the virus has undergone several antigenic variation cycles and the horse has responded to them all, the neutralizing antibody spectrum of the horse's serum becomes very broad, and viremia drops to a low level.

In addition to evading the immune response through repeated antigenic variation in its envelope protein, EIAV triggers immune-mediated tissue damage. Many of the antibodies produced by infected horses are not neutralizing. As a result, they bind to the virus but the virus remains infectious. These antibody-virus immune complexes persist in the circulation. The red cells of viremic horses adsorb the virus onto their surface. Antibodies and complement then bind to these coated red cells, as a result, complement is activated and the red cells are hemolyzed and cleared from the circulation resulting in severe anemia. These coated red cells are also readily phagocytosed by macrophages (Sentsui & Kono, 1987). Infected horses may also develop a membranoproliferative glomerulonephritis as a result of virus associated immune-complex deposition on their glomerular basement membranes.

Horses infected with EIAV appear to suffer from a transient phase of immunosuppression. Thus during viremic febrile episodes, their circulating lymphocytes have a significantly impaired response to mitogens such as phytohemagglutinin, concanavalin A, and pokeweed mitogen. This suppression could be induced by administering heat inactivated virus to experimental ponies suggesting that viral structural proteins are probably immunosuppressive (Newman et al., 1991).

Equine influenza

Equine influenza is caused by the influenza A virus. As in humans, the virus is transmitted by respiratory aerosols through coughing and nose-to-nose contact. The disease is most common in younger horses. They present with anorexia, fever, depression, a nasal discharge, coughing, and tachypnea. The disease has a high morbidity and a low mortality (Paillot, 2014).

Influenza viruses belong to the Orthomyxovirus family. They possess a single-stranded segmented RNA genome. The virus attacks and destroys epithelial cells in the trachea and bronchi, resulting in impaired mucus clearance and secondary bacterial invasion. Influenza viruses can stimulate the production of glucocorticosteroids, resulting in profound immunosuppression and secondary infections (Jamieson et al., 2010). It has been suggested, however, that variations in the severity of influenza may also be a result of the release of the proinflammatory cytokine interleukin-33 (Rozario et al., 2021).

Immunity to equine influenza involves both humoral and cell-mediated responses against the major viral antigens. Influenza A viruses express envelope proteins called hemagglutinins (H) and neuraminidases (N). There are at least 18 different hemagglutinins, and 9 neuraminidases found among the type A influenza viruses; they are identified according to a standard numbering system. The two subtypes of the equine influenza viruses are typified by A/equine/Prague/56, which has H7 and N7, and A/equine/Hong Kong/92, which has H3 and N8 (For more details, see Fig. 15.3).

As influenza viruses multiply, their RNA genome undergoes random mutation. As a result, they gradually change the structure of their hemagglutinins and neuraminidases. These changes alter the antigenicity of the virus. This gradual change is called antigenic drift. In horses, the rapid turnover of the population and the constant production of large numbers of susceptible young foals tends to ensure the persistence of influenza viruses without the necessity for extensive antigenic drift. As a result, the antigenic structure of equine influenza viruses has changed relatively slowly since they were first described. For example, the H3N8 equine influenza virus strains changed very little between 1963 and 1988. In 1989 they split into two clades. These two clades, one European and one American, differ in the structure of their hemagglutinin. Viruses of both clades can circulate in horse populations at the same time. Examples of the European clade include A/Italy/99 and A/Richmond/07. The American clade includes A/Ohio/03 and A/South Africa/03. The two clades are sufficiently antigenically different as to require both in vaccines. Both are distinctly different from the original strain A/Miami/1/63 (Lewis et al., 2011).

A serologic survey of horses in Mongolia has detected antibodies against the H5N1 bird flu virus in about 1% of animals suggesting that horses could potentially be infected with this widely distributed virus (Damdinjav et al., 2025). However, H5N1 seropositive horses have not been detected in North America as of January 2026.

Equine viral arteritis

Equine viral arteritis (EVA) is caused by a single-stranded RNA virus, the only member of the genus Alphaarterivirus in the subfamily Equarterivirinae. There is only one recognized viral serotype, but strains vary greatly in their virulence.

EVAV causes a systemic infection whose severity can vary from severe disease to asymptomatic infection. It commonly presents as anorexia, depression, and ventral edema. Pregnant mares may abort. Foals may also develop urticaria, rhinitis, dyspnea, and interstitial pneumonia. Most infections are inapparent (Holyoak et al., 2008). Its severity depends to a large extent on the age, breed, and sex of the horse. It tends to be endemic in Standardbreds, but only 5% of Thoroughbreds are seropositive.

Transmitted by aerosol, EVAV spreads rapidly within the lungs and then throughout the body. The virus can be detected in the bloodstream for 7–9 days, but then disappears as a result of the production of neutralizing antibodies. In most cases, the virus is eliminated by 28 days. However, a testosterone-dependent, persistent infection occurs in stallions.

As its name implies, EVA virus grows and destroys vascular endothelial cells, resulting in increased vascular permeability, hemorrhage, and edema, as well as the degeneration and necrosis of the arterial tunica media in small arteries. This is accompanied by a leukopenia and thrombocytopenia (Chirnside, 1992). Evidence from other species has demonstrated that arteriviruses bind to the neonatal immunoglobulin receptor, FcRn in order to invade cells. The virus uses this in association with the cell surface receptor CD163 (Shaw et al., 2024) (Chapter 10)

Horses can be divided into susceptible and resistant groups based on whether they possess a subpopulation of $CD3^+$ T cells that are susceptible to EAV

(Balasuriya et al., 2016). A comparison of susceptible and resistant stallions has indicated that EVA susceptibility is linked to an SNP found on chromosome ECA11. This SNP is located in exon 1 of the CXCL16 chemokine gene (Tallmadge et al., 2020). The CXCL16 chemokine exists as a cell membrane-bound form, and the EqCXCL16 transmembrane protein serves as a coreceptor for EVAV. EVAV therefore preferentially infects subpopulations of $CD14^+$ monocytes expressing this specific CXCL16 allele (Sarkar et al., 2016a). It is also expressed on equine $CD3^+$ T cells. As a result, stallions that possess this specific susceptibility gene retain these persistently infected T cells within the ampullae of their vas deferens and can act as long-term viral carriers (Balasuriya et al., 2016; Sarkar et al., 2016b).

In addition to infecting and destroying vascular endothelial cells, EVAV also grows well in macrophages. As a result, it can activate these cells and induce production of the inflammatory cytokines, IL-1β, IL-6, TNF-α, and CXCL8. This cytokine release plays a key role in determining the severity of the disease. However, the infection also has an immunosuppressive effect. Thus, investigations have shown that EAV-infected macrophages show reduced endocytosis and phagocytosis. In addition, EAV also suppresses the functions of monocyte-derived dendritic cells. Their antigen-presenting ability is impaired. They cannot stimulate T cells, and they undergo an early death by apoptosis (Moyo et al., 2023).

Viral encephalitis

The Togaviridae are subdivided into the Alphaviruses that cause diseases such as Eastern (EEE), Western (WEE), and Venezuelan equine encephalitides (VEE). and the Flaviviruses such as West Nile Virus (WNV). All these viruses can cause severe neurologic diseases in both humans and horses. These viruses are carried by birds. Many different bird species can act as reservoirs of these viruses. In the case of the Alphaviruses, they are transmitted to humans and horses by the bite of an infected mosquito, *Culiseta melanura*. When they infect horses, they cause a generalized febrile response, accompanied by colic, and neurologic changes such as blindness, head pressing, ataxia, and compulsive walking.

Local replication of the virus at the injection site is followed by lymphatic spread to the spleen and liver. This results in a short viremia when the virus crosses into the brain. It mainly affects the cerebrum. The brain lesions in EEE are associated with neutrophilic cuffing, whereas those in WEE cases are characterized by lymphocytic/plasmacytic cuffing.

Like other viruses, the alphaviruses suppress the horse's immune response. The viral non-structural protein nsP2 can suppress the host's interferon response. by inhibiting the cGAS-STING pathway. In addition, Alphaviruses avoid lymphoid organs. Thus, they do not grow in innate immune cells such as monocytes or dendritic cells and hence avoid triggering a strong type I interferon response (Parashar et al., 2025). They also inhibit gene transcription, thus suppressing T cell responses and downregulating MHC expression.

West Nile virus

West Nile fever is caused by a single-stranded RNA virus of the genus Flavivirus (WNV). It is transmitted to horses by the bite of culicine mosquitoes. Following local multiplication at the bite site, viremia begins 3–5 days later. The virus infects the brain in about 10% of cases. It causes a diffuse or multifocal encephalitis. This usually begins with depression and anorexia, weakness, ataxia, and neurologic signs such as narcolepsy or excitability. Mortality is estimated to be about 30%–40%. Equine susceptibility to this virus is associated with a haplotype comprising six SNPs. These susceptibility genotypes are associated with MHC and Ly49 alleles, although the precise locations of these genes have yet to be identified (Tallmadge et al., 2020).

WNV triggers both innate and adaptive immune responses that eventually lead to viral clearance. Activated macrophages show increased nitric oxide production. and express increased levels of type I and type II interferons. In addition, upregulation of TNF-α, IL-1β, CXCL10, TLRs, and MyD88 can be detected in lymphoid tissues (Bielefeldt- Ohmann et al., 2017). Cell mediated immunity plays a key role in disease recovery. For example, both $CD4^+$ and $CD8^+$ T cells invade the brain lesions. The $CD8^+$ T cells are responsible for viral clearance. West Nile virus induces a long-lasting memory T cell response to viral antigens that persists for at least a year (Tolnai et al., 2025)

Infected horses also mount an effective antibody-mediated response. Seroconversion occurs by 10 days, and peak antibody titers are reached by 21 days (Naveed et al., 2024). A study on the immunoglobulin isotypes induced by WNV in infected and vaccinated horses found that IgM responses were detected in infected horse sera but not in vaccinated animals. The natural antibody response induced by infection or vaccination was primarily composed of IgG1 subclass immunoglobulins (Khatibzadeh et al., 2015).

African horse sickness

African horse sickness (AHS) is caused by a double-stranded non-enveloped RNA Orbivirus belonging to the family Reoviridae. It is related to the Bluetongue virus in ruminants. AHS is not contagious but is spread between animals by biting Culicoides midges. It is enzootic in much of Africa and South Asia. It is genetically diverse with nine distinct serotypes due to variations in its seven structural protein genes. One of these proteins, VP2, is the majpr target of this antigenic variation (Barbour & Restrepo, 2000).

After transmission to a horse by a midge bite, the virus first moves to regional lymph nodes, and this is followed by a primary viremia. The virus subsequently reaches its target organs, specifically the lungs and lymphoid tissues. The disease varies greatly in its lethality, ranging from the peracute form, with 95% mortality, to "horse sickness fever", where the animals recover. It can also be classified into pulmonary, cardiac, and fever forms. Mules are less susceptible and have a 50%–70% mortality. Donkeys are resistant and usually develop subclinical disease.

Following primary replication, the subsequent viremia spreads the virus through the body. Like bluetongue virus, the virus spread may be facilitated by adsorption to erythrocytes. The virus then binds to, invades, and replicates in vascular endothelial cells. The resulting damage results in fluid leakage and edema as well as thrombosis, a leukopenia, and severe thrombocytopenia. As a result, it causes significant damage to the lungs and other target organs (Pretorius et al., 2012). Disseminated intravascular coagulation is also a significant cause of death in infected animals (Burrage & Laegreid, 1994). The resulting consumptive coagulopathy results in excessive hemorrhage in sick horses.

Given time, infected horses mount an effective immune response to the AHS virus. Protection is primarily mediated by antibodies directed against the serotype-specific outer capsid viral protein VP2. Antibodies target multiple epitopes on VP2. In addition, there is a cell-mediated response to the virus, and at least three different $CD8^+$ T cell epitopes have been identified on VP2 in addition to an IFN-γ response. Attenuated vaccines are usually administered annually in endemic areas (Dennis et al., 2019). Studies on the response to these vaccines show a secondary response involving both B and T cells. The T cells are $CD8^+$ and are assumed to be cytotoxic (Pretorius et al., 2012).

Equine serum hepatitis

On rare occasions, horses may develop lethal, acute hepatic necrosis 30–70 days after being treated with an immune globulin of equine origin. This is called equine serum hepatitis or Theiler's disease. Arnold Theiler noted hundreds of cases of hepatitis in horses following passive immunization with equine antiserum (Aleman et al., 2005; Panciera, 1969). It occurred in horses that had received antiserum against tetanus, botulism, *Strep. equi*, anthrax, influenza, or encephalitis, as well as pregnant mare serum and equine plasma. The disease has also occurred after active immunization against equine encephalitis and rhinopneumonitis when the vaccines were prepared using fetal equine cells. Certain serum mixtures or just a single vaccine batch have been associated with outbreaks of the disease. Occasional cases have been described in untreated horses living with affected animals, suggesting that the disease is transmissible (Hjerpe, 1964).

Four novel viruses have been identified in horses with Theiler's disease. Three of these are flaviviruses (Hepacivirus, Theiler's disease-associated virus, and Equine Pegivirus), and the fourth is Equine Parvovirus (EqPV-H) (Rasche et al., 2021).). Hepacivirus causes a transient hepatitis, although it may result in chronic hepatitis. Theiler's virus was identified during an outbreak of acute hepatitis in horses that had received equine botulinum antitoxin. In another example, 15 out of 17 (88%) horses injected with a specific lot of immune globulin were shown to be carrying the pegivirus. The disease was severe, with 53%–88% mortality. Clinical signs included anorexia, icterus, excessive sweating, and neurological abnormalities. Clinical chemistry confirmed severe liver damage with high liver enzyme levels, ammonia, and bilirubin. However, equine pegivirus has been' reported to be a common infection in horses in the United States and Europe and is not associated with hepatitis (Tomlinson et al., 2020)

In a more recent situation, a horse that died 65 days after receiving tetanus antitoxin was shown to be infected by a parvovirus. The virus was shown to be present in the tetanus antitoxin administered to this horse 9 weeks previously. This equine parvovirus-hepatitis (EqPV-H) virus belongs to the *Copiparvovirus* genus and is related to the bovine and porcine parvoviruses. Experimental inoculation of EqPV-H into two healthy adult horses resulted in the development of acute hepatitis 80–90 days later. Subsequent studies have demonstrated that EqPV-H was present in 18 consecutive cases of Theiler's disease, while the other viruses were not consistently present. EqPV-H appears to be endemic in some horse populations since 13% of a random sample had circulating antibodies against it. In another study, 9/10 horses with Theiler's disease and 20/37 in-contact horses were positive for EqPV-H by PCR (Tomlinson et al., 2020).

Commercial tetanus antitoxin is usually heated at 60°C for 1 hour, but parvoviruses are relatively heat-resistant. Some antitoxins have added phenol or thiomersal as preservatives, but while these may inactivate the flaviviruses, they may be insufficient to inactivate EqPV-H. Producers of equine blood products must ensure that their products are free of all these viruses.

Hendraviruses

Hendravirus is, as described in the chapter on vaccines, is a negative stranded RNA virus that causes an acute and fatal disease in horses in Eastern Australia. Its reservoir hosts are fruit bats. A successful subunit vaccine has been developed against it (Middleton et al., 2014).

DNA viruses

Viruses, if they are to survive, must evade the immune responses. They use many different mechanisms, including, but not limited to, severe immunosuppression. These may also result in significant immunopathology. The major DNA virus diseases affecting horses are caused by Equine herpesviruses-1 and -4. DNA viruses have a large genome and, as a result, can afford to devote many different genes to immune evasion. In large DNA viruses such as the equine herpesviruses, as much as half their total genome may be devoted to immunoregulatory genes (Haig, 2001).

Equine herpesvirus-1 and -4

Important horse diseases are caused by members of the family of equid alphaherpesviruses. Nine different equid herpesviruses have been identified. Five of these infect domestic equids, while two different viruses infect zebras. The most important of these is equine herpesvirus-1 (EHV-1). Its genome consists of linear double-stranded DNA of about 150 kilobase pairs. EHV-2 and EHV-5 are also found in horses with respiratory disease, but their significance is unclear. Both of these are classified as gammaherpesviruses (Fu et al., 1986). EHV-3 is the causal agent of equine coital exanthema (Allen et al., 1977). EHV-4 causes especially severe abortion outbreaks.

Equine herpesviruses type 1 (EHV-1) and type 4 (EHV-4) cause respiratory and neurologic disease and abortion. They are usually transmitted between horses through direct contact with infectious secretions or by inhalation of infectious aerosols genertated by caughing and sneezing. Both viruses cause upper respiratory tract disease with fever, lethargy, anorexia, nasal discharge, cough, and mandibular lymphadenopathy. Both EHV-1 and EHV-4 can cause abortion in naïve mares, weak nonviable foals, or a relatively infrequent paralytic neurologic disease (equine herpesvirus myeloencephalopathy, EHM).

Pathogenesis

When EHV-1 first invades a horse, it replicates in the epithelial cells of the upper respiratory tract (Laval et al., 2021). This induces a short-lived local inflammatory response characterized by the production of IFN-α. Other chemokines and cytokines, such as IL-10 and IFN-γ are also produced at this time. EHV-virions are resistant to the lethal effects of equine nasal defensins. The virus triggers a limited antibody response mainly involving IgG1, IgG4/7, and IgA production (Larson & Wagner, 2021). The infection causes mild respiratory symptoms as a result of epithelial cell destruction. Fig. 17.6.

EHV infection is mild and self-limiting in most cases since the virus moves elsewhere. For example, in some horses, the virus succeeds in crossing the epithelial

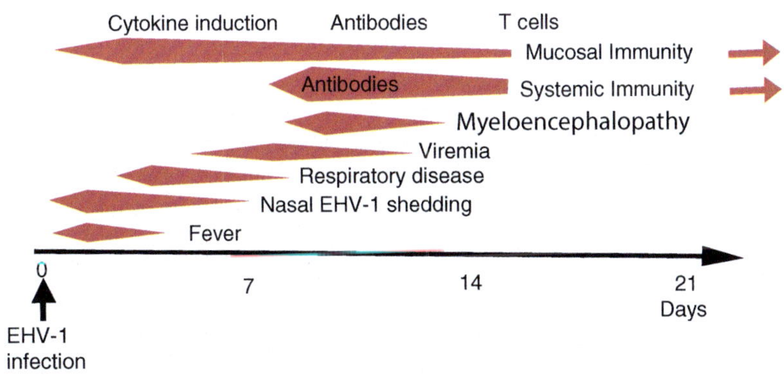

FIGURE 17.6

The timeline of onset and duration of clinical signs, viral shedding, cell-associated viremia and immunity after EHV-1 infection of a naive or susceptible horse.

- *From Larson, E. M., & Wagner, B. (2021). Viral infection and allergy—What immune responses can tell us about disease severity and infection.* Molecular Immunology, 135, *329–341.*

basement membrane, probably by the migration of infected leukocytes. From there, it reaches the bloodstream and the draining lymph nodes. Thus, there is a cell-associated viremia. The virus also enters nerve endings in the respiratory epithelium and reaches the trigeminal ganglion. The virus also establishes a latent infection in the lymphoid tissues. Once it has reached the bloodstream, the infected leukocytes bind to endothelial cells. The virus specifically targets endothelial cells in the pregnant uterus and the central nervous system.

Secondary replication of EHV-1 in the pregnant uterus causes vasculitis and local thrombosis that results in necrosis and edema of the endometrium and can lead to abortion. Secondary replication of the blood vessels in the CNS can cause vasculitis, thrombosis, and ischemic necrosis of brain tissue. Depending upon the extent of the damage, this can be fatal.

Like other herpesviruses, the EHVs establish a latent infection in horses, which then become asymptomatic carriers. Most horses are therefore re-infected multiple times during their lifetime, usually sub-clinically. Viral reactivation occurs when horses are stressed, resulting in a viremia and short-term viral shedding.

Initially, horses mount a local innate immune response associated with the production of the type I interferons, IFN-α and IFN-β. This is associated with the short duration of the infection of the respiratory epithelium and reduced viral shedding. Likewise, the local innate response is associated with upregulation of TLR-3 and TLR9 as well as the production of cytokines such as IL-1β, TNF-α, and IL-6, in addition to the production of chemokines CXCL-8, CCL2, CCL5, and MCP-1. Some of the EHV glycoproteins however, control the recruitment of leukocytes to the equine respiratory tract. One glycoprotein, (gG) can bind chemokines and so block the immigration of neutrophils in response to CXCL8 (Van de Walle et al., 2007). A second viral glycoprotein (gp2), has similar blocking properties, while a third protein, pUL56, downregulates MHC class I expression on infected cells and so enables the virus to evade cytotoxic T cell lysis (Soboll Hussey et al., 2014). It is of interest to note that transcriptomic analysis of infected and non-infected nasal mucosa has demonstrated upregulation of IFN-α in non-immune horses but not in the mucosa of immune horses (Holmes et al., 2024). It has also been demonstrated that EHV-1 infection can significantly downregulate endothelial cell expression of TLR3 and TLR4. It also blocks the downstream signaling of the JAK/STAT pathway. As a result, EHV-1 also downregulates the IFN-β response in equine endothelial cells (Oladunni et al., 2019).

In addition to the innate response, horses mount a local T cell response in the nasal mucosa. Many of these are double-positive cells ($CD4^+$ $CD8^+$). The T cells in the epithelial layer are primarily $CD4^+$, whereas $CD8^+$ cells predominate in the mucosa and submucosa. On stimulation with EHV-1, these mucosal T cells fail to produce IFN-γ (Holmes & Wagner, 2024).

A primary EHV-1 infection triggers an antibody response involving the production of IgG subclasses IgG1, IgG4/7, and IgG3/5. (In effect, reflecting both Th1 and Th2 responses.) However, prior sensitization with EHV-4 results in horses mounting a Th1-biased subclass response against subsequent EHV-1 infection involving only

IgG1 and IgG 4/7 (Bannai et al., 2011). High serum IgG4/7 antibody titers are associated with the prevention of viral shedding, viremia, and immunity. In immune horses, protective immunity is linked to the production of intranasal antibodies of the IgG4/7 subclass. They appear to be virus-neutralizing (Perkins et al., 2019).

When EHV-1 infects lymphocytes, its expression of the viral glycoproteins gC and gD is delayed; as a result, the infected cells continue to circulate as normal despite the presence of virus-neutralizing antibodies. EHV gains entrance to these cells by binding to the cell surface CD172a and then undergoing endocytosis (Laval et al., 2021). Subsequent abortion and neurologic disease develop when the virus spreads from the infected leukocytes to vascular endothelial cells. Given its extensive immune evasive mechanisms and tendency to develop latency, it is unsurprising that vaccines directed against EHV-1 are not as effective as desired (Kydd et al., 2006). Other equine herpesviruses may employ other immunoevasive techniques. For example, EHV-2 harbors a gene encoding an interleukin-10-like protein (Rode et al., 1993).

Some donkey viral diseases

Despite the fact that donkeys are a large and important component of the global equine population, there is not a lot of information regarding their susceptibility or immunity to the major equine viral diseases. In practice, horses and donkeys are susceptible to many of the same vital infections, but there are subtle differences that must be considered (Barrandeguy & Carossino, 2018). Donkeys are often permitted to live much longer than horses, and geriatric changes in their immune system must be taken into consideration (Chapter 25).

Equine infectious anemia

Infected donkeys tend to have very low levels of EIA viremia compared to horses. As a result, they rarely show clinical signs. Thus, in one study, the viral load in donkeys was approximately 1000 times lower than in horses. In this study, the monocytes of both species were equally susceptible in vitro, indicating that the difference is not related to the permissiveness of the host cells. The EIAV RNA appears to be translated into protein in horse cells more efficiently than in donkey cells (Camara et al., 2020). EIA has been reported to occur in mules. When donkeys and ponies were infected with two strains of EIAV known to cause disease in horses, the ponies sickened. The donkeys did not (Cook et al., 2001). They remained asymptomatic except for a transient decrease in their platelet counts.

Equine influenza

Influenza is the most common infectious respiratory disease in donkeys and cases have ben reported worldwide. Infected donkeys and mules show similar clinical signs to those seen in horses. However, influenza tendsto be more severe in donkeys with the subsequent development of bronchopneumonia. Thus, affected donkeys may require antibiotic and anti-inflammatory treatment. Reports from China indicate that influenza-infected donkeys have a higher mortality than do horses (Camara et al., 2020).

Equine viral arteritis

EVAV is a widely distributed disease capable of infecting donkeys and mules. Infected donkeys tend to have subclinical infections or show mild clinical signs (Mendoza et al., 2018). When they sicken, they develop fever and mild depression, as well as an ocular and nasal discharge. However, since they are mainly asymptomatic, they can serve as potential reservoirs of the virus. There are donkey-specific strains that are rarely tramsmitted to horses. Thus, donkey stallions are also involved in virus transmission.

Alphaviral encephalitis

Donkeys and mules develop similar clinical signs and have a similar susceptibility and case fatality rate to EEV and VEE infections as do horses (Camara et al., 2020). They are also susceptible to infection by WNV although it is unclear to what extent they develop clinical disease (Molini et al., 2021). WNV infection has been reported to be present in donkeys showing neurological signs. Following a brief remission, the animals developed liver failure (Camara et al., 2020). This has also been reported to occur in mules. Some surveys have reported widespread WNV seropositivity in donkey populations without evidence of disease.

African horse sickness

Experimental studies on African donkeys indicate that they are resistant to AHSV. They develop minimal lesions on experimental challenge and the disease is rarely fatal. They may become asymptomatic carriers of the virus (Camara et al., 2020). However, European donkeys appear to be highly susceptible and develop a fatal disease (Barrandeguy & Carossino, 2018).

Equine herpesviruses

Asinine herpesviruses (AHV-1 through AHV-8) also belong to the Alphaherpesvirus family. Like other herpesviruses they usually establish latent infections. As in horses, both AHV-1 and AHV-4 have been associated with abortion, respiratory, and neurologic disease in donkeys. AHV-4 and AHV-5 may be the causal agents of pulmonary fibrosis (Mendoza et al., 2018). The donkey and equine herpesviruses are closely related, with 55%–96% amino acid sequence identity. Some studies have indicated that there is a higher prevalence of herpesvirus in donkeys than in horses.

AHV-3 appears to be well-adapted to donkeys and only induces a mild rhinitis. (Barrandeguy & Carossino, 2018. There are currently no vaccines avaailable to protect donkeys against AHV. Equine herpesvirus EHV-8, has been reported to cause encephalitis in donkeys in China (Wang et al., 2022).

References

Alcami, A., & Koszinowski, U. H. (2000). Viral mechanisms of immune evasion. *Trends in Microbiology, 8*, 410–418.

Aleman, M., Nieto, J. E., Carr, E. A., & Carlson, G. P. (2005). Serum hepatitis associated with commercial plasma transfusion in horses. *Journal of Veterinary Internal Medicine, 19*, 120–122.

Allen, G. P., O'Callaghan, D. J., & Randall, C. C. (1977). Genetic relatedness of equine herpesvirus types 1 and 3. *Journal of Virology, 24*, 761–767.

Assil, S., Coléon, S., Dong, C., Decembre, E., et al. (2019). Plasmacytoid dendritic cells and infected cells form an interferogenic synapse required for antiviral responses. *Cell Host & Microbe, 25*, 730–745.

Bai, B., Zhang, X., Zhang, M., Ma, W., et al. (2025). EIAV encodes an accessory protein that antagonizes the host restriction factor equine tetherin. *Proceedings of the National Academy of Sciences*. https://doi.org/10.1073/pnas.2413703122

Balasuriya, U. B. R., Sarkar, S., Carossino, M., Go, Y. Y., et al. (2016). Host factors that contribute to equine arteritis virus persistence in the stallion: An update. *Journal of Equine Veterinary Science, 43*, s11–s17.

Bannai, H., Tsujimura, K., Kondo, T., Nemoto, M., et al. (2011). Induction of a Th1—Biased IgG subclass response against equine herpesvirus type 1 in horses previously infected with type 4 virus. *Virology, 73*(4), 535–539.

Barbour, A. G., & Restrepo, B. I. (2000). Antigenic variation in vector-borne pathogens. *Emerging Infectious Diseases, 6*, 449–456.

Barrandeguy, N. E., & Carossino, M. (2018). Infectious diseases in donkeys and mules: An overview and update. *Journal of Equine Veterinary Science, 65*, 98–105.

Bielefeldt-Ohmann, H., Bosco-Louth, A., Hartwig, A.-E., Uddin, M. J., et al. (2017). Characterization of non-lethal West Nile virus (WNV) infection of horses: Subclinical pathology and innate immune response. *Microbial Pathogenesis, 103*, 71–79.

Burrage, T. G., & Laegreid, W. W. (1994). African horse sickness: Pathogenesis and immunity. *Comparative Immunology, Microbiology & Infectious Diseases, 17*(3/4), 275–285.

Camara, R. J. F., Bueno, B. L., Resende, C. F., Balasuriya, U. B. R., et al. (2020). Viral diseases that affect donkeys and mules. *Animals*. https://doi.org/10.3390/ani10122203

Cardeti, G., Manna, G., Cersini, A., Nardini, R., et al. (2024). Horse innate immunity in the control of equine infectious anemia virus infection: A preliminary study. *Viruses*. https://doi.org/10.3390/v16121804

Carpenter, S., Evans, L. H., Sevoian, M., & Chesebro, B. (1987). Role of the host immune response in selection of equine infectious anemia variants. *Journal of Virology, 61*, 3783.

Chirnside, E. D. (1992). Equine arteritis virus: An overview. *British Veterinary Journal, 148*, 181–197.

Cook, S. J., Cook, R. F., Montelaro, R. C., & Issel, C. J. (2001). Differential responses of *Equus caballus* and *Equus asinus* to infection with two pathogenic strains of equine infectious anemia virus. *Veterinary Microbiology, 79*, 93–109.

Damdinjav, B., Raveendran, S., Mojsiejczuk, B., Ankhanbaatar, U., et al. (2025). Evidence of influenza A (H5N1) spillover infections in horses, Mongolia. *Emerging Infectious Diseases, 31*(1), 183–185.

de Amorin, Byron, M., Giudici, A. J. L., Chong, L., et al. (2023). Characterization of interferons in the equine conceptus and endometrium. *Journal of Equine Veterinary Science, 25*, Article 104764.

Dennis, S. J., Meyers, A. E., Hitzeroth, I. I., & Rybicki, E. P. (2019). African horse sickness: A review of current understanding and vaccine development. *Viruses*. https://doi.org/10.3390/v11090844

Detournay, O., Morrison, D. A., Wagner, B., Zarnegar, B., & Wattrang, E. (2013). Genome analysis and mRNA expression of equine type 1 interferon genes. *Journal of Interferon & Cytokine Research*. https://doi.org/10.1089/jir.2012.0130

Fischer, C. D., Wachoski-Dark, G. L., Grant, D. M., Bramer, S. A., & Klein, C. (2018). Interferon epsilon is constitutively expressed in equine endometrium and up-regulated during the luteal phase. *Animal Reproduction Science, 195*, 38–43.

Fu, Z. F., Robinson, A. J., Horner, G. W., Dickinson, L. G., et al. (1986). Respiratory disease in foals and the epizootiology of equine herpesvirus type 2 infection. *New Zealand Veterinary Journal, 34*, 152–155.

Haig, D. M. (2001). Subversion and piracy: DNA viruses and immune evasion. *Research in Veterinary Science, 70*, 205–219.

Hammond, S. A., Cook, S. J., Lichtenstein, D. L., Issel, C. J., & Montelaro, R. C. (1997). Maturation of the cellular and humoral immune responses to persistent infection in horses by equine infectious anemia virus is a complex and lengthy process. *Journal of Virology, 71*, 3840–3852.

Heinrich, A., Riethmuller, D., Gloger, M., Schusser, G. F., et al. (2009). RNA interference protects horse cells *in vitro* from infection with Equine Arteritis Virus. *Antiviral Research, 81*, 209=216.

Helbig, K. J., & Beard, M. R. (2014). The role of viperin in the innate antiviral response. *Journal of Molecular Biology, 426*, 1210–1219.

Hjerpe, C. A. (1964). Serum hepatitis in the horse. *Journal of the American Veterinary Medical Association, 144*, 734–740.

Holmes, C. M., Babasyan, S., Eady, N., Schnabel, C. L., & Wagner, B. (2024). Immune horses rapidly increase antileukoproteinase and lack type 1 interferon secretion during mucosal innate immune responses against equine herpesvirus type 1. *Microbiology Spectrum*. https://doi.org/10.1128/spectrum.01092-24

Holmes, C. M., & Wagner, B. (2024). Characterization of nasal mucosal T cells in horses and their response to equine herpesvirus type 1. *Viruses*. https://doi.org/10.3390/v16101514

Holyoak, G. R., Balasuriya, U. B. R., Broaddus, C. C., & Timoney, P. J. (2008). Equine viral arteritis: Current status and prevention. *Theriogenology*. https://doi.org/10.1016/j.theriogenology.2008.04.020

Iannello, A., Debbeche, O., Martin, E., et al. (2006). Viral strategies for evading antiviral cellular immune responses of the host. *Journal of Leukocyte Biology, 79*, 16–35.

Ichihashi, T., Asano, A., Usui, T., Takeuchi, T., & WatanabeY, Y. Y. (2013). Antiviral and antiproliferative effects of canine interferon-λ1. *Veterinary Immunology and Immunopathology, 156*, 141–146.

Jamieson, A. M., Yu, S., Annicelli, C. H., & Medzhitov, R. (2010). Influenza virus-induced glucocorticoids compromise innate host defense against a secondary bacterial infection. *Cell Host & Microbe, 18*, 103–114.

Khatibzadeh, S. M., Gold, C. B., Keggan, A. E., Perkins, G. A., et al. (2015). West Nile virus-specific immunoglobulin isotype responses in vaccinated and infected horses. *American Journal of Veterinary Research, 76*(1), 92–100.

Klotman, M. E., & Chang, T. L. (2006). Defensins in innate antiviral immunity. *Nature Reviews Immunology, 6*, 447–456.

Kydd, J. H., Townsend, H. G. G., & Hannant, D. (2006). The equine immune response to equine herpesvirus-1. The virus and its vaccines. *Veterinary Immunology and Immunopathology, 111*, 15–30.

Lanier, L. L. (2008). Evolutionary struggles between NK cells and viruses. *Nature Reviews Immunology, 8*, 259–268.

Larson, E. M., & Wagner, B. (2021). Viral infection and allergy—What immune responses can tell us about disease severity and infection. *Molecular Immunology, 135*, 329–341.

Laval, K., Poelaert, K. C. K., Cleemput, J. V., Zhao, j, et al. (2021). The pathogenesis and immune evasive mechanisms of equine herpesvirus type 1. *Frontiers in Microbiology*. https://doi.org/10.3389/fmicb.2021.662686

Lazear, H. M., Schoggins, J. W., & Diamond, M. S. (2019). Shared and distinct functions of type I and type III interferons. *Immunity, 50*, 907–923.

Lewis, N. S., Daly, J. M., Russell, C. A., Horton, D. L., et al. (2011). Antigenic and genetic evolution of equine influenza A (H3N8) virus from 1968 to 2007. *Journal of Virology, 85*, 12742–12749.

Lund, J. M., Alexopoulou, L., Sato, A., et al. (2005). Recognition of single-stranded RNA viruses by toll-like receptor 7. *Proceedings of the National Academy of Sciences of the United States of America, 101*, 5598–5603.

Maillard, P. V., Ciaudo, C., Marchais, A., Li, Y., Jay, F., Ding, S. W., & Voinnet, O. (2013). Antiviral RNA interference in mammalian cells. *Science, 342*, 235–238.

McGuire, T. C., Fraser, D. G., & Mealey, R. H. (2002). Cytotoxic T lymphocytes and neutralizing antibody in the control of equine infectious anemia virus. *Viral Immunology, 15*, 521–531.

Mendoza, F. J., Toribio, R. E., & Perez-Ecija, A. (2018). Donkey internal medicine—Part II: Cardiovascular, respiratory, neurologic, urinary, opthalmic, dermatology and musculoskeletal disorders. *Journal of Equine Veterinary Science, 65*, 86–97.

Middleton, D., Pallister, J., Klein, R., Feng, Y.-R., et al. (2014). Hendra virus vaccine, a one health approach to protecting horse, human, and environmental health. *Emerging Infectious Diseases, 20*(3), 372–379.

Molini, U., Franzo, G., Nel, H., Khaiseb, S., et al. (2021). West Nile virus seroprevalence in a selected donkey population in Namibia. *Frontiers in Veterinary Science*. https://doi.org/10.3389/fvets.2021.681354

Moyo, N. A., Westcott, D., Simmonds, R., & Steinbach, F. (2023). Equine arteritis virus in monocytic cells suppressed differentiation and function of dendritic cells. *Viruses*. https://doi.org/10.3390/v15010255

Muscat, K. E., Padalino, B., Hartley, C. A., Ficorilli, et al. (2018). Equine transport and changes in equine herpesvirus status. *Frontiers in Veterinary Science*. https://doi.org/10.3389/fvets.2018.00224

Naveed, A., EertinkLG, W. D., & Li, F. (2024). Lessons learned from West Nile virus infection: Vaccinations in equines and their implications for one health approaches. *Viruses*. https://doi.org/10.3390/v16050781

Newman, M. J., Issel, C. J., Truax, R. E., Powell, M. D., et al. (1991). Transient suppression of equine immune responses by equine infectious anemia virus (EIAV). *Virology, 184*(1), 55–66.

Oladunni, F. S., Sarkar, S., Reedy, S., Balasuriya, et al. (2019). Equid herpesvirus 1 targets the sensitization and induction steps to inhibit the type I interferon response in equine endothelial cells. *Journal of Virology*. https://doi.org/10.1128/JVL.01342-19

Paillot, R. (2014). A systematic review of recent advances in equine influenza vaccination. *Vaccines, 2*, 797–831.

Panciera, R. J. (1969). Serum hepatitis in the horse. *Journal of the American Veterinary Medical Association, 155*, 408–410.

Parashar, S., Malviya, R., Sridhar, S. B., Wadhwa, T., et al. (2025). Eastern equine encephalitis virus: Pathogenesis, immune response and clinical manifestations. *Infectious Medicine*. https://doi.org/10.1016/j.imj.2025.100167

Perkins, G., Babasyan, S., Stout, A. E., Freer, H., et al. (2019). Intranasal IgG4/7 antibody responses protect horses against equid herpesvirus 1 (EHV-1) infection including nasal virus shedding and cell-associated viremia. *Virology, 531*, 219–232.

Pretorius, A., Van Kleef, M., Van Wyngaardt, W., & Heath, J. (2012). Virus specific CD8+- T cells detected in PBMC in horses vaccinated against African horse sickness virus. *Veterinary Immunology and Immunopathology, 146*, 81–86.

Raabe, M. R., Issel, C. J., & Montelaro, R. C. (1998). Equine monocyte-derived macrophage cultures and their application for infectivity and neutralization studies of equine infectious anemia virus. *Journal of Virological Methods, 71*, 87–104.

Ranjan, P., Bowzard, J. B., Schwerzmann, J. W., Jeisy-Scott, V., Fujita, T., & Sambhara, S. (2009). Cytoplasmic nucleic acid sensors in antiviral immunity. *Trends in Molecular Medicine, 15*, 359–368.

Rasche, A., Lehmann, F., Goldmann, N., Nagel, M., et al. (2021). A hepatitis B virus causes chronic infections in equids worldwide. *Proceedings of the National Academy of Sciences*. https://doi.org/10.1073/pnas2013982118

Rigden, R. C., Carrasco, C. P., Summerfield, A., & McCullough, K. C. (2002). Macrophage phagocytosis of foot-and-mouth disease virus may create infectious carriers. *Immunology, 106*, 537–548.

Rode, H.-J., Janssen, W., Rosen-Wolff, A., Bugert, J. J., et al. (1993). The genome of equine herpesvirus type 2 harbors an interleukin-10 (IL-10) -like gene. *Virus Genes, 7*(1), 111–116.

Rozario, C., Martinez-Sobrino, L., McSorley, H. J., & Chauche, C. (2021). Could interleukin-33 (IL-33) govern the outcome of an equine influenza virus infection? Learning from other species. *Viruses*. https://doi.org/10.3390/v13122519

Sagan, S. M., & Sarnow, P. (2013). RNAi, antiviral after all. *Science, 342*, 207–208.

Sarkar, S., Bailey, E., Go, Y. Y., Cook, F., et al. (2016a). Equine arteritis virus uses equine CXCL16 as an entry receptor. *Journal of Virology, 90*, 3366–3384.

Sarkar, S., Bailey, E., Go, Y. Y., Cook, R. F., et al. (2016b). Allelic variation in CXCL16 determines CD3+ T lymphocyte susceptibility to equine arteritis infection and establishment of long-term carrier state in the stallion. *PLoS Genetics*. https://doi.org/10.1371/journal.pgen.1006467

Scalzo, A. A. (2002). Successful control of viruses by NK cells-a balance of opposing forces? *Trends in Microbiology, 10*, 470–474.

Sellon, D. C. (1993). Equine infectious anemia. *Veterinary Clinics of North America: Equine Practice, 9*(2), 321–336.

Sentsui, B., & Kono, Y. (1987). Complement-mediated hemolysis of horse erythrocytes treated with equine infectious anemia virus. *Archives of Virology, 95*, 53–66.

Shaw, T. M., Huey, D., Mousa-Bakky, M., Compaleo, J., et al. (2024). The neonatal Fc receptor (FcRn) is a pan-arterivirus receptor. *Nature Communications*. https://doi.org/10.1038/s41467.024-51142-x

Shekhar, S., & Yang, X. (2015). Natural killer cells in host defense against veterinary pathogens. *Veterinary Immunology and Immunopathology, 168*, 30–34.

Soboll Hussey, G., Ashton, L. V., Quintana, A. M., Van de Walle, G. R., et al. (2014). Equine herpesvirus type 1 pUL56 modulates immune responses of airway epithelial cells. *Virology, 46*, 76–86.

Stetson, D. B., & Medzhitov, R. (2006). Type I interferons in host defense. *Immunity, 25*, 373–381.

Tallmadge, R. L., Antczak, D. F., & Felippe, M. J. B. (2020). Genetics of immune disease in the horse. *Veterinary Clinics: Equine Practice, 36*, 273–288.

Tolnai, C., O'Sullivan, C., Lorincz, M., Karvouni, M., et al. (2025). Cellular immune response in horses after West Nile neuroinvasive disease. *Animals*. https://doi.org/10.3390/ani15162352

Tomlinson, J. E., Wolfisberg, R., Fahnoe, U., Sharma, H., et al. (2020). Equine pegiviruses cause persistent infection of bone marrow and are not associated with hepatitis. *PLoS Pathogens*. https://doi.org/10.1371/journal.ppat.1008677

Vail, K. J., Petri da Silveira, B., Bell, S. L., Cohen, N. D., et al. (2021). The opportunistic intracellular pathogen *Rhodococcus equi* elicits type I interferon by engaging cytosolic DNA sensing in macrophages. *PLoS Pathogens*. https://doi.org/10.1371/journal.ppat/1009888

Van de Walle, G. R., May, M. L., Sukhumavasi, W., von Einem, J., & Ostrander, N. (2007). Herpesvirus chemokine-binding glycoprotein G (gG) efficiently inhibits neutrophil chemotaxis in vitro and in vivo. *Journal of Immunology, 179*, 4161–4169.

Van der Meulen, K. M., Favoreel, H. W., Pensaert, B., & Nauwynck. (2006). Immune escape of equine herpesvirus-1and other herpesviruses of veterinary importance. *Veterinary Immunology and Immunopathology, 111*(1–2), 31–40.

Verhelst, J., Hulpiau, P., & Saelens, X. (2013). Mx proteins: Antiviral gatekeepers that restrain the uninvited. *Microbiology and Molecular Biology Reviews, 77*(4), 551–566.

Wang, T., Hu, L., Liu, M., Wang, T., et al. (2022). The emergence of viral encephalitis in donkeys by equid herpesvirus 8 in China. *Frontiers in Microbiology*. https://doi.org/10.3389/fmicb.2022.840754

Yin, X., Guo, M., Gu, Q., Wu, X., et al. (2014). Antiviral potency and functional analysis of tetherin orthologues encoded by horse and donkey. *Virology Journal, 11*, 152.

CHAPTER

Immunity to selected equine parasites

18

Infectious diseases, as pointed out earlier, rarely result from the deliberate activities of a malicious microorganism. In most cases, disease occurs because of the host's response to the infection or because the invader inadvertently causes damage to its host. Well adapted parasites do not make these mistakes. They exploit the host's resources without causing irreparable damage or triggering a destructive defensive response. A consistent feature of all parasite infestations, however, is that they block or delay host defenses so that they can survive for sufficient time to reproduce. Some parasites may simply delay their destruction until they complete a single life cycle. Other, well-adapted parasites may contrive to survive for the life of the horse, protected from immunological attack by highly evolved evasive mechanisms.

Ideally, a successful parasite will influence its host's immune responses by selectively suppressing only those responses that reduce parasite survival while at the same time allowing other responses to proceed and thus minimizing susceptibility to potential pathogens. In addition, many parasites use their host's cytokine-mediated control pathways for their own purposes. This sharing of cytokines by host and parasites reflects the long history of their association and their success in adapting to a parasitic lifestyle.

Immunity to protozoa

The mechanisms of innate resistance to protozoa in horses are similar to those that prevent bacterial and viral invasion, although species- and genetic influences may be of greater significance. Like other invaders, protozoa stimulate both antibody- and cell-mediated immune responses. In general, antibodies control extracellular parasites in blood and tissue fluids, whereas cell-mediated responses are directed against intracellular protozoa. Serum antibodies directed against protozoan surface antigens may opsonize, agglutinate, or immobilize them. Antibodies, together with complement and cytotoxic cells, may kill them, and some antibodies may inhibit their division. In order to evade this, protozoans employ many strategies to avoid destruction. For example, many hide within cells by employing host-mediated processes such as phagocytosis. Apicomplexans such as Babesia and Theileria, actively penetrate cells. Many hemoprotozoa are restricted to the equine bloodstream. They mainly employ sequential antigenic variation to avoid total elimination.

The Immunology of Horses and Donkeys. https://doi.org/10.1016/B978-0-443-44863-8.00018-1

Equine immune responses to parasitic protozoa often result in the development of hypersensitivity reactions. Type 2 cytotoxic reactions are of significance in piroplasmosis and trypanosomiasis, where they contribute to the development of severe anemia. In piroplasmosis, red cells express parasite antigens on their surfaces and are thus recognized as foreign and eliminated by complement-mediated hemolysis and phagocytosis. In some cases, excessive immune-complex formation can result in the development of a vasculitis or glomerulonephritis (type III hypersensitivity).

Equine piroplasmosis

The term Equine piroplasmosis encompasses three tick-borne diseases caused by the apicomplexan parasites, *Babesia caballi, Theileria equi,* and *Theileria haleyi.* They infect horses, donkeys, mules, and zebras. The parasites reside within erythrocytes and, as a result, cause hemolytic anemia (Wise et al., 2013). They differ in their pathogenesis since *B. caballi* only infects erythrocytes. whereas *T. equi* also infects peripheral blood mononuclear cells. Infected horses carry these parasites for a long time and are thus readily ingested by feeding ticks and transmitted to other equids. The diseases they cause vary greatly in severity. Generally, they cause fever, anorexia, hemolytic anemia, icterus, abortions, splenomegaly, hepatomegaly, and death (Mendoza et al., 2024). Horses can develop limited immunity against both Babesia and Theileria, although there are no vaccines currently available. *T. haneyi* causes a relatively mild form of equine piroplasmosis when compared to *T. equi* (Knowles et al., 2018).

Theileria equi

Once infected through a tick bite, horses may remain infected with *T. equi* for life. They mount an initial innate immune response mediated by neutrophils, macrophages, and NK cells. Splenic macrophages appear to play an especially important role since splenectomized horses develop a very high parasitemia (80%) and usually die, whereas intact horses usually recover (Onyiche et al., 2019). An intact spleen is to ensure complete recovery. Foals with severe combined immunodeficiency (SCID) and lacking both T and B cells are also unable to control the parasitemia and die (Chapter 23). Thus, adaptive immune responses, both antibody- and cell-mediated, play a critical protective role.

Blood lymphocytes proliferate in response to *T. equi* antigens. They develop a cell-mediated response as demonstrated by a delayed hypersensitivity skin response to injected *T. equi* antigens in infected donkeys. In addition, peripheral blood lymphocytes inhibit the growth of cells containing schizonts in vitro. *T. equi*-infected horses appear to express very low levels of proinflammatory cytokines, and there is no apparent correlation between cytokine levels and disease severity, although this is debated (Ramadan et al., 2024). However, the two regulatory cytokines, IL-10 and TGF-β are highly expressed in infected animals. Their expression appears to be linked to inhibition of antibody production (Onzere et al., 2024).

Antibodies directed against the dominant *T. equi* merozoite antigens generally appear around days 7–11 and reach maximum levels at 30–45 days. IgG4/7 specific antibodies increase during acute infections, whereas IgG3/5 predominates in animals with low parasitemia and chronic infections. Nevertheless, there is no correlation between antibody levels and parasitemia. These depend upon the stage of disease and vary between individual horses. Rarely, infected horses may become inapparent carriers of *T. equi*. On occasion, these carriers may develop disease in response to immunosuppressive stresses. Vaccination of horses with a conserved recombinant equine merozoite antigen (EMA-2) protein from *T. equi* generates an antibody response in which IgG3/5 predominates (Santos et al., 2021).

Babesia caballi

In the case of *B. caballi* infection, it is clear that maternal antibodies can protect young foals from infection for up to 9 months (Wise et al., 2013). Infected horses produce antibodies to rhoptry-associated protein-1 (RAP-1). In other *Babesia* species, immunity to RAP-1 is protective (Wise et al., 2013). Protected animals produce significant quantities of nitric oxide, TNF-α, and other cytokines. These originate in macrophages (Hanafusa et al., 1998). This mixture also contributes to the severity of the clinical disease: fever, dyspnea, and edema. For example, NO levels increase significantly before death even though parasitemia remains low. It is also likely that in adult horses, although the disease is self-limiting, this may be due to the persistence of small numbers of parasites (premunition). There is no cross-immunity between Theileria and Babesia, and horses can be infected with both organisms simultaneously!

Equine protozoal myeloencephalitis

Protozoal meningoencephalitis (EPM) occurs in horses across the Americas. It is caused by the coccidian parasite *Sarcocystis neurona*. Horses ingest the parasite by eating or drinking contaminated food or water. The organism is shed in the feces of its definitive host, the opossum (*Didelphis virginiana*). The parasite sporocysts invade the horses intestinal mucosa. Clinical disease occurs when the merozoite stages invade the horse's brain and spinal cord. As a result, affected horses typically develop asymmetrical ataxia and muscle atrophy.

Only a small proportion (0.5%–1%) of seropositive and presumably *S. neurona*-infected, horses develop brain disease resulting in clinical EPM (The prevalence of Sarcocystis seropositive horses is highly variable and averages 78% across the United States). Thus, there appears to be no association between the development of disease and the presence of serum antibodies reflecting antigen exposure (MacKay & Howe, 2022). Predisposed horses include the aged and those immunosuppressed by stresses, such as excessive exercise and transportation. However, experimental infection of immunodeficient horses with *S. neurona* does not inevitably result in neurologic disease despite a prolonged parasitemia (Sellon et al., 2004).

Analysis of the antibody responses in the serum and cerebrospinal fluid of diseased and asymptomatic horses has revealed that their mean IgG3/5 serum concentration and the IgG1:IgG3/5 ratio were significantly different between diseased and clinically normal horses. This suggests that the immune response to *S. neurona* in EPM affected horses may be skewed toward a Th1 cell-mediated response (Chapter 12) (Angwin et al., 2025).

There have been limited studies on equine immunity to EPM. A study of horses showing clinical signs and possessing specific antibodies against *S neurona* indicated that these horses had significantly higher numbers of $CD4^+$ T cells and neutrophils in their bloodstream. However, these lymphocytes had reduced mitogenic responses to pokeweed mitogen when compared to lymphocytes from clinically normal horses. Conversely, the antigen-specific proliferative responses to *S. neurona* merozoite antigens were increased. These changes may simply reflect alterations in the composition of the lymphocyte subsets in these horses (Yang et al., 2006).

It is interesting to note that horses diagnosed with equine protozoal myeloencephalitis also make autoantibodies against myelin protein 2. They appear to share a common antigenic determinant with the parasite. Conversely, horses suffering from the autoimmune disease, polyneuritis equi, may also possess antibodies against *S. neurona*. Thus, some cases of polyneuritis equi may, in fact, be caused by *S. neurona,* and possibly result from molecular mimicry between *S. neurona* and myelin (Ellison et al., 2015). The disease is diagnosed either by serology or by an RT-PCR assay on cerebrospinal fluid (Chapter 22).

Equine trypanosomiasis

Trypanosomes cause multiple diseases in horses, such as Dourine, Nagana, and Surra. Unlike bovine trypanosomiasis, however, relatively few studies have been undertaken on their immune responses to these agents. The two most significant equine pathogens are *Trypanosoma equiperdum* and *Trypanosoma evansi*. However, they are also susceptible to the tsetse fly-transmitted species such as *T. vivax* (Raftery et al., 2025).

Trypanosoma equiperdum

Dourine is a venereal form of trypanosomiasis caused by *T. equiperdum* (Gizaw et al., 2017). The parasite is present in genital secretions of both mares and stallions but rarely in the bloodstream. Affected horses develop genital edema, and cutaneous plaques together with anorexia, fever, and weight loss. A study has been conducted to identify the *T. equiperdum* antigens recognized by the equine immune system. It appears that infected horses recognize a mixture of low molecular weight proteins. Their size ranges from 16 to 35 kDa. The IgG antibodies first appear on day 17 of the infection. There is no evidence to date to suggest that this organism undergoes sequential antigenic variation like *T. evansi* although the disease is associated with periodic exacerbations and relapses (Luciani et al., 2013).

Trypanosoma evansi

T. evansi is a salivarian trypanosome that causes Surra, a widespread and unfortunately, common animal disease that occurs in Africa, Asia, and South America. It is transmitted by biting flies such as Tabanus and Stomoxys. Its principal hosts are horses and camels, but it can also infect other species including cattle, sheep, goats, capybaras, and vampire bats. *T. evansi* is closely related to the bovine trypanosome, *T. brucei* with which it shares 96% gene sequence similarity. The clinical disease includes weight loss, fever, weakness, ventral edema, anemia, paralysis, abortion, and death.

As in bovine trypanosomiasis, in horses with Surra, periods of high parasitemia alternate regularly with periods of low or undetectable parasitemia. Serum from infected horses contains antibodies against trypanosomes isolated prior to sampling but not against those that develop subsequently. Each period of high parasitemia corresponds to the expansion of a population of trypanosomes expressing new surface glycoprotein antigens. The elimination of this population by antibodies leads to a rapid fall in parasite numbers. However, the surviving parasites express new surface glycoproteins and thus grow back. As a result, a fresh trypanosome population arises to produce yet another high parasitemia. This cyclical parasitemia, with each peak resulting from the appearance of a trypanosome population expressing new surface glycoproteins, can continue for many months.

The major antigens of these trypanosomes are known as variant surface glycoproteins (VSGs). The VSGs form a coat on the surface of *T. evansi* that hides other cell surface antigens. VSGs are therefore targeted by host antibodies. As previous VSGs are recognized by the immune system and the organisms destroyed, new VSGs are produced, giving rise to waves of parasitemia. The VSGs produced early in *T. evansi* infections tend to develop in a predictable sequence (Jones & McKinnell, 1984). However, as the infection progresses, the production of VSGs becomes more random. When antigenic change occurs, the VSGs in the old coat are shed and replaced by a different VSG. Sequencing of the *T. evansi* genome has, however, found that the number of VSG genes is only 399, whereas *T. brucei* possesses 1496 (Zheng et al., 2019).

Antigenic variation in *T. evansi* is a result of changes in their DNA and the replacement of an active VSG gene with one from the silent gene pool. Each parasite expresses one VSG at a time. Early in infections, complete VSG gene replacement occurs. Subsequently, partial replacement and point mutations can create new antigenic specificities. In some cases, the expressed VSG gene can be a mosaic generated by several pseudogenes. The potential for recombination-based variation in *T. evansi* is therefore enormous.

T. evansi infections can trigger an enormous increase in IgM-secreting cells so that very high levels of polyclonal IgM develop in the blood of infected horses. Some of these antibodies are directed against autoantigens. These include rheumatoid factor-like molecules and antibodies against thymocytes, single-stranded DNA, red cells, and platelets. This polyclonal B cell activation appears to be triggered by the variant antigens (Diffley, 1983).

T. evansi are also profoundly immunosuppressive. For this purpose they inhibit multiple immune pathways. For example, they can block the classical complement pathway and so prevent their lysis in the bloodstream. They can control the polarization of host macrophages so that the cells develop a suppressive M2 phenotype. A trypanosome suppressive immunomodulating factor induces macrophage TNF-α and NO production by M1 cells that results in inhibition of T cell proliferation. This factor also downregulates the horse's type 2 immune responses. It also appears to upregulate the activities of regulatory DCs (Desquesnes et al., 2013). All this prolongs the parasitemia and increases its transmission opportunities.

Immunity to helminths

Multiple species of parasitic nematodes and cestodes infect horses. Intestinal helminths have coevolved with the bacterial populations in the gut and may be considered to be part of the normal microbiota. Thus, the bacteria and helminths interact with each other in addition to interacting with their host's immune system. Parasite antimicrobial peptides may control bacterial numbers. The host's bacteria will also colonize the worms guts. Their interactions with the host can influence intestinal inflammation and motility. The major defense against gastrointestinal helminths in horses and donkeys is a type 2, antibody-mediated allergic response, but the microbiota also plays an immunoregulatory role that may promote helminth colonization and survival.

The effectiveness of the host's defenses depends upon the animal's age, its nutritional status, its genetics, and the site of infection, as well as the species of worm involved and whether the infection is sudden and large, or a much slower trickle infection. One consistent feature of intestinal nematode infestations is the very wide variation in parasite load based on their management. Thus, most animals raised on pastures harbor few worms, but some individual horses and donkeys may harbor large numbers.

Adaptive immunity

Helminths present the equine immune system with a challenge. Most parasitic worms migrate through the tissues as larvae and eventually reach the intestine or lungs, where they develop into adults. Clearly, the mechanisms that destroy these migrating larvae must be very different from those used to expel large adult worms residing in the intestine or airways. The expulsion of adult worms requires a coordinated response by multiple cell types under the control of T-cell-derived cytokines. These cells, especially tuft cells, collectively trigger a strong type 2 immune response that results in mast cell degranulation, eosinophil infiltration, acute inflammation, and ideally, disconnection and expulsion of the adult worms (Díaz & Allen, 2007) (Fig. 18.1).

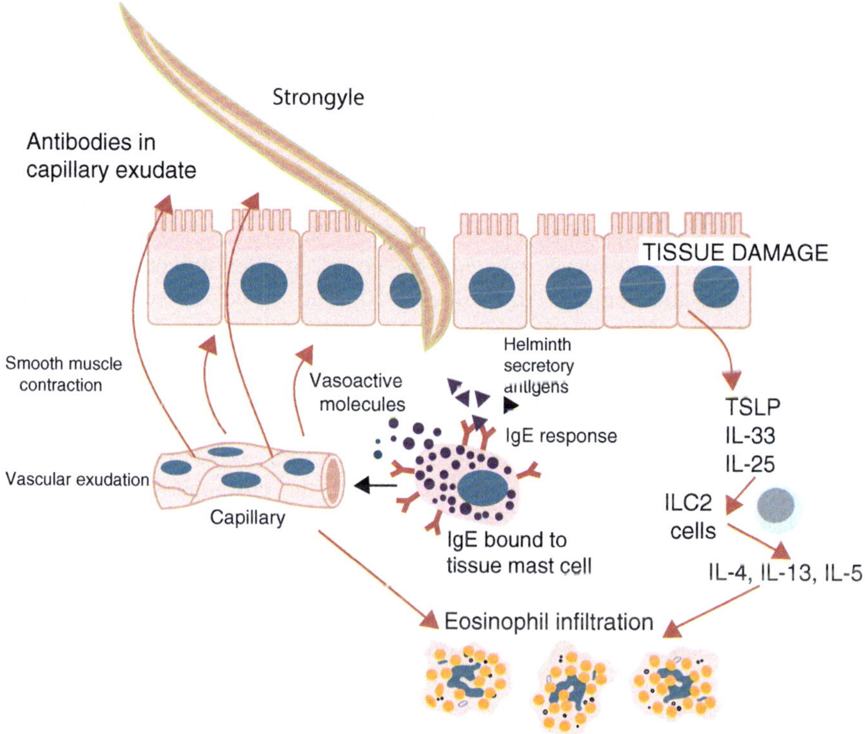

FIGURE 18.1 The mechanisms involved in resistance to adult helminths—a type 2 immune response.

Local mast cell dertanulation triggers a local inflammatory response that causes some parasitic worms to disengage and be expelled.

In general, antigens derived from larvae and adult worms within tissues trigger type 2 immune responses and, as a result, are attacked by eosinophils and basophils. Adult worms attached to mucosal surfaces are less vulnerable to direct attack but also trigger similar responses and so can be expelled by IgE and cytokine-mediated mechanisms. Type 1, cell-mediated responses are relatively less important. Type 2 immunity to helminths involves the production of IL-4, IL-5, IL-9, and IL-13. Because nematode antigens trigger type 2 responses, IgE levels and eosinophil numbers are usually elevated in parasitized animals. Additionally, many helminth infestations are associated with the characteristic signs of type 1 hypersensitivity responses, including edema, asthma, and urticarial dermatitis (Chapter 19).

Eosinophils and helminth destruction

Invading helminths such as *Strongylus vulgaris* and *Habronema* larvae trigger a type 2 immune response that results in Th2 cells producing multiple cytokines. Of these,

IL-5 is a potent eosinophil activator and attractant. Large numbers of eosinophils are therefore attracted to the sites of parasite entry. Eosinophils are also attracted by mast cell- and parasite-derived products, as well as by other cytokines and chemokines. IL-5 from Th2 cells and GM-CSF from Th17 cells mobilize bone marrow eosinophils, releasing large numbers into the circulation. Chemokines, such as the eotaxins, attract eosinophils to the invaders (Masure et al., 2013). Heavily parasitized horses develop an eosinophilia, but this is highly variable and differs greatly between parasite species. Thus, it peaks at 3 weeks in *Parascaris equorum* infestations and at 5 weeks with *S. edentatus* infections. It does not occur in horses suffering from cyathostomiasis (Brosnahan, 2020). The degree of tissue eosinophilia also varies between horses and parasites. Eosinophils exposed to helminth antigens increase their expression of MHC class II and may become antigen-presenting cells. These antigen-presenting eosinophils are highly effective in promoting Th2 responses against worm antigens. Eosinophils express many different pattern-recognition receptors, including TLRs1-5, TLR7, TLR9, NOD1, NOD2, as well as dectin-1. When these receptors are stimulated, the eosinophils activate their peroxidase, increase adhesiveness, and release IL-1β, IL-6, TNF-α, and GM-CSF as well as their cytotoxic granule contents.

Eosinophils employ Fc receptors to bind antibody-coated helminths; they then degranulate and release their granule contents directly onto the parasite cuticle. The granules contain oxidants, nitric oxide, lysophospholipase, and phospholipase D. Major basic protein, the crystalline core of the eosinophil-specific granules, can severely damage the cuticles of parasitic helminths. Eosinophil cationic protein and eosinophil neurotoxin are ribonucleases that are also lethal for helminths.

Eosinophil granules released from cells remain functional. These free granules express membrane receptors for IFN-γ, and eotaxins that, when triggered, stimulate the granules to secrete their contents. Thus, free eosinophil granules function autonomously to contribute to the defenses against helminths. Eosinophils can also generate extracellular traps using released mitochondrial DNA (Meeusen & Balic, 2000) (Fig. 18.2).

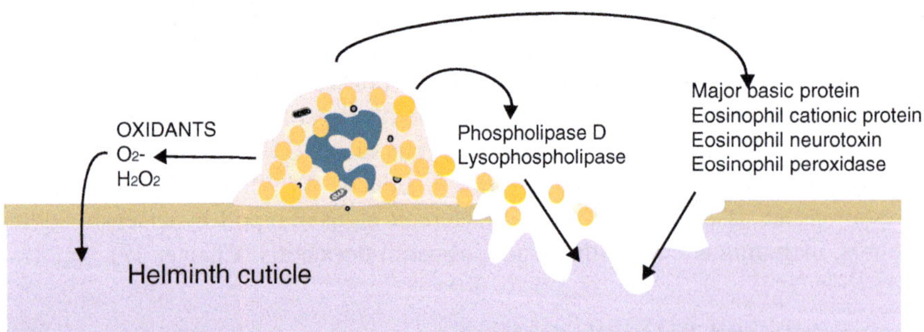

FIGURE 18.2 The mechanisms by which eosinophils damage helminth parasites.

Eosinophil granules contain numerous molecules that can damage helminth cuticles.

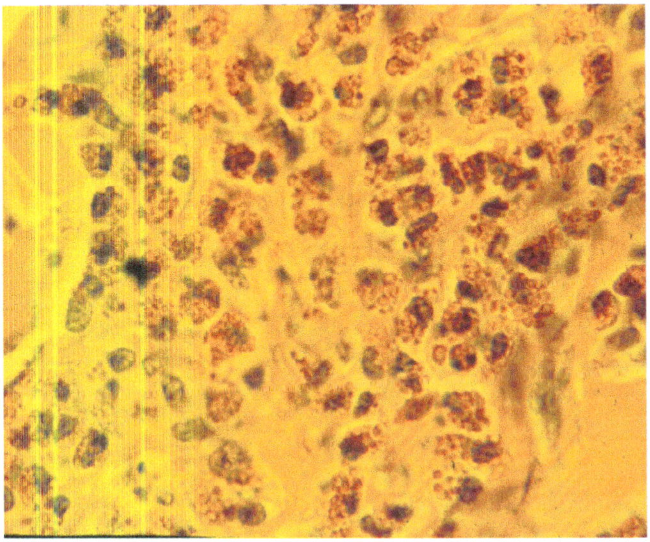

FIGURE 18.3 Photomicrograph of a lesion in horse skin caused by allergy to migrating parasitic helminth (*Habronema*) larvae.

The granular cells are eosinophils, and their presence indicates the occurrence of a type 1 hypersensitivity reaction.

Many nematodes are damaged or killed by eosinophil toxic products, supporting the idea that eosinophils serve a protective function. Nevertheless, this may not apply to all parasites (Fabre et al., 2009). Studies on *Anaplocephala perfoliata*, the horse tapeworm, show a correlation between worm count and tissue eosinophilia, whereas there is no correlation between tissue eosinophilia and *S. vulgaris* numbers (Rotting et al., 2008) (Fig. 18.3).

Although IgE-dependent eosinophil-mediated cytotoxicity is the most significant mechanism of resistance to larval helminths, other antibodies also play a protective role. The mechanisms involved include antibody-mediated neutralization of larval proteases, blocking of the anal and oral pores of larvae by immune complexes, and prevention of molting and inhibition of larval development by antibodies directed against exsheathing antigens. Antibodies directed against adult worms may block egg production or interfere with larval worm development.

Immunity to migrating larvae

Larvae and some adult worms are obliged to migrate through tissues, where they can be attacked by inflammatory cells and molecules. Unlike bacteria or protozoa, however, larval worms have a thick cuticle that protects their vulnerable hypodermal plasma membrane. As larvae develop and undergo periodic molts, the damaged cuticles are shed to be replaced with new ones. These cuticles cannot be penetrated by the terminal complement complex nor by T-cell perforins. Thus, eosinophils and macrophages are the key to destroying these migrating larvae. Both cell types express FcεRII (CD23) and can, therefore, bind and kill IgE-coated parasites. Chitinases are produced by mast cells, macrophages, and neutrophils and they can degrade helminth cuticles. Some chitinases may lack enzyme activity but can bind to helminth cuticles and serve as opsonins or chemoattractants (Reid et al., 2009).

If migrating worm larvae cannot be killed, at least they can be walled off. Activated M2 macrophages produce arginase. Arginase generates proline-rich polyamines. Proline and polyamines are made available for collagen synthesis and can induce local fibroblast proliferation. The granulomas that develop around tissue helminths, such as schistosomes or liver flukes, are driven by arginase from M2 macrophages (Adams et al., 2014).

Immunity to adult helminths

Adult parasitic worms attached to the intestinal wall by their mouthparts are relatively invulnerable to immune attack. As a result, they must be forced to disengage from the gut wall and be expelled in the feces. While embedded in the intestinal mucosa, adult worms secrete and excrete multiple antigens. and these stimulate the production of both IgA and IgE. IgE responses are probably more important than IgA since they play a key role in expelling adult worms from mucosal surfaces. The presence of adult worms and their excretory and secretory products in the intestinal wall can trigger some pattern recognition receptors in enterocytes. Some helminth products can also bind and activate TLRs and thus trigger secondary inflammatory cytokine release.

Parasite-mediated tissue damage triggers the release of all three Th2-stimulating cytokines, TSLP, IL-25, and IL-33, from enterocytes and tuft cells. These cytokines target both DC2 and ILC2 cells. For example, TSLP activates dendritic cells. IL-25 stimulates the production of type 2 cytokines by ILC2 cells and facilitates the differentiation of Th2 cells. IL-33 acts on Th2 cells, ILC2 cells, basophils, and mast cells through its ST2 receptor to drive their production of IL-4, IL-5, and IL-13 and hence promote Th2 responses (Humphreys et al., 2008).

In response to this flood of cytokines, T cells release their effector cytokines. For example, T cells in the intestinal epithelium produce IL-4 and IL-25. Likewise, Th2 cells produce more IL-4 in a positive feedback loop, generating the other Th2 cytokines as well as IL-25. The IL-4 activates STAT6, which upregulates the transcription factor, GATA3, which causes differentiation into Th2 cells and suppresses Th1 responses. IL-6 acts with TGF-β to induce Th17 responses. IL-13 repairs epithelia, enhances mucus production, and together with IL-9 recruits and activates mucosal mast cells. Both IL-4 and IL-13 activate enterocytes, smooth muscle cells, and macrophages. Increased enterocyte proliferation and turnover may cause the worms to disengage (Cliffe et al., 2005). These cytokines also increase intestinal permeability and fluid secretion. The Th2 cytokines stimulate Paneth cells, and the consequent increase in intestinal defensins may damage helminth cuticles. The cytokines also stimulate goblet cells to produce a resistin-like molecule that interferes with worm feeding (Gerbe & Jay, 2016). Mucins and other goblet cell products may also promote worm expulsion. IL-4 and IL-13 as well as IL-9 promote increased smooth muscle contractility (Zaph et al., 2014). They also stimulate goblet cell secretion.

Mast cells and basophils

Mast cells and basophils are also required for helminth expulsion. They can be activated directly by PAMPs through PRRs, although it is unclear which parasite PAMPs do this. In response, the mast cells produce IL-4, IL-13, and IL-5 plus chemotactic factors. Mast cell proteases degrade tight junctions and allow fluid efflux into the intestine. Some mast cell products, such as chitinases, may be directly toxic to helminths. Basophils are also attracted to attached worms and are a major source of IL-4. Eosinophils are attracted to these worms by IL-5 plus the eotaxins, as described above (Voehringer, 2009) (Fig. 18.4).

Tuft cells

Tuft cells are a specialized population of chemosensory cells found among the epithelial cell layer of the nasal mucosa, trachea, salivary glands, stomach, and intestine (Grencis & Worthington, 2016). Tuft cells are the so-called because they have a tuft of long microvilli at their outer pole that extends into the intestinal lumen (Fig. 18.4). These cells play a key role in detecting the presence of intestinal parasites and then initiating type 2 immune responses. Tuft cells apparently use their microvilli to sense succinate, produced by intestinal helminths (Poveda et al., 2023). In response, they produce large amounts of IL-25. In the presence of parasitic helminths, IL-25 promotes the proliferation of tuft cells and mucus-producing goblet cells. Tuft cell IL-25 also recruits eosinophils and activates Th2 cells, ILC2, and ILC3 cells (Schneider et al., 2019; Xu et al., 2025). These cells, in turn, produce IL-4 and IL-13. These cytokines act on intestinal stem cells to promote the differentiation of goblet cells and tuft cells. Thus, equine tuft cells grown in vitro in organoid cultures are stimulated to differentiate by exposure to IL-4 and IL-13. They also differentiate on exposure to the larvae of *Parascaris univalens* or *S. vulgaris* (Hellman et al., 2024). The tuft cells also produce pharmacologically active chemicals, including leukotrienes, prostaglandins, and acetylcholine. The acetylcholine acts on nearby epithelial cells to induce chloride release and so cause helminths to disengage (Billipp et al., 2024). The acetylcholine also appears to have direct anthelmintic properties (Roberts et al., 2021).

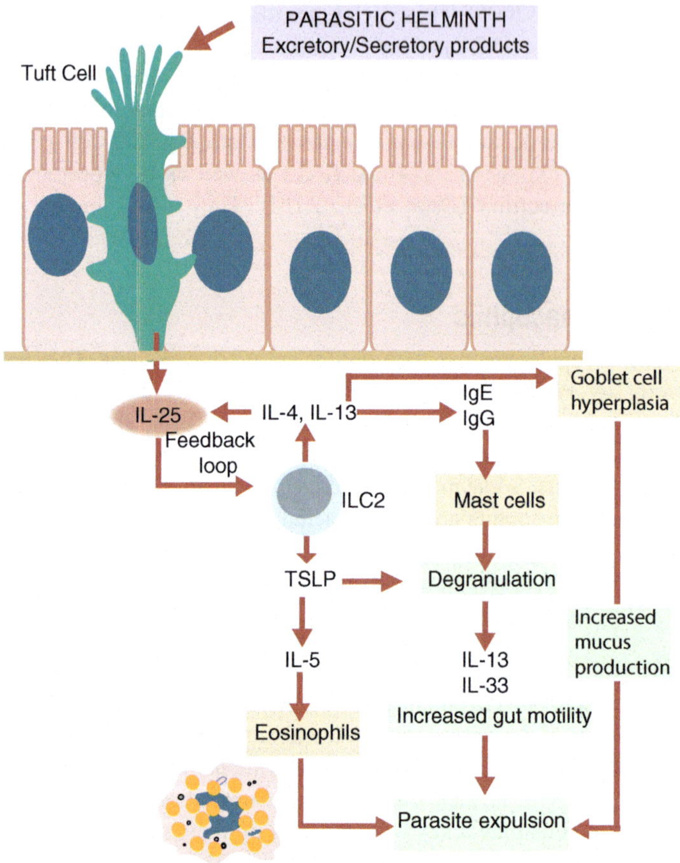

FIGURE 18.4 The mechanisms by which tuft cells participate in intestinal parasite expulsion.

The tuft cells produce IL-25 that activates ILC2s. These cells in turn produce IL-4 and IL-13 that promotes a strong type 2 immune response that results in tuft and goblet cell hyperplasia.

ILC2 cells

Type 2 innate lymphoid cells (ILC2 cells) are also a major source of acetylcholine and prostaglandin E_2 during parasitic nematode infections of the gastrointestinal tract. Their production is triggered by exposure to the activating cytokines, IL-33 and IL-25, from Tuft cells. IL-13 and IL-4 from ILC2 cells stimulate further tuft cell proliferation and IL-25 production. ILC2 cells are also an important source of IL-5, IL-9, and IL-13 (Coakley & Harris, 2020). IL-13 and IL-4 from the activated ILC2 cells also increase gut motility and mucus production (Gronke & Diefenbach, 2016).

Evasion of the immune response

Although there are multiple mechanisms whereby horses resist helminth infection, it is obvious that these defenses are not very effective. Successful helminth parasites survive and reproduce in the presence of a fully functional host immune system. In general, helminths are most vulnerable to immunological attack while migrating through tissues. Thus, most evasion strategies work at the larval stage.

Evasion of innate responses

Many helminth larvae express surface antioxidants such as superoxide dismutase, glutathione peroxidase, and glutathione S-transferase, that neutralize the host's oxidative burst and protect their surfaces from oxidation. Many parasites also interfere with the complement system. For example, schistosomes can neutralize the alternative complement pathway by inserting decay-accelerating factor (CD55) from their host into their outer lipid bilayer. Tapeworms can secrete sulfated proteoglycans, which prematurely activate complement in the tissue fluid.

Evasion of adaptive responses

Parasitic helminths become progressively less antigenic as they evolve in the presence of a functioning immune system. Presumably, natural selection favors the survival of individual worms with reduced antigenicity. Larval helminths living within tissues may also reduce their antigenicity by adsorbing host antigens onto their surface and thus masking parasite antigens. This occurs in some tapeworm infestations, where their cysticerci are coated with IgG. Cysticerci can also adsorb host MHC molecules to their surface.

Another mechanism of immune evasion is the use of sequential antigenic variation. Although helminths have not evolved a system as complex as that in trypanosomiasis, gradual antigenic variation is recognized. The cuticular antigens of *T. spiralis* larvae change after each molt. Even during their growth phase, these larvae change the expression of surface antigens. Some parasites, such as *Fasciola hepatica,* shed their glycocalyx and hence, their surface antigens when exposed to antibodies. Some worms can interfere with antigen processing. Macrophages from schistosome-infested animals are incompetent antigen-presenting cells. Filarial worms secrete inhibitors that block macrophage proteases.

Immunosuppression is a consistent feature of parasitized animals. This may be due to the production of immunosuppressive molecules. For example, *F. hepatica* secretes proteases that destroy immunoglobulins. These proteases generate Fab fragments that then bind and mask parasite antigens.

Specific equine helminths

The significance and strength of antihelminth immune responses in horses are highly variable. They vary between breeds, as well as between horses of different ages. Much depens upon the size and duration of the parasite challenge.

Trematodes

Despite being considered relatively resistant, horses that share pastures with sheep and cattle may become infested with the liver fluke, *F. hepatica*. Fluke infestations have been recorded in horses in much of Europe, including both England and Ireland, as well as in Australia. For example, 8.7% of UK horses are seropositive for fluke infections (Howell et al., 2020). Additionally, donkeys appear to be a more permissive host. Fasciola infects about 10% of donkeys in the United Kingdom, and fluke infestations are especially common in donkeys in Ethiopia, Bolivia, and Egypt (Williams & Hodgkinson, 2017). When juvenile *F. hepatica* invades an animal, it triggers both B-cell and T-cell responses. The newly excysted flukes are recognized by pattern recognition receptors, and the three master cytokines, IL-33, IL-25, and TSLP, are produced by sentinel cells. Eosinophil counts rise over the next few weeks. Eosinophils can bind to the surface of juvenile *F. hepatica*, degranulate, and cause obvious damage to the parasites. However, much of the fluke surface is covered by a protective layer of dense flocculent material to which eosinophils cannot bind (Glauert et al., 1985).

Likewise, equine macrophages are activated by the presence of the flukes. However, the flukes appear to be able to manipulate this activation pathway so that the macrophages are of the M2 phenotype. A secreted antioxidant from *F. hepatica* called peroxiredoxin activates arginase-1 and IL-10, causing alternative activation of macrophages. This results in high arginase activity, low nitric oxide, low IFN-γ, and high IL-10 production. This, plus elevated IL-4, IL-5, and IL-13 production, promotes Th2 responses. These are much less damaging to the flukes than cytotoxic T cells or activated M1 macrophages. *F. hepatica* also secretes cathepsins that can destroy immunoglobulins. These proteases generate Fab fragments that bind and mask parasite antigens. Juvenile *F. hepatica* can readily shed their glycocalyx and hence their surface antigens when exposed to these antibodies.

Immune evasion

F. hepatica produces numerous excretory and secretory molecules that can suppress both innate and adaptive responses. These can inhibit T cell mitogenicity and reduce the oxidative burst in neutrophils. In addition, *F. hepatica* tegumental protein suppresses the production of IFN-γ and IL-12 by acting directly on dendritic cells and possibly suppressing signaling by NF-κB. These enzymes can also cleave

CD4. This results in the suppression of both Th1 and Th17 responses. It also causes a delay in IFN-γ production (Flynn & Musah-Eroje, 2020).

Parasitic helminths secrete a family of immunomodulatory peptides called helminth defense molecules (HDMs) that resemble mammalian cathelicidins. One of these molecules produced by *F. hepatica* can be endocytosed by host macrophages and prevents endosomal maturation, impedes antigen presentation, and inhibits antigen carriage to the cell surface in conjunction with MHC class II molecules (Flynn & Mulcahy, 2008). HDMs bind to lipopolysaccharides as well as to membrane lipids and so prevent activation of inflammasomes and the production of IL-1β (Flynn & Musah-Eroje, 2020).

A transforming growth factor (TGF)-like molecule (TLM) is produced by juvenile *F. hepatica*. Like TGF-β it is immunosuppressive since it binds to the host TGF receptors with high affinity. On binding to these receptors on fibroblasts, it slows cell growth and hence slows wound healing. This probably facilitates the migration of these immature larval stages through tissues. When it binds to the TGF receptors on macrophages, it causes an increase in expression of the T-cell inhibitory receptors PD-1 and the mannose receptor. It also increases the expression of the suppressive cytokine, IL-10. TLM reduces macrophage ADCC activity by suppressing macrophage NO production. TLM production appears to be fluke life-stage-specific (Sulaiman et al., 2016).

Cestodes

A. perfoliata is the commonest tapeworm in horses. The adult tapeworm attaches to the wall of the horse's cecum close to the ileocecal junction and causes significant local inflammation(Gasser et al., 2005). In horses infested by large numbers of worms, this can result in severe or even lethal intussusception or cecal perforation. Analysis of this inflammatory response by the use of RT-PCR has demonstrated increased levels of IL-13 and TGF-β in the early-stage infection. However, in late-stage infections, there is also a drop in the expression of IL-4, IL-13, and Interferon transcripts, while TGF-β, IL-10, and Foxp3 transcription is elevated. *A. perfoliata* produces secretory products that induce T-cell apoptosis, premature death of concanavalin A-stimulated blood leukocytes, and inhibition of their transcription of both IL-1β and IL-2. Thus, *A. perfoliata* effectively downregulates a horse's T cell responses (Lawson et al., 2019). The horse does, however, mount an antibody response to the excretory/secretory (E/S) antigens of the worm, but this differs significantly between horses of different ages, probably reflecting the size of the worm burden (Proudman et al., 1997). Analysis of these E/S antigens has identified multiple protein sequences homologous to known helminth immune modulators. At least 49 of these immune modulators have been detected on the surface of extracellular vesicles produced by the tapeworm, in addition to being released in soluble form. Presumably, these proteins also serve to moderate any immune response mounted by the horse (Wititkornkul et al., 2021).

Nematodes

Parascaris equorum

P. equorum is a roundworm found in horses worldwide. While 2–4 week-old foals are relatively susceptible to experimental *P. equorum* infection, foals that are 6–12 months of age are considerably more resistant. Each group was administered a standard dose of larvae, but in the older animals, many fewer worms succeeded in reaching the small intestine (Clayton & Duncan, 1979). Horses appear to develop relatively strong immunity to *P. equorum.* Apparently healthy donkeys infected with *P. equorum* show significant upregulation of both TNF-α and IL-1β in their intestinal tract. This may reflect local macrophage activation, although it likely simply reflects a degree of inflammation in the mucosae of the parasitized intestine. The cytokine levels correlate with the number of collected worms (Attia et al., 2022).

Strongylus vulgaris

Strongyles are the most important and pathogenic parasitic nematodes in horses. This is because of the severe damage they cause to the mesenteric arteries during larval migration. Immunity to strongyles is slow to develop and relatively ineffective. Third-stage larvae are picked up while grazing. These larvae exsheath and shed their L2 cuticle before they penetrate the intestinal mucosa and submucosa. They enter the arterioles and migrate through the mesenteric arteries. They leave the tissues when they reach the cecum and proximal colon. Here, they persist and mature for several months and can cause severe arteritis before molting into mature adults (L5) and emigrating into the lumen. This damage may be reflected by attacks of colic. The adults attach to the gut wall and complete their sexual development. This life cycle takes about 6 months. In immune horses, many of the migrating larvae are killed when they enter the mucosa (Klei, 2000).

Repeated experimental challenge of pony foals that were not treated with ivermectin resulted in persistent eosinophilia. presumably as a result of the production of IL-5. Treatment with ivermectin significantly reduced blood eosinophil numbers. Both treated and untreated ponies produced IgG antibodies against *S. vulgaris* antigens. The mitogenic T cell responses to phytohemagglutinin and concanavalin A did not differ between the treated and untreated groups. These results suggest that killing of strongyle larvae by ivermectin treatment causes no significant alterations in the immune responses to these nematodes (Dennis et al., 1992).

Oral vaccination of ponies using radiation-attenuated L3 larvae induces a drop in larval burdens, prevents the verminous arteritis, and reduces clinical disease when the animals are challenged. The vaccinated ponies produce *S. vulgaris*-specific antibodies directed against soluble adult worm antigen. These antibodies belong to the IgG1, IgG4/7, and IgG3/5 classes (Swiderski et al., 1999). The IgG3/5 levels show the greatest increase. The migrating larvae are killed by antibody-dependent cytotoxicity. This vaccination induces a strong type 2 immune response in peripheral blood mononuclear cells as reflected by increased levels of the type 2 cytokines, IL-4 and IL-5. These cytokines are produced by $CD4^+$ T cells (Horohov, 2000). The expression of both IL-4 and IL-13 in serum are increased in horses with high strongyle fecal egg counts (Yalavarthi et al., 2025).

The vaccinated ponies also develop eosinophilia that begins on day 4 and peaks on day 9. The levels of IL-5 increase significantly by day 15. There are also statistically significant decreases in IFN-γ levels in the unvaccinated control group. A much smaller decline is seen in the vaccinated animals. All groups exhibit a decline in IL-10 production. Activated eosinophils can kill the L3 larvae through ADCC. This does not happen with L4 larvae, which appear to be antigenically different. Thus, in vitro studies on the responses to migrating strongyle larvae have shown that the L3 larvae induce a different cytokine profile than the L4 larvae. Molting of larvae from the L3 to L4 stage is accompanied by high expression of IL-4 and IL-5, whereas IL-4 larvae induce an IFN-γ response only (Hellman et al., 2024). As a result, horses may be persistently infected with strongyles.

When L3 larvae of *S. vulgaris* are exposed to a mixture of buffy coat leukocytes in the presence of immune serum, eosinophils are the predominant adherent cell type. They are also the only cell type capable of immobilizing these larvae. This reaction appears to be mediated by complement (Klei et al., 1992).

Cyathostomes

These small strongyles trigger a degree of resistance in horses that increases with age (Klei & Chapman, 1999). Thus, young horses develop a higher parasite burden than old horses. Horses slowly develop resistance to reinfection. For example, horses that were previously sensitized and challenged had lower numbers of mucosal worms. This resistance appears to be directed at all stages of the parasite life cycle. The level of serum antibodies against adult worm antigens is not correlated with their resistance. A type 2 immune response is also involved in this resistance. A "self-cure" response has been observed in a pony that underwent a spontaneous expulsion of luminal cyathostomes. Its fecal egg content went from 483 to 50 over a period of 5 weeks. The IL-4 content in its cecal lymph nodes was eightfold greater than in a control pony (Horohov et al., 1997).

Lungworms

Dictyocaulus arnfeldi is a worm that invades the lungs of horses, donkeys, mules, and zebras. The infestation can cause severe respiratory distress in horses. Donkeys appear to be resistant to this parasite and rarely exhibit clinical disease. They can therefore act as healthy carriers (Mendoza et al., 2018). The severity of the disease depends on their number and location within the respiratory tract (Ibrahim, 2017). Given that irradiated lungworm vaccines are very effective in cattle, it is probable that they would also be effective in horses and donkeys should economics permit.

Immunity to arthropods

When arthropods such as ticks, fleas, midges, or mosquitoes bite a horse, they inject saliva. Their saliva contains digestive enzymes that assist the parasite in obtaining its meal; either cellular debris or blood. The saliva also contains components that have evolved to minimize host responses; however, many are also antigenic. As a result, they can trigger a local or systemic immune response. This can result in the development of allergies. Consequently, horses with insect bite hypersensitivity can develop severe pruritus, leading to extreme discomfort and altered behavior (Chapter 19).

Host immune responses to injected arthropod salivary antigens are of three types. Some salivary components are of low molecular weight. They can, however, bind covalently to skin proteins such as collagen, and then act as haptens, stimulating Th1 responses. On subsequent exposure, these haptens may induce delayed hypersensitivity responses. Other salivary antigens may bind to epidermal Langerhans cells and induce cutaneous basophil hypersensitivity (Cox & Stewart, 2023). This is a Th2 response associated with the production of IgG antibodies and a basophil infiltration. If these basophils are destroyed by anti-basophil serum, resistance to biting arthropods is reduced (Eberle & Voehringer, 2016). The third type of response to arthropod saliva is a Th2 response, leading to eosinophil infiltration, IgE production, mast cell degranulation, and type 1 hypersensitivity. This response may induce local inflammation, leading to urticaria, pain, and pruritus. Each of these three types of response may modify the skin in such a way that the feeding of the offending arthropod is impaired, and the animal becomes a less attractive source of food. Unfortunately, natural selection and evolution ensure that the biting arthropod is well able to withstand such responses (Wilson, 2014). By far the most significant arthropod-mediated disease is cutaneous hypersensitivity to the bites of Culicoides midges. This is discussed in the next chapter.

Tick bites

Ticks transmit equine piroplasmosis as well as *Anaplasma phagocytophilum* (Previously known as *E. equi*) (Cocco et al., 2023). They are also the vectors of *Borrelia burgdorferi*, the cause of Lyme disease. Ticks are unique among arthropods in that they attach and feed from their hosts for several days. This provides time for innate and adaptive immune responses to occur and for ticks to employ countermeasures. Thus, tick saliva contains components that suppress pain and itch, hemostasis, inflammation, adaptive immunity, and wound healing. Because tick salivary proteins are antigenic, they would be expected to induce adaptive immune responses that impair a tick's ability to feed. Ticks, however, have evolved immunosuppressive and anti-inflammatory countermeasures that permit them to feed more effectively. Tick saliva impairs macrophage function and suppresses T cell responses to mitogens, as well as the production of IL-1β and the Th1 cytokines IFN-γ and IL-2. It suppresses NK cell activity and macrophage oxidant production. It is abundantly clear that ticks have evolved many mechanisms to prevent immunological attacks while they are feeding. Evasins are tick salivary proteins that inhibit mammalian chemokines and effectively inhibit leukocyte recruitment (Bhusal et al., 2020).

Mange

Chorioptic mange cause by *Chorioptes bovis* is the commonest form of equine mange and tends to occur on the legs of heavy draft breeds. While these mites are normally inocuous, clinical mange may develop in immunocompromized horses. Aninals develop pruritus, inflammation, crusting and alopecia. This may be the result of a local type 1 hypersensitivity response to mite allergens. It has been linked to the development of equine pastern dermatitis with imbalances in the skin microbiota (Gerber et al., 2023).

Demodectic Mange caused bt *Demodex* spp. is rare in horses. The mange mites live within hair follicles and sebaceous glands. Under normal circumstances, innate immune responses regulate mite populations and prevent mite overgrowth. Immunosuppressive agents such as prolonged steroid therapy may predispose animals to the development of generalized demodicosis.

Sarcoptic mange is also rare in horses, but when it develops, it may be severe. *Sarcoptes scabeiequi* mites burrow into the horse's epidermis. They reach the lower stratum corneum where they can trigger both antibody- and cell-mediated immune responses. Hypersensitivity to saliva and feces may cause intense pruritus. This may lead in turn to scratching, extensive hair loss, and crusting.

Horse botflies

Botfly larvae parasitize horses worldwide. The two main species involved are *Gasterophilus intestinalis* and *Gasterophilus nasalis*. The fly lays its eggs on the hairs of the forelimbs of horses, donkeys, and mules. The first instar larvae migrate to the mouth and develop in the tongue tissue. Second instar larvae are swallowed and attach to the nonglandular surface of the stomach, where they mature into third instar larvae. These larvae then pass out of the horse in its feces. The attached larvae cause inflammation, erosions, and ulcerations. The larvae suppress the horse's immune system. Transcriptome analysis indicates that they downregulate the expression of the S100 proteins S100-A8 and S100-A9 (calprotectin). They also downregulate the toll-like receptor pathway (Hu et al., 2022).

Botfly larvae must evade the horse's xenograft response. In warble fly infestations in cattle, the proteases secreted by these larvae can inhibit the host's responses to mitogens and reduce IL-2 production, probably by destroying cell surface receptors (Wikel, 1999). Likewise, in flystrike in sheep, variants of the TLR9 gene influence disease severity. Resistant sheep also mount a greater inflammatory response and produce more fluid exudate when injected with larval excretory and secretory products. On the other hand, larval proteases inhibit complement activation and degrade immunoglobulins. T and B cells also recognize antigens in maggot saliva and respond to them. Thus, in horses with botfly infestations, serum antibodies are directed against second and third-instar larvae. Their levels are significantly higher in horses with moderate or severe infection compared to healthy horses. Both IgG and IgA antibodies to botfly larvae can be detected in horse serum and saliva (Pawlas-Opiela et al., 2022).

References

Adams, P. N., Aldridge, A., Vukman, K. V., Donnelly, S., & O'Neill, S. M. (2014). *Fasciola hepatica* tegumental antigens indirectly induce an M2 macrophage-like phenotype in vivo. *Parasite Immunology, 36*, 531–539.

Angwin, C. J., de Assis Rocha, I., Reed, S. M., Morrow, J. K., et al. (2025). Analysis of igG responses to *Sarcocystis neurona* in horses with equine protozoal myeloencephalitis (EPM) suggests a Th1-biased immune response. *Veterinary Immunology and Immunopathology*. https://doi.org/10.1016/j.vetimm.2025.111009

Attia, M. M., Soliman, S. M., Salaeh, N. M. K., Salem, H. M., et al. (2022). Evaluation of the immune responses and oxidative stress in donkeys: Immunological studies provoked by *Parascaris equorum* infection. *Saudi Journal of Biological Sciences, 29*, 2173–2179.

Bhusal, R. P., Eaton, J. R. O., Chowdhury, S. T., Power, C. A., et al. (2020). Evasins: Tick salivary proteins that inhibit mammalian chemokines. *Trends in Biochemical Sciences*. https://doi.org/10.1016/j.tibs.2019.10.003

Billipp, T. E., Fung, C., Webeck, L. M., Sargent, D. B., et al. (2024). Tuft cell-derived acetylcholine promotes epithelial chloride secretion and intestinal helminth clearance. *Immunity, 57*, 1243–1259.

Brosnahan, M. M. (2020). Eosinophils of the horse: Part II: Eosinophils in clinical diseases. *Equine Veterinary Education, 32*(11), 590–602.

Clayton, H. M., & Duncan, J. L. (1979). The development of immunity to Parascaris equorum infection in the foal. *Research in Veterinary Science, 26*(3), 383–384.

Cliffe, L. J., Humphreys, N. E., Lane, T. E., et al. (2005). Accelerated intestinal epithelial cell turnover: A new mechanism of parasite expulsion. *Science, 308*, 1463–1465.

Coakley, G., & Harris, N. L. (2020). The intestinal epithelium at the forefront of host-helminth interactions. *Trends in Parasitology, 36*(9), 761–772.

Cocco, R., Rizzo, M., Carta, C., Arfuso, F., et al. (2023). Immune and inflammatory responses of donkeys (*Equus asinus*) tested positive for tick-borne pathogens. *Journal of Equine Veterinary Science*. https://doi.org/10.1016/j.jevs.2022.104190

Cox, A., & Stewart, A. J. (2023). Insect bite hypersensitivity in horses: Causes, diagnosis, scoring and new therapies. *Animals*. https://doi.org/10.3390/ani13152514

Díaz, A., & Allen, J. E. (2007). Mapping immune response profiles: The emerging scenario from helminth immunology. *European Journal of Immunology, 37*, 3319–3326.

Dennis, V. A., Klei, T. R., Miller, M. A., Chapman, M. R., & McClure, J. R. (1992). Immune responses of pony foals during the repeated infections of *Strongylus vulgaris* and regular ivermectin treatments. *Veterinary Parasitology, 42*, 83–99.

Desquesnes, M., Holzmuller, P., Lai, D.-H., Dargantes, A., et al. (2013). *Trypanosoma evansi* and Surra: A review and perspectives on origin, history, distribution, taxonomy, morphology, hosts and pathogenic effects. *BioMed Research International*. https://doi.org/10.1155/2013/194176

Diffley, P. (1983). Trypanosomal surface coat variant antigen causes polyclonal lymphocyte activation. *Journal of Immunology, 131*(4), 1863–1986.

Eberle, J. U., & Voehringer, D. (2016). Role of basophils in protective immunity to parasitic infections. *Seminars in Immunopathology, 38*(5), 605–613.

Ellison, S. P., Kennedy, T., Li, A., & Schweiss, L. (2015). Serum antibodies against a reactive site of equine myelin protein 2 linked to polyneuritis equi found in horses diagnosed with EPM. *International Journal of Applied Research in Veterinary Medicine, 13*(3), 164–181.

Fabre, V., Beitin, D. P., Bliss, S. K., et al. (2009). Eosinophil deficiency compromises parasite survival in chronic nematode infection. *Journal of Immunology, 182*, 1577–1583.

Flynn, R. J., & Mulcahy, G. (2008). Possible role for toll-like receptors in interaction of *Fasciola hepatica* excretory/secretory products with bovine macrophages. *Infection and Immunity, 76*, 678–684.

Flynn, R. J., & Musah-Eroje. (2020). Evasion of host immunity during Fasciola hepatica infection. From. In M. Cancela, & Maggioli (Eds.), *Fasciola hepatica: Methods and protocols. Methods in molecular biology*. https://doi.org/10.1007/978-1-0716-0475-5

Gasser, R. B., Williamson, R. M. C., & Beverige, I. (2005). Anaplocephala perfoliata in horses—Significant scope for further research, improved diagnosis and control. *Parasitology, 131*(Pt 1), 1–13.

Gerbe, F., & Jay, P. (2016). Intestinal tuft cells: Epithelial sentinels linking luminal cues to the immune system. *Mucosal Immunology, 9*, 1353–1359.

Gerber, V., Kaiser-Thom, S., & Oesch, S. (2023). Equine pastern dermatitis: A narrative review on clinical presentation, diagnosis, risk factors, prevention and therapeutic approaches. *Journal of the American Veterinary Medical Association, 261*(S1), s58–s65.

Gizaw, Y., Megersa, M., & Fayera, T. (2017). Dourine: A neglected disease of equids. *Tropical Animal Health and Production, 49*, 887–897.

Glauert, A. M., Lammas, D. A., & Duffus, W. P. H. (1985). Ultrastructural observations on the interaction in vitro between bovine eosinophils and juvenile *Fasciola hepatica*. *Parasitology, 91*, 459–470.

Grencis, R. K., & Worthington, J. J. (2016). Tuft cells: A new flavor in innate epithelial immunity. *Trends in Parasitology, 32*, 583–585.

Gronke, K., & Diefenbach, A. (2016). Tuft cell-derived IL-25 activates and maintains ILC2. *Immunology & Cell Biology, 94*, 221–223.

Hanafusa, Y., Cho, K. O., Kanemaru, T., Wada, R., et al. (1998). Pathogenesis of *Babesia caballi* unfection in experimental horses. *Journal of Veterinary Medical Science, 60*, 1127–1132.

Hellman, S., Martin, F., Tyden, E., Sellin, M. E., et al. (2024). Equine enteroid-derived monolayers recapitulate key features of parasitic intestinal nematode infection. *Veterinary Research*. https://doi.org/10.1186/s13567-024-01266-1

Horohov, D. W. (2000). Equine T cell cytokines: Protection and pathology. *Veterinary Clinics of North America: Equine Practice, 16*(1), 1–14.

Horohov, D. W., Swiderski, C. E., Robinson, J. A., & Klei, T. R. (1997). Cytokine production in equine disease. In V. E. C. J. Schijns, & M. C. Horzinek (Eds.), *Cytokines in veterinary medicine* (pp. 167–176). CAB International.

Howell, A. K., Malalana, F., Beesley, N. J., Hodgkinson, J. E., et al. (2020). Fasciola hepatica in UK horses. *Equine Veterinary Journal, 52*, 194–199.

Hu, D., Tang, Y., Wang, C., Qi, Y., et al. (2022). The role of intestinal microbial metabolites in the immunity of equine animals infected with horse botflies. *Frontiers in Veterinary Science*. https://doi.org/10.3389/fvets.2022.832062

Humphreys, N. E., Xu, D., Hepworth, M. R., et al. (2008). IL-33, a potent inducer of adaptive immunity to intestinal nematodes. *Journal of Immunology, 80*, 2443–2449.
Ibrahim, N. (2017). Equine lung worm: A systematic review. *Global Journal of Medical Research, 17*(2). ISSN: 0975-5888.
Jones, T. W., & McKinnell, C. D. (1984). Antigenic variation in *Trypanosoma evansi*. Isolation and characterization of variable antigen type populations from rabbits infected with a stock of T. evansi. *Tropenmedizin und Parasitologie, 35*(4), 237–241.
Klei, T. R. (2000). Equine immunity to parasites. *Veterinary Clinics of North America: Equine Practice, 16*(1), 69–78.
Klei, T. R., & Chapman, M. R. (1999). Immunity in quine cyathostome infections. *Veterinary Parasitology, 85*, 123–136.
Klei, T. R., Chapman, M. R., & Dennis, V. A. (1992). Role of the eosinophil in serum-mediated adherence of equine leukocytes to infective larvae of *Strongylus vulgaris*. *The Journal of Parasitology, 78*(3), 477–484.
Knowles, D. P., Kappmeyer, L. S., Haney, D., Herndon, D. R., et al. (2018). Discovery of a novel species, *Theileria haneyi* n. sp., infective to equids, highlights exceptional genomic diversity within the genus Theileria: Implications for apicomplexan parasite surveillance. *International Journal for Parasitology, 48*(9–10), 679–690.
Lawson, A. L., Pittaway, C. E., Sparrow, R. M., Balkwill, E. C., et al. (2019). Analysis of caecal mucosal inflammation and immune modulation during *Anoplocephala perfoliata* infection of horses. *Parasite Immunology*. https://doi.org/10.1111/pim.12667
Luciani, M., Di Pancracio, C., Di Febo, T., Tittarelli, M., et al. (2013). IgG antibodies from dourine infected horses identify a distinctive *Trypanosoma equiperdum* antigenic pattern of low molecular weight molecules. *Veterinary Immunology and Immunopathology, 151*, 140–146.
MacKay, R. J., & Howe, D. K. (2022). Equine protozoal myeloencephalitis. *Veterinary Clinics of North America: Equine Practice, 38*, 249–268.
Masure, D., Vlaminck, J., Wang, T., Chiers, K., et al. (2013). A role for eosinophils in the intestinal immunity against infective *Ascaris suum* larvae. *PLoS Neglected Tropical Diseases, 7*(3). https://doi.org/10.1371/journal.pntd.0002138
Meeusen, E. N. T., & Balic, A. (2000). Do eosinophils have a role in the killing of helminth parasites? *Parasitology Today, 16*, 95–101.
Mendoza, F. J., Perez-Ecija, A., Rappmeyer, L. S., Suarez, C. E., & Bastos, R. G. (2024). New insights in the diagnosis and treatment of equine piroplasmosis: Pitfalls, idiosyncracies and myths. *Frontiers in Veterinary Science*. https://doi.org/10.3389/fvets.2024.1459989
Mendoza, F. J., Toribio, R. E., & Perez-Ecija, A. (2018). Donkey internal medicine—Part II: Cardiovascular, respiratory, neurologic, urinary. opthalmic, dermatology and musculoskeletal disorders. *Journal of Equine Veterinary Science, 65*, 86–97.
Onyiche, T. E., Suganuma, K., Igarashi, I., Yokoyama, N., et al. (2019). A review on equine piroplasmosis: Epidemiology, vector ecology, risk factors, host immunity, diagnosis and control. *International Journal of Environmental Research and Public Health*.
Onzere, C. K., Bastos, R. G., Bishop, R. P., Suarez, C. E., & Fry, L. M. (2024). Expression of IL-10 and TGF-β1 in horses experimentally infected with T. equi merozoites is associated with antibody production but not modulation of pro-inflammatory responses. *Frontiers in Immunology*. https://doi.org/10.3389/fimmu.2024.1370255
Pawlas-Opiela, M., Jawor, P., Galli, J., Zak-Bocheenek, A., et al. (2022). The relationship between the intensity of *Gasterophilus intestinalis* infection and the serum and salivary

humoral immune response in horses. *Scientific Reports*. https://doi.org/10.1038/s41598-022-21482-z

Poveda, M. C., Britton, C., Devaney, E., McNeilly, T. N., et al. (2023). Tuft cells: Detectors, amplifiers, effectors, and targets in parasite infection. *Cells*. https://doi.org/10.3390/cells12202477

Proudman, C. J., Holmes, M. A., Sheoran, A. S., Edwards, S. E. R., & Trees, A. J. (1997). Immunoepidemiology of the equine tapeworm *Anaplocephala perfoliata*: Age intensity profile and age-dependency of antibody subtype responses. *Parasitology, 114*, 89–94.

Raftery, A. G., Gummery, L., Garcia, K., Mohite, D., et al. (2025). Equine trypanosomiasis, a systematic review: Disease management. *Equine Veterinary Journal*. https://doi.org/10.1002/evj.70136

Ramadan, R. M., Taha, N. M., Auda, H. M., Elsamman, E. M., et al. (2024). Molecular and immunological studies on Theileria equi and its vector in Egypt. *Experimental & Applied Acarology, 83*, 439–458.

Reid, C. J., Thompson, L., Donnelly, S., Deaton, C. M., et al. (2009). The activity and expression of chitinase in the equine lung and its activity in normal horses and animals with recurrent airway obstruction. *Research in Veterinary Science, 87*(1), 20–25.

Roberts, L. B., Schnoeller, C., Berkachy, R., Darby, M., et al. (2021). Acetylcholine production by group 2 innate lymphoid cells promotes mucosal immunity to helminths. *Science Immunology, 6*, Article eabd0359.

Rotting, A. K., Freeman, D. E., Constable, P. D., Moore, R. M., et al. (2008). The effects of *Strongylus vulgaris* parasitism on eosinophil distribution and accumulation in equine large intestinal mucosa. *Equine Veterinary Journal, 40*, 379–384.

Santos, A. C., Nogueira, E. W., Moraes, B. S. S., Müller, V., et al. (2021). Immune responses of adult horses, pregnant mares and foals to an experimental vaccine with recombinant EMA-2 protein of *Theileria equi*. *Research in Veterinary Science, 239*, 186–192.

Schneider, C., O'Leary, C. E., & Locksley, R. M. (2019). Regulation of immune responses by tuft cells. *Nature Reviews Immunology, 19*(9), 584–593. https://doi.org/10.1038/s41577-019-0176-x

Sellon, D. C., Knowles, D. P., Greiner, E. C., Long, M. T., et al. (2004). Infection of immunodeficient horses with *Sarcocystis neurona* does not result in neurologic disease. *Clinical and Diagnostic Laboratory Immunology, 11*(6), 1134–1139.

Sulaiman, A. A., Zolnierczyk, K., Japa, O., Owen, J. P., et al. (2016). A trematode parasite derived growth factor binds and exerts influences on host immune functions via host cytokine receptor complexes. *PLoS Pathogens, 12*(11), Article e1005991.

Swiderski, C. E., Klei, T. R., Folsom, R. W., Pourciau, S. S., et al. (1999). Vaccination against Strongylus vulgaris in ponies: Comparison of the humoral and cytokine responses of vaccinates and nonvaccinates. *Advances in Veterinary Medicine, 41*, 389–404.

Voehringer, D. (2009). The role of basophils in helminth infection. *Trends in Parasitology, 25*, 551–556.

Wikel, S. K. (1999). Modulation of the host immune system by ectoparasitic arthropods: Blood-feeding and tissue-dwelling arthropods manipulate host defenses to their advantage. *BioScience, 49*(4), 311–320.

Williams, D. J. L., & Hodgkinson, J. E. (2017). Fascioliasis in horses: A neglected re-emerging disease. *Equine Veterinary Education, 29*(4), 202–204.

Wilson, A. D. (2014). Immune responses to ectoparasites in horses, with a focus on insect bite hypersensitivity. *Parasite Immunology, 36*, 560–572.

Wise, L. N., Kappmeyer, L. S., Mealey, R. H., & Knowles, D. P. (2013). Review of equine piroplasmosis. *Journal of Veterinary Internal Medicine, 27*, 1334–1346.

Wititkornkul, B., Hulme, B. J., Tomes, J. J., Allen, N. R., et al. (2021). Evidence of immune modulators in the secretome of the equine tapeworm *Anoplocephala perfoliata*. *Pathogens*. https://doi.org/10.3390/pathogens10070912

Xu, H., Wang, Y., Guo, X., et al. (2025). ILC3s promote intestinal tuft cell hyperplasia and anthelmintic immunity through RANK signaling. *Science Immunology*. https://doi.org/10.1126/sciimunol.adn1491

Yalavarthi, G., Sabbineni, H., Kosuri, P., Amalaradjou, M., et al. (2025). Influence of housing patterns and fecal egg count on cytokine profiles (IL-4 and IL-13) in equines. *Journal of Equine Veterinary Science*. https://doi.org/10.1016/j.jevs.2025.105547

Yang, J., Ellison, S., Gogal, R., Norton, H., et al. (2006). Immune response to *Sarcocystis neurona* infection in naturally infected horses with equine protozoal myeloencephalitis. *Veterinary Parasitology, 138*, 200–210.

Zaph, C., Cooper, P. J., & Harris, N. L. (2014). Mucosal immune responses following intestinal nematode infection. *Parasite Immunology, 36*, 439–452.

Zheng, L., Jiang, N., Sang, X., Zhang, N., et al. (2019). In depth analysis of the genome of *Trypanosoma evansi*, an etiological agent of surra. *Science China Life Sciences*. https://doi.org/10.1007/s11427-018-9473-8

CHAPTER

Equine anaphylaxis and allergic diseases

19

Adverse inflammatory reactions triggered by the immune system are classified into four major types based on their pathogenesis. Type I hypersensitivity reactions are acute inflammatory diseases that result from the rapid release of the biologically active contents from mast cell, and basophil cytoplasmic granules. This granule release is triggered when antigens bind to IgE on the surface of mast cells or basophils. The granule contents consist of a mixture of potent vasoactive molecules that trigger inflammation and attract eosinophils. This inflammatory response plays an important role in resistance to parasitic helminths and arthropods. It is also, however, a cause of unwanted disease and thus of major significance in Veterinary Medicine. Immunoglobulin E production is a key feature of these type 1 hypersensitivity responses. Disease severity and the organs involved depend on the number and location of mast cells, the degree of sensitization of an animal, the amount of allergen involved, and its route of administration.

Immunoglobulin E

IgE, like the other equine immunoglobulins, is produced by B cells and plasma cells. These are readily detected in tissues such as the skin and lungs. The function of IgE is to trigger an acute inflammatory response that serves to eliminate parasites, especially helminth parasites, from the tissues and the gastrointestinal tract. Like other equine antibodies, the IgE gene is located within the IGH locus on chromosome ECA24. There is a single IgE heavy chain gene located between the IgG5 gene and the IgA gene. This gene consists of four exons, each encoding a single immunoglobulin domain. At least four different IGHE alleles exist in the horse (Wagner, 2009). These involve sequence differences in the immunoglobulin heavy chains. It is unclear to what extent these result in functional differences.

IgE is a typical Y-shaped, four-chain immunoglobulin with four constant domains in each of its ε heavy chains and a molecular weight of 190 kDa. Each heavy chain contains six potential N-glycosylation sites. IgE is readily destroyed by mild heat treatment. It does not activate complement. The average concentration of IgE in normal healthy horse serum has been reported to be 84 ± 90.9 mg/mL. However, there is great individual variation. In parasitized animals, it may rise to 109 ± 69 mg/mL. It has a half-life in serum of about 2 days (Wagner, 2009). This short half-life is a result of its removal from the bloodstream and its high-affinity binding to the Fc receptors on tissue mast cells.

The Immunology of Horses and Donkeys. https://doi.org/10.1016/B978-0-443-44863-8.00004-1

IgE does not act simply by binding and coating antigens, as do the other immunoglobulins. IgE acts as a signal-transducing molecule. When two mast cell-bound IgE molecules are cross-linked by an allergen molecule on the surface of a mast cell, they trigger receptor activation, leading to the rapid release of mast cell granules and inflammatory mediators into the tissues. The resulting acute inflammation enhances local defenses and helps eliminate invaders, especially helminths and arthropods (Hellman et al., 2017). Because of its very short half-life, IgE it must be produced continuously in order to maintain its serum levels. Most of the body's IgE is firmly bound to high-affinity FcεRI receptors on the surface of tissue mast cells. As a result, the IgE serum concentration does not reflect its total amount in the body (Tizard, 2022).

Given the effectiveness of Fc receptors and their role in transferring maternal antibodies from a mare's serum to her colostrum, it is unsurprising that IgE is also transferred. IgE is actively transported into the mammary gland and is therefore present in mare's colostrum. As a result, IgE is found in foal serum immediately after suckling. It peaks 2–5 days later before progressively declining. It has all gone by 2–4 months. Endogenous production of IgE by a young horse does not begin until 9–11 months of age (Wagner, Flaminio, et al., 2006).

Mast cells

Mast cells play a crucial role in both allergic diseases and innate immunity (Voehringer, 2013). They act as sentinel cells. They recognize PAMPs and DAMPs through their PRRs and in response, release a complex mixture of inflammatory cytokines and other chemical mediators. This release normally occurs in a controlled manner and ensures that the severity and type of inflammation are appropriate to the body's immediate needs—but not always!

Equine mast cells are large, ovoid cells (15–20 μm in diameter) scattered throughout the body in connective tissue, under the skin, in mucosal surfaces in the intestine and airways and around nerves. Structurally, they are similar to the mast cells seen in other mammals. Thus, they are round or oval cells containing many large, electron-dense granules together with a few mitochondria. Their granules stain strongly with dyes such as toluidine blue. These granules often mask the bean-shaped nucleus. Horses have two types of mast cell granules that differ in their structure. Type 1 granules contain a reticulum of coarse, dense, interlacing strands. Type 2 granules are less dense and larger (Mair et al., 1988). Fig. 19.1.

IgE receptors

Horse mast cells express two types of IgE receptors on their surface: high-affinity FcεRI and low-affinity FcεRII (CD23). They are expressed on both mast cells and basophils and play a critical role in IgE-mediated responses.

The equine high-affinity mast cell IgE receptor FcεR1 has been cloned and sequenced. It consists of four peptide chains: one α, one β, and two γ chains

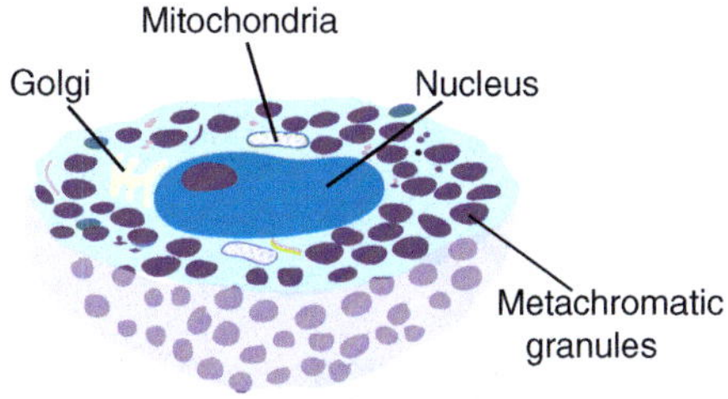

FIGURE 19.1 The structure of a typical equine mast cell.

Its cytoplasm is densely packed with large metachromatic granules.

(αβγγ). The α chain binds IgE, the β chain stabilizes the complex, and the γ chains serve as signal transducers. (This same γ chain is also a signal transducer in FcγRI, FcγRIII, and γ/δ TCR.) The α chain consists of 230 amino acids (McAleese et al., 2000). The β- and γ-chains have also been cloned. The γ-chain is highly conserved between species, but the β-chain is highly variable and shorter than in any other mammal species sequenced to date (McAleese & Miller, 2003). FcεRI is expressed on mast cells, basophils, neutrophils, and eosinophils.

The affinity of FcεRI for IgE is very high (10^{-10} M), so they bind almost irreversibly and thus ensure that mast cells are constantly coated with IgE. An important feature of these receptors is their range of expression. Once expressed on the mast cell surface, the receptor half-life is about 24 hours. Some are recycled, while most are internalized and degraded. In the absence of IgE, there are about 8000 FcεRI per cell (on circulating basophils). Binding of IgE to these receptors stabilizes them, slows their degradation, and reduces their turnover. As a result, receptor numbers can climb to as high as 250,000/cell in allergic individuals. Receptor numbers cannot, however, keep pace with IgE production, and they may be swamped by high levels of non-antigen-specific IgE.

A second form of FcεRI contains only three chains: one α- and two γ-chains (αγγ). It is expressed on antigen-presenting dendritic cells and equine peripheral blood monocytes. These are IgE^{+}/MHC II^{high}/$CD14^{low}$ cells (Larson et al., 2020). Their numbers are moderately positively correlated with serum IgE levels. Their numbers appear to be similar in healthy horses and horses suffering from insect bite hyperensitivity. On cross-linking of FcεRI with IgE, these monocytes and DCs produce IL-10, suggesting that they may play an immune regulatory role. Fig. 19.2.

The second type of IgE receptor, FcεRII (also classified as CD23), is a selectin expressed on B cells, NK cells, macrophages, dendritic cells, eosinophils, and platelets. In addition to binding IgE, FcεRII binds to the complement receptor CR2 (CD21). Thus, B cells expressing FcεRII can link to CR2 on other B cells, T cells, and dendritic cells. By linking B cells to dendritic cells, FcεRII enhances B cell survival and promotes IgE production. This receptor has also been cloned and sequenced in the horse (Watson et al., 2000). It contains 327 amino acids.

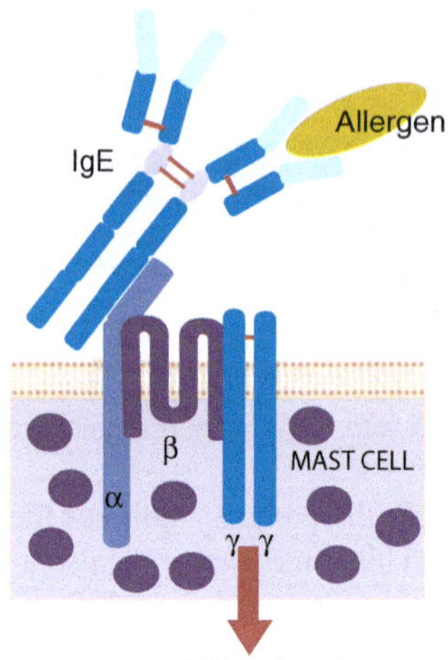

FIGURE 19.2 The structure of the FcεRI receptor.

This is the receptor through which T cells are triggered to degranulate.

Degranulation and mediators

Mast cells release their preformed mediators within minutes of their receptors bindin to an antigen. Although there are numerous ways by which mast cells can be induced to degranulate, the most important is that triggered by an antigen when it cross-links two IgE molecules bound to two high-affinity FcεRI receptors. The receptors aggregate, and this aggregation triggers degranulation. The β and γ chains of FcεRI each have an immunoreceptor tyrosine-based activation motif (ITAM) that is needed for signal transduction. Immediately after antigen cross-links two FcεRI by binding to their α chains, aggregation occurs, the two tyrosine kinases, Lyn and Syc are activated, and the ITAMS are phosphorylated. This, in turn, activates phospholipase C, leading to the production of diacylglycerol and inositol triphosphate. These two mediators then trigger a rise in cytosolic Ca^{++}, cytoskeletal rearrangements such as microtubule polymerization and actin depolymerization. The rise in Ca^{++} triggers protein kinase activation. The protein kinases phosphorylate myosin in the cytoskeleton so that the mast cell granules migrate to the cell surface. The granule membranes then fuse with the plasma membrane, and their contents are released into the extracellular fluid. During degranulation, the granules can also move along microtubules from the interior of the mast cell toward the plasma membrane. The granules thus create a "degranulation channel," and their contents are released in all directions.

Cross-linking and aggregation of two IgE-FcεRI complexes by an antigen also activates phospholipase A. This acts on cell membrane phospholipids to generate arachidonic acid. Cyclooxygenases and lipoxygenases then convert the arachidonic acid to leukotrienes and prostaglandins. Additionally, the protein kinases promote the transcription of genes encoding many different cytokines and chemokines. Fig. 19.3.

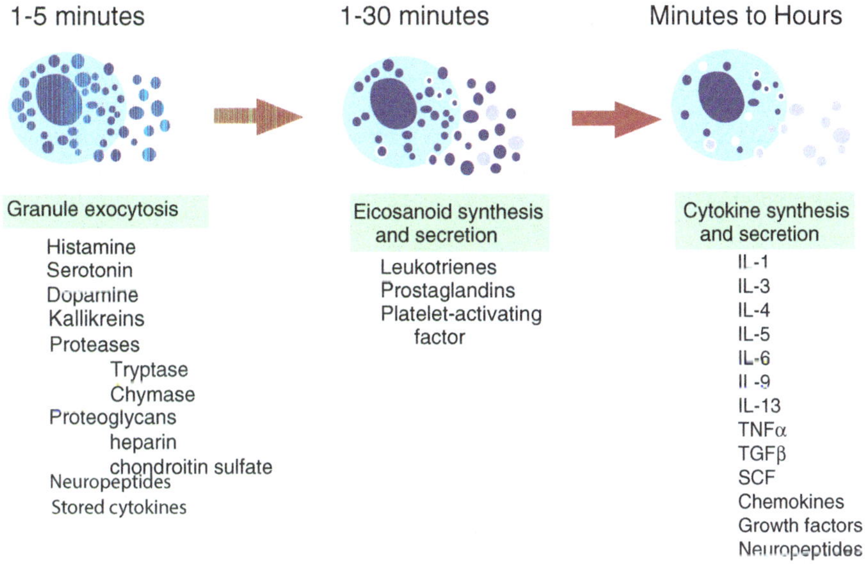

FIGURE 19.3 The process of mast cell degranulation.

Granule contents and cytokines are released within minutes but the process continues for several hours after degranulation.

Mast cell granules contain three classes of biologically active molecules. First, they are loaded with preformed inflammatory mediators. These include vasoactive amines such as histamine and serotonin. Since the granules are modified lysosomes, they also contain a mixture of lysosomal proteinases. Equine mast cells have been shown to possess at least two proteinases. One is very similar to human tryptase (85% amino acid identity), consisting of 34–36 kDa subunits. The other protease, a chymase, shows 95% identity to human granzyme H (Pemberton et al., 2001).

Proteoglycans (heavily glycosylated proteins) are also major granule components. They have a serine-glycine rich backbone (serglycin) with glycosamino side chains and thus a very high anionic charge. One such proteoglycan, heparin, is a major granule component that plays an important role in packaging histamine and the proteases. The proteoglycans bind strongly to cationic molecules such as toluidine blue and the Romanowsky combination dyes and are therefore responsible for the metachromatic staining of mast cell granules.

Mast cell granules store large quantities of growth factors and cytokines such as TNF-α, IL-4, IL-5, IL-6, and IL-15, as well as vascular endothelial growth factor (VEGF) and some chemokines. Mast cells can also capture and store IL-17 by endocytosis. Mast cell granules are not homogeneous; some granules contain serotonin and cathepsin D, while others contain histamine and TNF-α. Mast cells also produce chitinases (Patel & Goyal, 2017). Chitin is a complex carbohydrate characteristically found in insects, fungi, and helminths. The production of chitinases supports the suggestion that allergic reactions may have evolved, in part, to combat these invaders. Chitin itself is a key allergen in equine hypersensitivity dermatitis (Komi et al., 2018).

In addition to the release of preformed mediators, mast cells, once activated, synthesize and secrete proinflammatory lipids such as prostaglandins and leukotrienes. They also begin the synthesis and release of a diverse mixture of cytokines, chemokines, and growth factors.

Basophils

Equine basophils are functionally and phenotypically similar to mast cells. Basophils originate in the bone marrow, circulate as mature cells within the bloodstream, and are recruited to inflammatory sites in tissues. Unlike mast cells, which are long-lived and may divide, basophils are short-lived, non-dividing cells. They die by apoptosis in tissues after participating in inflammatory reactions. They play an important role in IgE-mediated skin inflammation. They mature as they circulate in the bloodstream and have a lifespan of only 60–70 hours. Equine basophils are smaller than mast cells, with multilobular nuclei and fewer, smaller cytoplasmic granules (Raza et al., 2021). They are IgE+, $MHCII^{high}$, and $CD14^{-}$ (Wagner et al., 2010).

Eosinophils

Horse tissues undergoing type I hypersensitivity reactions are characteristically infiltrated by large numbers of eosinophils. These eosinophils are attracted to sites of mast cell degranulation, where they also release their granule contents. Equine eosinophils are polymorphonuclear leukocytes, slightly larger than neutrophils or basophils (12–17 μm in diameter), with cytoplasmic granules that stain intensely with the red dye eosin. They normally originate from granulocytic precursors in the bone marrow and spend about 30 minutes circulating in the bloodstream before migrating into the tissues, where they have a half-life of about 12 days. The proportion of eosinophils among the blood leukocytes varies greatly since it is affected by the presence of parasites. Normal values range from about 4%–7% of the blood leukocytes in horses. However, this number varies between age, breed, stress (exercise), and is very much a reflection of the animal's parasite burden. There are also diurnal and seasonal variations in these numbers (Brosnahan, 2020a). Eosinophils tend to favor certain equine tissues. Thus, they are prominent throughout the intestinal tract, especially the small intestine and colon. The great majority of a horse's eosinophils are located in the mucosae of the gastrointestinal tract (Rotting et al., 2008). They are also present in the spleen and reproductive tracts of normal healthy horses.

Horses possess two distinct eosinophil subsets as determined by their size and granule numbers. The small cells are $CD49d^{+}$ cells that are associated with the transition to an allergic state. The second subset is $CD49d^+$, and $CD49f^+$. These are larger cells with more granules. They are found within the lesions and are probably more toxic. These two subsets may simply reflect developmental stages as the eosinophils mature (Pantelyushin et al., 2020).

Activation

Eosinophils develop from bone marrow stem cells under the influence of IL-3, GM-CSF, and especially IL-5. They share a common progenitor with basophils and mast cells. Both Th2 cells and mast cells produce IL-5 and the chemokine known as eotaxin (CCL11) that stimulates the release of eosinophils from the bone marrow through its receptor CCR3. IL-25, IL-33, and TSLP all induce IL-5 production (Brosnahan, 2020b). Thus, Th2 cells mobilize eosinophils while promoting IgE responses. These eosinophils are attracted to sites of mast cell degranulation by eotaxins, histamine, and its breakdown product imidazolacetic acid, leukotrienes C4 and B_4, and by platelet-activating factor (PAF) (Foster et al., 1992). Eosinophils are especially attracted by CXCL8 (IL-8) complexed to IgA. Some allergens directly activate eosinophils, stimulating their chemotaxis and upregulating CCR3 expression. The mobilization and activation of eosinophils enhance their ability to kill parasites and support the belief that one major function of the IgE-mediated responses is the generation of type 2 responses, resulting in the control of helminth parasites. Some activated eosinophils also express MHC class II molecules and may serve as antigen-presenting cells.

Mast cells and eosinophils interact. Thus, eosinophil major basic protein causes mast cells to release histamine. Mast cells in turn, release eosinophil chemotactic agents, activate eosinophils, and enhance the expression of eosinophil receptors. Mast cells can synthesize and secrete IL-3, IL-5, and GM-CSF, all of which promote eosinophil accumulation, degranulation, and survival.

Degranulation and mediators

Eosinophils express many PRRs that recognize PAMPs and DAMPs. When triggered, the eosinophils release multiple cytokines and chemokines, as well as their granule contents. Although eosinophils can phagocytose small particles, they are much more suited to the extracellular destruction of large parasites since they can degranulate into the surrounding fluid. Eosinophils may release intact granules by exocytosis or, more commonly, undergo piecemeal degranulation. In this process, small vesicles bud off the secondary granules and are released into the extracellular tissues. This occurs in response to IgE-coated parasites, many chemokines, platelet-activating factor, and C5a. Once free in the extracellular fluid, eosinophil granules can function as independent structures capable of releasing their proteins in response to IFN-γ or CCL11. Activated eosinophils can also eject extracellular traps containing mitochondrial DNA and granule cationic proteins. They do this in response to bacterial products such as endotoxins. The release of these traps is not accompanied by cell death.

The biological role of eosinophils is to release their granule contents at an appropriate time and location, and hence destroy foreign antigens associated with pathogens or parasites. Horse eosinophils contain multiple large cytoplasmic granules. These contain alkaline phosphatase, peroxidase, ribonuclease, arylsulfatase, cathepsin, acid phosphatase, β-glucuronidase, and α- and β-mannosidases. They do not contain lysozyme (Acharya & Ackerman, 2014; Brosnahan, 2020a). Eosinophils also produce lipid mediators such as leukotrienes and platelet-activating factors. Eosinophil granule proteins can kill helminths and bacteria and are important mediators of tissue pathology. They all, for example, damage the respiratory epithelium. The production by eosinophils of multiple Th2 cytokines, as well as indoleamine dioxygenase, inhibits local Th1 responses and ensures that a "Th2 environment" is maintained where eosinophils accumulate.

In addition to their role as antiparasitic cells, eosinophils play multiple other defensive roles in horses. For example, they tend to be increased in the blood of horses with non-infectious respiratory disease (Chapter 20). They are often abundant in the skin of horses with allergic skin diseases, such as insect bite hypersensitivity. Horses also suffer from several "eosinophil-associated diseases," especially diseases affecting the gastrointestinal tract (Brosnahan, 2020b). An eosinophilic synovitis in an American Quarter horse has been attributed to *Borrelia burgdorferi*, the cause of equine Lyme disease (Serpa et al., 2025).

In summary, type 1 hypersensitivity reactions are mediated by IgE and recruit three key cells, mast cells, basophils and eosinophils to participate in the reaction. Their biological role is to mediate anti-parasite responses, but they also mediate allergic diseases.

Multisystemic eosinophilic epitheliotropic disease

Multisystemic eosinophilic epitheliotropic disease (MEED) is a rare equine disease of unknown etiology (Bosseler et al., 2013). Young Standardbred horses are most prone to develop it. It may be an acute or chronic condition with a reported duration from 5 days to 9 months. Affected horses suffer from massive multifocal to diffuse eosinophilic and lymphocytoplasmic infiltrations of body organs. It may affect multiple body systems, including the gastrointestinal tract, skin, liver, lymph nodes, and lungs. In many cases, the lesions may be restricted to the intestine, resulting in gastritis and colitis (Pucheu-Haston & Del Piero, 2013). The most frequent presenting signs are weight loss and diarrhea. Many affected animals also exhibit cutaneous lesions such a pruritic exfoliative dermatitis with diffuse alopecia and crusting. There is limited evidence that some cases of MEED are caused by parasites. Other cases may result from an allergic response to unknown antigens. Some cases are associated with the presence of a lymphosarcoma. (In other species, it is associated with the development of T cell neoplasia and the consequent overproduction of eosinophil-activating cytokines such as interleukin-5.) Many equine cases have no obvious cause. The disease has a poor prognosis.

Equine anaphylaxis

In the equine respiratory tract, mast cells are found in the greatest numbers in the nasopharynx. The majority of these (57%–94%) are located in the lamina propria. while up to 20% are associated with the mucosal glandular tissue. Only small numbers are present in the surface epithelium or in the nasal lymphoid tissues. In equine lungs, 20% of the mast cell population is associated with the small airways, 25% with the pleura, and 32% with small blood vessels (Mair et al., 1988). These distributions are of importance since they determine the extent and severity of equine anaphylactic shock.

Anaphylaxis is a life-threatening, acute, immediate hypersensitivity reaction occurring as a result of the rapid release of inflammatory mediators from large numbers of pulmonary mast cells. Affected horses develop acute respiratory distress, and cardiovascular collapse, that may be lethal. The major shock organs of horses are the lungs and the intestines. During anaphylaxis, bronchial and bronchiolar constriction leads to coughing, dyspnea, and eventually apnea. On necropsy, severe pulmonary emphysema and peribronchiolar edema are commonly seen. In addition to the lung lesions, edematous hemorrhagic enterocolitis may result in severe diarrhea. Fig. 19.4.

Experimental anaphylaxis in ponies sensitized by inoculation of whole bovine serum exhibited a characteristic pattern. Within 2 minutes of beginning the allergen infusion, there was a severe drop in carotid artery pressure accompanied by a rise in pulmonary arterial blood pressure and a brief fall in vena caval pressure. The animals then went through alternating phases of apnea and dyspnea. By 3 minutes, the vena

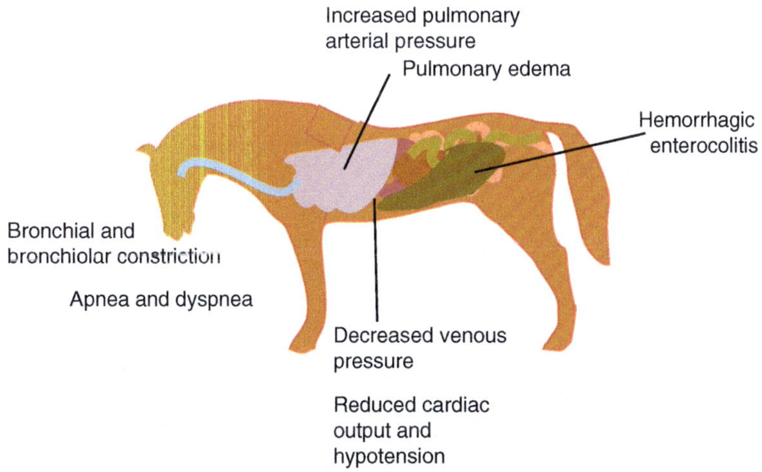

FIGURE 19.4

The signs of equine anaphylaxis.

caval pressure increased transiently, coinciding with a period of apnea. After about 8–10 minutes, the venous pressure returned to normal. The carotid pressure returned to normal by 15 minutes, and pulmonary artery pressure normalized after 20–25 minutes (Eyre & Lewis, 1973). In other experimental anaphylaxis studies in ponies, the initial apnea was followed by 2–3 minutes of rapid breathing. There was another period of apnea lasting 3–4 minutes, and after a short period of shallow, rapid breathing, respiration returned to normal by 12 minutes. Unsensitized ponies receiving the same dose of antigen did not exhibit any measurable adverse responses.

During the shock phase of this reaction, there was also a marked hemoconcentration accompanied by a leukopenia, thrombocytopenia, and increased plasma potassium. The total leukocyte count decreased within 5–10 minutes but returned to normal by 30–40 minutes. This decrease involved neutrophils and monocytes while lymphocyte numbers remained unchanged. At the same time, there was a severe thrombocytopenia with the platelet count dropping to around 25% of normal. Mast cells in the pleura, omentum, liver capsule, and subcutaneous tissues demonstrated some dispersal of their cytoplasmic granules into the surrounding tissues.

In these experimental ponies, there was a five-to six-fold increase in plasma histamine levels 2–4 minutes after the beginning of the allergen infusion. This dropped by half at 10 minutes but remained at that level for 20 minutes. The highest concentrations of histamine coincided with the most severe periods of dyspnea. At the same time as the histamine levels rose, there was a four-fivefold rise in blood kinin levels. These peaked at 5 minutes and declined to normal by 10 minutes. Serotonin levels declined during the first 5 minutes but had returned to normal by 20 minutes.

On necropsy of shocked ponies, the lungs were found to be severely congested and edematous. There was significant alveolar emphysema and bronchiolar edema. The peribronchiolar edema fluid contained mononuclear cells as well as neutrophils. There were also erythrocytes in the alveoli. In addition, there were inflamed, congested, edematous areas in the large colon and cecum. The kidneys, spleen, and liver were also engorged (Eyre & Lewis, 1973).

Insect bite hypersensitivity

Bloodsucking insects such as mosquitoes, black flies, and horseflies, as well as midges, are important causes of allergic diseases in horses, sheep, and cattle. Hypersensitivity to insect bites may cause a seasonal allergic dermatitis, variously called, according to geographical location, Gulf Coast itch, summer eczema, Queensland itch, or sweet itch. This is the most common allergic disease of horses. The insects involved include midges (*Culicoides* species), black flies (*Simulium* species), stable flies (*Stomoxys* and *Haematobia*), mosquitoes, and stick-tight fleas (*Echidnophaga gallinacea*). Some of these species have been incriminated because their saliva triggers a positive inflammatory response in an intradermal skin test, but this may simply be a result of antibody cross-reactivity (Schaffartzik et al., 2012).

Biology

Insect bite hypersensitivity (IBH) is a common pruritic dermatitis primarily caused by hypersensitivity responses to allergens in Culicoides saliva. Culicoides are very small, blood-feeding midges, about 1–3 mm in length. (This is about the same size as a flea)! As in mosquitoes, only the females feed on blood. These Culicoides midges are smaller than mosquitoes but much more abundant. Fig. 19.5.

There are multiple Culicoides species and subspecies found worldwide. *C. obsoletus* is the most common species affecting horses in North America and Europe. *C. nubeculosis* is found in Europe. *C. variipennis* is also found in North America. All three of these species can act as vectors for viral diseases such African Horse Sickness (and Bluetongue). Because of their diversity, it is not uncommon for more than one species of Culicoides to feed on a single horse. They do not suck blood like mosquitoes, they bite! These bites are painful and very annoying to the targeted horse. There is no evidence for the preexistence of a skin barrier defect in IBH-affected horses. The mouthparts of Culicoides midges are well able to penetrate the skin barrier. Female midge mouthparts consist of two serrated blades that they push into the skin and then cut with a backward stroke. They either insert them directly into a capillary or into a pool of extravasated blood. At the same time, they inject a saliva that is both anticoagulant and vasodilatory and may even have

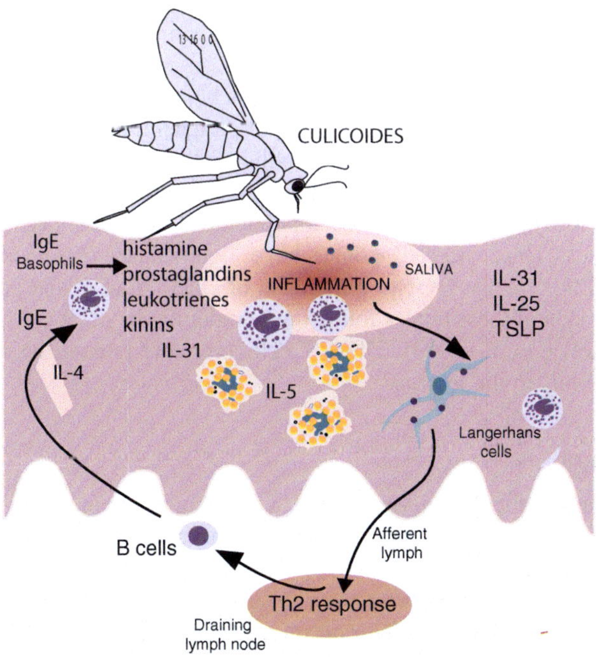

FIGURE 19.5

The basic pathways involved in Culicoides hypersensitivity.

anesthetic properties. The enzymes in saliva break down connective tissue in the epithelial tissues. Some horses react to these injected foreign proteins by mounting both antibody and cell-mediated immune responses. Culicoides hypersensitivity may therefore be a mixture of type I and type IV hypersensitivity responses. It is also influenced by both genetic and local environmental factors.

Allergens

The severity of the IBH response is determined by Th2 cells and the balance between Th2 and Treg activity. At least 21 salivary allergens have been identified as being relevant to IBH. For example, the saliva of *Culicoides nubeculosus* contains 11 characterized allergens,—Cul n 1 to Cul n 11. Four salivary allergens from the blackfly, *Simulium vittatum*, Sim v 1–4 are also bound by equine IgE, but these may simply be a result of cross-reactions with Culicoides. Not all horses, of course, react to all allergens. Their reactivity ranges from 13% to 56%, depending on the allergen tested. On average, each horse reacts to about four allergens (range 1–10). Cul n 1 and Sim v 1 share sequence homology with an allergenic protein in wasp venom, and Cul n 2 is a hyaluronidase related to a major allergen in bee venom. A mixture of *C. obsoletus* allergens used in an ELISA assay had a sensitivity of 92% and a specificity of 85% when compared to intradermal skin testing. Total IgE, in contrast, is not significantly increased in horses affected by IBH when compared to healthy control animals (Wagner, Miller, et al., 2006).

Affected horses show a significant increase in blood eosinophils, monocytes, and basophils. Analysis of the in vitro functions of peripheral blood leukocytes in *Culicoides*-sensitive horses indicated that basophils are the major source of IL-4 in these cases. Thus, these cells may play a significant role in the induction of this disease (Raza et al., 2021). The lymphocyte subpopulations have also been characterized in these horses. Thus, affected ponies have significantly increased numbers of $CD5^+$ and $CD4^+$ T cells. Increased numbers of $CD3^+$ T cells and eosinophils are present in the skin of these horses following intradermal inoculation of a Culicoides extract (McKelvie et al., 1999). These T cells probably release the cytokines that attract eosinophils to the lesions.

Epidemiology

Like mosquitoes, Culicoides midges breed in standing water, including salt marshes, ponds, lakes, and even wet manure. They are not strong fliers, so they do not fly long distances and cannot fly against the wind. They prefer still, warm nights, and fly at dawn and dusk when large swarms may be seen. While globally widespread, local environmental conditions affect their prevalence and behavior. Culicoides hypersensitivity may or may not be seasonal, depending on the prevalence of the midges. Clinical signs do not generally appear until a horse has reached 2–4 years of age, and then gradually worsen. The lesions generally appear during the summer months when the flies are biting but may improve somewhat over the cooler winter months. The disease appears to be more common in Icelandic horses and some lines of Swiss warmbloods. It occurs more frequently in some horse families than in others, and its severity is associated with some equine MHC antigens such as ELA-Aw7. Its heritability appears to range from 0.08 to 0.30 (Viluma et al., 2017). Other studies have demonstrated that an ELA class II allele, *COR112:274,* is associated with disease susceptibility in both Icelandic horses and Exmoor ponies. Homozygosity across the entire MHC class II region is also associated with a significantly higher risk of developing insect bite hypersensitivity (Andersson et al., 2012).

Clinical disease

The severity of IBH lesions depends on the number of bites, the stage of the disease, the intensity of the pruritus, and the degree of secondary infection. The initial lesions include many papules, tufted hair, pruritic urticaria and skin sensitivity. The intense pruritus is often followed by self-mutilation resulting in excoriation, erosion, ulceration, hair loss, and skin thickening. Subsequent secondary infections may mask the original allergic nature of the lesion. Fig. 19.6.

Culicoides preferred feeding sites are located along the dorsal midline at the tail base, the withers, and the mane. Less commonly, they attack the head, ears, and legs. Likewise, some Culicoides species may cause a ventral midline dermatitis. Chronic lesions result in alopecia with skin lichenification and scaling that may develop into transverse ridges.

The course of the disease is readily divided into two phases. Thus, it is induced by a type I hypersensitivity reaction mediated by Th2 cells, the production of IgE and mast cell degranulation. Horses have a relatively high level of IgE in their blood. They average about 84.0 mg/mL. As usual, however, there is enormous variability in IgE levels between individual horses. As a result, total serum IgE is not a useful assay for the confirmation of allergic disease (Wilson et al., 2006). IgE^{+} B cells can be readily detected in biopsies from acute skin lesions. Some evidence suggests that *Culicoides*-specific IgG3/5 is also produced by affected horses and may contribute to disease pathogenesis. The key mast cell mediators of these IBH reactions are histamine, which may be largely responsible for the pruritus, leukotrienes, and platelet-activating factor (PAF), as well as interleukin-31. Infiltrating eosinophils and neutrophils also contribute to the development of the itch (Fettelschloss-Gabriel et al., 2021). The chemokine CXCL8 (IL-8) may also play a significant role in lesion development. Histamine can be detected in the plasma of horses with acute lesions. Intradermal injection of platelet-activating factor results in local masr cell degranulation and the development of lesions similar to those induced by Culicoides. Experimentally, leukotrienes and histamine can also be released from Culicoides-stimulated equine leukocytes. Thus, 78% of allergic horses and 3% of control animals released leukotrienes after their leukocytes were exposed to *C. nubeculosus* allergens in vitro.

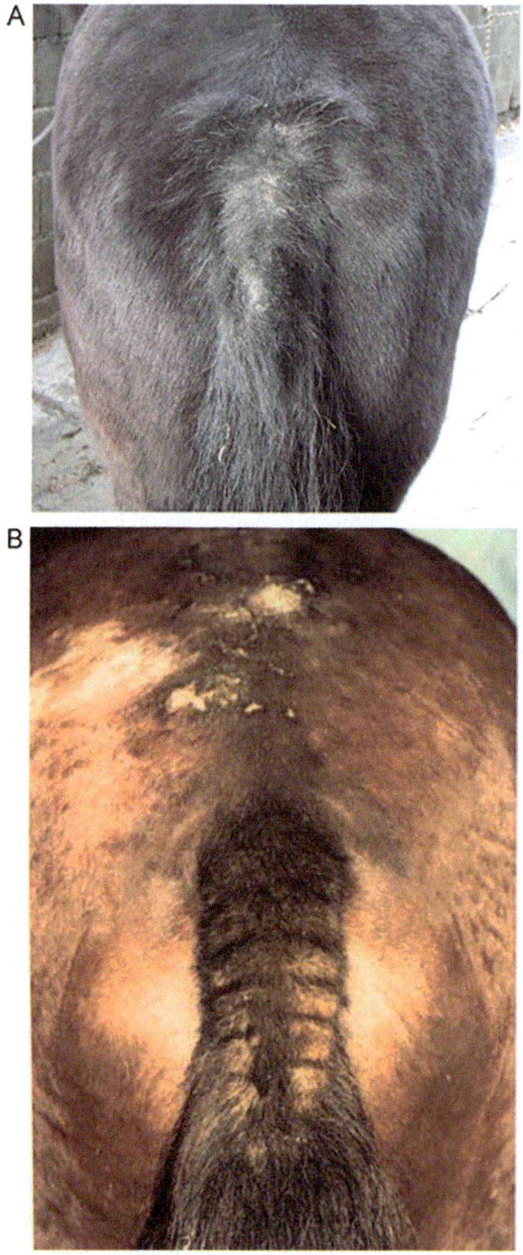

FIGURE 19.6 Clinical signs of insect bite hypersensitivity (IBH).

(A) Localized hair loss and excoriations at the tail. (B) More severe form of IBH with lichenification of the skin, a "rat-tail", and affected areas on the croup.

- With permission Schaffartzik et al. (2012).

The gene expression profile in lesional skin has been compared to the expression profile in normal equine skin. Thus, the upregulation of IL-1Ra, CCR5, IFN-γ, and IL-31Rα was strongly correlated with the severity of the hypersensitivity. Elevated IL-31 and IL-33 levels, on the other hand, tended to be associated with milder forms of the disease. The blood basophil counts were strongly correlated with IL-31Rα, IL-5, IL-5Rα, IFN-γ, HRH2 (histamine receptor H2), HRH 4, CCR3, CCR5, IL-12β, IL-10, IL-1β and CCL26 mRNA expression in skin punch biopsies (Jebbawi et al., 2024).

IL-31 is a major mediator of the itch associated with IBH lesions. Measurement of IL-31 in skin punch biopsies of insect-bite hypersensitive horses and in allergen-stimulated mononuclear cells in vitro demonstrated its presence in significant amounts (Craig et al., 2024).

Some studies have detected evidence that a T cell-mediated delayed hypersensitivity response to injected allergens also occurs in IBH. However, this is inconsistent, and its significance is unclear. Lesional skin of IBH-affected horses contains large numbers of $CD4^+$ T cells and few $CD8^+$ T cells (Cox & Stewart, 2023).

On histopathology, the insect bite lesions consist of a perivascular dermatitis and subepidermal edema. The cellular infiltrate consists of mononuclear cells, but this is often associated with a perivascular or diffuse eosinophil infiltration, especially in acute cases. Tryptase-positive mast cells may accumulate at the dermo-epidermal junction. Langerhans cells also accumulate here. Some horses may develop an eosinophilic folliculitis, epidermal pustules or even eosinophilic granulomas. Old lesions show epidermal hyperplasia, hyperkeratosis and lichenification, and dermal fibrosis.

As in so many allergic diseases, more than one allergic response may develop simultaneously in a single individual. While the most obvious lesions and symptoms are associated with inflammatory reactions at the insect bite sites, insect bite hypersensitivity also has systemic effects. For example, IBH may be accompanied by severe equine asthma syndrome (Chapter 20). The presence of IBH in a horse is associated with airway hypersensitivity and decreased arterial oxygenation (Verdon et al., 2019).

In general, the development of IBH precedes the development of severe asthma in a manner reminiscent of the human "allergic march." The immunological challenge presented by IBH may well redirect the immune system as a whole to alter its normal balance and move toward a Th2-biased state. Studies on horses with IBH have shown that their pO_2 is decreased compared to normal horses, even in the absence of overt respiratory disease. While there is an association between IBH and equine asthma, this may not be IgE-mediated. Thus, horses affected by both IBH and asthma do not have higher IgE concentrations than horses affected by each condition alone. However, as pointed out previously, measurement of IgE levels alone is of limited value since they do not take IgE specificity and mast cell receptor affinity into account. Presumably, the degranulation of multiple mast cells in the horse's skin and the presence of increased levels of vasoactive mediators in the bloodstream means that airway smooth muscle is at least partially contracted and dyspnea may result (Lanz et al., 2017).

Diagnosis and treatment

Diagnosis of equine IBH is based on clinical signs, history, seasonality, location (pasture close to standing water), and absence of fly control. Allergy skin testing using whole Culicoides extracts may be useful, but even clinically healthy horses may give positive results in both in vivo and in vitro testing. These crude whole-body extracts are not standardized, and the amount of salivary allergens in them may therefore be minimal (Van der Meide et al., 2013). False-positive and false-negative results are common. Detection of IgE denotes exposure, not necessarily disease. Some horses may not have detectable IgE if they mount a cell-mediated, type IV hypersensitivity response. Indeed, healthy horses of all age groups may have detectable IgE antibodies to Culicoides on their skin mast cells without showing any clinical signs (Wagner et al., 2009). Presumably, the concentration of these antibodies is insufficient to permit cross-linking between IgE receptor molecules and triggering mast cell degranulation (Peeters et al., 2013).

Treatment involves avoidance! This is the only safe and effective method of prevention. There are many different fly repellents available in the form of sprays, wipes, and spot-on products. These usually contain pyrethrins or permethrin. Lightweight blankets are the easiest and most common method of protection. They should be put on before dusk and removed well after dawn. Reduction of the acute inflammation and pruritus through the use of topical or systemic steroids may make animals much more comfortable. Immunotherapy has yet to yield significant positive benefits, probably because only crude fly extracts are available (Fettelschloss-Gabriel et al., 2021).

Vaccines

Given that the lesions of IBD result from the activities of eosinophils, and that these eosinophils are attracted and activated by cytokines such as IL-5 and IL-31, it makes sense to seek to reduce disease severity by specifically neutralizing these cytokines. For example, a vaccine against IBH has been developed. The vaccine consists of equine IL-5 covalently linked to a virus-like particle derived from cucumber mosaic virus containing a universal tetanus toxoid epitope. The vaccine has been tested in susceptible Icelandic horses. The vaccine was well tolerated and produced an antibody response against IL-5 in 17 of 19 horses. This resulted in a statistically significant drop in CBH clinical lesion scores in the vaccinated animals compared to the scores in unvaccinated control horses. Analysis showed that their eosinophil counts, but not the IgE levels, correlated with disease severity. Interestingly, the vaccine did not appear to affect blood lymphocyte counts, but greatly reduced the numbers of eosinophils in the lesions (Fettelschloss-Gabriel et al., 2018). However the vaccine was slow to take effect and reduced the blood basophil counts in horses with Culicoides hypersensitivity, but only in the third year of the study (Rhiner et al., 2022).

In a separate study, a vaccine has also been developed against equine interleukin-31. IL-31 derived from Th2 cells, also contributes to the inflammatory response. The vaccine was formulated in the same way as the IL-5 vaccine described above, namely, equine IL-31 was coupled to virus-like particles from cucumber mosaic virus (Birkmann et al., 2024). It successfully induced autoantibodies against IL-31 and has reduced the severity of IBH lesion scores as determined by double-blind, placebo-controlled studies (Olomski et al., 2020).

Donkeys and mules can also develop Culicoides hypersensitivity. They differ however in the location of the lesions which generally develop on their legs and head rather than on the animal's back.

Equine allergies

Like the other domestic mammals, horses can develop allergies to diverse foreign allergens. For example, they may become allergic to inhaled airborne particles, including pollens and other plant particles, molds, and arthropod-derived dusts. In these cases, the allergens are absorbed through the skin, the respiratory tract, or the gastrointestinal tract and stimulate IgE production. Once sensitized, subsequent exposure to these allergens will trigger mast cell degranulation, histamine release, and perhaps an eosinophil infiltration. Allergies may also be triggered in horses by some drugs and vaccines. The sum of the external factors that an individual horse is exposed to throughout its lifetime (the exposome) includes factors such as humidity, diet, behavior, pollution, and allergens; and host factors such as the animal's skin microbiota. Given its location, the skin is the organ that directly interacts with the exposome and where environmental influences would be expected to have the greatest influence.

Inhaled allergens

Horses, especially those living in dusty, moldy stables, inhale numerous airborne allergens. These allergens include organic dusts containing mold spores, bacterial endotoxins, tree and plant pollens, and arthropods and, as a result, many cases are seasonal. These horses often spend much of the day in an enclosed stable with poor air circulation. The development of allergies to inhaled allergens is therefore common. It usually involves simultaneous allergies to multiple allergens. Equine allergic responses fall into two main categories, respiratory disease and skin disease. Respiratory signs include a chronic nasal discharge with greenish mucus; chronic, persistent sneezing and coughing, irritated eyes with a chronic discharge from the tear duct (watery eyes), exercise intolerance, heaves, and RAO. Respiratory allergies are described and discussed in Chapter 20.

Allergic dermatitis

Allergic (or atopic) dermatitis encompasses several equine skin diseases that typically present with pruritic rashes. Signs of skin allergies include hives—large, raised welts, itching, and irritation. Affected horses may develop patchy hair loss due to chronic itching and scratching. Secondary infections of self traumatized areas are not uncommon. The syndrome is frustrating to treat because it is influenced by many different environmental factors. At its simplest, it may be considered to be a local skin hypersensitivity response to environmental allergens. However, it is made vastly more complex and difficult to treat because of the interactions with other factors that determine its progression and outcome (Fig. 19.7) (Marsella et al., 2023).

Allergic dermatitis develops as a result of a type I hypersensitivity reaction mediated by allergen-specific IgE and mast cells. An inappropriate type 2 immune response can also cause the release of cytokines such as IL-5, IL-6, IL-13, and IL-31. The relative importance of these cytokines is unclear, but IL-31 plays a major role in the disease (Olomski et al., 2020). IL-31 is increased in allergen-stimulated peripheral blood mononuclear cells in the skin lesions of horses with insect bite hypersensitivity. An intradermal injection of IL-31 induces pruritus in normal horses (Craig et al., 2020).

The development of some forms of allergic dermatitis in horses is probably secondary to the influx of environmental or food allergens as a result of epithelial barrier dysfunction. In other words, the primary defect is in the skin permeability barrier and is followed by influx of allergen and a subsequent IgE response resulting in mast cell degranulation. (*The outside-inside theory*). An alternative explanation suggests that there is a process associated with the allergic state in which the allergic response in the skin results in secondary barrier defects—*the inside-outside theory.* Of course, both theories could be correct and simply reflect two different disease endotypes. Once AD develops, by whatever route, then the skin response becomes a self-perpetuating cycle of inflammation, itch, and skin damage.

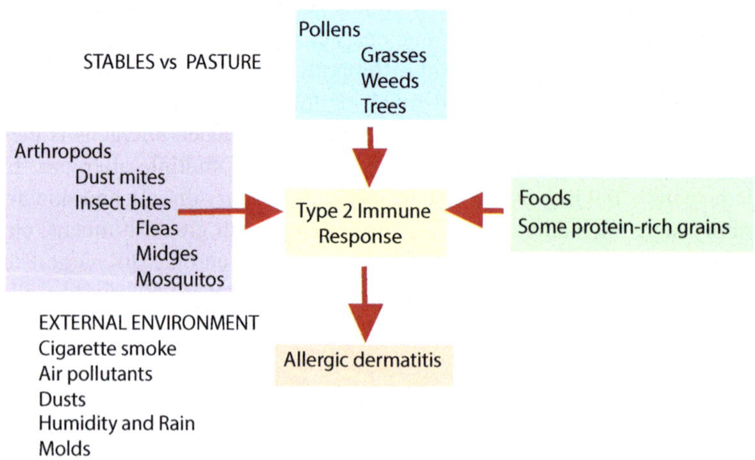

FIGURE 19.7

The environmental and other allergens that can influence and trigger equine atopic dermatitis.

Allergens

Many horses are sensitized against pollen-derived allergens. This sensitization is usually directed against plants that rely on the wind to spread their pollen long distances. Most pollens and mold spores are about 20–60 μm in diameter and tend to lodge in the eyes and nasal passages. Smaller airborne particles around 10 μm in diameter can be inhaled and penetrate to the lower respiratory tract. Pollen grain allergens are usually glycoproteins found within the pollen protoplast but are released when the pollen lands on a moist surface and rehydrates. In addition to their glycoproteins, pollens may also release lipids that can bind to toll-like receptors, activate NKT cells, and also promote type 2 immune responses. These lipids include saturated and unsaturated fatty acids and glycophospholipids, as well as lipopolysaccharides from the microbiota on the pollen surface. It is evident, therefore, that simple aqueous pollen extracts may not contain all the biologically active substances released by pollen grains and may therefore underestimate their allergenicity when used for skin testing or immunotherapy. Many grass and tree pollens also contain proteases that can disrupt the skin epithelial barrier by degrading the proteins in tight junctions.

The major allergenic tree pollens originate from box elder (*Acer negundo*), cedar, and oak trees. As with other plants, their prevalence varies seasonally and regionally. Tree pollination usually occurs in spring (between December and April) and tends to be brief. Tree pollen allergies seem to be most significant in temperate climate zones. However, they are becoming a greater problem in subtropical climates as well.

Wind-pollinated grasses such as Bermuda grass, Johnson grass, Rye grass, and Kentucky bluegrass release large amounts of pollen during spring and summer (May through July), the growing season. Seasonal patterns are more obvious in northern regions. Maximum pollen levels occur in the afternoons on hot, dry, windy days.

Wind-borne weed pollens are generally produced by non-colorful annual flowers that do not attract insects. Weed pollination generally occurs from late summer through October. In the United States, the pollen from common ragweed (*Ambrosia* spp.) is the single most important cause of allergies. It predominates in the central plains and in agricultural areas in the eastern US. A single plant can release a million pollen grains daily, and these can be detected up to 400 miles away. Pollen release is highly seasonal, with peak pollen counts occurring in late September. Other important pollen sources include sagebrush (*Artemesia*), English plantain (*Plantago*), yellow dock (*Rumex*), lambsquarters (*Chenopodium*), and pigweed (*Amaranthus*). These, of course, differ between countries and regions.

Molds

Mold spores are also common aeroallergens. They are especially significant in horses housed in dusty stables. Those fungi that form hyphae may be specialized to produce reproductive spores that are dispersed by wind, water, or insects. Some molds sporulate under low humidity conditions, while others prefer high humidity to achieve maximal dispersal. Mold allergies are generally subject to acute exacerbations as a result of temporary high concentrations of these airborne spores. Examples include exposure to freshly mown grass or working in poorly vented barns. Some sources of important mold allergens include *Alternaria, Fusarium, Cladosporium, Aspergillus,* and *Penicillium.* The reported level of sensitization to fungal allergens is highly variable, reflecting animal housing, geographical differences, and a lack of standardization.

Dust mites

Another major source of airborne allergens is derived from common but microscopic environmental mites, especially dust mites and storage mites. The most important of these mites are *Dermatophagoides fariniae* and *D. pteronyssinus*. While dust mites are a significant cause of allergies in dogs, they can also cause problems in horses. They may be difficult to find in barn dust, but large numbers of dust mites may be present in horse rugs and saddle blankets. Rugs and blankets should be washed regularly in very hot water to eliminate this problem. Likewise, storage mites feed on grains and commonly infest stored horse food. They may therefore be present in horse feeds, especially in bulk storage (Wallace & Vogelnest, 2010).

Susceptibility factors

Skin barrier defects

It is now generally accepted that the pathogenesis of many forms of AD begins with a skin barrier defect manifested by dry, itchy skin and associated with changes in the cutaneous microbiota. Rather than being a consequence of allergic dermatitis, skin barrier defects may well be its major predisposing cause. Defects in either the skin barrier protein filaggrin or in skin lipids such as the ceramides permit loss of water as well as the penetration of allergens and microbes and increase the chances of interactions between the skin immune system and environmental irritants (Marsella, 2025). One way to measure the integrity of the skin lipid barrier is to determine transepidermal water loss (TEWL). TEWL is increased in the skin of allergic horses when compared to control horses. This is especially evident in skin locations prone to AD and is greater in younger than in older animals. TEWL is also increased in both lesional and non-lesional skin in natural cases of AD (Marsella, 2025). Fig. 19.8.

Environmental allergens and bacteria breaching the skin barrier trigger the expression of pro-inflammatory cytokines, including TSLP and IL-33, and, as a result, activate Th2 cells as well as degranulating basophils and mast cells. This local immune response generates IL-31, a key mediator of itch. These responses eventually result in the development of dermatitis. The dermatitis is initially erythematous and edematous and is described as an urticarial type. Urticarial lesions are extremely

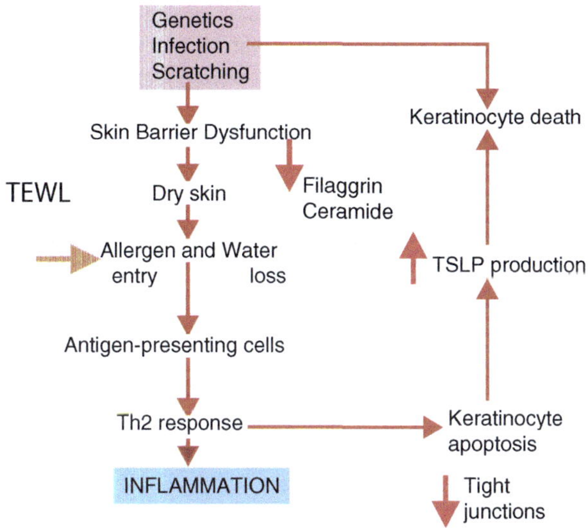

FIGURE 19.8

The pathogenesis of allergic dermatitis.

pruritic; consequently, scratching may mask the true nature of the lesion. The inflammatory cell infiltrate in these urticarial lesions is typical of allergic inflammation. The lesions are infiltrated with B cells, macrophages, and mast cells while expression of IL-4, IL-13, and TSLP is increased compared to non-lesional skin.

Skin lipid defects

keratinocytes, together with the highly hydrophobic lipids in the stratum corneum, form a physical barrier that serves to keep water in and invaders out. In addition, the keratin within these cells is bundled together by a protein called filaggrin to form a dense protein-lipid matrix. Horse epidermis may contain much less lipid than human skin, perhaps because of the additional protection afforded by hair (Marsella, 2025).

The vulnerability of horses to the development of AD may be increased by alterations in their skin lipid content (Marsella et al., 2014). As in other domestic mammals, loss of lipids increases transepidermal water loss. Horses with AD have an altered serum phospholipid profile when compared to healthy horses (Hallamaa et al., 2014). They have lower levels of phosphatidyl choline and sphingomyelin. Changes in sphingomyelin correlated with alterations in clinical disease, suggesting that it may play an active role in the course of insect bite hypersensitivity (Hallamaa & Batchu, 2016).

Provided the skin lipid barrier is intact, it will minimize water evaporation and block the ingress of environmental allergens. In many cases of equine AD, the initial lesion appears to be a defect in the epithelial lipid barrier, leading to a decrease in its thickness. IL-4 and IL-13 interfere with the activities of fatty acid elongases in the skin. In atopic skin, the lipid lamellae in the barrier may be thinner and fragmented or discontinuous, while spaces between the corneal cells may be wider. An electron microscope study suggested that the continuity and thickness of the intercellular lamellae were decreased in non-lesional atopic equine skin as compared to normal skin (Marsella et al., 2014). Another feature of atopic skin is the presence of bands of variable density in the lipid layers of the skin. It is suggested that these bands may reflect fluctuating levels of ceramide associated with acute inflammatory episodes. A ceramide defect occurs in human AD, and it is regarded both as a primary causal defect and also a secondary consequence of AD. A study on the epidermal ultrastructure of normal and allergic horses documented the presence of amorphous intracellular lipids in the stratum corneum from allergic horses. This is similar to the findings in atopic humans and dogs (Marsella, 2025).

Protein defects

One of the most important proteins in the cornified layers of the skin is filaggrin. Filaggrin is a histidine-rich filament-associated protein involved in cross-linking keratin fibers so that they become densely packed. It is therefore a major component of the skin barrier. Filaggrin is first synthesized as a large polyprotein tetramer containing four filaggrin monomers called profilaggrin. In addition to filaggrin, several other tightly crosslinked, insoluble proteins are key components of the corneocyte barrier. These include envoplakin, periplakin, and involucrin. Defects in the genes encoding any of these can also impair skin barrier function. Antimicrobial peptides, including both the defensins and cathelicidins, are also delivered to the intercellular sites by secretion from the contents of lamellar bodies (Chapter 13).

It is possible to extract RNA from tissue samples and sequence it. This provides a snapshot of which genes are turned on in that tissue at the time of sampling. Thus, studies on the transcriptome of the epidermis from normal and allergic horses have identified downregulation of the genes encoding tight junction proteins and keratins, as well as upregulation of serine proteases and IL-13 (Cvitas et al., 2020). Keratinocytes harvested from horses with insect bite hypersensitivity also show upregulation of IL-31 gene expression (Cvitas et al., 2022).

Diagnosis

Allergic dermatitis is a progressive, life-long disease, and intervention is necessary to control it and positively affect the animal's quality of life. Constant scratching makes both horses and owners uncomfortable. It can be controlled but rarely cured. There is no single diagnostic test or clinical feature that definitively indicates a diagnosis of AD., It is primarily diagnosed by intradermal skin testing. Thus, injection of the offending allergen into the skin results in local mast cell degranulation, histamine release, and the development of a local immediate hypersensitivity reaction. It is important to rule out other causes of itch, such as insect bite dermatitis, and mange, as well as adverse food reactions and Malassezia dermatitis.

In an extensive survey of intradermal skin testing results in normal horses and horses with atopic dermatitis, Lorch and her colleagues found that atopic horses had a significantly increased number of positive reactions compared to normal horses (Lorch et al., 2001). This applied to every allergen group (weeds, grasses, trees, and insects) but not to molds. The greatest number of positive reactions in horses with atopic dermatitis was observed in response to black ant extract, grain mill dust, grain smut dust, horse fly, and cocklebur extracts. Of horses with atopic dermatitis tested at 4 hours, 20% responded to grass, 45% responded to weeds, 21% responded to trees, 15% responded to molds, and 60% responded to insect extracts. (Interestingly, of non atopic horses, 11% responded to grass, 25% to weeds, 9% to trees, 12% to molds and 22% to insect extracts). Fig. 19.9.

While total IgE is elevated in the blood of atopic horses, much of the normal IgE in serum consists of low-affinity antibodies directed against abundant environmental allergens. In contrast to total IgE, allergen-specific IgE levels often correlate well with disease presence and severity. This forms the rational basis for treating these animals by specific immunotherapy.

Equine chronic urticaria

Chronic urticaria (hives) is not uncommon in horses. It occurs in horses of all ages and may be pruritic. Thoroughbreds and Arabians appear to be predisposed

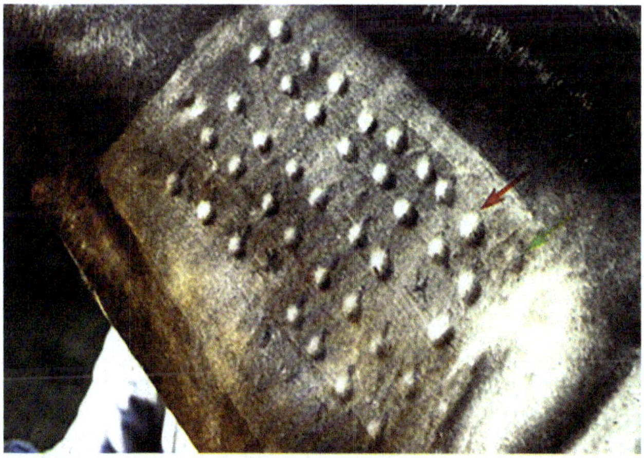

FIGURE 19.9 Multiple positive intradermal test reactions at 30 minutes.

Saline negative-control and histamine positive control.

- With permission Scott and Miller (2011).

(Akucewich & Kunkle, 2007, pp. 100–109). Lesions appear suddenly and often disappear within 24 hours. Animals develop well-defined raised bumps with lumps, wheals, or rings of variable sizes in the superficial dermis. If severe, they may result in swelling of the animal's head. They are believed to be caused by mast cell degranulation. resulting in the release of histamine, leukotrienes, and prostaglandins. leading to a local increase in vascular permeability. Histology may show perivascular or diffuse accumulations of lymphocytes and eosinophils.

The mechanisms involved in this mast cell degranulation may be immunologic in origin or not. Thus, it may be a result of a generalized allergic response. Horses with urticaria had significantly more IgE-positive cells in the subepidermal dermis when compared to control animals. They also had fewer mast cells in the subepidermal, and deep dermis compared to animals with insect bite hypersensitivity (Rufenacht et al., 2005).

The cause or causes of chronic urticaria are unknown, and no single obvious trigger has been identified. Presumed triggers include insects, environmental allergens such as pollens or molds, foods, drugs, and vaccines. Lorch and her colleagues skin tested seven horses with recurrent urticaria and found that 15% responded to grass, 40% to weeds, 13% to trees, 11% to molds and 40% to insect extracts (Lorch et al., 2001).

Drugs are probably the commonest cause of chronic urticaria. It may also be caused by specific dietary components. Thus, it has generally been assumed to be IgE-mediated and results from mast cell degranulation and mediator release. Urticaria has occasionally been linked to infectious agents as well as intestinal parasites. Urticaria in racehorses has been attributed to psychogenic factors. As discussed above, urticaria results from mast cell degranulation in the skin. Thus, while the commonest cause is likely IgE-mediated, anything else that triggers mast cell degranulation, including chemicals, hormones, or trauma, may have the same effect. In cases of nonseasonal urticaria, eosinophils appear to play an important role in its pathogenesis. Thus, they are present in about 50% of these cases. A reduction in eosinophil counts by blocking IL-5 receptor binding has resulted in clinical improvement (Birkmann et al., 2024). Horses with urticaria usually respond favorably to treatment with glucocorticoids or antihistamines. However, if the cause is unknown, the lesions may reappear once treatment is stopped.

Food allergies

Pruritic food allergies have been reported to occur in horses but are probably uncommon and not well understood. They are also somewhat controversial. Thus, while often suspected, they are rarely confirmed (Littlewood & Jackson, 2022). Their true incidence is unknown. Many reported cases may simply be adverse reactions to food components. There is also very little hard data on the subject. Most reports are anecdotal, and there are very few papers published on the subject in refereed journals. There have, however, been some significant papers published on the subject

(Favrot & Olivry, 2022). For example, chronic urticaria was observed to be highly prevalent in racehorses at Chantilly, France (Francqueville & Sabbah, 1999; Volland-Franqueville & Sabbah, 2004). These horses had received high amounts of concentrated feed during training. The individual ingredients of this diet were crushed, solubilized, and used for intradermal skin testing in the affected horses. At least one positive intradermal skin response was observed in 21 of the 22 horses involved in the study. The positive skin test responses included seven to hays, eight to oats, eight to alfalfa, three to commercial food supplements, two to barley, two to straw, and two to a commercial and vitamin mix. Nineteen of the horses showed visible clinical improvement within 3 days of a diet change, and no relapses occurred in 17 of the 19 horses. Specific dietary components have been implicated in the development of pruritus and urticaria, sometimes associated with gastrointestinal problems such as chronic colic or diarrhea. These are all very nonspecific. Oats, barley, wheat bran, chicory, potatoes, white clover, dry garlic (Miyazawa et al., 1991), and alfalfa have all been reported to be allergens in this species, but dietary trials have not been undertaken (Fadok, 2013). Reported clinical signs are very variable, but they usually consist of a pruritic urticaria, but this is by no means specific to food allergies and is readily confused with insect bite dermatitis. Simultaneous hypersensitivities to multiple unrelated food allergens are probably not uncommon. Serologic tests are not reliable in diagnosing equine food allergies (Dupont et al., 2016). Neither are intradermal skin tests. The only reliable diagnostic procedure is the use of an elimination diet. This involves feeding the horse a diet consisting of new foods and supplements to which it has not been previously exposed. Grazing animals should be moved to a new pasture or isolated indoors away from a pasture. The trial diet should be fed for up to 10 weeks. If the allergy signs resolve during this time, then previously fed foods should be returned, one at a time. If the condition recurs, then that food is the likely cause. If removed a second time, and the condition improves again, then this food is likely the culprit.

Drug allergies

Penicillin-induced hemolytic anemia is not uncommon in horses. This can be suspected based on recent treatment with penicillin and improvement in the anemia when its use is discontinued. It may also be possible to detect antibodies against penicillin or penicillin-coated red cells in these animals. In the case of equine responses to procaine penicillin, the procaine is rapidly dissociated from the penicillin in the bloodstream. As a result, the adverse events may simply be due to the toxic effects of the procaine on the brain and central nervous system and may not be immune-mediated. However, horses may also develop urticaria and anaphylaxis in response to the water-soluble sodium or potassium salts of penicillin (Olsen et al., 2007). Other drugs that have been associated with the development of allergic responses in horses include trimethoprim sulfa. phenylbutazone, ivermectin, as well as some diuretics, and phenothiazines (Scott & Miller, 2011).

References

Acharya, K. R., & Ackerman, S. J. (2014). Eosinophil granule proteins: Form and function. *Journal of Biological Chemistry, 289*, 17406–17415.

Akucewich, L., & Kunkle, G. U. (2007). *Compendium equine edition.*

Andersson, L. S., Swinbune, J. E., Meadows, J. R. S., Brostrom, H., et al. (2012). The same ELA class II risk factors confer equine insect bite hypersensitivity in two distinct populations. *Immunogenetics, 64*, 201–208.

Birkmann, K., Jebbawi, F., Waldern, N., Hug, S., et al. (2024). Eosinophils play a surprising leading role in recurrent urticaria in horses. *Vaccines*. https://doi.org/10.3390/vaccines12060562

Bosseler, L., Verryken, K., Bauwens, C., de Vries, C., et al. (2013). Equine multisystemic. Eosinophilic epitheliotropic disease: A case report and review of the literature. *New Zealand Veterinary Journal, 61*, 177–182.

Brosnahan, M. M. (2020a). Eosinophils of the horse: Part 1: Development, distribution, structure and biochemical mediators. *Equine Veterinary Education, 32*(10), 545–552.

Brosnahan, M. M. (2020b). Eosinophils of the horse: Part II: Eosinophils in clinical diseases. *Equine Veterinary Education, 32*(11), 590–602.

Cox, A., & Stewart, A. J. (2023). Insect bite hypersensitivity in horses: Causes, diagnosis, scoring and new therapies. *Animals*. https://doi.org/10.3390/ani13152514

Craig, N. M., Munguia, N. S., Trujillo, A. J., Chan, A. M., et al. (2024). Interleukin 31 mediates pruritus in horses. *American Journal of Veterinary Research*. https://doi.org/10.2460/ajvr.24.05.0144

Craig, N., Wilkes, R., Munguia, N. S., & Marsella, R. (2020). IL-31: A mediator of pruritus in horses. *Veterinary Dermatology, 31*(S1), 87.

Cvitas, I., Oberhansli, S., Leeb, T., Dettwiler, et al. (2020). Investigating the epithelial barrier and immune signatures in the pathogenesis of equine insect bite hypersensitivity. *PLoS One, 15*, e0232189.

Cvitas, I., Oberhansli, S., Leeb, T., & Marti, E. (2022). Equine keratinocytes in the pathogenesis of insect bite hypersensitivity: Just another brick in the wall? *PLoS One, 17*, e0266263.

Dupont, S., De Spiegeleer, A., Liu, D. J. X., Lefere, L., et al. (2016). A commercially available immunoglobulin E-based test for food allergy gives inconsistent results in healthy ponies. *Equine Veterinary Journal, 48*, 109–113.

Eyre, P., & Lewis, A. J. (1973). Acute systemic anaphylaxis in the horse. *British Journal of Pharmacology, 48*, 426–437.

Fadok, V. A. (2013). Update on equine allergies. *Veterinary Clinics: Equine Practice, 29*, 541–550.

Favrot, C., & Olivry, T. (2022). On the possible role of food allergy in chronic urticaria in racing horses. *Veterinary Dermatology, 33*, 103–104.

Fettelschloss-Gabriel, A., Birkmann, K., & Pantelyushin, S. (2021). Molecular mechanisms and treatment modalities in equine Culicoides hypersensitivity. *The Veterinary Journal*. https://doi.org/10.1016/j.tvjl.2021.105741

Fettelschloss-Gabriel, A., Fettelschloss, V., Thoms, F., Giese, C., et al. (2018). Treating insect-bite hypersensitivity in horses with active vaccination against IL-5. *The Journal of Allergy and Clinical Immunology*. https://doi.org/10.1016/j.jaci.2018.01.041

Foster, A. P., Lees, P., & Cunningham, F. M. (1992). Platelet activating factor is a mediator of equine neutrophil and eosinophil migration in vitro. *Research in Veterinary Science, 53*, 223–229.

Francqueville, M., & Sabbah, A. (1999). Chronic urticaria in sports horses. *Allergie et Immunologie, 32*, 212–213.

Hallamaa, R. E., & Batchu, K. C. (2016). Phospholipid analysis in sera of horses with allergic dermatitis and in matched healthy controls. *Lipids in Health and Disease*. https://doi.org/10.1186/s12944-016-0209-4

Hallamaa, R. E., Batchu, K. C., & Tallberg, T. (2014). Phospholipids in sera of horses with summer eczema. Lipid analysis of the autoserum preparation used in therapy. *Equine Veterinary Journal, 46*, 322–327.

Hellman, L. T., Akula, S., Thorpe, M., & Fu, Z. (2017). Tracing the origins of IgE, mast cells, and allergies by studies of wild animals. *Frontiers in Immunology*. https://doi.org/10.3389/fimmu.2017.01749

Jebbawi, F., Chmenitzer, A., Dietrich, M., Pantelyushin, S., et al. (2024). Cytokines and chemokines skin gene expression in correlation with immune cells in blood and severity in equine insect bite hypersensitivity. *Frontiers in Immunology*. https://doi.org/10.3389/fimmu.2024.1414891

Komi, D. E., Sharma, L., & Dela Cruz, C. S. (2018). Chitin and its effects on inflammatory and immune responses. *Clinical Reviews in Allergy and Immunology, 54*, 213–223.

Lanz, S., Brunner, A., Graubner, C., Marti, E., & Gerber, V. (2017). Insect bite hypersensitivity in horses is associated with airway hyperreactivity. *Journal of Veterinary Internal Medicine, 31*, 1877–1883.

Larson, E. M., Babasyan, S., & Wagner, B. (2020). Phenotype and function of IgE-binding monocytes in equine *Culicoides* hypersensitivity. *PLoS One*. https://doi.org/10.1371/journal.pone.0233537

Littlewood, J. D., & Jackson, H. A. (2022). On the possible role of food allergy in chronic urticaria in racing horses. *Veterinary Dermatology, 33*, 179.

Lorch, G., Hillier, A., Kwochka, K. W., Saville, W. A., & LeRoy, B. E. (2001). Results of intradermal tests in horses without atopy and horses with atopic dermatitis or recurrent urticaria. *American Journal of Veterinary Research, 62*(7), 1051–1059.

Mair, T. S., Stokes, C. R., & Bourne, F. J. (1988). Distribution and ultrastructure of mast cells in the equine respiratory tract. *Equine Veterinary Journal, 20*(1), 54–58.

Marsella, R. (2025). Skin barrier in normal and allergic horses: What do we know? *Veterinary Sciences*. https://doi.org/10.3390/vetsci12020091

Marsella, R., Johnson, C., & Ahrens, K. (2014). First report of ultra structural cutaneous abnormalities in equine atopic dermatitis. *Research in Veterinary Science, 97*, 382–385.

Marsella, R., White, S., Fadok, V. A., Mueller, R., et al. (2023). Equine allergic skin diseases: Clinical consensus guidelines of the World Association for Veterinary Dermatology. *Veterinary Dermatology*. https://doi.org/10.1111/vde.13168

McAleese, S. M., Halliwell, R. E. W., & Miller, H. R. P. (2000). Cloning and sequencing of the horse and sheep high-affinity IgE receptor α chain cDNA. *Immunogenetics, 51*, 878–881.

McAleese, S. M., & Miller, H. R. P. (2003). Cloning and sequencing of the equine and ovine high-affinity IgE receptor β-chain and γ-chain cDNA. *Immunogenetics, 55*, 122–125.

McKelvie, J., Foster, A. P., Cunningham, F. M., & Hamblin, A. S. (1999). Characterization of lymphocyte subpopulations in the skin and circulation of horses with sweet itch (Culicoides hypersensitivity). *Equine Veterinary Journal, 311*(6), 466–472.

Miyazawa, K., Ito, M., & Ohsaki, K. (1991). An equine case of urticaria associated with dry garlic feeding. *Journal of Veterinary Medical Science, 53*(4), 747–748.

Olomski, F., Fettelschloss, V., Jonddottir, S., Birkmann, K., et al. (2020). Interleukin -31 in insect bite hypersensitivity -alleviating clinical symptoms by active vaccination against itch. *Allergy, 75*, 862–871.

Olsen, L., Ingvast-Larsson, C., Bostrom, H., Larsson, P., & Tjalve, H. (2007). Clinical signs and etiology of adverse reactions to procaine penicillin and sodium/potassium penicillin in horses. *Journal of Veterinary Pharmacology and Therapeutics, 30*, 201–207.

Pantelyushin, S., Rhiner, T., Jebbawi, F., Sella, F., et al. (2020). Interleukin-5 dependent inflammatory eosinophil subtype involved in allergic insect bite hypersensitivity of horses. *Allergy*. https://doi.org/10.1111/all.15869

Patel, S., & Goyal, A. (2017). Chitin and chitinase: Role in pathogenicity, allergenicity and health. *International Journal of Biological Macromolecules, 97*, 331–338.

Peeters, L. M., Janssens, S., Godderis, B. M., De Keyser, K., Wilson, A. D., Kaufmann, C., et al. (2013). Evaluation of an IgE ELISA with *Culicoides* Spp. Extracts and recombinant salivary antigens for diagnosis of insect bite hypersensitivity in Warmblood horses. *The Veterinary Journal, 198*, 141–147.

Pemberton, A. D., McEuen, A. R., & Scudamore, C. L. (2001). Characterization of tryptase and a granzyme H-like chymase isolated from equine mastocytoma tissue. *Veterinary Immunology and Immunopathology, 83*, 253–267.

Pucheu-Haston, C. M., & Del Piero, F. (2013). Equine multisystemic eosinophilic epitheliotrophic disease. *Equine Veterinary Education, 25*, 614–617.

Raza, F., Babasyan, S., Larson, E. M., Freer, H. S., et al. (2021). Peripheral blood basophils are the main source of early interleukin-4 secretion upon in vitro stimulation with Culicoides allergen in allergic horses. *PLoS One*. https://doi.org/10.1371/j0urnal.pone.0252243

Rhiner, T., Fettelschloss, V., Schoster, A., Birkmann, K., & Fettelschloss-Gabriel. (2022). Targeting eosinophils by active vaccination against interleukin-5. Reduces basophil counts in horses with insect bite hypersensitivity in the 2nd year of vaccination. *The Veterinary Journal*. https://doi.org/10.1016/j.tvjl.2022.105896

Rotting, A. K., Freeman, D. E., Constable, P. D., Eurell, J. A. C., & Wallig, M. A. (2008). Mucosal distribution of eosinophilic granulocytes within the gastrointestinal tract of horses. *American Journal of Veterinary Research, 69*(7), 874–879.

Rufenacht, S., Marti, E., Von Scharner, C., Doherr, M. D., et al. (2005). Immunoglobulin E-bearing cells and mast cells in skin biopsies of horses with urticaria. *Veterinary Dermatology, 16*, 94–101.

Schaffartzik, A., Hamza, E., Janda, J., Crameri, R., Marti, E., & Rhyner, C. (2012). Equine insect bite hypersensitivity: What do we know. *Veterinary Immunology and Immunopathology, 147*, 113–126.

Scott, D. W., & Miller, W. H. (2011). *Equine dermatology* (2nd ed.). St. Louis, Missouri: Elsevier Saunders.

Serpa, P. B. S., Bogers, S., Byron, C., Cardona, G., & Patton, M. (2025). Presumptive Lyme disease -associated eosinophilic synovitis in a horse. *Journal of Equine Veterinary Science*. https://doi.org/10.1016/j.jevs.2025.105595

Tizard, I. R. (2022). *Allergies and hypersensitivity diseases in domestic animals*. St Louis: Elsevier.

Van der Meide, N. M., Roders, N., Oldruitenborgh- Oosterbaan, M. M., Schaap, P. J., van Oers, M. M., & Leribold, W. (2013). Cloning and expression of candidate allergens from *Culicoides obsoletus* for diagnosis of insect bite hypersensitivity in horses. *Veterinary Immunology and Immunopathology, 153*, 227–239.

Verdon, M., Lanz, S., Rhyner, C., Gerber, V., & Marti, E. (2019). Allergen-specific immunoglobulin E in sera of horses affected with insect bite hypersensitivity, severe equine asthma or both conditions. *Journal of Veterinary Internal Medicine, 33*, 266–274.

Viluma, A., Mikko, S., Hahn, D., Skow, L., et al. (2017). Genomic structure of the horse major histocompatibility complex class II region resolved using PacBio long-read sequencing technology. *Scientific Reports*. https://doi.org/10.1038/srep45518

Voehringer, D. (2013). Protective and pathological roles of mast cells and basophils. *Nature Reviews Immunology, 13*, 362–375.

Volland-Franqueville, M., & Sabbah, A. (2004). Recurrent or chronic urticaria in thoroughbred racehorses. *European Annals of Allergy and Clinical Immunology, 36*, 9–12.

Wagner, B. (2009). IgE in horses: Occurrence in health and disease. *Veterinary Immunology and Immunopathology, 132*, 21–30.

Wagner, B., Flaminio, J. B. F., Hillegas, J., Liebold, W., et al. (2006). Occurrence of IgE in foals: Evidence for transfer of maternal IgE by the colostrum and late onset of endogenous IgE production in the horse. *Veterinary Immunology and Immunopathology, 110*, 269–278.

Wagner, B., Miller, W. H., Erb, H. N., Lunn, D. P., & Antczak, D. F. (2009). Sensitization of skin mast cells with IgE antibodies to Culicoides allergens occurs frequently in clinically healthy horses. *Veterinary Immunology and Immunopathology, 132*, 53–61.

Wagner, B., Miller, W. H., Morgan, E. E., Hillegas, J. M., et al. (2006). IgE and IgG antibodies in skin allergy of the horse. *Veterinary Research, 37*, 813–825.

Wagner, B., Stokol, T., & Ainsworth, D. M. (2010). Induction of interleukin-4 production in neonatal IgE+ cells after crosslinking of maternal IgE. *Developmental & Comparative Immunology, 34*, 436–444.

Wallace, J. C., & Vogelnest, L. J. (2010). Evaluation of the presence of house dust mites in horse rugs. *Veterinary Dermatology, 21*(6), 602–607.

Watson, J. L., Jackson, K. A., King, D. P., & Scott, J. L. (2000). Molecular cloning and sequencing of the low-affinity IgE receptor (CD23) for horse and cattle. *Veterinary Immunology and Immunopathology, 73*, 323–329.

Wilson, A. D., Harwood, L., Torsteinsdottir, S., & Marti, E. (2006). Production of monoclonal antibodies specific for native equine IgE and their application to monitor total serum IgE responses in Icelandic and non-Icelandic horses with insect bite dermal hypersensitivity. *Veterinary Immunology and Immunopathology, 112*, 156–170.

CHAPTER

20 Immune complex and other hypersensitivity diseases in horses

In 1966, two British Immunologists, Philip Gell and Robin Coombs, were the first to classify the hypersensitivity responses generated by the immune system into four types based on their pathogenesis. This classification has withstood the test of time with only minor revisions. Type 1 hypersensitivity mediated by the activities of mast cell-bound IgE was discussed in the previous chapter. The three other types of hypersensitivity reactions that occur in horses are discussed in this chapter.

Type II hypersensitivity

The second type of lesion generated by an immune response involves the destruction of target cells by the activities of antibodies and complement. This is classified as Type II hypersensitivity. The most obvious of these responses is the destruction of foreign erythrocytes in animals that have received incompatible blood transfusions. However, other significant type II hypersensitivity diseases can occur in horses and donkeys. Examples of these diseases include neonatal erythrolysis in foals, immune-mediated hemolytic anemia, and immune-mediated thrombocytopenia. Immune-mediated anemias are associated with equine clostridial and streptococcal infections, purpura hemorrhagica, and equine infectious anemia, as well as penicillin allergies (Swiderski, 2000). Equine infectious anemia virus also causes an immune-mediated thrombocytopenia when viral antigens plus complement are deposited on platelet surfaces. The coated platelets are subsequently removed by the immune system.

Reactions to drugs

Red cells may be destroyed as a result of drug hypersensitivities by two mechanisms. In some cases, the drug and antibody may combine directly and activate the complement system. As a result, nearby red cells are destroyed in a bystander effect. More commonly, some drugs may simply bind to red cell surface glycoproteins. For example, penicillin, quinine, L-dopa, aminosalicylic acid, and phenacetin can all bind to red cells. Since these coated cells are structurally modified, they are recognized by the immune system as foreign and eliminated by an anti-drug antibody response, resulting in a hemolytic anemia. This condition can be suspected based

The Immunology of Horses and Donkeys. https://doi.org/10.1016/B978-0-443-44863-8.00023-5

on recent treatment with penicillin and improvement in the anemia when its use is discontinued. It may also be possible to detect antibodies against penicillin or penicillin-coated red cells in these horses (McConnico et al., 1992; Thomas & Livesey, 1998).

Sulfonamides, phenylbutazone, aminopyrine, phenothiazine, and possibly chloramphenicol may also cause agranulocytosis by binding to granulocytes. Phenylbutazone, quinine, chloramphenicol, and sulfonamides can cause thrombocytopenia if they bind to platelet glycoproteins (Warkentin, 2007). If the cells of affected animals are examined using a direct antiglobulin test, antibodies may be demonstrated on their surface. If these antibodies are eluted, they can be shown to be directed against the offending drug rather than the target cell (Robbins et al., 1993).

Infectious diseases

Just as drugs can be adsorbed onto red cells and render them immunologically foreign, so too can bacterial antigens such as the lipopolysaccharides, or bacteria such as *Anaplasma*, viruses such as equine infectious anemia virus, and protozoan antigens such as those from the trypanosomes and *Babesia*. These antigen-coated red cells are regarded as foreign by the immune system and are therefore either lysed by antibodies and complement or phagocytosed and destroyed by mononuclear phagocytes. Clinically severe anemia is, therefore, characteristic of all these infections.

Type III hypersensitivities

Immune complexes formed by the combination of antibodies with an antigen activate the classical complement pathway. As a result, when these complexes are deposited in tissues, the activated complement generates chemotactic peptides that attract neutrophils. The accumulated neutrophils may then release oxidants and enzymes, causing acute inflammation and tissue damage. Lesions generated in this way are classified as type III or immune-complex–mediated hypersensitivity reactions. Fig. 20.1.

The severity and significance of type III hypersensitivity reactions depend, as might be expected, on the amount and site of deposition of the immune complexes. For example, one form of reaction occurs locally when immune complexes are generated within tissues. Another form results when large quantities of immune complexes are produced within the bloodstream. This can occur, for example, when an antigen is administered intravenously to an immune recipient, immune complexes generated within the bloodstream are filtered out by the glomeruli in the kidney, and so the development of glomerular lesions (glomerulonephritis) is characteristic of this type of hypersensitivity. If the complexes bind to blood cells, anemia, leukopenia, or thrombocytopenia may result. Immune complexes may

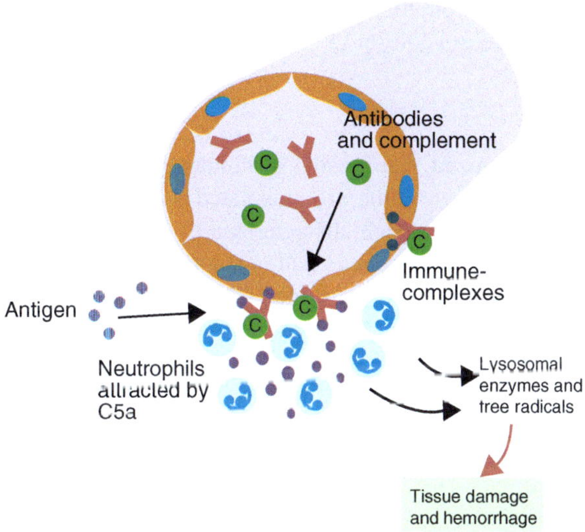

FIGURE 20.1

The pathogenesis of a type III hypersensitivity reaction where immune complexes deposited in tissues, especially in blood vessel walls, cause local inflammation.

also be deposited in blood vessel walls and so cause vasculitis, or in joints to cause arthritis.

It might reasonably be pointed out that the combination of an antigen with an antibody always produces immune complexes. However, the occurrence of clinically significant type III hypersensitivity reactions results from the formation of excessive amounts of these immune complexes in the wrong places over a long time. Minor and transient immune-complex-mediated lesions probably develop relatively frequently following an antibody response but resolve without causing clinically significant disease or tissue damage.

Respiratory diseases

The respiratory tract is an organ where the defenses of the body come into direct contact with inhaled antigens and pathogens. They are an especially critical site in the horse, a species that relies on speed and endurance to avoid predators. Their lungs are large and able to exchange high volumes of inhaled and exhaled air at a very rapid rate. As such, they also require well-tuned defenses that can handle inhaled pathogens and other airborne antigens efficiently and rapidly. Nevertheless, the combination of large quantities of foreign antigens, such as those derived from bacteria, molds, plants, and arthropods present in the air of dusty stables, together with an effective antibody response, results in increased vulnerability of horses to both type I and type III respiratory hypersensitivities. Collectively, these can induce significant lung damage in addition to respiratory distress. Fig. 20.2.

Equine asthma

It has long been recognized that asthma in humans consists of several distinctly different disease syndromes. Some are associated with high eosinophil counts in bronchoalveolar washes, others are characterized by high neutrophil counts. Some human cases involve both neutrophils and eosinophils, while others have neither. A similar spectrum and complexity are seen in equine asthma (Lavoie-Lamoureux et al., 2012). Thus, two major forms of chronic obstructive respiratory disease are recognized in horses. They consist of recurrent airway obstruction or "heaves" and inflammatory airway disease (Bond et al., 2018; Couëtil et al., 2016). It is also appropriate to point out that there appear to be allergic (Th2) and non-allergic (non-Th2) phenotypes of equine asthma (Bond et al., 2018). Fig. 20.3.

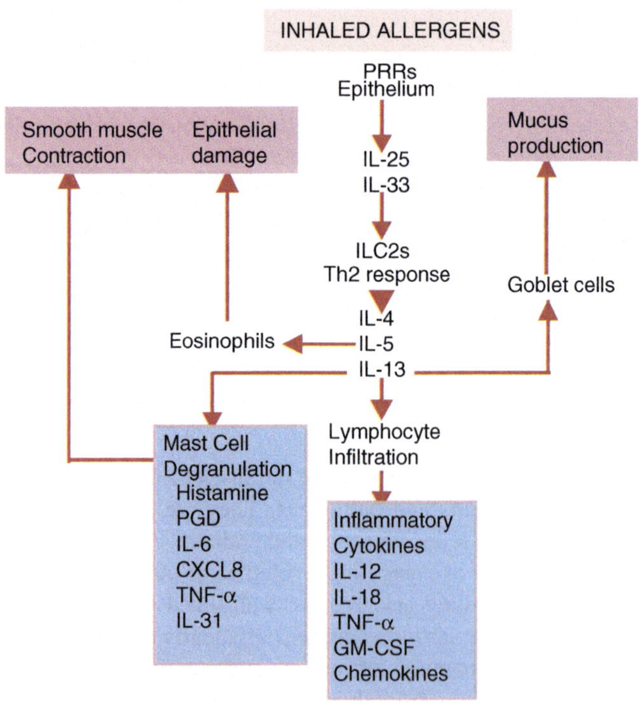

FIGURE 20.2

The pathogenesis of the inhalant allergic diseases in horses.

SEVERE (Recurrent airway obstruction)	MILD (Inflammatory airway disease)
Respiratory distress at rest	No respiratory distress at rest
Coughing Increased breathing effort	Coughing and underpeformance Exercise intolerance
Heave line Nasal discharge Bronchospasm Emphysema Bronchiolitis	Excessive mucus Nasal discharge Cough
Type 2 cytokines Some Il-17 response	Type 1 cytokines
Neutrophil infiltration	Neutrophilic, eosinophlic, mastocytic, or mixed infiltration

FIGURE 20.3

The differences between the two major forms of equine asthmatic disease.

Inflammatory airway disease

Inflammatory airway disease (IAD) is a relatively mild respiratory disease of horses in which breathing appears normal at rest. Affected animals develop minimal clinical signs such as a nasal discharge, cough, and decreased performance. IAD may affect up to 30% of young horses (<5 years old) in training. Although commonly linked to bacterial or viral infections, in many cases, no infectious agent can be isolated. Horses with IAD show impaired performance, exercise intolerance, and a chronic intermittent cough. Excessive airway mucus production is also apparent. Cytological evaluation of their bronchiolar lavage fluid shows evidence of inflammation reflected by a mild neutrophilia, lymphocytosis and monocytosis (Moore et al., 1995). Eosinophil and mast cell numbers are usually not elevated. (Although a subset of IAD horses may show an eosinophilia.) $CD4^+$ T cell and B cell numbers are reduced. Cytokine transcripts show elevated IL-1β, IL-5, IL-6, IL-8, IL-10, IL-17, and -23 as well as TNF-α and IFN-γ in affected horses compared to controls. However, these differences are influenced by the presence of mast cells, eosinophils, or neutrophils. Thus, in bronchial washes with high neutrophil numbers, IL-17 is also elevated while IL-4 is depressed compared to those with high mast cell numbers.

Although its pathogenesis is uncertain, IAD is commonly associated with the inhalation of organic dusts, molds, storage mites and other aeroallergens, and may be seasonal (Couetil et al., 2007). Affected animals have elevated levels of IgG3/5 directed against these allergens, confirming the occurrence of a type 2 immune response (Jentsch et al., 2024; Schnabel et al., 2023).

It is relevant to point out here that exercise-induced pulmonary hemorrhage is not uncommon in Thoroughbreds and Standardbreds after racing. The pathogenesis of this syndrome remains unclear. However it appears that the bronchiolar damage associated with allergic lung disease may predispose horses to this condition

(Derksen et al., 1992). The newly formed blood vessels in inflammatory sites are fragile and prone to rupture (Moore, 1996).

It should also be pointed out that mild lower airway inflammation is common in apparently healthy racehorses showing neither respiratory signs nor exercise intolerance. Exercise alone does increase blood CXCL8 levels but there were no differences in inflammatory cytokine gene expression detected in racehorses after racing (Taylor et al., 2021).

Recurrent airway obstruction

Equine recurrent airway obstruction (RAO) resembles severe asthma in humans (Sheats et al., 2019). It includes obstructive pulmonary disease seen in stabled horses and summer pasture-associated obstructive pulmonary disease. It is defined as a severe, debilitating disease characterized by coughing, a nasal discharge, and an increased respiratory effort due to bronchoconstriction, airway hyperreactivity, neutrophil infiltration, and excess mucus accumulation in the airways. Characteristically, horses with RAO suffer from labored breathing while at rest. It has been estimated that it may affect as many as 20% of horses in the Northern hemisphere (Hotchkiss et al., 2007).

RAO is also known as "heaves". RAO resembles severe asthma in humans since it results from chronic lower airway inflammation, airway hyperresponsiveness, and bronchoconstrictive episodes that involve the entire lung parenchyma (Sheats et al., 2019). As a result of the effort required to breathe, the external oblique abdominal muscle hypertrophies. This can be seen as a "heave line" across the lower flanks of affected horses (Gehlen et al., 2008).

RAO is typically occurs in horses over 9–12 years of age. Its clinical signs range from mild exercise intolerance to serious respiratory distress. The condition is initially mild but worsens with time. Affected animals suffer from episodes of severe respiratory distress triggered by inhalation of airborne antigens. During these episodes, horses develop airflow obstruction as a result of bronchospasm, increased mucus production, airway hyperplasia, and airway hyper-responsiveness. Neutrophil recruitment is apparent by 4–6 hours after antigen challenge and precedes the development of airway obstruction. Th2 cytokines appear to contribute to the recruitment and activation of these neutrophils as well as the release of extracellular NETS (Chapter 4) (Henriquez et al., 2014). During remissions, horses may be clinically normal, and their airway function and bronchial cytology appear normal (Leguilette, 2003). Airway remodeling can occur in chronic RAO cases, and their airway smooth muscles may become hypertrophied.

RAO occurs most obviously in horses that inhale large amounts of organic dust, such as those generated in dusty stables and on a hay diet. Fungal spores, endotoxins, storage mites (*Dermatophagoides* sp), bacterial, and mold antigens, as well as grass pollens and other plant debris, can trigger the disease (Costa et al., 2006). Some of the major triggers are the proteins of *Aspergillus fumigatus* (Jentsch et al., 2024). Other important mold spores are derived from Penicillium, Cladosporum, Mucor,

Fusarium and Alternaria. Many result from the molds that grow in hay stored under damp conditions.

RAO is a hypersensitivity disease with a mixed cytokine profile implicating enhanced Th1, Th2, and Th17 responses as well as extensive neutrophilic infiltration. This likely implies that several different RAO disease endotypes are occurring in horses. Thus, horses with RAO have elevated levels of IgE in their bronchiolar lavage fluid as well as in their serum. Lung biopsies show significant increases in type 2 cytokines, IL-1β, IL-8 (CXCL8), TNF-α, and TGF-β as well as TLR4 and NF-κB transcripts (Woodrow et al., 2022). Similar but less marked trends occur in IL-17 and IFN-γ concentrations. High concentrations of the chemokine CXCL8 (IL-8) are found in the bronchoalveolar washings of affected animals (Lavoie-Lamoureux et al., 2012). Exposure of cultured equine bronchial epithelial cells to hay dust components or lipopolysaccharide increases their CXCL-8, CXCL2, and IL-1β expression (Franchini et al., 2000). The percentage of $CD4^+$, $Foxp3^+$ Treg cells increases in the bronchoalveolar washings of horses with RAO, suggesting that these also influence the course of this disease (Ainsworth et al., 2009). Some cases of RAO may resemble hypersensitivity pneumonitis clinically. (See below)

An analysis of the gene expression profiles in the mediastinal lymph nodes of horses with RAO also implicates the pro-inflammatory cytokine IL-17 in the disease process (Korn et al., 2015). This would be expected given the prevalence of neutrophils in bronchoalveolar fluid. IL-17 expression is greatly enhanced in these lymph nodes and is linked to the downregulation of IL-4 expression.

Inflammatory cells

Unlike IAD where eosinophil numbers are commonly elevated, BALF from RAO cases commonly shows a marked increase in neutrophil numbers as well as decreased alveolar macrophage and lymphocyte counts.

Neutrophils predominate in the bronchial inflammatory exudate in most cases of RAO. They have been shown to undergo NETosis and enhanced migratory capacity, a process that contributes to the proinflammatory environment (Vargas et al., 2017). These changes in neutrophil behavior appear to be in response to the strong Th17 response (Sage et al., 2024). Elevated levels of NETs can be readily detected in bronchoalveolar lavage fluid from horses with severe asthma. Their levels are correlated with disease severity and they are not found in horses with mild asthma (Janssen et al., 2022).

Affected animals usually have large numbers of neutrophils in their small bronchioles and high titers of antibodies to equine influenza in their bronchial secretions. The significance of the latter is unclear. It has been suggested that continuous, prolonged activation of bronchoalveolar epithelial cells by dust particles and air-borne endotoxins leads to excessive production of neutrophil-attracting chemokines. These neutrophils then cause local tissue damage by releasing proteases, peroxidases, and oxidants. Figs. 20.4 and 20.5.

Neutrophils are not the only leukocytes present in the respiratory exudate. Basophils are also present. These basophils are sensitized with IgE. The basophils from

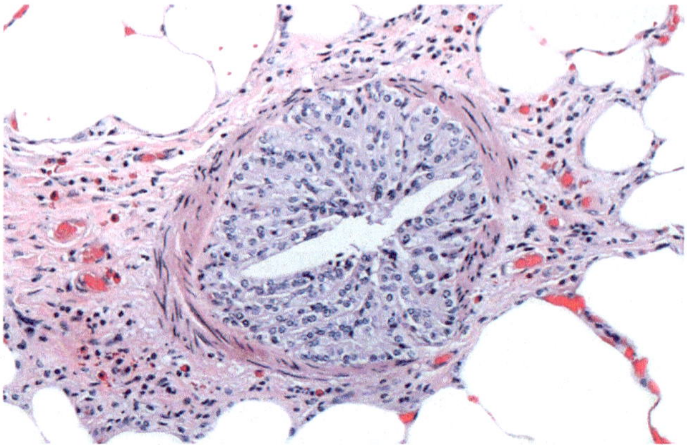

FIGURE 20.4 Histologic lesion from a horse lung suffering from RAO. ×20.

Note how the airway is almost blocked by infiltrating inflammatory cells.

- Courtesy of Dr. Brian Porter.

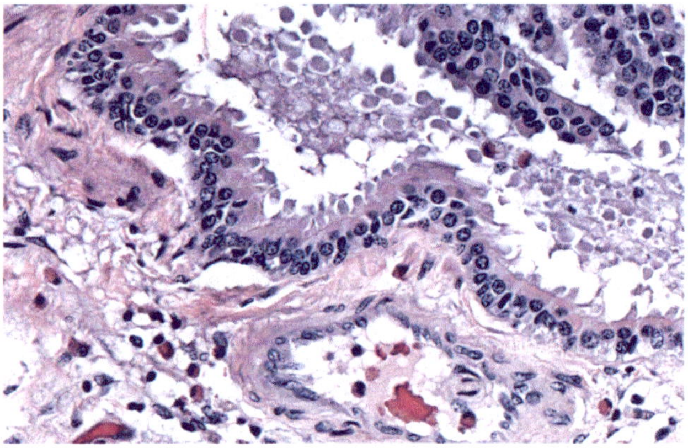

FIGURE 20.5

Higher power view of the cellular inflitrate in the lungs of a horse with RAO. ×40.

- Courtesy of Dr Brian Porter.

RAO horses readily degranulated when exposed to allergens from environmental fungi such as *Mucor mucedo* and *Mucor spinosus* (Dirscherl et al., 1993).

Alveolar macrophages

Alveolar macrophages also participate in the inflammatory response associated with RAO (Tamarinde et al., 2006). Thus, macrophages from susceptible horses isolated 6 and 12 hours after challenge with *Apergillus fumigatus* produce high levels of TNF-α, IL-1β, and CXCL8 compared to control nonsusceptible animals. Analysis of the macrophages present in BALF from asthmatic horses also showed that these cells were $CD14^+$ and $CD16^+$. A decreased percentage of $CD16^+$ macrophages was found in horses with severe disease compared to animals with moderate or mild disease (Gressler et al., 2022). In a separate study, the alveolar macrophages in BALF were shown to be $CD163^+$ and $CD206^+$ following challenge with moldy hay (Kang et al., 2021; Laan et al., 2006).

Mast cells

Mast cells are frequently encountered in the BALF of horses with RAO. Transcriptome analysis has shown that these mast cells are of the "classical" mucosal phenotype and are rich in tryptase but lack chymase or carboxypeptidase. They express the genes encoding the α and γ chains of FcRε1 but not the β chain genes. The significance of this is unclear. Other activated genes include those such as CD1 involved in lipid antigen presentation, as well as the gene for C1q involved in complement activation (Akula et al., 2022; Woodrow et al., 2022).

Diagnosis and treatment

Removal of affected horses to air-conditioned, dust-free stalls usually results in clinical improvement, but this is reversed if the horses are returned to dusty stables. In some cases, the RAO may persist even when horses are moved to low-dust environments, probably as a consequence of chronic airway remodeling (Miskovic et al., 2007). Combination therapy with bronchodilators and corticosteroids is the most effective form of treatment. The bronchodilators provide immediate relief while the corticosteroids suppress the pulmonary inflammation (Rush, 2001).

Horses with RAO may show positive skin reactions to intradermal inoculation of actinomycete and fungal extracts (such as *Rhizopus nigricans*, *Candida albicans*, *S. rectivirgula, Aspergillus fumigatus, Mucor* spp, and *Geotrichum deliquescens*). Affected horses may also respond to aerosol challenge with extracts of these organisms by developing dyspnea. Clinical signs may resolve on removal of the moldy hay and reappear on re-exposure (DeLuca et al., 2008), There is, however, no evidence of significant IgE involvement in RAO and little correlation between skin test results and severity of disease. For example, airway wall eosinophilia is not a feature of equine heaves (Dubuc & Lavoie, 2014). Extensive intradermal skin testing of horses with mild asthma (IAD) and severe asthma (RAO) has indicated that the most severe immediate (4 hours) skin reactions in both cases were triggered by insect-derived allergens, mite allergens, and canine epithelium (Feudo et al., 2021).

There is also, however, evidence for a genetic predisposition to RAO (Couetil et al., 2020). The prevalence of RAO is increased threefold when one parent is affected and fivefold when both parents are affected (Houtsma et al., 2015). There is a clear genetic susceptibility to RAO among horses and differences among different horse breeds. The genes involved have been located in two chromosome regions on ECA13 and ECA15 (Simões et al., 2022). The region on ECA13 containing the IL-4 receptor gene has been associated with the disease in a family of Swiss Warmbloods. A gene influencing the production of hydrogen peroxide in the respiratory epithelium (*TXNDC1*) is also located in this region. The region on ECA15 has been linked to a different family of the same breed (Swinburne et al., 2009).

RAO also occurs in donkeys, although it may not be identified if the donkeys are not exercised. Generally, coughing and dyspnea are only noted on exercise.

Hypersensitivity pneumonitis

As described above, Type III hypersensitivity reactions occur in horse lungs when sensitized animals inhale large quantities of foreign antigens. It is well recognized as a problem in humans (farmer's lung). In the case of RAO, it affects horses housed in dusty stables and their riders spending prolonged periods in dusty barns and riding schools (Moore et al., 2004). Normally, these dust particles are relatively large and are trapped in mucus in the nasal passages and the upper respiratory tract and eliminated. If, however, hay is stored when damp, bacterial growth and metabolism will result in heating. As a result of this warmth, mold spores and thermophilic actinomycetes will grow on the plant material. One of the most important of these thermophilic actinomycetes is *Saccharopolyspora rectivirgula*, an organism that produces large numbers of very small spores (~1 μm diameter). When inhaled by a horse, these spores can penetrate as far as the alveoli. If horses are fed moldy hay for long periods, constant inhalation of *S. rectivirgula* spores will result in the development of high-titered serum antibodies to *S. rectivirgula* antigens. Eventually, inhaled spore antigens will encounter these antibodies within the alveolar walls, and the resulting immune complexes and complement activation will cause a pneumonia (or pneumonitis), the basis of which is a type III hypersensitivity reaction (Spagnolo et al., 2015). If untreated, the chronic inflammation can lead to pulmonary fibrosis. It is often misdiagnosed as an infectious pneumonia.

Hypersensitivity pneumonitis (or allergic alveolitis) consists of an acute alveolitis together with vasculitis and exudation of fluid into the alveolar spaces. The alveolar septa may be thickened, and the entire lesion is infiltrated with inflammatory cells. Since many of these cells are eosinophils and lymphocytes, it is clear that the response is not a pure type III reaction. In animals inhaling small amounts of an antigen over a long period, a proliferative bronchiolitis and fibrosis may also develop.

Clinically, hypersensitivity pneumonitis presents as a pneumonia occurring between 5 and 10 hours after acute exposure to grossly moldy hay. The animal may have difficulty breathing and develop a severe cough. In chronically affected animals, the dyspnea may be continuous. The most effective method of managing this condition is by removing the source of the antigen. Administration of steroids may be beneficial.

In one reported outbreak, the dust generated from chickens housed together with the horses resulted in the development of this form of hypersensitivity pneumonitis (Mansmann et al., 1975). Hay sickness ("Heyseki") is a hypersensitivity pneumonitis seen in horses in Iceland that appears to be an equine equivalent of farmer's lung (Asmundsson et al., 1983). Thus, out of a group of 15 horses with hay sickness, all the animals had precipitating antibodies to *S. rectivirgula*. Two had precipitins against *Rhizopus* species and *Aspergillus fumigatus*. The disease has also been described in Swiss horses (Pauli et al., 1972). These animals had an eosinophilia in their blood and nasal secretions, they gave positive skin test responses to allergens from food and bedding, and they possessed precipitins to *S. rectivirgula* and *Aspergillus fumigatus*. Pathologically, they had an acute interstitial pneumonitis and a mononuclear cell infiltration in the lung. As the disease became chronic, these horses developed epithelial hyperplasia and fibrosis of the lung parenchyma (Pauli et al., 1972).

Immune-mediated vasculitis

Inflammation and damage to blood vessel walls may be the result of infections, toxins, or tumors. It is often a direct consequence of targeting by the pathogen, such as African Horse Sickness virus or Equine Viral Arteritis virus, infecting vascular endothelial cells. A secondary form of vasculitis occurs when circulating immune complexes are deposited in blood vessel walls. The endothelial cell damage in turn results in local clot formation—immunothrombosis. Immune complexes are deposited in the blood vessels of horses in cases of equine infectious anemia, cutaneous vasculitis, and foal polysynovitis. However, the most important cause of such a vasculitis is associated with infections with *Streptococcus equi* (Bozorgmanesh, 2024). The clinical manifestations of these vasculitides depend in large part on their location. The immune complexes may be deposited in arteries, veins, or capillaries. However, immune complex deposition tends to be greatest in vessels with the highest intravascular pressure. Fig. 20.6.

Leukocytoclastic vasculitis is a necrotizing inflammatory reaction involving the walls of small blood vessels. Its pathogenesis is complex, and there are likely many causative factors and endotypes. Its clinical manifestations depend upon the severity and extent of the inflammatory lesions as well as their distribution. It results from type III hypersensitivity responses mediated by immune complexes deposited in blood vessel walls. As a result, interference with local blood flow can lead to edema, hemorrhage, immunothrombosis, and purpura. Skin necrosis and ulceration may follow. Both cutaneous and systemic forms occur as a result of impaired small blood vessel function.

Numerous triggers of leukocytoclastic vasculitis have been identified, and a careful history including recent drug treatments is needed if the trigger is to be identified. The commonest cause of these vasculitides in horses is a type III hypersensitivity reaction, but many vasculitis cases are idiopathic. Lesions can develop at any site on the body, including the oral cavity and mucus membranes. These lesions evolve, so that ulcers may develop several days after the first appearance of lesions.

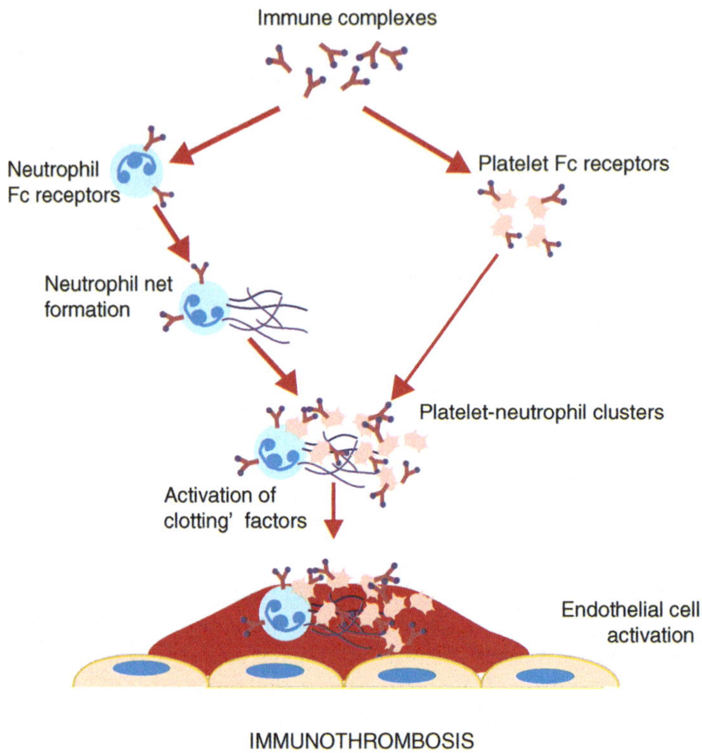

FIGURE 20.6

The pathogenesis of immune complex-mediated immunothrombosis and vasculitis.

Purpura hemorrhagica

Two to 4 weeks following an acute *Strep. equi* infection (or vaccination against *Strep. equi*), horses may develop urticaria, followed by severe subcutaneous edema, especially involving the limbs, and the development of hemorrhages in the mucosa and subcutaneous tissues. Affected horses are anorexic and depressed and have a high fever. Immune complexes containing *Strep. equi* antigens are found in the bloodstream of affected animals (Galan & Timoney, 1985). These immune complexes cause an acute vasculitis as well as a type I mesangioproliferative glomerulonephritis (Delph et al., 2019; Divers et al., 1992).

Purpura hemorrhagica is a leukocytoclastic vasculitis of horses that develops following infections in which suppuration is present in some region of the body. Other triggers of purpura hemorrhagica include infections with *Corynebacterium pseudotuberculosis*, *Rhodococcus equi,* equine influenza virus, and equine herpesvirus type 1. In some cases, purpura may develop in the absence of any obvious prior bacterial or viral infection. Horses usually recover when aggressively treated with systemic glucocorticosteroids (Pusterla et al., 2003). This condition is also termed anaphylactoid purpura (Gunson & Rooney, 1977).

Biopsies of affected skin show the presence of a severe leukocytoclastic vasculitis with a marked neutrophilic infiltration around affected blood vessels. This vasculitis may be associated with necrosis of the infarcted muscle. Immune complexes are found in the serum of affected horses and consist of streptococcal M or R protein complexed with IgM or IgA. These immune complexes are deposited in the kidneys and cause a membranoproliferative glomerulonephritis with resulting proteinuria and azoturia. Deposition of these complexes in blood vessel walls results in vasculitis, edema, immunothrombosis, and hemorrhage. Complement components may also be deposited in association with the antigen-antibody complexes. Preexisting high serum antibody levels to *Strep. equi* may predispose horses to this condition. Affected horses may also have unusually high blood IgA levels (Gunson & Rooney, 1977).

There are great variations in thr severity and clinical course of purpura hemorrhagica, ranging from a mild transient reaction to fatal disease. The most prominent signs include severe subcutaneous edema on all four limbs and the ventral abdomen. Petechial or ecchymotic hemorrhages develop on the visible mucous membranes. Other signs may include depression and reluctance to move, fever, anorexia, tachycardia and tachypnoea, colic, epistaxis, and weight loss. The edema may result in skin exudation, ulceration, crusting, and sloughing. Severe edema of the head may compromise breathing and eating. Other abnormalities include anemia, neutrophilia, hyperglobulinemia, elevated muscle enzymes (due to rhabdomyolysis), and hyperproteinemia. The vasculitis may also affect the gastrointestinal tract, lungs, and muscles. In severe cases, some horses develop a generalized leukocytoclastic vasculitis that may lead to thrombosis and infarction (Kaese et al., 2005). Small-intestinal intussusception may complicate the disease, as does muscle infarction. There may be hemorrhage and necrosis of skeletal muscle. Infarctive purpura hemorrhagica is a rare and highly fatal form of the disease. The vascular lesions are either cell-poor or lymphohistiocytic.

Equine pastern vasculitis

Pastern vasculitis is a disease primarily encountered in adult draft horses. Lesions appear on the non-pigmented caudal aspects of the pasterns but may extend as far as the cannon bone. They are often bilateral. The hindlimbs are most commonly affected. The lesions are red and swollen. They may develop into ulcers or fissures with exudation and crusting. The lesions vary in severity from mild to an exudative form, to a chronic proliferative form, and probably reflect several distinct causes. For example it may be a manifestation of Chorioptic mange (Chapter 18). Secondary

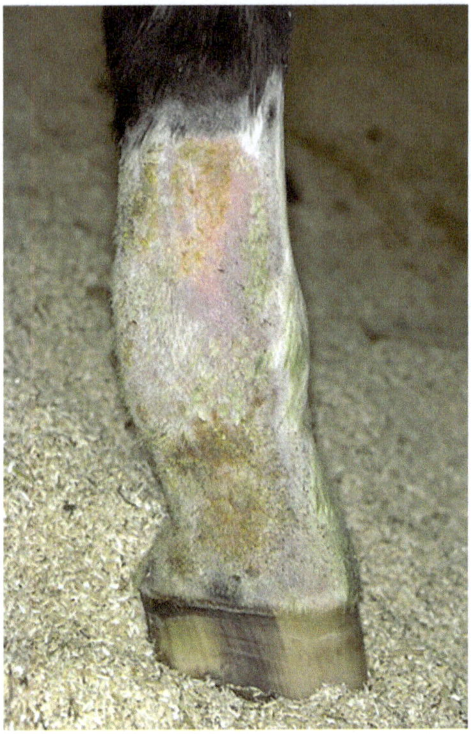

FIGURE 20.7

A case of pastern vasculitis.

- With permission Psalla et al. (2013).

bacterial and fungal infections are also common. The predisposing lesion appears to be a vasculitis. Biopsies of affected skin show a deep dermal neutrophil leukocytoclastic arteritis with nuclear dust, thickening, and edema of the blood vessel walls, with microhemorrhages. The etiology of the lesion is unknown, although photoactivation appears to be a trigger factor, and the prognosis is guarded (Psalla et al., 2013). Fig. 20.7.

Other equine vasculitides

Horses have been reported to develop other forms of vasculitis. About half are of unknown etiology. The others may be secondary to a photo-aggravated dermatitis (confined to the non-pigmented areas of the skin). Drug-induced vasculitis has been reported to occur in response to penicillin, potentiated sulfonamides, rifampin, and acepromazine. It is not clear what the mechanisms are in these drug-induced diseases. The diagnosis is usually made based on the association between drug administration and lesion development. A vasculitis may also develop in horses suffering from systemic lupus erythematosus. While very rare, it presents as erythema, alopecia, and depigmentation (Bozorgmanesh, 2024). This is almost certainly a consequence of the massive overproduction of immune complexes in horses with SLE (Chapter 22). A single case of a vasculitis developing in a horse with a diffuse lymphoma (paraneoplastic vasculitis) has been reported. This is a well recognized complication in humans (Williams et al., 1995).

Glomerulonephritis

When circulating immune complexes are deposited in the vessels of the renal glomeruli, they cause basement membrane thickening and stimulate glomerular cells to proliferate. Any or all of the three glomerular cell populations, epithelial cells, endothelial cells, and mesangial cells, can proliferate. The lesion is therefore called membranoproliferative glomerulonephritis (MPGN). MPGN lesions are classified based on the site of immune complex deposition (Sethi & Fervenza, 2012) Fig. 20.8.

MPGN is caused by immune-complex deposition in glomerular blood vessels. The complexes can usually penetrate the vascular endothelium, but not the basement membrane, and are therefore trapped on the luminal surface of the vessel where they stimulate endothelial cell swelling and proliferation (Slauson & Lewis, 1979). Experimentally, if an animal is given repeated injections of small doses of an antigen over a long period, continued damage to the glomerular cells by immune complexes leads to the local production of transforming growth factor-β (TGF-β). This cytokine stimulates nearby cells to produce fibronectin, collagen, and proteoglycans. This results in a thickening of the basement membrane to form a so-called "wire loop" lesion (also called a membranous glomerulonephritis). Alternatively, the immune complexes and complement may be deposited in the mesangial region of glomeruli. Mesangial cells are modified smooth muscle cells. As such, they can respond to immune complexes by proliferating and producing IL-6 and TGF-β. The IL-6 stimulates autocrine growth of the mesangial cells. The TGF-β stimulates the production of extracellular matrix. The resulting cell growth eventually interferes with glomerular function. By using immunofluorescence, it can be shown that lumpy aggregates of immune complexes are deposited in capillary walls and on the epithelial side of the glomerular basement membrane. Fig. 20.9.

MPGN develops when prolonged antigenemia persists in the presence of antibodies. As a result, it is a feature of many chronic infectious diseases. These include viral diseases such as equine infectious anemia. It also occurs in parasitic diseases such as piroplasmosis. It also develops in chronic bacterial diseases such as metritis, chronic pneumonia, and recurrent staphylococcal pyoderma. In many equine cases, the etiology of the glomerular lesions is unknown (Waldvogel et al., 1983).

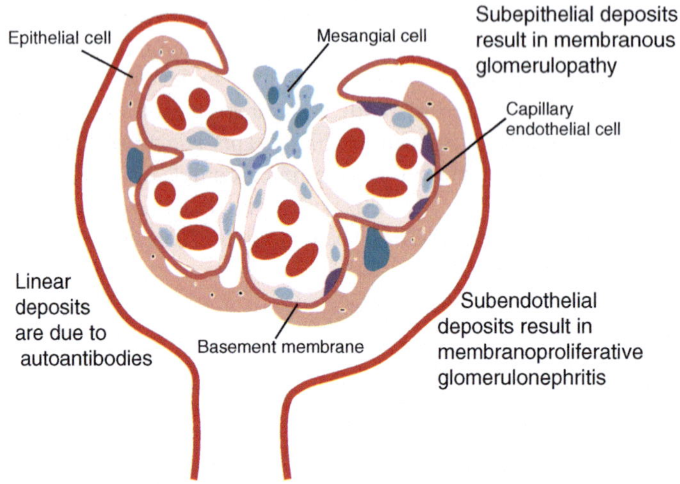

FIGURE 20.8

The pathogenesis of immune complex-mediated glomerulonephritis.

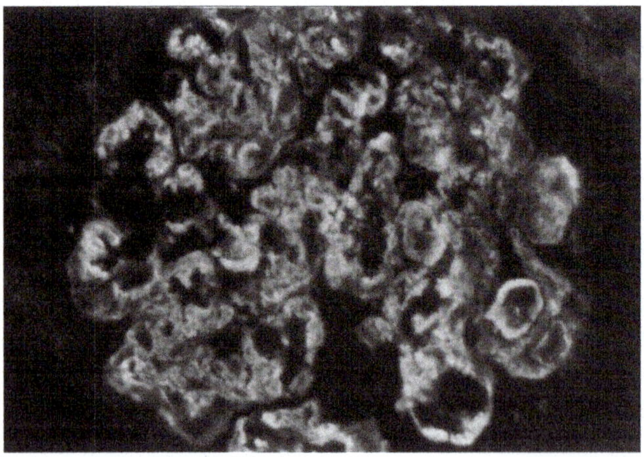

FIGURE 20.9 An immunofluorescence photomicrograph of a glomerulus from a horse with renal failure stained with anti-equine IgG. It shows the presence of "lumpy" deposits of IgG-containing immune complexes within the capillary walls and mesangium.

The antigen involved comes from group C streptococci.

- With permission Divers et al. (1992).

In a typical example, a 12-year-old thoroughbred gelding developed a global glomerulonephritis 3 months after it had suffered from a respiratory infection caused by *Strep. zooepidemicus*. Analysis demonstrated that the glomerulonephritis was the result of immune complexes involving IgG antibodies and group-C streptococcal antigen being deposited on its glomerular basement membranes (Fig. 20.9). The dense, coarse granular deposits resulted in marked thickening of the glomerular capillary walls. Similar deposits were found in the glomerular mesangium (Divers et al., 1992).

In some animals suffering from cancer, large amounts of tumor antigen may be shed into the bloodstream, filtered out in the kidneys and thus result in the development of MPGN. This has been associated with lymphosarcomas, osteosarcomas, and mastocytomas. Under some circumstances, horses may also make autoantibodies to their glomerular basement membrane (Chapter 22) (Banks, 1979).

Clinical consequences

The presence of immune complexes within glomeruli stimulates neutrophils, mesangial cells, macrophages, and platelets to release thromboxanes, nitric oxide, and platelet activating factor. These increase basement membrane permeability so that plasma proteins, especially albumin, are lost in the urine. This loss, if severe, may exceed the ability of the horse to replace the protein. As a result, albumin levels drop, the plasma colloid osmotic pressure falls, fluid passes from blood into tissue spaces, and the animal may become edematous and ascitic. The loss of fluid into tissues results in a reduction of blood volume, a compensatory increase in secretion of antidiuretic hormone, increased sodium retention, and accentuation of the edema. The decreased blood volume also results in a drop in renal blood flow, reduction in glomerular filtration, retention of urea and creatinine, azotemia, and hypercholesterolemia. Although all these may occur as a result of immune-complex deposition in glomeruli, the development of this nephrotic syndrome is not inevitable. Many horses may remain clinically normal despite the presence of immune complexes in their glomeruli, and immune complexes are commonly observed in old, apparently healthy horses. The most common initial signs are anorexia and weight loss (Scarratt & Sponenberg, 1984). They may also develop extensive subcutaneous edema. Polyuria and polydipsia occur when about two-thirds of the glomeruli are destroyed. It has been usual to treat affected animals with corticosteroids and immunosuppressive drugs, but the rationale and effectiveness of this treatment are unclear, except when the glomerulonephritis is associated with concurrent autoimmune disease such as systemic lupus erythematosus (Geor et al., 2005). The glomerular lesion is not inflammatory, and although the lesion contains immunoglobulins, there is no evidence to suggest that it is caused by hyperactivity of the immune system.

Type IV hypersensitivity

Delayed hypersensitivity responses

Some antigens, when injected into the skin of sensitized animals, only provoke inflammation at the injection site after a delay of 12–24 hours. These delayed hypersensitivity reactions are classified as type IV hypersensitivities and result from interactions between the injected antigen and T cells. Delayed hypersensitivity reactions can be considered T-cell-mediated inflammatory responses directed against organisms that are resistant to elimination by conventional antibody responses. Antibody-mediated inflammatory skin responses develop rapidly. Cell-mediated responses are much slower to develop (hence their name).

Tuberculin testing

An important example of a delayed hypersensitivity reaction is the tuberculin response. This is an inflammatory response that develops in the skin of an animal infected with tuberculosis following intradermal injection of a bacterial extract called tuberculin. A delayed hypersensitivity response has long been used to diagnose tuberculosis,—the tuberculin test (Hodgin et al., 1978). Tuberculosis is relatively unommon in horses. When it does occur it is usually caused by *Mycobacterium bovis* acquired from infected cattle. A classical tuberculin skin test in the horse involves injecting purified protein derivative (PPD) tuberculin from *M. bovis* intradermally in the neck of the horse and examining the injection site 48 hours later for a respones in the form of a firm swelling. When 300 healthy horses were tested in this way however, 70% appeared to be positive at 48 hours and 45% at 72 hours. Tuberculosis was not found in any of these horses on necropsy (Konyha & Kreier, 1971). The false positive responses were largely a result of sensitization to *M.avium*. As a result, the tuberculin test is not considered reliable in horses. Diagnosis of tuberculosis in horses is best achieved by microbiological culture.

Equine sarcoidosis

Equine sarcoidosis is a rare generalized disease syndrome characterized by the development of granulomatous inflammation of multiple organ systems, the development of skin lesions, and weight loss. It may occur in localized, partially generalized, or generalized forms. The skin lesions consist of an exfoliative and granulomatous dermatitis. A similar granulomatous disease occurs in humans, where it is called sarcoidosis. Simply put, the lesions that develop closely resemble those associated with tuberculosis, but there are no obvious bacteria present in the lesions (Axon et al., 2004). In humans, sarcoidosis is attributed to a chronic exaggerated Th1 helper cell response within the affected organs. The cause of this response is unknown, but it is assumed to be a hypersensitivity response to an unknown allergen or infectious agent, perhaps associated with a genetic predisposition (Wimmer-Scherr & Schwarz, 2025). In affected horses with the generalized form, granulomas develop in the skin, lungs, heart, liver, gastrointestinal tract, and mesenteric lymph nodes. They are commonly found on the lower limbs and associated with laminitis.Application of modern diagnostic techniques using the nested polymerase chain reaction has detected Mycobacterial DNA in some (but not all) equine organ and skin samples (Oliveira-Filho et al., 2012). Human studies have reported that 25%–40% of sarcoid cases test positive for Mycobacterial DNA. Other cases have tested positive for an unrelated bacterium, *Propionibacterium acnes*. Some equine cases have also been associated with herpesvirus infection and even with hairy vetch (*Vicia villosa*) poisoning (Wimmer-Scherr & Schwarz, 2025). These results suggest that there may be multiple forms of the disease, probably triggered by many different antigens. Treatment involves the administration of immunosuppressive doses of corticosteroids. Despite its name, sarcoidosis is not related to the skin cancers called sarcoids, caused by infection with bovine papilloma virus (Chapter 22).

Contact dermatitis

When some reactive chemicals come into contact with the skin of a horse, they may bind to skin proteins and alter them. As a result, the chemically altered proteins may become antigenic and are rejected by T cells in the same way as a foreign skin graft is rejected. This causes an inflammatory response called allergic contact dermatitis. The incidence of contact dermatitis in humans is rising, especially in industrialized countries. Chemically induced skin diseases are now the second most common form of occupational disease. The skin is the protective barrier that excludes chemicals from the body, and interactions between these reactive chemicals and the body's defenses often occur first in the skin.resulting in contact dermatitis. Fig. 20.10.

It is important to note that there are two distinctly different forms of contact dermatitis; Irritant contact dermatitis simply results when an irritating chemical encounters a horse's skin. For example, the sap of the buttercup is highly irritating and induces a vesicular dermatitis on the muzzle of horses. This reaction is, however, not immunologically mediated.

Allergic contact dermatitis (ACD) is also a chemically induced inflammatory skin response. However, rather than being simply due to the toxic effects of the chemical, the response is immunologically mediated. The chemical induces a defensive T cell response that is expressed as an acute cutaneous inflammatory reaction. This antigen-specific response develops within hours or days following contact of the skin with a specific chemical sensitizer. Allergic contact dermatitis reactions are, in effect, the equivalent of drug-mediated adverse events. As such, they are idiosyncratic and are not dose-dependent. Some chemical sensitizers, such as nickel, are

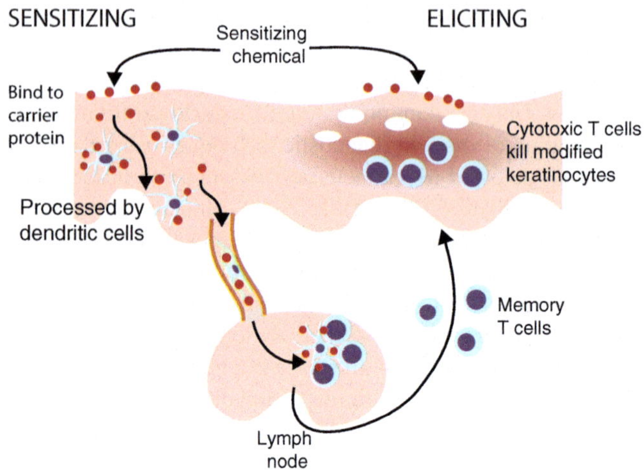

FIGURE 20.10 The pathogenesis of allergic contact dermatitis in horse skin.

A T cell response is directed against chemically modified keratinocytes.

not just contact irritants, but also immunogenic. Some reactive chemicals may also trigger inflammation by binding to PRMs and inflammasomes. For example, TLR4 is a PRM that can bind multiple contact sensitizers, including nickel and trinitrochlorobenzene. They therefore trigger dermatitis by releasing IL-1β and TNF-α. It may be difficult to distinguish clinically between irritant contact dermatitis and allergic contact dermatitis.

Contact sensitizers

Contact sensitizers are chemically reactive compounds that covalently bind to proteins on epithelial cells. Unlike some drug responses where the chemical binds covalently to soluble proteins and thus triggers an antibody response, these chemicals bind to cell surface proteins and therefore trigger a T cell-mediated response that resembles the graft rejection process. As with many drugs, most skin sensitizing chemicals are too small to be immunogenic on their own. They must therefore first bind covalently to epidermal cell proteins to create antigenic hapten-protein complexes. Most known contact sensitizers are small molecules such as cations or metals. They are delivered to the skin as drugs, oils, or skin creams. Many do not bind to the conventional MHC antigen binding sites. However, the non-polymorphic MHC-related molecule CD1a can bind and present hydrophobic molecules, especially lipids, to T cells. The chemicals that induce allergic contact dermatitis are usually highly reactive. They tend to be lipophilic so that they can readily penetrate the skin. Their upper size limit is about 500 Da if they are to pass through the stratum corneum.

Contact sensitizers come from a wide variety of sources. Many are natural products derived from plants. Thus, the reactive oils (urushiols) of the poison ivy plant (*Rhus radicans*) are major contact allergens in humans (but not in horses). Contact dermatitis in horses has also been attributed to organophosphate insecticides (fly sprays), heavy metals, aniline dyes, topical antinicrobials, such as neomycin, and a variety of feedstuffs (Swiderski, 2000). Horses may develop a contact dermatitis to contaminants on their bedding or preservatives in leather tack (bridle allergy). The leather in bridles, harnesses and saddles. may contain several potential contact allergens, including tanning agents such as chromium salts, glues such as butylphenol-formaldehyde resin, antifungal agents such as mercaptobenzothiazole derivatives and dimethyl fumarate, in addition to dyes such a cobalt salts (Herman et al., 2019).

Pathogenesis

Allergic contact dermatitis is a T cell-mediated cytotoxic response to chemically modified skin cells. As a result it is characterized by the development of a vesicular dermatitis. It is slow to develop, antigen-specific, and is primarily mediated by $CD8^+$ cytotoxic T cells. It can be conveniently divided into two distinct phases, sensitization and elicitation.

The development of ACD first requires sensitization of an animal against a specific chemical. This sensitization phase develops over a period of weeks to months following first exposure to the chemical. There are two mechanisms by which a horse may become sensitized. Compounds that bind covalently to cell proteins are treated as endogenous antigens. That means that they are processed and presented by MHC class II molecules. The second mechanism is used for lipid sensitizers. Lipids are processed and then bound to CD1a. CD1a is abundantly expressed on Langerhans cells and dermal dendritic cells. It rapidly binds its ligands without the need for complex antigen processing pathways. CD1a binds small hydrophobic oily molecules. For example, it readily binds urushiol from the poison ivy plant. The chemically modified proteins are first taken up by epidermal Langerhans cells. The Langerhans cells then migrate to the draining lymph nodes. Here, they mature into dendritic cells that process the hapten-carrier conjugate and then present it to T cells. They also release the pro-inflammatory cytokines and chemokines that costimulate the helper cell response. They prime the T cells, promoting their clonal expansion and differentiation into $CD8^+$ and $CD4^+$ cells. The migration of hapten-bearing antigen-presenting cells to the draining lymph node is essential for memory T cells to develop.

Once an animal has been sensitized, it may take six to 12 months after priming before the dermatitis develops. The memory T cells generated during the sensitization phase will mount a response when they encounter the chemically modified epidermal cells a second time and trigger a pruritic inflammatory response. The Langerhans cells activate both Th1 and Th17 cells. These helper cells, in turn, produce large amounts of IFN-γ and IL-17 and promote the activities of $CD8^+$ cytotoxic T cells. Primed cytotoxic $CD8^+$ T cells emigrate from the local lymph nodes into the bloodstream and eventually reach the site of chemical exposure on the skin. These primed T cells carry a skin-homing marker called cutaneous lymphocyte antigen that is a ligand for E-selectin, an adhesive cell surface protein expressed in chronically inflamed skin. This allows the T cells to specifically target the lesional site in the skin. This marker also induces the release of pro-inflammatory cytokines and the expression of adhesion molecules by keratinocytes and Langerhans cells. This attracts and activates yet more T cells. The $CD8^+$ T cells trigger chemokine production in the epidermis, which, as a result, attracts large numbers of neutrophils as well.

Following exposure to the sensitizing chemical, macrophages and $CD8^+$ T cells infiltrate the dermis. They take about 24–48 hours to do this. The cytotoxic T cells target and kill any skin cells that express the chemically modified proteins. The cytotoxic T cells will also release IFN-γ which activates keratinocytes and enhances their expression of IL-33, IL-25, and TSLP. In addition to killing the chemically modified keratinocytes, the cytotoxic T cells will also kill any dendritic cells carrying the chemical. Eventually, these cytotoxic T cells kill so many altered cells that gaps form, and intraepithelial vesicles develop. This destructive T cell response, together with the production of IL-33 and accompanying inflammatory cytokines, results in an intensely pruritic inflammatory skin reaction. Other cell types, such as ILC1 cells, NK cells, B cells, mast cells, neutrophils, and NKT cells, also participate in the reaction. The inflammation is eventually moderated by IL-10 and TGF-β produced by Treg cells.

Mast cells are found in close proximity to infiltrating T cells in ACD. As a result, the two cell types signal to each other. For example, T cell-derived IL-3, MIP-1α, and MCP-1 signal from T cells to mast cells. Conversely, activated mast cells signal to T cells. They may attract T cells by releasing lymphotactin, IL-16, or leukotriene B_4. They may bind the T cells through E-selectin, ICAM-1, and VCAM-1. Since mast cells can release both IL-4 and IL-13, they may also polarize some T cells and convert them to Th2 cells. The intense pruritus associated with ACD is probably not mediated directly by T cells but by mast cell derived mediators. A molecule called proadrenalomedullin, produced in lesional ACD skin, activates mast cells. This results in the production of tryptase, leukotrienes, and serotonin, all of which contribute to the itch sensation.

Erythema multiforme

A mucocutaneous disorder called erythema multiforme has been reported to occur in horses (Oryan et al., 2010). Erythema multiforme is characterized by sudden onset of urticaria, vesicle and papule formation, patchy skin loss, and low morbidity. The lesions gradually expand while there is central healing. As a result, this results in donut-shaped skin lesions developing. Scaling and crusting are not usual features, nor are the lesions pruritic. It appears to result from a T cell attack on skin cells. Affected animals develop vesicles, shed large areas of epidermis, and develop skin ulcers caused by widespread keratinocyte apoptosis. The apoptosis is believed to result from drugs or their metabolites binding to the epidermal keratinocytes, triggering their destruction by cytotoxic T cells. In equine cases, horses develop erythematous macules, raised papules, and non-pruritic plaques from the lateral aspect of the neck and shoulders to the rump. Histology shows scattered apoptotic keratinocytes, edema and a mixed infiltration with eosinophils, macrophages, lymphocytes, and plasma cells. The skin lesions are infiltrated mainly by $CD8^+$ T cells. The eosinophils may be present in large numbers. The horse may undergo spontaneous remission within a few months. The disease is typically mild and self-limiting and life-threatening secondary infections are not common (Marshall, 1991). The cause of erythema multiforme in horses is unknown. (In other domestic mammals, such as dogs, it is usually triggered by drug allergies, infections, or neoplasia) There are no reported age, breed, or gender predilections in the horse.

References

Ainsworth, D. M., Matychak, M., Reyner, C. L., et al. (2009). Effects of in vitro exposure to hay dust on the gene expression of chemokines and cell-surface receptors in primary bronchial epithelial cell cultures established from horses with chronic recurrent airway obstruction. *American Journal of Veterinary Research, 70*, 365–372.

Akula, S., Riihimaki, M., Waern, I., Abrink, M., et al. (2022). Quantitative transcriptome analysis of purified equine mast cells identifies a dominant mucosal mast cell population with possible inflammatory functions in airways of asthmatic horses. *International Journal of Molecular Sciences*. https://doi.org/10.3390/ijms232213976

Asmundsson, T., Gimnarsson, E., & Johannesson, T. (1983). "Haysickness" in Icelandic horses: Precipin tests and other studies. *Equine Veterinary Journal, 15*, 229–232.

Axon, J. E., Robinson, P., & Lucas, J. (2004). Generalized granulomatous disease in a horse. *Australian Veterinary Journal, 82*(1–2), 48–51.

Banks, K. L. (1979). Animal model: Antiglomerular basement membrane antibody in horses. *American Journal of Pathology, 94*(2), 443–446.

Bond, S., Leguillette, R., Richard, E. A., Couetil, L., et al. (2018). Equine asthma; integrative biologic relevance of a recently proposed nomenclture. *Journal of Veterinary Internal Medicine, 32*, 2088–2098.

Bozorgmanesh, R. (2024). Immune-mediated equine vasculopathies. *Veterinary Clinics of North America: Equine Practice, 40*, 253–261.

Costa, L. R. R., Johnson, J. R., Baur, M. F., & Beadle, R. E. (2006). Temporal clinical exacerbation of summer pasture-associated recurrent airway obstruction and relationshipo with climate and aeroallergens in horses. *American Journal of Veterinary Research, 97* (9), 1635–1642.

Couetil, L., Cardwell, J. M., Leguillette, R., Mazan, M., et al. (2020). Equine asthma: Current understanding and future directions. *Frontiers in Veterinary Science*. https://doi.org/10.3389/fvets.2020.00450

Couëtil, L. L., Cardwell, J. M., Gerber, V., Lavoie, J. P., et al. (2016). Inflammatory airway disease of horses–Revised consensus statement. *Journal of Veterinary Internal Medicine, 30*, 503–515.

Couetil, L. L., Hoffman, A. M., Hodgson, J., et al. (2007). Inflammatory airway disease of horses. *Journal of Veterinary Internal Medicine, 21*, 356–361.

Delph, K. M., Beard, L. A., Trimble, A. C., Sutter, M. E., et al. (2019). Strangles, convalescent *Streptococcus equi* subspecies *equi* M antibody titers and the presence of complications. *Journal of Veterinary Internal Medicine, 33*, 275–279.

DeLuca, L., Erb, H. N., Young, J. C., et al. (2008). The effect of adding oral dexamethasone to feed alterations on the airway cell inflammatory gene expression in stabled horses affected with recurrent airway obstruction. *Journal of Veterinary Internal Medicine, 22*, 427–435.

Derksen, F. J., Slocombe, R. F., Gray, P. R., & Robinson, N. E. (1992). Exercise-induced pulmonary hemorrhage in horses with experimentally induced allergic lung disease. *American Journal of Veterinary Research, 53*(1), 15–21.

Dirscherl, P., Grabner, A., & Buschmann. (1993). Responsiveness of basophil granulocytes mof horses suffering from chronic obstructive pulmonary disease to various allergens. *Veterinary Immunology and Immunopathology, 38*, 217–227.

Divers, T. J., Timoney, J. F., Lewis, R. M., & Smith, C. A. (1992). Equine glomerulonephritis and renal failure associated with complexes of Group-C streptococcal antigen and IgG antibody. *Veterinary Immunology and Immunopathology, 32*, 93–102.

Dubuc, J., & Lavoie, J.-P. (2014). Airway wall eosinophilia is not a feature of equine heaves. *The Veterinary Journal, 202*, 387–389.

Feudo, C. M. L., Stucci, L., Alberti, E., Conturba, B., et al. (2021). Intradermal testing results in horses affected by mild-moderate and severe equine asthma. *Animals*. https://doi.org/10.3390/ani11072086

Franchini, M., Gill, U., von Fellenberg, R., & Bracher, V. D. (2000). Inteleukin-8 concentration and neutrophil chemotactic activity in bronchoalveolar lavage fluid of horses with chronic obstructive pulmonary disease following exposure to hay. *American Journal of Veterinary Research, 61*, 1369–1374.

Galan, J. E., & Timoney, J. F. (1985). Immune complexes in purpura hemorrhagica of the horse contain IgA and M antigen of *Streptococcus equi*. *Journal of Immunology, 135*, 3134–3137.

Gehlen, H., Oey, L., Rohn, K., et al. (2008). Pulmonary dysfunction and skeletal muscle changes in horses with RAO. *Journal of Veterinary Internal Medicine, 22*, 1014–1021.

Geor, R. J., Clark, E. G., Haines, D. M., & Napier, P. G. (2005). Systemic lupus erythematosus in a filly. *Journal of the American Veterinary Medical Association, 197*, 1489–1492.

Gressler, A. E., Lubke, S., Wagner, B., Arnold, C., et al. (2022). Comprehensive flow cytometric characterization of bronchoalveolar lavage cells indicates comparable phenotypes between asthmatic and healthy horses but functional lymphocyte differences. *Frontiers in Immunology*. https://doi.org/10.3389/fimmu.2022.896255

Gunson, D. E., & Rooney, J. R. (1977). Anaphylactoid purpura in a horse. *Veterinary Pathology Online, 14*, 325–331.

Henriquez, C., Perez, B., Morales, N., Sarmiento, J., et al. (2014). Participation of T regulatory cells in equine recurrent airway obstruction. *Veterinary Immunology and Immunopathology, 158*, 128–134.

Herman, A., Goossens, A., Tennstedt, D., Bergendorff, O., et al. (2019). The preservative 2-(thiocyanomethylthio) benzothiazole: A potential allergen in leather products. *Contact Dermatitis*. https://doi.org/10.1111/cod.13295

Hodgin, E. C., McGuire, T. C., Perryman, L. E., & Grant, B. D. (1978). Evaluation of delayed hypersensitivity responses in normal horses and immunodeficient foals. *American Journal of Veterinary Research, 39*(7), 1161–1167.

Hotchkiss, J. W., Reid, S. W. J., & Chrisley, R. M. (2007). A survey of horse owners in Great Britain regarding horses in their care. Part 1: Horse demographic characteristics and management. *Equine Veterinary Journal, 39*, 294–300.

Houtsma, A., Bedenice, D., Pusterla, N., Pugliese, B., et al. (2015). Association between inflammatory airway disease of horses and exposure to respiratory viruses: A case control study. *Multidisciplinary Respiratory Medicine, 10*, 33–40.

Janssen, P., Tosi, I., Hego, A., Maréchal, P., et al. (2022). Neutrophil extracellular traps are found in bronchiolar lavage fluids of horses with severe asthma and correlate with asthma severity. *Frontiers in Immunology*. https://doi.org/10.3389/fimmu.2022.921077

Jentsch, M. C., Lübke, S., Schrödl, W., Volke, D., et al. (2024). Immunoproteomics enable broad identification of new *Aspergillus fumigatus* antigens in severe equine asthma. *Frontiers in Immunology*. https://doi.org/10.3389/fimmu.2024.1347164

Kaese, H. J., Valberg, S. J., Hayden, D. W., et al. (2005). Infarctive purpura hemorrhagica in five horses. *Journal of the American Veterinary Medical Association, 226*, 1893–1898.

Kang, H., Bienzle, D., Lee, G. K. C., Piche, E., et al. (2021). Flow cytometric analysis of equine bronchoalveolar lavage cells in horses with and without severe equine asthma. *Veterinary Pathology*. https://doi.org/10.1177/03009858211042588

Konyha, L. D., & Kreier, J. P. (1971). The significance of tuberculin tests in the horse. *American Review of Respiratory Disease, 103*(1), 91–99.

Korn, A., Miller, D., Dong, L., Buckles, E. L., et al. (2015). Differential gene expression profiles and selected cytokine protein analysis of mediastinal lymph nodes of horses with chronic recurrent airway obstruction (RAO) support an interleukin-17 immune response. *PLoS One*. https://doi.org/10.1371/journal.pone.0142622

Laan, T. T. J. M., Bull, S., Pirie, R., et al. (2006). The role of alveolar macrophages in the pathogenesis of recurrent airway obstruction in horses. *Journal of Veterinary Internal Medicine, 20*, 167–174.

Lavoie-Lamoureux, A., Leclere, M., Lemos, K., Wagner, B., & Lavoie, J. P. (2012). Markers of systemic inflammation in horses with heaves. *Journal of Veterinary Internal Medicine, 26*, 1419–1426.

Leguilette, R. (2003). Recurrent airway obstruction—Heaves. *Veterinary Clinics: Equine Practice, 19*, 63–86.

Mansmann, R. A., Osburn, B. I., Wheat, J. D., & Frick, O. (1975). Chicken hypersensitivity pneumonitis in horses. *Journal of the American Veterinary Medical Association, 166*(7), 673–677.

Marshall, C. (1991). Erythema multiforme in two horses. *Journal of the South African Veterinary Association, 62*(3), 133–136.

McConnico, R. S., Roberts, M. C., & Tompkins, M. (1992). Penicillin-induced immune mediated hemolytic anemia in a horse. *Journal of the American Veterinary Medical Association, 201*, 1402–1403.

Miskovic, M., Couetil, L. L., & Thompson, C. A. (2007). Lung function and airway cytologic profiles in horses with recurrent airway obstruction maintained in low-dust environments. *Journal of Veterinary Internal Medicine, 21*, 1060–1066.

Moore, B. R. (1996). Lower respiratory tract disease. *Veterinary Clinics of North America: Equine Practice, 12*(3), 457–472.

Moore, B. R., Krakowka, S., Robertson, J. T., & Cummins, J. M. (1995). Cytologic evaluation of bronchoalveolar lavage obtained from Standardbred horses with inflammatory airway disease. *American Journal of Veterinary Research, 56*(5), 562–567.

Moore, J. E., Matsuda, M., Yamamoto, S., Buckley, T., & Millar, B. C. (2004). Hypersensitivity pneumonitis in the horse: An underdiagnosed condition? *Journal of Equine Veterinary Science*. https://doi.org/10.1016/j.jevs.2004.11.003

Oliveira-Filho, J. P., Monteiro, L. N., Delfiol, D. J. Z., Sequeira, J. L., et al. (2012). Mycobacterium DNA detection on liver and skin of a horse with generalized sarcoidosis. *Journal of Veterinary Diagnostic Investigation, 24*(3), 596–600.

Oryan, A., Ghane, M., & Ahmadi, N. (2010). Erythema multiforme and its clinicopathological disorders in a horse. *Comparative Clinical Pathology, 19*, 179–184.

Pauli, B., Gerber, H., & Schatzmann, U. (1972). Farmer's lung beim pferde. *Pathology Microbiology, 38*, 200–214.

Psalla, D., Rufenacht, S., Stoffel, M. H., Chiers, K., et al. (2013). Equine pastern vasculitis: A clinical and histopathological study. *The Veterinary Journal*, 524–530.

Pusterla, N., Watson, J. L., Affolter, V. K., et al. (2003). Purpura haemorrhagica in 53 horses. *The Veterinary Record, 153*, 118–121.

Robbins, R. L., Wallace, S. S., Brunner, C. J., et al. (1993). Immune-mediated hemolytic disease after penicillin therapy in a horse. *Equine Veterinary Journal, 25*, 462–465.

Rush, B. (2001). International workshop on equine chronic airway disease: Corticosteroid therapy. *Equine Veterinary Journal, 33*(1), 5–19.

Sage, S. E., Leeb, T., Jagannathan, V., & Gerber, V. (2024). Single-cell profiling of bronchoalveolar cells reveals a Th17 signature in neutrophilic severe equine asthma. *Immunology, 171*, 549–565.

Scarratt, W. K., & Sponenberg, D. P. (1984). Chronic glomerulonephritis in two horses. *Journal of Equine Veterinary Science, 4*(6), 252–255.

Schnabel, C. L., Jentsch, C., Lübke, S., Kaiser-Thom, S., et al. (2023). Immunoproteomics reveal increased serum IgG3/5 binding to *Dermatophagoides* and to yeast protein antigens in severe equine asthma in a preliminary study. *Frontiers in Immunology*. https://doi.org/10.3389/fimmu.2023.1293684

Sethi, S., & Fervenza, F. C. (2012). Membranoproliferative glomerulonephritis—A new look at an old entity. *New England Journal of Medicine, 366*, 1119–1131.

Sheats, M. K., Davis, K. U., & Poole, J. A. (2019). Comparative review of asthma in farmers and horses. *Current Allergy and Asthma Reports*. https://doi.org/10.1007/s11882-019-0882-2

Simões, J., Batista, M., & Tilley, P. (2022). The immune mechanisms of severe equine athma current understanding and what is missing. *Animals*. https://doi.org/10.3390/ani12060744

Slauson, D. O., & Lewis, R. M. (1979). Comparative pathology of glomerulonephritis in animals. *Veterinary Pathology Online, 16*, 135–164.

Spagnolo, P., Rossi, G., Cavazza, A., et al. (2015). Hypersensitivity pneumonitis: A comprehensive review. *Journal of Investigational Allergology & Clinical Immunology, 25*(4), 237–250.

Swiderski, C. E. (2000). Hypersensitivity disorders in horses. *Veterinary Clinics of North America: Equine Practice, 16*(1), 131–151.

Swinburne, J. E., Bogle, H., Klukowska-Rotzler, J., Drogemuller, M., Leeb, T., et al. (2009). A whole genome scan for recurrent airway obstruction in Warmblood sports horses indicates two positional candidate regions. *Mammalian Genome, 20*, 504–515.

Tamarinde, T., Laan, J. M., Bull, S., Pirie, R., & Fink-Gremmels, J. (2006). The role of alveolar macrophages in the pathogenesis of recurrent airway obstruction in horses. *Journal of Veterinary Internal Medicine, 20*, 167–174.

Taylor, S. D., Ivester, K. M., Stewart, C., Page, A. E., et al. (2021). The effect of lower airway inflammation on inflammatory cytokine gene expression in bronchoalveolar lavage fluid and whole blood in racing Thoroughbreds. *Veterinary Immunology and Immunopathology*. https://doi.org/10.1016/2021.110266

Thomas, H. L., & Livesey, M. A. (1998). Immune-mediated hemolytic anemia associated with trimethotrim-sulphamethoxazole administration in a horse. *Canadian Veterinary Journal, 39*, 171–173.

Vargas, A., Boivin, R., Cano, P., Murcia, Y., et al. (2017). Neutrophil extracellular traps are downregulated by glucocorticosteroids in lungs in an equine model of asthma. *Respiratory Research, 18*, 207.

Waldvogel, A., Wild, P., & Wegmann, C. (1983). Membranoproliferative glomerulonephritis in a horse. *Veterinary Pathology Online, 20*, 500–503.

Warkentin, T. E. (2007). Drug-induced immune-mediated thrombocytopenia—From purpura to thrombosis. *New England Journal of Medicine, 356*(9), 891–893.

Williams, M. A., Dowling, P. M., Angarano, D. W., et al. (1995). Paraneoplastic bullous stomatitis in a horse. *Journal of the American Veterinary Medical Association, 207*(3), 331–334.

Wimmer-Scherr, C. M., & Schwarz, C. (2025). A narrative literature review of equine sarcoidosis. *Equine Veterinary Education, 37*, 44–51.

Woodrow, J. S., Hines, M., Sommardaht, C., Flatland, B., et al. (2022). Initial investigation of molecular phenotypes of airway mast cells and cytokine profiles in equine asthma. *Frontiers in Veterinary Science*. https://doi.org/10.3389/fvets.2022.997139

CHAPTER

Equine cancer immunology and immunotherapy

21

Horses are not commonly considered ideal subjects for studies on cancer immunology. Nevertheless, they are valued animals that can live into old age. As cancer prevalence increases with age, so do aged horses develop multiple forms of cancer. About 50% of equine cancers develop in the skin. Some of these have unique immunological features, which means that they are prospective targets for newly developed immunotherapy techniques.

Normal cellular functions depend on the regulation of cell division. When cells multiply, it is essential that they do so only as and when required. Unfortunately, as a result of mutations triggered by chemicals, radiation, or viruses, cells may break free of these constraints. The essential difference between a normal cell and a cancer cell is thus a loss of control of cell growth as a result of multiple mutations. These mutations may also result in cancer cells expressing abnormal proteins. These abnormal proteins may be recognized by T cells and trigger cytotoxic T cell responses. These immune responses may be protective. Recent innovations in the area of immunotherapy have developed new and unique methods of promoting anticancer T cell immunity and have yielded very encouraging results, not least in horses.

Tumors as allografts

When organ transplantation became a common procedure as a result of the development of potent immunosuppressive drugs, it was found that patients with prolonged graft survival were also more likely to develop certain cancers than non-immunosuppressed individuals. It was therefore suggested that the immune system was responsible for the prevention of cancer. For example, tumors developed in 22% of cats that received cyclosporine to prevent renal allograft rejection, and about half of these were B-cell lymphomas. Immunosuppressed cats were 6 times more likely to develop cancer than normal cats (Wormser et al., 2016). From this suggestion, the concept of immune surveillance emerged. This theory proposed that cell mutation is a common event. When a mutation occurs, the protein coded by the mutated gene is altered. This alteration may make this new protein antigenic. The recognition of these new antigens by cytotoxic T cells therefore results in the elimination of most abnormal cells. Theory suggests that cancer can only result if cancer cells somehow evade destruction by T cells.

The Immunology of Horses and Donkeys. https://doi.org/10.1016/B978-0-443-44863-8.00025-9

Tumor neoantigens

Cancer cells develop as a result of multiple mutations. These mutations may generate molecules that are unique to the cancer cells (tumor-specific antigens) or, more commonly, abnormal or unusual molecules (tumor-associated antigens). To distinguish between normal and cancer cells, host T cells must recognize these new antigens. Several major types of tumor antigen have been identified. Thus, there are differentiation antigens associated with specific stages in the development of a cell type. For example, some cancer cells express the products of developmental genes that are turned off in adult cells and are only expressed early in an individual's development. These proteins are called oncofetal antigens. Examples include tumors of the gastrointestinal tract that produce a glycoprotein called carcinoembryonic antigen (CEA; classified as CD66e), normally found only in the fetal intestine. The presence of CEA in serum may indicate the presence of a colon or rectal adenocarcinoma (Hässig et al., 1991). Alpha-fetoprotein produced by hepatoma cells is normally expressed only in the fetal liver (Sorensen et al., 1990). Likewise, squamous cell carcinoma cells may possess antigens normally restricted to fetal liver and skin. These oncofetal antigens are usually poor immunogens and do not provoke protective immunity. However, their detection may be useful for diagnosis and for monitoring the progress of a tumor.

Second, there are mutated forms of normal cellular proteins. For example, melanoma cells may express the products of mutated oncogenes on their surface. Some tumor antigens are recognized because they are abnormally glycosylated. Chemically induced tumors may express surface antigens unique to the tumor and not to the inducing chemical. Because carcinogenic chemicals can produce many different mutations, tumors induced by a single chemical in different animals may be antigenically different. Even within a single chemically induced tumor mass, distinct antigenic subpopulations of cells exist. As a result, immunity to one chemically induced tumor may not prevent the growth of a second tumor caused by the same chemical.

Tumors caused by viruses may express antigens characteristic of the inducing virus. These antigens, although coded for by a viral genome, are not part of a virion. Examples include the FOCMA antigens found on the neoplastic lymphoid cells of cats infected with feline leukemia virus and Marek's cancer-specific antigens found on Marek's disease tumor cells in chickens. (Both of these are virus-induced, naturally occurring, T cell tumors.) Studies on these mutations and the neoantigens they generate suggest that they are not widely shared but are tumor-specific. Their production also differs between tumor types. Thus, neoantigen expression tends to be very high in human melanomas, lung, stomach, and colorectal tumors, and low in many leukemias.

Inflammation and cancer

The tumor microenvironment often determines the development and fate of cancer cells. Cancer cells can communicate with nearby cells, especially fibroblasts and inflammatory cells. As a result, the survival of cancer cells is determined in part by the presence of inflammation (Coussens & Werb, 2002). Chronic inflammatory diseases increase the risk for developing many types of cancer; conversely, the use of non-steroidal anti-inflammatory drugs reduces tumor susceptibility (Mantovani et al., 2008). Even the limited degree of inflammation caused by influenza vaccination may be sufficient to trigger neoplastic transformation in some horses (Kannegieter et al., 2010). Mutations in oncogenes such as *ras* and *myc* are closely linked to these inflammatory pathways. Inflammatory cytokines, chemokines, and cells are present in the microenvironment of early tumors and influence their blood supply, metastasis, and survival. Inflammatory cytokines, such as tumor necrosis factor-α (TNF-α), and macrophages are often required if tumor cells are to develop and spread (Hagemann et al., 2007).

Cancer cells exploit signals from their microenvironment (Wong & Reiter, 2011). Stromal cells such as fibroblasts, macrophages, and endothelial cells can generate IL-6, which promotes tumor growth and angiogenesis. Inflammatory cells such as macrophages, mast cells, and tumor-infiltrating lymphocytes can promote tumor growth by remodeling tissues, stimulating angiogenesis, and suppressing local immune responses. As a result, more than half of the mass of some tumors may consist of supporting cells, including fibroblasts, macrophages, and vascular endothelial cells. Cancers cannot spread and metastasize without the support of these cells (Li et al., 2005).

If a metastasizing tumor does not invade lymphoid organs, it may escape immune surveillance. On the other hand, tumors that invade lymph nodes can be divided into strongly and weakly immunogenic types. Strongly immunogenic tumors elicit a T cell response following processing by dendritic cells. Weakly immunogenic tumors tend to grow as walled-off nodules that may not be processed in sufficient amounts to trigger their destruction. Tumors that fail to generate inflammation may simply be ignored by the rest of the immune system.

Cellular defenses

Natural killer cells

NK cells can detect and kill some cancer cells. As described in Chapter 10, they use two major types of receptors: First, receptors that can respond to the absence of MHC class I molecules on a cell surface by killing these abnormal cells; and second, receptors that can recognize stress-induced proteins on cell surfaces and, as a result, kill stressed cells. Thus, NK cells effectively kill two types of cellular targets: cells that fail to express MHC class I molecules and cells that express stress-related proteins. Both conditions commonly apply to cancer cells. As a result, NK cells play a significant role in the destruction of many tumors. Fig. 21.1.

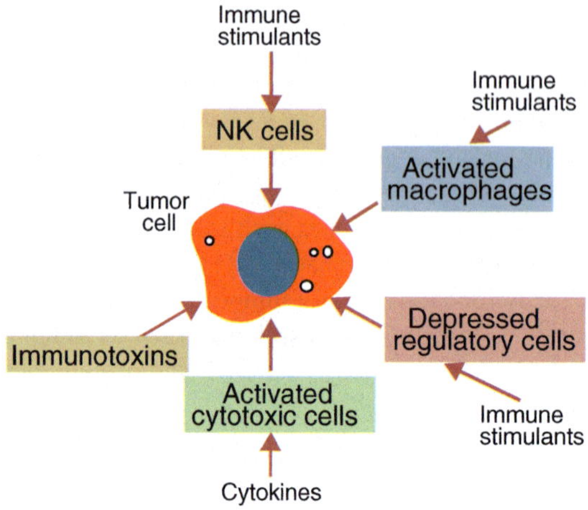

FIGURE 21.1 The major cell types that participate in tumor cell destruction and methods of stimulating that activity.

Cytotoxic T cells

T cells also have the potential to destroy cancer cells. They possess receptors that can recognize antigen-MHC complexes expressed on all nucleated cells. The immense diversity of the T cell antigen receptor repertoire enables them to identify and respond to unique new antigens made by cancer cells (Zamora et al., 2018).

Tumor-infiltrating $CD8^+$ cytotoxic T cells are found in many cancers. Their presence tends to be associated with a better prognosis. Some success has been achieved in humans by isolating these lymphocytes from excised tumors and growing them in tissue culture. Infusion of tumor-infiltrating lymphocytes, some of which are cytotoxic, may also benefit some cancer patients. These cultured cells are transfused into the patient and may induce remission. Similar results may be obtained with lymphokine-activated killer (LAK) cells. LAK cells are generated by taking the patient's peripheral blood lymphocytes, activating them in vitro with interleukin-2, and then returning them intravenously to the patient. Horses are known to possess LAK cells whose activity is stimulated by the presence of interleukin-2. These LAK cells have been shown to be cytotoxic for both MHC^- and MHC^+ cellular targets (Vivieros & Antczak, 1999).

The products of mutated genes or abnormally expressed cellular proteins may be processed and presented to T cells. As a result, lymphocytes from some tumor-bearing animals may kill cancer cells cultured in vitro. For example, a protein called cyclin B1 that regulates mitosis is barely expressed in normal cells but overexpressed in many tumors, where it can stimulate T cell cytotoxicity. Implicit in this is the fact that these T cells must recognize some antigenic peptides presented by the MHC I receptors expressed on malignant cells. These antigens may be normal cellular proteins to which tolerance is weak, or they may be neoantigens, peptides that are not present in normal animals but are newly created by tumor-specific mutations.

Macrophage-mediated immunity

Solid tumors may be infiltrated by macrophages attracted by pro-inflammatory cytokines and prostaglandins. M2 macrophages may promote cancer cell proliferation and metastasis by releasing growth factors such as TGF-β, PDGF, and FGF. These M2 macrophages may also suppress T and NK cell responses, promote angiogenesis, and enhance cancer cell infiltration (Meeremans et al., 2025). Conversely, M1 macrophages may secrete cytotoxic molecules, including potent oxidants. Non specific activation of macrophages by bacillus Calmette-Guérin (BCG) or *Propionibacterium acnes* results in enhanced production of IL-1 or TNF-α and subsequent enhancement of helper T cell and NK cell activity. IL-1β has a cytostatic effect on some tumors, and TNF-α may have potent antitumor activity.

Failure of immunity to cancer cells

The fact that tumors tend to occur in older horses testifies to failures in their immunological protective mechanisms. Studies of tumor-bearing animals have indicated several mechanisms by which the immune systems fail to reject tumors. Fig. 21.2.

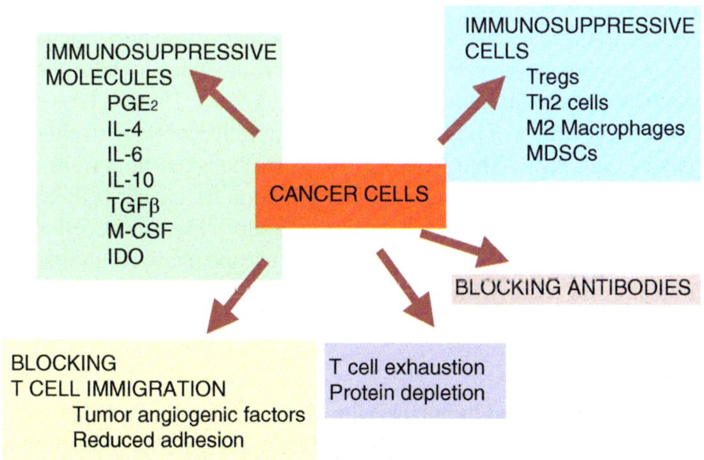

FIGURE 21.2 Some of the mechanisms by which cancer cells evade immune destruction.

Cancer cell selection

Cancer cells do not usually become malignant in a single step. Rather, they gradually go from normal to benign to malignant in a stepwise process called tumor progression. The process occurs through a series of mutations that switch genes on and off. These mutations do not necessarily alter the immunogenicity of cancer cells or do so in small steps. Thus, their immunogenicity may not change until the cells are irreversibly committed to malignancy.

There are two other selection mechanisms by which developing cancer cells can evade the host's immune response and so enhance their own survival. One method of cancer cell evasion is "sneaking through," the process by which malignant cells may not trigger an immune response until the tumor has reached a size at which it cannot be controlled by the host. Thus, in experimental tumors, small numbers of cancer cells may grow after subcutaneous inoculation, although large numbers may not. It may be that the cancer cells may not reach the lymph nodes and trigger an immune response until the tumor burden is too large to be controlled. Even a very small tumor may contain an enormous number of cells. For example, a 10 mm tumor contains about 10^9 cells.

The second immune evasion mechanism involves "immunoediting" cancers. Thus, the immune system may indeed eliminate some cancer cells, especially those that express neoantigens and trigger T cell cytotoxicity. If, however, mutations are subtle and their immunogenicity is low, some cancer cells may escape T cell destruction. These variants may then grow to produce clinical cancers. This may also result in tumors that contain multiple different cancer cell populations. Cancers with high intratumor heterogeneity tend to be associated with poor immunogenicity. Immunoediting consists of three phases: elimination, equilibrium, and escape. Immune elimination usually occurs early in tumor growth at a time when the tumor is small. If effective, the tumor cells are wiped out. If, however, some tumor cells may avoid destruction, the response moves into the equilibrium phase, where the tumor becomes established while immunological attack continues. There is ongoing elimination of some cancer cells, but non-immunogenic variants continue to emerge that can survive, persist, and grow. Thus, there is a balance between tumor elimination and tumor growth. Eventually, however, ongoing selection for cancer cells with minimal immunogenicity permits the tumor to escape. The surviving cancer cells are resistant to immunological attack. Tumors are often in the escape phase when first diagnosed, so that clinical cases usually fail to mount effective immune responses.

Immunosuppression

It is commonly observed that tumor-bearing animals are immunosuppressed. This is most clearly seen in animals with lymphoid tumors. For example, B cell tumors tend to suppress antibody formation, whereas T cell tumors suppress cell-mediated immune responses and NK cell activity.

Some tumor-derived molecules may redirect immune functions so that they promote tumor growth. Thus, tumor-derived IL-4, IL-6, IL-10, TGF-β, prostaglandin E_2, and macrophage colony-stimulating factor can deactivate or suppress the activation of both M1 macrophages and Th1 cells. The TGF-β can convert antitumor effector cells into Treg cells. Many tumors produce indolamine 2,3-dioxygenase (IDO), a potent immunosuppressive agent and a suppressor of NK cell function (Chapter 2).

T cell dysfunction

Within the tumor microenvironment, numerous factors may act together to suppress T cell function. A combination of hypoxia, nutrient shortage, acidic pH, suppressive cytokines such as TGF-β and IL-10, and lipids like PGE_2 suppresses the activities of tumor-infiltrating T cells. T cell cytotoxicity may be blocked by upregulating PD-L1 expression as a result of hypoxia, by IDO production suppressing T cell functions, or by excessive Treg activity. Cytotoxic T cells must be able to contact cancer cells to kill them. Tumor-derived angiogenic factors such as vascular endothelial growth factor (VEGF) and endothelin-1 can block the expression of the endothelial cell adhesion molecules so that T cells may be unable to leave tumor blood vessels and reach the cancer cells. Tumor vascular endothelium may express immunosuppressive molecules such as IDO and PGE_2. Tumor endothelium can also express ligands such as TRAIL that may kill T cells as they cross the vascular endothelium.

CD95 ligand

CD95 ligand (CD95L) is normally expressed on cytotoxic T cells and NK cells. When it binds to the death receptor CD95 on target cells, it triggers their apoptosis. CD95L has also been detected on some leukemic T cells and NK cells, colon adenocarcinoma cells, melanomas, and hepatocellular carcinomas. Since cytotoxic T cells may also express CD95, cytotoxicity may work in reverse, and the $CD95L^+$ tumor cells may kill the T cells. At the same time, these cancer cells may downregulate their own CD95 so that they become resistant to cell-mediated cytotoxicity.

Regulatory cells

Much of the immunosuppression that develops in in tumor-bearing individuals is due to the activities of regulatory cells. These may be $CD8^+$ Treg cells, IL-10-secreting Th2 cells, M2 macrophages, or even Breg cells. Enhanced regulatory cell activity can be detected in many tumor-bearing animals, including sarcoid-bearing horses (Wilson & Hicks., 2016).

Myeloid-derived suppressor cells

Myeloid-derived suppressor cells (MDSC) are immature myeloid cells that normally develop into macrophages, granulocytes, and dendritic cells (Zhang et al., 2021). They are generated by soluble factors from cancer cells and are attracted by chemokines or hypoxia to the tumors. Once inside tumors, MDSCs suppress cytotoxic T cell responses by expressing the inhibitory surface protein PD-L1, and by secreting immunosuppressive mediators such as arginase, IL-10, TGF-β, and reactive oxygen species. MDSCs also produce arginase that impairs T cell function by reducing expression of CD3ζ. Some MDSCs promote the production of Treg cells. MDSCs may also enhance cancer cell survival by promoting the switch from M1 to M2 cells. MDSCs have been identified in tumor-bearing dogs where they suppress lymphocyte proliferation (Goulart et al., 2012).

Tumor immunotherapy

For many years, immunologists have attempted to treat cancers by vaccination or other forms of immunotherapy. Initially, progress was distressingly slow. Successes were limited to rare cancers, and even when immunotherapy worked, results were unpredictable and inconsistent. That has now changed. Vaccines against cancers are still at an early stage in their development, but new techniques involving both passive and active immunotherapy have begun to yield encouraging results. Progress has not been confined to human cancers. Encouraging results are increasingly being obtained in the treatment of cancers in our domestic animals, including horses (Bergman, 2018).

Active immunotherapy

In active immunotherapy, the horse's own immune system is stimulated to respond to the tumor. In passive immunotherapy, immune cells or their products are administered.

Several approaches have been used in attempts to cure or modify tumor growth through immunotherapy. The simplest is to stimulate the immune system nonspecifically. Any improvement in an animal's immune capabilities will tend to enhance its resistance to tumors, although a cure may be expected only if the tumor mass is small or is surgically excised. The most widely used immune stimulant is the attenuated strain of *Mycobacterium bovis*, BCG. This organism activates macrophages and stimulates cytokine release, thus promoting T cell activity. It may be given systemically or injected directly into the tumor mass.

The immune response modifier Imiquimod (Aldara) has been widely used to treat many skin cancers, most notably equine sarcoids (Hollis, 2022). This drug activates TLR7 and, as a result, stimulates cells to secrete IFN-α, TNF-α, and IL-6. These cytokines activate Langerhans cells as well as inducing local innate immune responses. Imiquimod also activates the opioid growth factor receptor, which has antiproliferative effects. It also appears to activate NK cells, macrophages, and B cells (Miller et al., 1999).

Passive immunotherapy

Cytokine therapy

Many attempts have been made to treat human cancer patients by administering individual cytokines, but with limited success. Interferons, for example, are effective only against selected tumors. Thus 70%–90% of human patients with hairy cell leukemia treated with IFN-α show complete or partial remission. On the other hand, administration of IL-2 to melanoma and renal cell cancer patients induces partial or complete remission in only 15%–20% of cases. Low doses of recombinant human IL-2, when injected locally into papillomas or carcinomas of the vulva in cattle, induced remissions in 83% of treated animals. Some complete regressions were observed. IL-2 therapy produced 63% complete remissions in cattle with ocular squamous cell carcinomas (Hill et al., 1994).

Adoptive cell transfer

Limited success has been obtained in treating melanomas in gray horses by immunotherapy. For example, administration of a plasmid expressing IL-13 directly into metastases produced significant regression in 60% of cases and appeared to be safe. In dogs with melanomas, plasmids containing DNA coding for the herpesvirus thymidine kinase gene were able to sensitize transfected cells to ganciclovir. (Ganciclovir is a potent anti-herpesvirus drug.) The treatment induced substantial regression. A similar therapy, given in association with a subcutaneous autologous killed cancer vaccine, appeared to work well in a horse (Finocchiaro et al., 2009).

Monoclonal antibodies

A major advance in cancer immunotherapy has been the development of bioengineered monoclonal antibodies directed against specific tumor cell antigens or against molecules that promote tumor growth. There are now more than 75 FDA-approved monoclonal antibodies used in the treatment of human cancers. For example, in 1987, the FDA approved rituximab, a monoclonal antibody directed against the B-cell surface antigen CD20. Rituximab has revolutionized the treatment of B-cell lymphomas in humans. The anti-CD20 binds to the malignant B cells and triggers their apoptosis.

Initially, these monoclonal antibodies were derived exclusively from mice. However, as monoclonal antibody technology has improved, it has proved possible to "humanize" the murine antibodies by attaching the mouse antigen-binding region to a human immunoglobulin backbone. A similar process can produce "equinized" monoclonal antibodies for use in horses. These monoclonal antibodies can be directed against the cancer cells in order to destroy them through the process of antibody-dependent cellular cytotoxicity. Alternatively, monoclonal antibodies may be used to block growth-promoting factors or their receptors, or they may enhance the activity of immune cells.

Immune checkpoint therapy

Recent encouraging advances in the treatment of some human cancers have also resulted from the use of monoclonal antibodies that prevent T cell inhibition by checkpoint molecules. Checkpoint molecules are T cell surface receptors and their ligands that normally regulate immune responses by suppressing excessive T cell proliferation and cytotoxicity (Waldman et al., 2020).

The most important defense pathway against tumors employs cytotoxic, $CD8^+$ T cells. These T cells can kill cancer cells provided that they can recognize the cancer cell neoantigens and respond accordingly. However, these T cells are readily exhausted by prolonged, low-level immune stimulation. Once exhausted, these T cells take on an immunosuppressive function. They persist within the tumor microenvironment and suppress nearby effector T cells. Exhausted $CD8^+$ T cells express high levels of two inhibitory checkpoint molecules called programmed cell death-1 (PD-1) and cytotoxic T lymphocyte-associated protein-4 (CTLA4). These two proteins normally prevent excessive T cell cytotoxicity. Their increased expression has been detected in exhausted T cells from many human tumors and is associated with increased tumor aggressiveness. Fig. 21.3.

PD-1

Programmed death-1 (PD-1) is a receptor normally expressed on effector T cells. When stimulated by its ligands (PD-L1 and PD-L2), it suppresses T cell functions. Signaling through PD-1 thus normally prevents T cells from generating excessive cytotoxic signals and damaging surrounding tissues. It suppresses T cell cytotoxicity and triggers T cell apoptosis. Thus, if cancer cells produce PD-1 ligands, they will not be attacked by cytotoxic T cells. Additionally, some cancer cells induce PD-1 expression on activated T cells. This also results in a loss of T cell function and eventual T cell "exhaustion" (Boussiotis, 2016). T cell exhaustion is also the fate of some T cells in response to persistent antigenic stimulation in cancer patients. These cells lose their effector functions as a result of the excessive production of inhibitory receptors. Fig. 21.4.

Research into equine melanomas has demonstrated that many express high levels of PD-L1. Thus, in 77 melanistic tumors from horses, 59.7% contained more than 50% of PD-L1-positive cells. Out of 38 melanomas classified as malignant, 24 contained more than 50% of cells expressing PD-1, 13 tumors had 25%–50% expression, and one malignant tumor contained less than 10% of labeled cells (Pimenta et al., 2024). Of the 39 benign tumors investigated, 22 contained more than 50% PD-L1-positive cells, nine contained 25%–50%, three contained 10%–25%, two

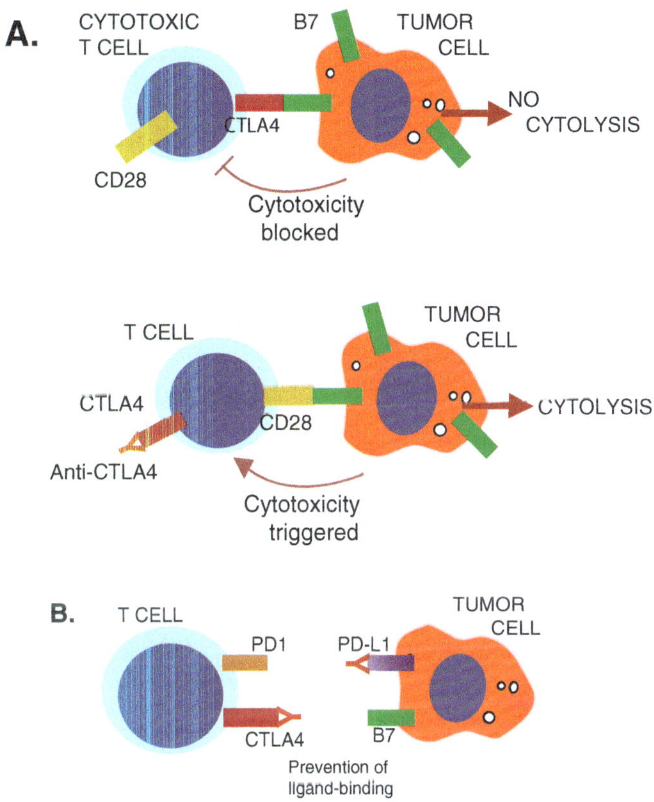

FIGURE 21.3 The principles of immune checkpoint therapy

(A) CTLA-4 is an inhibitory receptor expressed on T cells. Its ligand is B7 expressed on tumor cells. Blocking of CTLA-4 binding by monoclonal antibodies permits cytotoxic T cells to exercise their full activity against the tumor cells. (B) Alternatively (or additionally), PD-1 also blocks tumor cell killing by binding to its ligand PD-L1. Blockage of this interaction also allows T cell cytotoxicity to proceed.

had less than 10% and three benign tumors did not express detectable PD-L1. There was no association between PD-L1 expression and tumor location, and the expression was not equal among different tumors from the same horse.

It has also proved possible to study the effects of immune checkpoint blockade on equine melanomas. Equine melanomas contain cells that express both PD-1 and its ligand, PD-L1. A monoclonal antibody directed against bovine PD-L1 was shown to bind to equine PD-L1 and block its binding to PD-1. (Equine PD-1 is 69% homologous to bovine PD-1, while equine PD-L1 is 80.9% homologous to bovine PD-L1). An in vitro study confirmed that PD-L1 blockade enhanced the production of Th1

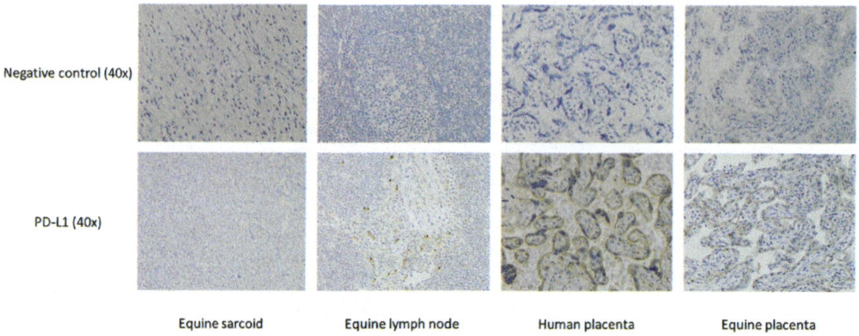

FIGURE 21.4 The expression of PD-L1 on equine cells

Positive and negative staining comparing the presence of PD-L1 in human and horse tissues including equine sarcoid cells. ×40.

- With permission Benvegnen et al. (2020).

cytokines (IFN-γ and IL-2) by equine T cells. It appears that immune checkpoint therapy may be of benefit in some equine melanoma cases (Ganbaatar et al., 2020).

Studies on humans have also demonstrated that blockade of PD-1 or PD-L1 binding by monoclonal antibodies results in recovery of T cell cytotoxic activity and a renewed anti-tumor response. Treatment with anti-PD-1 or anti-PD-L1 monoclonal antibodies has produced dramatic and prolonged remissions in humans with melanomas, renal cell carcinomas, and non-small cell lung cancers. PD-L1 blockade is therefore a feasible therapy to use in horses for tumors such as melanomas (Ganbaatar et al., 2020). Interestingly, PD-L1 is not expressed on equine sarcoid cells (Benvegnen et al., 2020). There is a similar situation in equine penile squamous cell carcinomas, where the PD-L1 gene was expressed in only 3/20 cases while the PD-1 gene was not detected in any of the cases (Porcellato, Brachelente, et al., 2021; Porcellato, Mecocci, et al., 2020).

CTLA-4

A second T cell inhibitory receptor is Cytotoxic T-lymphocyte-Associated protein-4 (CTLA-4). CTLA-4 is expressed on T cell surfaces following their activation (Chapter 12). Its ligands are CD80 and CD86, expressed on antigen-presenting cells. Like PD-1, its function is to prevent uncontrolled T cell activation. Ligands acting through CTLA-4 deliver suppressive signals to the T cells and inhibit their activation. Conversely, if CTLA-4 signaling is blocked, then T cell responses will recover. CTLA-4 blockade in tumor-bearing animals, therefore, results in a significant increase in T-cell-mediated tumor cytotoxicity and the development of new antitumor T cells. Studies on humans have shown that administration of a monoclonal antibody against CTLA-4 (Ipilimumab) results in a significant increase in T cell antitumor activity and dramatic remissions in many (but not all) patients. It has been demonstrated that CTLA-4-positive T cells are present in all equine penile squamous cell carcinomas tested, but their numbers are very low, and they are not highly expressed (Porcellato, Brachelente, et al., 2021; Porcellato, Mecocci, et al., 2020).

Other checkpoint molecules that are potential targets for monoclonal antibody therapy include lymphocyte activation protein 3 (LAG-3) found on both CD4 and CD8 T cells and NK cells; T cell immunoglobulin and mucin domain-containing -3 (TIM-3) found on T cells; T-cell immunoreceptor with Ig and ITIM domains (TIGIT) also found on lymphocytes; and the NK cell inhibitory receptor NKG2A.

Checkpoint inhibitors have achieved remarkable success in the treatment of human metastatic melanomas, kidney and lung tumors, and hematologic cancers (Teng et al., 2016). A combination of anti-PD-1 and anti-CTLA-4 appears to be exceptionally effective in permitting T cell cytotoxicity to proceed and results in long-term remissions. Unfortunately, not all cancers respond to checkpoint inhibitors. In some patients, T cells may be irreversibly exhausted or so exhausted that their function may only be restored temporarily, and the disease redevelops after an early response.

Checkpoint inhibitors can also be used in combination with other chemotherapeutic agents, such as tyrosine kinase inhibitors or therapeutic vaccines (Sharma et al., 2023). Unfortunately, checkpoint therapy is not without its problems. The activation of suppressed T cells can trigger some autoimmune diseases or immune responses against the commensal microbiota (Hu et al., 2022).

Checkpoint therapy is still in its infancy, and results should steadily improve as experience is gained.

Active immunization

Therapeutic vaccination against cancer is a very active research area, and many promising cancer vaccines are under development. These include adjuvanted purified antigens, DNA vaccines, mRNA vaccines, vector-based vaccines, tumor cell vaccines, and dendritic cell vaccines.

Tumor vaccines trigger adaptive immunity against tumor-associated antigens administered in such a way that they stimulate a potent cytotoxic T cell response while overcoming tumor-mediated immunosuppression. They have the great advantage that they can circumvent the resistance of tumor cells to cytotoxic drugs. Additionally, they are highly specific, have low toxicity, and have a long-lasting effect as a result of memory responses.

These tumor-associated antigens belong to two broad categories. There are tumor-specific shared antigens expressed on more than one type of tumor cell, and that may also be expressed on normal tissues. The other category includes unique molecules expressed by cancer cells because of mutations resulting from carcinogen exposure.

These tumor antigens can be obtained from either autologous sources (the cancerous animal itself) or from allogeneic sources (other animals). They can include whole cell lysates or purified tumor peptides or even defined tumor cell antigens.

Many different potential antigens have been tested, including vaccines containing proteins, peptides, cell extracts, and whole tumor cells. It is also possible to make DNA vaccines expressing the genes encoding specific tumor antigens. These can be delivered directly as DNA plasmids or inserted into appropriate recombinant viral or bacterial vectors. In theory, injected tumor antigens should induce both memory and effector T cells. As a result, immunity should persist and control tumor growth indefinitely.

Many attempts have been made to produce tumor vaccines for animals. Thus, a canine lymphoma vaccine was first investigated in the 1980s. These early attempts used whole cell vaccines consisting of irradiated or lysed tumor cells together with an adjuvant. These early vaccines were, however, poorly defined, and it was difficult to produce a standardized product.

The lack of success of these early vaccines may also have resulted from immunosuppressive mechanisms acting within the tumor microenvironment, as well as the activation of regulatory T cells and the blocking of activation signals. As described above, these suppressive signals are mediated by checkpoint molecules such as CTLA-4, PD-1, and its ligand PD-L1.

Autologous tumor vaccines

It is, of course, possible to excise part of a tumor and prepare an inactivated vaccine to be injected back into the patient. The best example of this approach is the production of autogenous vaccines against bovine fibropapillomas. These papillomas may develop on the teats or other inconvenient sites on cattle. They are caused by members of a large family of bovine papillomaviruses (BPV). Vaccines are available that can be used for both prevention and treatment, but success depends on the specific papillomavirus involved. There are several ways of making these vaccines. For example, the papillomas can be surgically excised, and small pieces stored in 10% buffered formalin. After cleaning, selected pieces are suspended in saline and homogenized. A preservative or antibiotics are then added to inhibit bacterial growth. After filtration, more formalin may be added to ensure viral inactivation. The vaccine is administered subcutaneously in three doses at 1-week intervals. This vaccination is often quite effective for the treatment of small warts (Terziev et al., 2015).

Selected equine tumors

Equine sarcoids

Sarcoids are the most commonly diagnosed skin cancers in equids and a significant problem in these species (Ogluszka et al., 2021). They occur in horses, donkeys,

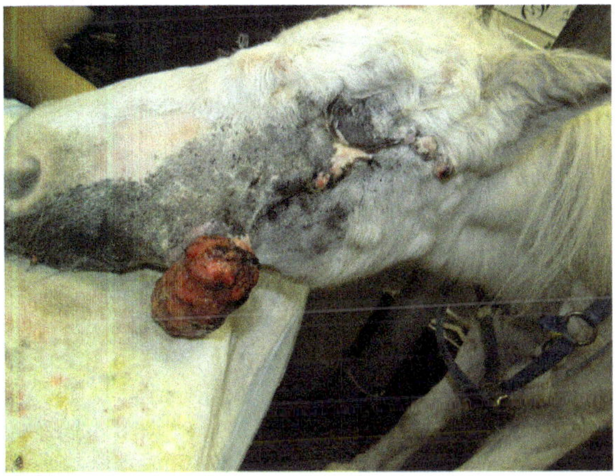

FIGURE 21.5 An equine sarcoid.

- Courtesy of Dr Leslie Easterwood.

mules, and zebras. They are locally aggressive but benign fibroblastic tumors associated with abortive infection by bovine papillomavirus (BPV) type 1 and, less frequently, BPV-2. Subsequently, BPV13 has been detected in sarcoids in Brazil and Europe (Jindra et al., 2021). BPV-14 has also been associated with the disease. While not metastatic, sarcoids are persistent and often recur following surgery. Histology shows an increased density of dermal fibroblasts when compared to normal skin. There is increased proliferation of interlacing bundles of spindle-shaped fibroblasts. There is also significant extracellular matrix deposition while the overlying epidermis is hyperplastic and hyperkeratotic. Fig. 21.5.

Bovine papillomaviruses trigger the development of equine sarcoids. In cattle, the papillomas caused by these viruses can regress spontaneously as the animals mount an immune response. This is not the case in horses. Horses appear to be unable to mount an effective neutralizing response to BPV. BPVs are small double-stranded DNA viruses belonging to the Papillomaviridae family. They contain genes encoding three early proteins, E5, E6, and E7, that can transform cells and are the key oncoproteins that promote sarcoid development. BPV is present in equine sarcoids. The viral nucleic acid is consistently present in sarcoid fibroblasts. Its presence in the normal skin of these animals has been reported inconsistently. BPV mRNA is also detectable in these sarcoids and contains the E protein transcripts. Conflicting results have been obtained in determining whether BPV production occurs in these horses. It may be abortive in many cases. Electron microscopy has been unable to detect the presence of intact BPV virions in sarcoid tissues. Sequencing has also suggested that there may be a specific BPV subtype involved in the pathogenesis of equine sarcoids. Experimental inoculation of foals with BPV results in a transient viremia followed by the development of localized sarcoid-like granulomas at the injection site (Jindra et al., 2022).

The invasiveness of sarcoid cells appears to be linked to dysregulation of the animal's matrix metalloproteases (MMPs). Thus BPV viral E7 protein overstimulates their expression. As a result, MMP-1 and MMP-8 are elevated. These enzymes degrade basement membranes and thus permit tumor cell spread through the surrounding tissues.

There are great variations in the size and complexity of sarcoids in equine patients. This suggests that the genetics of the horse have a significant influence on viral growth and disease severity. Analysis of affected horse populations has revealed that genes located on chromosomes ECA20 and ECA22 may be linked to sarcoid progression (Staiger et al., 2016). The location of the genes on ECA20 has been identified as an intron in the DQA1 gene in the ELA class II region. This gene encodes a protein involved in antigen presentation. This may well imply that susceptible horses have defects in their immune responses. The SNP on ECA22 identified a 200 kb region containing four possible genes. The implicated genes are *PROCR, EDEM2, EIF6*, and *MMP24*. Their possible links to sarcoid progression are unclear and speculative. In the Arabian breed, it has been demonstrated that susceptibility to sarcoids is not only associated with MHC class II but also with the MHC class I KLRA polymorphic markers. This suggests that NK cells may also play an important role in the pathogenesis of equine sarcoids (Vychodilova et al., 2025).

Vaccination

Sarcoids are amenable to immunotherapy. For example, they are characteristically infiltrated by large numbers of $CD8^+$ and $CD4^+$ T cells. Many of these T cells are double-positive, expressing both CD4 and CD8 in addition to FoxP3. As described in Chapter 12, FoxP3 is the key transcription factor employed by regulatory T cells (Tregs). Transcription studies have shown that compared to healthy skin, sarcoids show increased transcription of FoxP3 as well as the gene encoding the regulatory cytokine TGF-β. Transcription of the IL-17 gene is also elevated in sarcoids. In contrast, transcription of the effector cytokines, IL-2, IL-4, and IFN-γ is not increased. Likewise, the transcription of the antiviral proteins IFN-α and IFN-β is not increased compared to normal equine skin. Horses cannot mount an effective antiviral response to BPV in sarcoid tissues (Wilson & Hicks, 2016).

Natural humoral immunity to BPV in horses also appears to be poor. For example, studies on sarcoid-affected horses showed that they lacked measurable antibodies to BPV L1. In another study, serum from sarcoid-affected horses was examined for the presence of antibodies. Six out of 12 sarcoid-affected horses had antibodies to these autologous sarcoid cells (Gysens et al., 2023). This partially explains how sarcoids persist in this species. BPV may simply escape the attention of the equine immune system because of its localization within skin cells and by the ability of its E5 protein to inhibit MHC class I-mediated antigen presentation (Marchetti et al., 2009). The E5 protein causes the MHC class I molecules to be retained within the Golgi apparatus and prevents their transport to the cell surface (Marchetti et al., 2002).

Recombinant papillomavirus capsid proteins can spontaneously assemble into virus-like particles in vitro. As a result, these virus-like particles may be used for immunization. They do not contain viral DNA and are thus very safe. However, they are very immunogenic and induce high levels of virus-neutralizing antibodies. Fourteen horses were vaccinated with BPV-1 L1 papillomavirus-like particles plus adjuvant. Forty-two days later, the horses were challenged with BPV virions. All the unvaccinated control horses developed pseudosarcoids at every inoculation site. Thirteen of the vaccinated horses, in contrast, were completely protected. One vaccinated horse developed seven very small (2 mm) tumors that completely regressed by 5 weeks. The vaccination resulted in the animals developing BPV neutralizing antibodies, and this was protective against experimental BPV-1-induced disease (Hainisch et al., 2013). Similar results have been obtained in donkeys with sarcoids. Animals immunized with BPV L1 and E7 showed a tendency toward tumor regression (Hainisch et al., 2023).

A second experimental anti-BPV vaccine involved the use of an influenza virus A and B vectors expressing BPV-1 antigens (Jindra et al., 2021). The flu virus vector incorporated a truncated NS1 gene. (iNS1). It also carried the genes for BPV1, E6, and E7 antigens. The NS1 gene is a potent interferon inducer. In a clinical trial of sarcoid-affected horses, at least one lesion was directly inoculated with the vaccine and the animal subsequently boosted with iNSA/E6E7 equ or iNSN/E6E7 equi. This resulted in the synchronous regression of both injected and non-injected lesions. Complete tumor regression was achieved in 10 of 29 horses. However, six horses with a history of unsuccessful therapy either did not respond or responded transiently. Encouraging preliminary results have also been obtained using a recombinant baculovirus vector vaccine expressing the L1 protein of BPV.

Immunostimulation

Given that innate immune responses are the first line of defense against pathogens, it makes sense to enhance innate immunity to sarcoids by stimulating TLR responses. These receptors respond to PAMPs and DAMPs. One very effective TLR stimulant is the tuberculosis vaccine consisting of avirulent *Mycobacterium bovis* BCG. Murphy and his colleagues first showed that equine sarcoids were responsive to treatment with mycobacterial cell-wall fractions (Murphy et al., 1979). They injected BCG vaccine directly into the lesions. Their results showed that 73% of sarcoid cases underwent complete regression, and the remainder experienced partial regression. The longest period of remission was 24 months, while the shortest was 9 months.

If the BCG vaccine is infiltrated into the tissues between the tumor and normal skin, it stimulates an aggressive innate immune response by activating the local TLRs. These in turn activate local T cell responses and, as a result, they then attack and destroy the sarcoid fibroblasts. Unfortunately, BCG sensitizes horses to tuberculin and thus potentially interferes with the diagnosis of tuberculosis (Chapter 20). Related immunostimulants, such as purified Mycobacterial cell walls, have also been used to treat this tumor. They activate T cells, NK cells, and M1 macrophages. These may have direct cytotoxic effects or release proinflammatory cytokines such as TNF-α. Once activated, the cytotoxic T cells have persistent antitumor activity. They possess the advantage of not rendering an animal tuberculin positive. These immunostimulants are inoculated directly into the tumor mass to ensure local, in situ activation. The rate of regression depends on the size of the tumor (surgical debulking may be required to remove most of the tumor mass), and multiple treatments are usually necessary for a complete cure. Periocular sarcoids appear to be most susceptible to this form of immunotherapy (Theon, 1998). Regression after BCG therapy appears to be related to size since larger tumors give a poorer response. Likewise, tumors on the limbs respond less well. Horses that have a positive tuberculin test before treatment respond more favorably (Klein et al., 1986).

One such immunostimulant that has received USDA approval for use in horses is Immunocidin. Immunocidin consists of a purified protein fraction extracted from Mycobacteria. Since it is purified, its actions are predictable and adverse side effects fewer. It is administered intralesionally, but the immune response is, of course, generalized so that sarcoids at remote sites also regress. Animals are given 2–6 injections at 2-week intervals, depending upon the horse's response. As the T cells attack the tumor cells and the body rejects the tumor cells through drainage tracts, the tumor itself swells, goes necrotic, and sloughs.

The immune response modifier Imiquimod (Aldara) has both antiviral and antitumor activities. It is used in humans for the treatment of genital warts and superficial basal cell tumors. It is also a TLR activator. It activates TLR7, resulting in the local release of IL-6 and TNF-α (Jindra et al., 2023). It activates Langerhans cells as well as NK cells. Imiquimod has been used to treat equine sarcoids topically with encouraging results (Nogueira et al., 2006). It causes severe local reactions (exudation, erythema, erosions, depigmentation, and alopecia), and the treatment may be required for many weeks. Selected superficial lesions have a reported response rate (reduction in size by greater than 75%) of 60%–84%. Some achieve complete remission, but the recurrence rate is about 7.4% (Hollis, 2022). Sarcoids are also responsive to other immunostimulants such as killed *Propionobacterium acnes*, the complex carbohydrate acemannan, and the antiviral drug acyclovir (Hollis, 2022).

Equine lymphomas

Equine lymphomas are predominantly T-cell in origin, although some equine B-cell lymphomas are T-cell rich (Durham et al., 2012). Horses with lymphosarcomas are commonly immunosuppressed. This usually involves T cells, but B-cell function may also be impaired. Equine B-cell neoplasms generally cause a monoclonal gammopathy. A case of a horse with a lymphosarcoma with suppressor cell activity has been described. The animal presented with signs of immunodeficiency and was found to be deficient in IgM. Equine T cell lymphomas have been associated with immune-mediated anemia and thrombocytopenia (Taintor & Schleis, 2011).

Equine melanomas

Melanomas are some of the most common tumors in horses. Approximately 15% of equine skin tumors are melanocytic. Of these, about 90% are initially benign, but about 66% may eventually metastasize. While they occur in horses of all colors, gray horses are especially prone to developing these tumors. There is an 80% prevalence in gray horses over 15 years of age (Pimenta et al., 2023). As their name implies, these tumors result from the neoplastic transformation of melanocytes, the pigment-bearing cells in the skin and eyes. Fig 21.6.

It has been shown that these tumors have a moderate heritability in gray horses. For example, in the Lipizzaner breed, the heritability is estimated to be about 0.36. Breeds such as Arabians, Lipizzaners, Thoroughbreds, and Andalusians appear to be predisposed to developing melanomas. The gray phenotype is an autosomal dominant trait related to progressive hair depigmentation.

Melanomas are uniquely immunogenic tumors, and several melanoma-associated antigens have been identified. In horses, a S100 protein is consistently expressed on melanoma cells. The enzyme tyrosinase is also consistently expressed. Likewise, these cells consistently express a melanocyte differentiation antigen, gp100 (Ramos-Vara et al., 2014). Further analysis of equine melanoma cells has been conducted in an effort to identify potentially immunogenic proteins that may serve as vaccine antigens. Thus, PNL2, PGP9.5, and S100 protein could be detected in all equine melanomas. PNL 2 was not expressed on non-melanocytic equine tumors such as sarcoids, carcinomas, and sarcomas, nor in normal tissues.

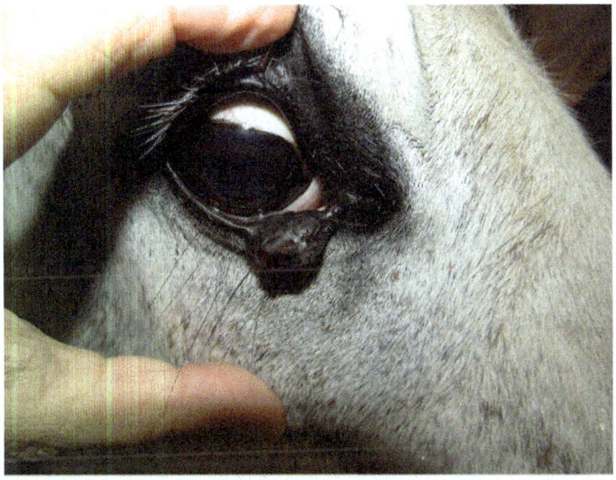

FIGURE 21.6 A periorbital equine melanoma.

- Courtesy of Dr Leslie Easterwood.

As with sarcoids, multiple immunotherapeutic approaches have been investigated in the horse. One such approach has simply been the direct inoculation of cytokines such as IL-2, IL-18, or IFN-γ into the tumor masses. The intention of this approach is simply to activate cytotoxic T cells, generate IFN-γ, and trigger tumor cell apoptosis. Encouraging remissions have been obtained by injecting IL-12 and IL-18 encoding plasmids (Heinzerling et al., 2001; Muller et al., 2011).

A second approach is to inject TLR-activating PAMPs to trigger inflammation. Thus, complete Freund's adjuvant, a mixture of mineral oil and heat-killed mycobacteria, injected directly into the tumor masses, resulted in tumor remission in 5/11 treated horses (Carroll et al., 2021).

A similar microbial experimental vaccine consisted of DNA plasmids encoding the *Strep pyogenes, EMM55* gene. EMM55 is a highly antigenic priming protein, and thus it was expected to trigger a strong local antibody response. This was injected into the melanoma by needleless injection. Following treatment, the size of the injected lesions was reduced by 40% and the antimelanoma antibody response was enhanced (Brown et al., 2014)

A third approach involves the treatment of horses by active immunization. For example, autologous vaccines can be made from excised tumors. Results have been mixed. An anti-melanoma DNA vaccine (Oncept, Boehringer Ingelheim) has been developed and approved for use in dogs. This vaccine contains an *Escherichia coli* plasmid engineered to express the gene encoding human tyrosinase. Once inside a cell nucleus, the DNA plasmid transcribes and translates the tyrosinase gene, and as a result, cells produce this enzyme within the recipient. Tyrosinase catalyzes the hydroxylation of tyrosine to dihydroxyphenylalanine, a key step in melanin production.) This human tyrosinase is, however, only 90% homologous to the equine protein. This difference is such that vaccinated horses will mount immune responses against the human protein. These responses include the production of both antibodies and T cells and result in the destruction of the melanoma cells (Pellin, 2022). While originally conceived for use in dogs, Oncept has been used successfully for the treatment of equine melanomas. In a preliminary trial involving eight horses with melanomas, Oncept caused tumor stagnation and shrinkage in four of the horses. Of the remaining four, in three it had no apparent effect, and one showed accelerated tumor growth. It was well tolerated with minimal adverse effects (Brunner et al., 2024).

Encouraging results have also been obtained by inoculation of plasmid DNA encoding interleukin 12 and IL-18 alone or in combination with human tyrosinase or glycoprotein. This resulted in an average decrease of 79% in tumor volume and was investigated as a possible vaccine antigen.

Limited success has been obtained in treating melanomas in gray horses by immunotherapy. For example, administration of a plasmid expressing IL-13 directly into tumor metastases produced significant regression in 60% of cases and appeared to be safe. In dogs with melanomas, plasmids containing DNA coding for the herpesvirus thymidine kinase suicide gene were able to sensitize transfected cells to ganciclovir. (Ganciclovir is a potent anti-herpesvirus drug.) (Porcellato, Brachelente, et al., 2021; Porcellato, Mecocci, et al., 2020). The treatment induced substantial regression. A similar therapy, given in association with a subcutaneous autologous killed cancer vaccine, appeared to work well in a horse.

Squamous cell carcinomas

Squamous cell carcinomas are not uncommon in horses. One of the most common forms involves the eye. These tumors are locally invasive and may require major surgery. They do not tend to metastasize. Immunotherapy has been applied to these tumors with some success. Thus, horses were vaccinated topically in the form of eye drops, with a liposomal-TLR ligand complex (LTC therapy). These contain TLR3 and TLR9 nucleic acid ligands and have been engineered to bind strongly to epithelial cells and, by delivering the ligands, trigger a strong Toll-like receptor response. This, in turn, induces a high level of interferon production by the horse leukocytes. As a result, the squamous cell carcinoma growth is suppressed. In a study involving nine eye tumors in eight horses, it resulted in a positive response rate of 67%. This regression was durable and well tolerated clinically (Wotman et al., 2023).

Equine papilloma virus type 2 is considered a risk factor for genital squamous cell carcinomas in the horse. These tumors are common in older horses and usually have a poor prognosis. In a study, the EqPV-2-L1RNA was detected in 18/20 samples. The tumors were infiltrated with $CD3^+$ lymphocytes, macrophages, plasma cells, and $FoxP3^+$ T cells. Some samples contained elevated expression of TGF-β1, IFN-γ, and IL-2 (Porcellato et al., 2020). Given the similarity of this immune infiltrate to that observed in equine sarcoids, this type of tumor may respond well to immunotherapy. Trials are currently underway using LTC immunotherapy as described above.

References

Benvegnen, J., De Breuyn, B., Gerber, V., Rottenberg, S., & Koch, C. (2020). Immunohistochemical analysis of programed death ligand 1 expression in equine sarcoids. *Journal of Equine Veterinary Science*. https://doi.org/10.1016/j.jevs.2020.103338

Bergman, P. J. (2018). Veterinary oncology immunotherapies. *Veterinary Clinics of North America: Small Animal Practice, 48*, 257–277.

Boussiotis, V. A. (2016). Molecular and biochemical aspects of the PD-1 checkpoint pathway. *New England Journal of Medicine, 375*, 1767–1778.

Brown, E. L., Ramiya, V. K., Wright, C. A., Jerald, M. M., et al. (2014). Treatment of metastatic equine melanoma with a plasmid vaccine encoding Streptococcus pyogenes EMM55 protein. *Journal of Equine Veterinary Science, 34*, 704–708.

Brunner, S., Furst, A. E., & Jackson, M. A. (2024). Retrospective study of the effectiveness of human tyrosinase vaccination in eight horses. *Schweizer Archiv fuer Tierheilkunde, 166* (12), 648–656.

Carroll, C. S. E., Andrew, E. R., Malik, L., Elliott, K. F., et al. (2021). Simple and effective bacterial-based intratumoral cancer immunotherapy. *Journal for Immunotherapy of Cancer, 9*, Article e002688.

Coussens, L. M., & Werb, Z. (2002). Inflammation and cancer. *Nature, 420*, 860–867.

Durham, A. C., Pillitteri, C. A., San Myint, M., & Valli, V. E. (2012). Two hundred three cases of equine lymphoma classified according to the World Health Classification (WHO) classification criteria. *Veterinary Pathology Online*. https://doi.org/10.1177/0300985812451603

Finocchiaro, L. M., Riveros, M. D., & Glikin, G. C. (2009). Cytokine-enhanced vaccine and suicide gene therapy as adjuvant treatments of metastatic melanoma in a horse. *The Veterinary Record, 164*, 278–279.

Ganbaatar, O., Konnai, S., Okagawa, T., Nojima, Y., et al. (2020). PD-L1 expression in equine malignant melanoma and functional effects of PD-L1 blockade. *PLoS One*. https://doi.org/10.1371/journal.pone.0234218

Goulart, M. R., Pluhar, G. E., & Ohifest, J. R. (2012). Identification of myeloid derived suppressor cells in dogs with naturally occurring cancer. *PLoS One*. https://doi.org/10.1371/journal.pone.0033274

Gysens, L., Depuydt, E., Patruno, M., Haspeslagh, M., et al. (2023). Immunogenicity analysis of BPV-1 positive equine sarcoid-derived cultured fibroblasts. *Veterinary Immunology and Immunopathology*. https://doi.org/10.1016/j.vetimm.2023.110547

Hagemann, T., Balkwill, F., & Lawrence, T. (2007). Inflammation and cancer: A double-edged sword. *Cancer Cell, 12*, 300–301.

Hainisch, E. K., Abel, H., Shafti-Keramat, S., Kirnbauer, R., & Brandt, S. (2013). Vaccination with virus-like particles protects horses from experimental BPV-1 infection. *Equine Veterinary Journal, 45*(Suppl. 44), 2–19.

Hainisch, E. K., Jindra, C., Kimbauer, R., & Brandt. (2023). Papilloma-like particles in equine medicine. *Viruses*. https://doi.org/10.3390/v15020345

Hässig, M., Casal, M., von Beust, B., Nussbaumer, M., & Rusch, P. (1991). CEA test in domestic animals. *Schweizer Archiv fuer Tierheilkunde, 133*(7), 311–313.

Heinzerling, L. M., Feige, K., Rieder, S., Akens, M. K., et al. (2001). Tumor regression induced by intratumoral injection of DNA coding for human interleukin-12 into melanoma metastases in gray horses. *Journal of Molecular Medicine, 78*, 692–702.

Hill, F. W. G., Klein, W. R., Hoyer, M. J., et al. (1994). Antitumor effect of locally injected low doses of recombinant human interleukin-2 in bovine vulval papilloma and carcinoma. *Veterinary Immunology and Immunopathology, 41*, 19–29.

Hollis, A. R. (2022). Management of equine sarcoids. *Veterinary Journal*. https://doi.org/10.1016/j.tvjl.2022.105926

Hu, Z. I., Link, V. M., Lima-Junior, D. S., Delaleu, J., et al. (2022). Immune checkpoint inhibitors unleash pathogenic immune responses against the microbiota. *Proceedings of the National Academy of Sciences, 119*(26). https://doi.org/10.1073/pnas.2200348119

Jindra, C., Hainisch, E. K., & Brandt, S. (2023). Immunotherapy of equine sarcoids_ from early approaches to innovative vaccines. *Vaccines*. https://doi.org/10.3390/vaccines11040769

Jindra, C., Hainisch, E. K., Rummele, A., Wolsek, M., et al. (2021). Influenza virus vector iNS1 expressing bovine papillomavirus 1 (BPV-1) antigens efficiently induces tumor regression in equine sarcoid patients. *PLoS One*. https://doi.org/10.1371/journal.pone.0260155

Jindra, C., Kamjunke, A.-K., Jones, S., & Brandt, S. (2022). Screening for bovine papillomavirus type 13 (BPV13) in a European population of sarcoid-bearing equids. *Equine Veterinary Journal, 54*, 662–669.

Kannegieter, N. J., Schaaf, K. L., Lovell, D. K., et al. (2010). Myofibroblastic fibrosarcoma with multifocal osseous metaplasia at the site of equine influenza vaccination. *Australian Veterinary Journal, 88*, 132–136.

Klein, W. R., Bras, G. E., Misdoro, W., Steerenberg, P. A., et al. (1986). Equine sarcoid: BCG immunotherapy compared to cryosurgery in a prospective randomized clinical trial. *Cancer Immunology, Immunotherapy, 21*, 133–140.

Li, Q., Withoff, S., & Verma, I. M. (2005). Inflammation-associated cancer: NF-kappa B is the lynchpin. *Trends in Immunology, 26*, 318–325.

Mantovani, A., Allavena, P., Sica, A., & Balkwill, F. (2008). Cancer-related inflammation. *Nature, 454*, 456.

Marchetti, B., Ashrafi, G. H., Tsirimonaki, E., O'Brien, P. M., & Campo, M. S. (2002). The bovine papillomavirus oncoprotein E5 retains MHC class I molecules in the Golgi apparatus and prevents their transport to the cell surface. *Oncogene, 21*, 7808–7816.

Marchetti, B., Gault, E. A., Cortese, M. S., Yuan, Z., et al. (2009). Bovine papillomavirus type 1 oncoprotein E5 inhibits equine MHC class I and interacts with equine MHC I heavy chain. *Journal of General Virology, 90*, 2865–2870.

Meeremans, M., Devriendt, B., Bairot, S., van Poucke, M., et al. (2025). Equine monocyte-erived macrophages revisited: Isolation and comprehensive characterization of pro- versus anti-inflammatory polarization. *Veterinary Quarterly*. https://doi.org/10.1080/01652176.2026.2593367

Miller, R. L., Gerster, J. F., Owens, M. L., Slade, H. B., & Tomai, M. A. (1999). Review article: Imiquimod applied topically: A novel immune response modifier and new class of drug. *International Journal of Immunopharmacology, 21*(1), 1–14.

Muller, J. M. V., Feige, K., Wunderlin, P., Hodl, A., et al. (2011). Double-blind placebo-controlled study with interleukin-18 and interleukin-12 encoding plasmid DNA shows antitumor effect in metastatic melanoma in gray horses. *Journal of Immunotherapy, 34*, 58–64.

Murphy, J. M., Severin, G. A., Lavach, J. D., Hepler, D. I., & Lueker, D. C. (1979). Immunotherapy in ocular equine sarcoid. *Journal of the American Veterinary Medical Association, 174*(3), 269–272.

Nogueira, S. A. F., Torres, S. M. F., Malone, E. D., Diaz, S. F., et al. (2006). Efficacy of imiquimod 5% cream in the treatment of equine sarcoids: A pilot study. *Veterinary Dermatology, 17*(4), 259–265.

Ogluszka, M., Starzynski, R. R., Pierzchala, M., Otrocka-Domagala, I., & Ras, A. (2021). Equine sarcoids,—Causes, molecular changes and clinicopathological features: A review. *Veterinary Pathology Online, 58*(3), 472–482.

Pellin, M. A. (2022). The use of Oncept melanoma vaccine in veterinary patients: A review of the literature. *Veterinary Sciences*. https://doi.org/10.3390/vetsci9110597

Pimenta, J., Prada, J., & Cotovio, M. (2023). Equine melanocytic tumors: A narrative review. *Animals*. https://doi.org/10.3390/ani13020247

Pimenta, J., Prada, J., Pires, I., & Cotovio, M. (2024). Programed cell death ligand-1 (PD-L1) immunohistochemical expression in equine melanocytic tumors. *Animals*. https://doi.org/10.3390/ani14010048

Porcellato, I., Brachelente, C., Cappelli, K., Menchetti, L., et al. (2021). FoxP3, CTLA-4 and IDO in canine melanocytic tumors. *Veterinary Pathology Online, 58*(1), 42–52.

Porcellato, I., Mecocci, S., Brachelente, C., Cappelli, K., et al. (2021). PD-L1/PD-1 and CTLA-4 expression in equine penile squamous cell carcinomas. *Animals*. https://doi.org/10.3390/ani11072121

Porcellato, I., Mecocci, S., Mechelli, L., Cappelli, K., et al. (2020). Equine penile squamous cell carcinomas as a model for human disease: A preliminary investigation on tumor immune microenvironment. *Cells*. https://doi.org/10.3390/cells9112364

Ramos-Vara, J. A., Frank, C. B., DuSold, D., & Miller, M. A. (2014). Immunohistochemical expression of melanocyte antigen PNL2, Melan A, S100, and PGP 9.5 in equine melanocytic neoplasms. *Veterinary Pathology Online, 51*(1), 161–166.

Sharma, P., Goswami, S., Raychaudhuri, D., Siddiqui, B. A., et al. (2023). Immune checkpoint therapy-current perspectives and future directions. *Cell, 186*, 1652–1669.

Sorensen, K., Neely, D. P., Read, W., & Grappell, P. M. (1990). Measurement and clinical significance of equine fetal protein in pregnant mares serum. *Journal of Equine Veterinary Science, 10*(6), 417–421.

Staiger, E. A., Tseng, C. T., Miller, D., Cassano, J. M., et al. (2016). Host genetic influences on papilloma-induced tumors in the horse. *International Journal of Cancer, 139*(4), 784–792.

Taintor, J., & Schleis, S. (2011). Equine lymphoma. *Equine Veterinary Education, 23*(4), 205–213.

Teng, M. W., Khanna, R., & Smyth, M. J. (2016). Checkpoint immunotherapy: Picking a winner. *Cancer Discovery, 6*, 818–820.

Terziev, G., Roydev, R., Kalkanov, I., Borissov, I., & Dinev, I. (2015). Papillomatosis in heifers. Comparative studies on surgical excision and autogenous vaccine therapies. *Trakia Journal of Sciences, 13*, 274–279.

Theon, A. P. (1998). Intralesional and topical chemotherapy and immunotherapy. *Veterinary Clinics of North America: Equine Practice, 14*(3), 659–671.

Vivieros, M. M., & Antczak, D. F. (1999). Characterization of equine natural killer and IL-2 stimulated lymphokine activated killer cell populations. *Developmental & Comparative Immunology, 23*, 521–532.

Vychodilova, L., Plasil, M., Futas, J., Kopeka, A., et al. (2025). Genetic susceptibility to sarcoid in Arabian horses: Associations with MHC class II and compound MHC class I/KLRA genotypes. *Veterinary Research Communications*. https://doi.org/10.1007/s11259-025-10748-2

Waldman, A. D., Fritz, J. M., & Lenardo, M. J. (2020). A guide to cancer immunotherapy: From T cell basic science to clinical practice. *Nature Reviews Immunology, 20*, 651–668.

Wilson, A. D., & Hicks, C. (2016). Both tumor cells and infiltrating T-cells in equine sarcoids express FOXP3 associated with an immune-suppressed cytokine environment. *Veterinary Research*. https://doi.org/10.1186/s13567-016-0339-8

Wong, S. Y., & Reiter, J. F. (2011). Wounding mobilizes hair follicle stem cells to form tumors. *Proceedings of the National Academy of Sciences of the United States of America, 108*, 4093–4098.

Wormser, C., Mariano, A., Holmes, E. S., Aronson, L. R., & Volk, S. W. (2016). Post-transplant malignant neoplasia associated with cyclosporine-based immunotherapy: Prevalence, risk factors and survival in feline renal transplant recipients. *Veterinary and Comparative Oncology, 14*(4), e126–e134.

Wotman, K. L., Chow, L., Martabano, B., Pezzanite, L. M., & Dow, S. (2023). Novel ocular immunotherapy induces tumor regression in an equine model of ocular surface squamous neoplasia. *Cancer Immunology Immunotherapy, 72*, 1185–1198.

Zamora, A. E., Crawford, J. C., & Thomas, P. G. (2018). Hitting the target: How T cells detect and eliminate tumors. *Journal of Immunology, 200*, 392–399.

Zhang, J., Hodges, A., Chen, S. H., & Pan, P. Y. (2021). Myeloid-derived suppressor cells as cellular immunotherapy in transplantation and autoimmune diseases. *Cellular Immunology.* https://doi.org/10.1016/j.cellimm.2021.104300

CHAPTER

Equine autoimmune diseases

22

The function of the immune system is to detect, attack, and destroy any microorganisms, such as bacteria, viruses, or parasites, that invade the body. Once a microbe invades, its antigens have to be identified as foreign. Thus, the success of the immune system depends in large part, upon its ability to discriminate between normal body components and antigens from invading foreign organisms. Once the invader is identified as foreign, it is destroyed as rapidly and completely as possible. However, molecules identified as normal body components are usually ignored. This distinction is not absolute, and on occasion, a misdirected immune response can cause serious damage to normal body tissues, resulting in disease and death.

Tolerance

Horse B cells and T cells possess receptors for foreign antigens. When appropriately activated by these foreign antigens, they respond by generating protective type 1 and type 2 immune responses and attack the invaders. If, perchance, the T cells or B cells express antigen receptors that can also bind antigens from normal body cells or tissues, then they may attack these as well and so cause autoimmune disease. This is normally prevented by the development of immune tolerance. Tolerance is the name given to the state in which the cells of the adaptive immune system cannot respond to a specific antigen. Tolerance is primarily directed against self-antigens from normal tissues. If tolerance fails, then autoimmunity develops.

Tolerance develops because most immature T and B cells that express receptors for self-antigens are killed within the thymus or the bone marrow before they can develop into functional cells. This "negative-selection" results in central tolerance. In addition, just to be safe, regulatory pathways also operate after cells leave the thymus and prevent any surviving self-reactive T or B cells from responding when they encounter a self-antigen. These regulatory pathways, therefore, promote peripheral tolerance. If either form of tolerance is lost, self-reactive T and B cells may develop and cause disease. Maintenance of central and peripheral tolerance is therefore essential to the prevention of autoimmunity.

Despite the generation of both central and peripheral tolerance, autoimmune diseases are relatively common. They are also highly diverse and can potentially damage or destroy any organ in the body. Broadly speaking, autoimmune diseases result from a breakdown of tolerance that results in the emergence of clones of "rogue"

The Immunology of Horses and Donkeys. https://doi.org/10.1016/B978-0-443-44863-8.00014-4

lymphocytes. These rogues may either be B cells that make autoantibodies directed against normal body components or T cells with a similar specificity for normal cells. Tolerance in B and T cells is regulated by multiple mechanisms. These control mechanisms often overlap so that the development of self-reactive rogue clones does not usually occur suddenly. It likely takes multiple accumulated defects, acting in diverse regulatory pathways, to cause a loss of control of lymphocyte proliferation. As a result of these defects in multiple control systems, autoimmune diseases usually have a multistep pathogenesis and, in general, occur in older horses.

Given the ubiquity of foreign antigens, especially those resulting from the presence of the normal microbiota on body surfaces, lymphocytes are under constant pressure to respond. Much of the complexity of the immune system results from the need to keep this unwanted and unneeded lymphocyte proliferation in check. The initial trigger that leads to a breakdown of self-tolerance probably involves the recognition of molecular patterns, especially nucleic acids, by pattern recognition receptors. This recognition results in the activation of sentinel cells, the release of proinflammatory cytokines, the development of an inflammatory environment, and the secondary activation of dendritic cells, resulting in B and T cell activation. While both B and T cells can mediate autoimmune disease, like any other form of immune response, helper T cells are required for the response to proceed.

The random generation of antigen-binding receptors in the developing animal ensures that many lymphocytes are produced by the bone marrow with receptors that can bind self-antigens. It has been estimated that as many as 50% of newly produced T cells and B cells may possess receptors that can bind self-antigens with high affinity. These cells are never completely eliminated. They are, however, usually rigorously suppressed. However, the reasons why some horses eventually develop autoimmune diseases while others do not remain unclear. Many factors influence susceptibility to autoimmunity. These include sex, breed, and age, genetic background, as well as environmental effects such as alterations in the microbiota and virus infections. We also know that the development of autoantibodies is a relatively common event that, by itself, does not inevitably lead to autoimmune disease. Indeed, some autoantibodies serve a physiological function such as, for example, the removal of aged erythrocytes.

Autoimmune diseases are also diverse. Self-reactivity of the immune system ranges from a very low "background" level that helps maintain lymphocyte homeostasis, to autoimmune responses with detectable autoantibodies with lymphocyte infiltration in tissues but no clinical consequences, to severe organ damage resulting in clinical disease and death. These diseases can involve not only aberrant adaptive responses but often abnormal innate responses as well. These so-called autoinflammatory diseases can result in the development of uncontrolled inflammation. Thus, in practice, immune-mediated diseases generally result from a combination of inappropriate innate and adaptive responses. The relative contributions of each vary between individual diseases.

Autoimmune endocrine diseases

Equine diabetes mellitus

In humans as well as dogs and cats, type 1 diabetes mellitus is an autoimmune disease. Islet cells in the pancreas are destroyed by an autoimmune attack. Type 2 diabetes in these species is not immune-mediated but reflects islet cell exhaustion in older individuals. While horses do develop diabetes mellitus, it most closely resembles type 2 diabetes mellitus and is not immune-mediated. Thus, it is associated with equine metabolic syndrome, and, as in humans, is associated with obesity, a high carbohydrate diet, and lack of exercise. There is no evidence that diabetes mellitus is immune-mediated in this species.

Lymphocytic hypophysitis

Autoimmune attack on cells of the pituitary gland is a cause of Cushing's disease in humans. Multifocal lymphocytic hypophysitis has also been reported in horses. One such case occurred in an Appaloosa gelding with clinically diagnosed pituitary pars intermedia dysfunction (PPID). On necropsy, the horse had a moderate multifocal lymphoplasmacytic hypophysitis. Subsequent surveys showed that 10 out of 25 equine PPID cases had a few and small scattered lymphocyte foci scattered throughout the gland. Staining for CD3, showed that many of these scattered cells were T cells. The presence of small numbers of scattered T lymphocytes appears to be a normal feature of the equine pituitary gland. Thus, in general, most cases of equine PPID syndrome are probably not immune-mediated (Grau-Roma et al., 2016) (Chapter 23).

Autoimmune eye diseases

Equine recurrent uveitis

The most common cause of blindness in horses is equine recurrent uveitis (ERU) (also called periodic ophthalmia, moon blindness, or iridocyclitis). It affects horses worldwide with an estimated prevalence of 10%–25%. (2%–25% have been reported to be affected in the USA, but only 1%–2% of horses suffer serious disease that significantly affects their vision). Affected horses suffer from repeated episodes of ocular inflammation, mainly involving the anterior uveal tract, followed by periods of remission. In acute cases, they develop severe ocular pain, blepharospasm, lacrimation, corneal changes such as edema and vascularization, aqueous flare, and photophobia. Some horses develop a persistent low-grade uveitis without overt signs of ocular discomfort, while others develop a severe posterior uveitis, including vitritis and retinitis, resulting in photoreceptor destruction. After repeated attacks, horses may develop cataracts, intraocular adhesions, retinal detachment, secondary glaucoma, and eventual loss of vision associated with a shrunken, non-functional eye.

ERU is an immune-mediated disease (Kingsley et al., 2023). The healthy uveal tract has a good blood supply protected by vascular barriers that exclude invading cells. However, once these blood-ocular barriers have been disrupted, perhaps by infection or trauma, then T cells and antibodies may invade the eye. They may do this repeatedly and as a result, trigger recurrent inflammatory episodes Fig. 22.1.

$CD4^+$ T cells in ERU-affected horses appear to lack a cell surface molecule called septin 7. The septins are cytoskeletal proteins involved in regulating cell shape and movement (cytokinesis). A deficiency of septin 7 therefore increases lymphocyte cytoplasmic fluidity so they can efficiently squeeze through small pores (Wiedemann et al., 2020). A septin 7 deficiency in ERU may allow these flexible T cells to penetrate the blood-eye barrier (Degroote et al., 2014). As a result, the ciliary body, choroid, and retina of affected horses are infiltrated with T cells. About half of these cells are $CD4^+$ Th1 cells, and about 20% are $CD8^+$ cytotoxic T cells. The $CD4^+$ cells are activated and produce large amounts of both IL-2 and IFN-γ (Horohov, 2000). Th17 cells and their stimulating cytokine IL-23 are also present in the infiltrate and contribute to the chronic inflammatory process (Saldinger et al., 2020). Neutrophils are also present in large numbers within these eye lesions. They are significantly activated (Weigand et al., 2021). They contribute to the local tissue

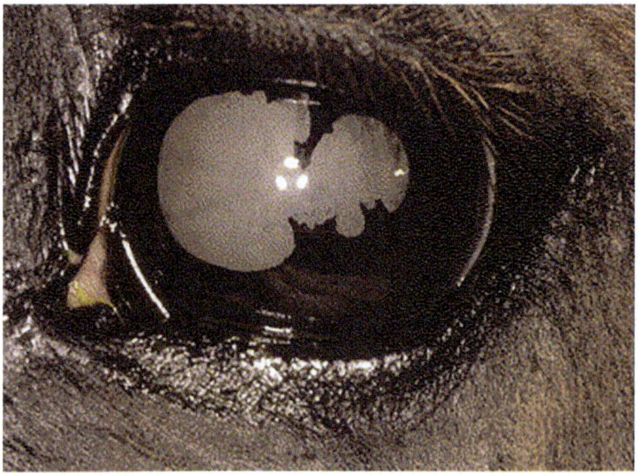

FIGURE 22.1 Chronic equine recurrent uveitis.

A horse with secondary late immature cataract formation and posterior synechiae as a result of ERU.

- With permission Keller and Hendrix (2005).

damage by releasing NETs that are deposited on the blood-retinal barrier. The NETs accumulate and cause local vascular damage. Their numbers correlate with disease severity as well as the presence of invading Leptospira (Fingerhut et al., 2022).

ERU-affected horses make a diversity of autoantibodies directed against retinal antigens (Deeg et al., 2001). These are directed against antigens that are normally hidden behind the blood-ocular barrier. Their B cells are considered "ignorant" regarding eye antigens. As a result, peripheral tolerance is weak, and the some B cells may express receptors that can be activated if they encounter these novel eye antigens. The dominant autoantigen in the equine eye is the interphotoreceptor retinoid-binding protein (IRBP), with subsequent epitope spreading to the retinal S-protein (also called arrestin-1). Other autoantibodies detected in ERU horses include those directed against recoverin, cellular retinaldehyde-binding protein, synaptotagmin-1, and malate dehydrogenase. Their significance in the pathogenesis of ERU is probably not great. These autoantibodies may not be detectable in affected horse serum but are present in the vitreous fluid.

ERU commonly develops as a result of infection with *Leptospira interrogans*. Following natural outbreaks of leptospirosis, most surviving horses developed ERU within 18–24 months. Affected horses develop circulating antibodies to three lipoproteins found on the inner leaflet of the outer membrane of *Leptospira interrogans* called Lru A, B, and C. The titer of these antibodies tends to rise during disease flares and drop when in remission. These Leptospiral lipoproteins show strong antigenic cross-reactivity with atigens in the equine lens, ciliary body, and retina. If horses are experimentally immunized with either equine cornea cells or with certain serovars of killed *L. interrogans*, they develop corneal opacity 10 days later when antibodies appear in their bloodstream. Partial antigenic cross-reactivity also exists between the equine cornea and the *L. interrogans* lipoproteins. *L. interrogans* serovar Pomona is the primary organism triggering ERU in North America, whereas *L. kirschneri* serovars Grippotyphosa, Pomona, and Bratislava are most prevalent in Europe (Dwyer et al., 1995).

Other infections have also been associated with the development of ERU. These include, *Strep equi, Rhodococcus equi*, and *Toxoplasma gondii*. Some cases may also be associated with *Borrelia burgdorferi* infection or with the nematode *Onchocerca cervicalis*. In the latter case, dead or dying worms may release cross-reactive antigens. Numerous other environmental antigens have been suggested as the initiating triggers through molecular mimicry. For example, rotaviruses possess an antigen that cross-reacts with retinal S-antigen, as does the dietary component, α_2-casein. Both of these can induce experimental autoimmune uveitis when used to immunize laboratory rats.

Some horse breeds appear to be predisposed to developing ERU. These include Appaloosas, German Warmbloods, and American Quarter horses.Three single-nucleotide polymorphisms (SNPs) in Appaloosa horses are correlated with the development of ERU (Fritz et al., 2014). One such SNP is strongly associated with the Leopard Complex gene locus on chromosome ECA1. This complex determines the size and number of pigmented spots on the animal's coat. Homozygosity at this locus further increases the risk of developing the disease. A nearby gene modifier called *PATN1* is also associated with increased ERU risk. The other two SNPS are associated with the equine MHC region (ELA) on chromosome ECA20. In German Warmbloods, the ELA-A9 haplotype is associated with increased susceptibility. Other genes involved include those regulating Th17 activity and an SNP on chromosome ECA18 associated with cataract formation. A single SNP located on chromosome ECA11 located within the gene that encodes metalloprotease 2, has also been implicated in the development of uveitis in Icelandic horses (Hack et al., 2022).

Clinical disease

Horses may develop ERU at any age, but peak prevalence is between 4 and 6 years of age. The disease is not gender specific. ERU has been subdivided into three clinical forms.—Classic, insidious, and posterior (Rockwell et al., 2019).

In the most common, classic disease, horses suffer from recurrent acute inflammatory episodes of uveitis separated by periods of relative remission. The inflammatory process may affect the anterior uveal structures, such as the iris, ciliary body, and the posterior choroid and retina. Clinical signs include severe photophobia, ocular pain, blepharospasm, increased lacrimation, corneal edema, aqueous flare, hypopyon, a vitreous haze, and a chorioretinitis. These acute episodes last 10–21 days. Each attack gets progressively more severe and gradually spreads to involve other eye tissues until complete blindness results (Gerding & Gilger, 2016).

In the insidious form of the disease, chronic low-grade uveitis over time results in severe damage and blindness. This form is not obviously painful. The most serious chronic type is seen in Leptospira-infected Appaloosas. In one series of cases, all affected horses lost vision in one eye, and 50% became completely blind. Of non-Appaloosas with chronic ERU, only 34% became blind in one eye and 6% became totally blind.

The posterior form of ERU primarily affects the posterior ocular structures, including the vitreous and the retina. It results in vitreous opacity, retinitis, and eventual degeneration. This form is most common in Warmblood and European horses.

Diagnosis and treatment

Diagnosis of ERU involves exclusion of other causes such as infectious agents (other than Leptospirosis), trauma, or neoplasia. The primary acute form should be distinguished from the chronic recurrent form. Hematology and Leptospira serology should be performed in endemic areas. Aggressive systemic, local, and topical corticosteroid therapy using prednisolone or dexamethasone is an effective treatment. Dexamethasone is used most often since it is available as an ointment and relatively inexpensive. In severe cases, placement of a subpalpebral lavage system for more frequent application of ophthalmic suspensions and solutions may be warranted. These steroids will usually bring the ocular inflammation under control, although the disease often recurs. Encouraging results have been obtained by the use of suprachoroidal sustained-release cyclosporine implants (Malalana et al., 2015).

Equine immune-mediated keratitis

Horses and donkeys may also develop an immune-mediated, non-ulcerative keratitis (IMK). Its clinical signs appear to vary geographically. In North America, reported cases develop chronic corneal opacity without ulceration, uveitis, or overt ocular discomfort. In Europe, however, horses develop severe blepharospasm, uveitis, and corneal ulceration. The lesions are usually unilateral, and their severity depends on the depth of the corneal lesion. The lesions are classified on the basis of the affected layers within the cornea. For example, they may be epithelial, superficial stromal, mid-stromal, or endothelial. Almost half of the cases are superficial stromal. About a quarter are mid-stromal and another quarter are endothelial, while epithelial keratitis is rare (Preston et al., 2023).

The epithelial and stromal forms of the disease are characteristically infiltrated by lymphocytes with a few neutrophils. They have varying degrees of vascularization and fibrosis (Knickelbein & Lassaline, 2024). Epithelial IMK is characterized by the development of punctate opacities in the ventral corneal epithelium. Superficial IMK is a relapsing-remitting corneal opacity consisting of a subepithelial yellow-white infiltrate surrounded by superficial corneal vascularization. Midstromal disease differs from the superficial disease in its location. It tends to have a denser cellular infiltrate and less vascular branching. Endothelial IMK shows a slowly progressive, diffuse ventral area of corneal edema. An endothelial cellular infiltrate may be apparent at the edge of the edematous lesion (Pate et al., 2012). In general, the endothelial form does not respond well to immunosuppressive medications and has a poor prognosis. On the other hand, horses with the more superficial forms of IMK may respond well to topical anti-inflammatory therapy (Matthews & Gilger, 2009).

In superficial stromal IMK, the cellular infiltrate consists predominantly of T cells with some plasma cells, macrophages, and few neutrophils. Both $CD4^+$ and $CD8^+$ T cells are present, as are IgG, IgM, and IgA deposits. The most damaging form of IMK is endothelitis in which the cornea becomes markedly edematous. Autoantibodies have been shown to be directed against a protein called maspin (Serpin B5). Maspin is expressed on corneal stromal keratocytes and as a serine protease inhibitor, is responsible for inhibiting corneal vascularization, cell migration, and adhesion to the intracellular matrix during wound healing (Braus et al., 2017). No breed or gender predisposition has been noted. Diagnosis is based on the exclusion of other causes, such as infections and the presence of concomitant uveitis. Treatment consists of topical steroids and/or cyclosporine. Surgical removal of the lesion (keratectomy) may be effective for persistent superficial or mid-stromal lesions.

Equine keratoconjunctivitis sicca

Keratoconjunctivitis sicca is a form of conjunctivitis resulting from a failure of the lacrimal glands to produce sufficient tears. In other species, the lacrimal tissue destruction is often immune-mediated. It has been reported to occur in horses

(Reilly & Beech, 1994). For example, a 3-year-old animal presented with bilateral ulcerative keratoconjunctivitis and improved clinically with ophthalmic cyclosporine therapy. The lacrimal glands showed an eosinophil infiltration with lesser numbers of lymphocytes, plasma cells, and macrophages. Although this suggests an immunological origin for the disease, it must be pointed out that nonimmunological mechanisms, such as facial nerve damage, can prevent blinking and so result in corneal dryness.

Autoimmune neurologic disease

Polyneuritis equi

Equine polyneuritis (neuritis of the cauda equina) is an uncommon disease syndrome affecting the cranial, sacral, and coccygeal nerves that results from the production of demyelinating autoantibodies to a peripheral myelin basic protein P2. Affected horses show hyperesthesia followed by progressive paralysis of the tail, rectum, and bladder. Loss of sensation in sacral dermatomes may be accompanied by hyperesthesia in the surrounding skin. In about 80% of cases, the disease also affects the cranial nerves. It mainly attacks the vagus nerve and so causes dysphonia. This is also associated with facial and trigeminal paralysis. Although sacral and lumbar involvement is usually bilateral, the cranial nerve involvement is often unilateral. The cranial nerve problems often precede the development of the sacral lesions (Yvorchuk-St Jean, 1987).

Affected nerves are thickened and discolored. Early lesions are characterized by infiltration with lymphocytes, multinucleated giant cells, and plasma cells. The predominant lymphocytes in the infiltrate are $CD8^+$ cytotoxic T cells with some B cells and plasma cells (Hahn, 2008) Fig. 22.2.

These are gradually replaced by abundant neutrophils and macrophages (van Galen et al., 2008). Affected nerves develop demyelination of the sacrococcygeal and lumbosacral nerve roots (Fig. 22.2). Chronic granulomatous inflammation eventually develops in the region of the extradural nerve roots. Perineural fibrosis and perivascular lymphocyte cuffs with hemorrhage are found in the affected nerves. Areas of demyelination and remyelination are present. There is a loss of myelinated axons; so that in severe cases, the nerve trunks are almost totally destroyed.

The etiology of polyneuritis equi is unknown, but it is probably triggered by an infection through molecular mimicry. Candidate triggers include Campylobacter, equine adenovirus 1, and equine herpesvirus-1 (Edington et al., 1984). Another possible contributor is *Sarcocystis neurona*. Horses diagnosed with equine protozoal myeloencephalitis caused by *S. neurona* also make autoantibodies against myelin basic protein 2. They appear to share a common antigenic determinant. Thus, polyneuritis may reflect molecular mimicry between *S. neurona* and myelin. Conversely, some horses diagnosed with polyneuritis equi may also possess

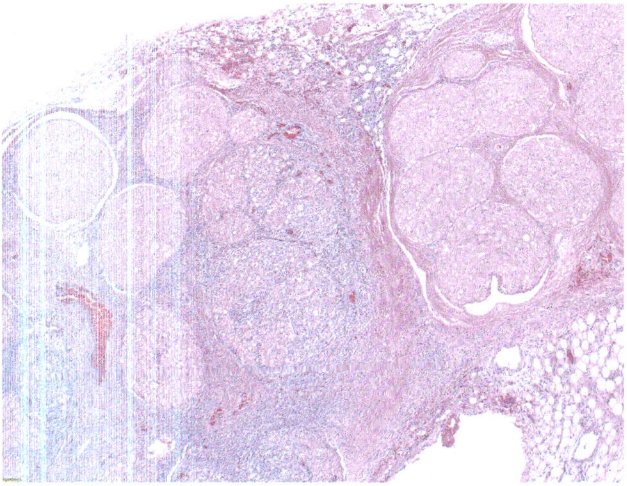

FIGURE 22.2 Nerve lesions from a case of polyneuritis equi.

Note the massive peri- and intraneuronal mononuclear cell infiltrate. Original magnification ×4. H&E stain.

- Courtesy of Dr. Brian Porter.

antibodies against *S. neurona*. Thus, some cases of polyneuritis equi may, in fact, be caused by *S. neurona* (Ellison et al., 2015).

Clinical disease

Polyneuritis has been reported in adult horses of many breeds. It presents as a slowly progressive paralysis of the tail, rectum, anus, and bladder. Hindlimb weakness and ataxia develop progressively. This may result in urine scalding, as well as hyperesthesia and hind muscle fasciculations. Muscle atrophy may result, but this is variable. When cranial nerves are involved, the lesions are often asymmetric. It generally affects nerves V, V11, and VIII. This may be reflected in facial muscle paralysis, head tilt, nystagmus, tongue paralysis, and dysphagia (Wright et al., 1987).

Diagnosis and treatment

Diagnosis of polyneuritis is based on clinical signs, history, and exclusion of other possibilities. While affected horses have autoantibodies against myelin basic protein P2, this assay is not available commercially. Serum chemistry may show evidence of chronic inflammation, such as elevated C-teactive protein (CRP) levels. While not specific, these CRP levels may be useful in following the disease course. Cerebrospinal fluid analysis may show xanthochromia and elevated protein and cell counts (neutrophil pleocytosis). Definitive diagnosis is based on necropsy findings.

Palliative treatment includes managing the cystitis, urinary and fecal incontinence, and urinary scalding. If the dysphagia is severe, horses may require tube feeding. Because of the severity of the nerve damage, immunosuppressive or anti-inflammatory therapy is rarely successful. The disease is progressive, and the prognosis is poor (Aleman et al., 2009).

Autoimmune skin diseases

Autoimmune skin diseases are relatively rare in horses. In some of these diseases, the autoantibodies directly target the skin. In others, the skin lesions are a secondary response to lesions elsewhere in the body (Rosenkrantz, 2013).

Equine pemphigus foliaceus

The pemphigus group of diseases are characterized by the development of flaccid vesicles, pustules, and erosions on the skin and mucus membranes. These vesicles may be very superficial and rupture readily, while others form deep within the epidermis, where they remain intact for longer. The autoantibodies produced in pemphigus are directed against target antigens in the desmosomes located in different skin layers Fig. 22.3.

Pemphigus foliaceus (PF) (From the Latin *folium*, a leaf) is the commonest form of pemphigus in horses and donkeys (Zabel et al., 2005). It is a superficial vesicular disease in which the lesions develop in the subcorneal epidermis as a result of the

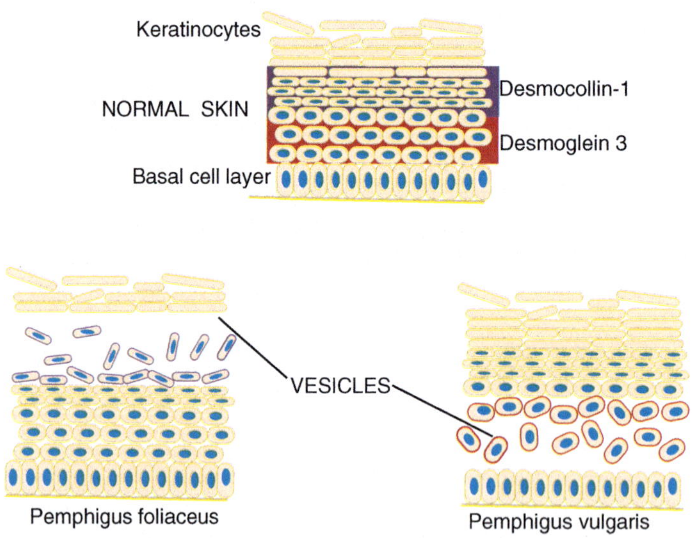

FIGURE 22.3 The pemphigus group of autoimmune skin diseases are conveniently divided into two major subgroups based upon the depth of the vesicles that form.

Superficial vesicles that form shallow vesicles are typical of pemphigus foliaceus. The diseases that form deep vesicles are typified by pemphigus vulgaris.

actions of IgG autoantibodies directed against keratinocyte desmosomal proteins. As a result, the desmosomes break down, and the keratinocytes separate and are considered acantholytic. Because they form so close to the surface, pemphigus foliaceus blisters are very fragile and rupture readily, leaving crusting, shallow erosions rather than ulcers as well as alopecia. When they are intact, they fill with inflammatory cells, primarily neutrophils, and are described as pustules. IgG is the dominant serum autoantibody. In humans, the major autoantigens in PF are desmogleins. or desmocollins Fig. 22.4.

The pustules tend to be bilateral and symmetrical. They generally affect the periocular and muzzle area (nostrils, eyelids, and lips) as well as the lower extremities. PF lesions rarely develop on mucosal surfaces such as in the oral cavity. Pruritus is not usually a feature of equine PF, but secondary bacterial infections, anorexia, fever, and depression may occur in horses with widespread lesions (Vandenabeele et al., 2004).

Diagnosis of PF must be confirmed by histopathology. Subcorneal vesicles are associated with marked acantholysis. Acantholytic keratinocytes are found in impression smears of the bullae. Neutrophils and occasional eosinophils are also found in large numbers within the blister fluid. Histology in the early stages of the disease shows subcorneal vesicles. However, these develop into subcorneal pustules. Direct fluorescent antibody (FA) or immunoperoxidase staining can detect the

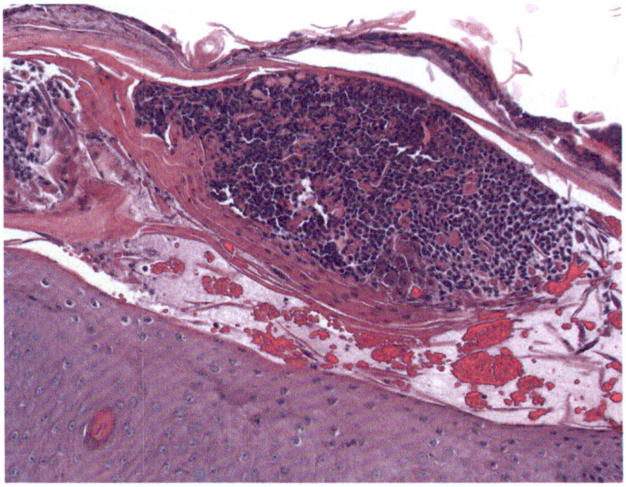

FIGURE 22.4 Histology of a pemphigus foliaceus vesicle.

Note its shallow location and the fact that it is packed with acantholytic cells. It is, in effect, a pustule.

- With permission Marsella (2024).

presence of immunoglobulins in the epidermis, bound to the intercellular cement in a "chicken-wire pattern". Indirect FA assays may be used to test the serum of affected animals for its ability to bind to mouse skin sections or cultured keratinocytes in a similar pattern.

Pemphigus foliaceus is the most common autoimmune disease in horses (Marsella, 2024). It appears that Appaloosas may be predisposed, but this is not consistent. There is no gender predilection. Affected animals cover a very wide age range, from 6 months to 25 years. Animals develop multifocal lesions. Because of the fragility of the pustules, they readily rupture so that generalized crusting, scaling, and alopecia develop. Lesions usually begin on the face or legs, but if left untreated, may spread to become generalized over a few months. Sometimes animals develop ventral edema as well as systemic signs such as fever, depression, and lethargy. Some of these lesions may be painful or pruritic (Fadok, 1995).

Equine pemphigus vulgaris

A more severe form of Pemphigus—pemphigus vulgaris. is very rare in horses (Tham et al., 2020). It has been definitively diagnosed in a 9-year-old Welsh pony stallion (Winfield et al., 2013). The animal had developed crusts and scales around its tail-head. There were multiple intact vesicles on its muzzle. This disease affected its oral cavity and the pony developed an ulcerated tongue. As a result, it salivated profusely and refused to eat. Despite treatment, the pony's condition continued to deteriorate, and it had to be euthanized. Postmortem examination also showed the presence of lesions on the cardia of its stomach. Pemphigus vulgaris results from an autoimmune attack on desmosomes. Because the targeted desmosomes are located deeper at the dermoepidermal junction than on pemphigus foliaceus, the vesicles are more severe, as are the ulcers. Histology confirmed that the skin lesions in this pony originated in the suprabasilar layer of the epidermis. The vesicles were filled with acantholytic keratinocytes. Direct immunofluorescence revealed IgG deposits between the cells. The animal possessed circulating antikeratinocyte IgG antibodies. Desmoglein 3 was identified as the targeted autoantigen (Marsella, 2024).

Bullous pemphigoid

Another related autoimmune skin disease that affects horses is bullous pemphigoid. This is caused by autoantibodies that target hemidesmosomes located under the dermal-epidermal junction in the skin and mucosa; thus, it causes subepidermal detachment of skin layers, resulting in bulla formation. As in the other related diseases, these bullae rupture readily and thus result in skin ulceration. It too is rarely observed in horses. Clinically, it closely resembles pemphigus vulgaris. Like PV horses, affected animals may develop ulcerative lesions within the oral cavity (Michutta et al., 2011). Analysis of equine bullous pemphigoid has determined that the targeted autoantigen is a linear epitope of collagen XVII (Olivry et al., 2000).

Paraneoplastic pemphigus is not related to either PF or PV. Instead, it is a manifestation of an autoimmune syndrome that develops in association with lymphoid or solid tumors. A case of a bullous disease affecting the oral cavity of a horse with cancer has been reported. This was considered to be a very rare case of paraneoplastic pemphigus (Williams et al., 1995).

Equine vitiligo

Vitiligo is a chronic condition that manifests itself as a patchy whitening of the skin and hair. It appears to be an autoimmune disease resulting from the production of antibodies to melanin and related pigments. Autoantibodies to melanin are commonly present in humans and dogs with vitiligo; however, NK cells and cytotoxic $CD8^+$ cells have also been implicated in its pathogenesis (Tham et al., 2019).

In horses, vitiligo has been reported in multiple breeds, including Gelderlands, Spanish Thoroughbreds, and Belgian horses. In Arabian horses, it is sufficiently common to be called "Arabian fading syndrome" or "Pinky Syndrome" (Mosos et al., 1991). The autoantibodies are directed primarily against the melanocyte-specific enzyme, tyrosinase, as well as two tyrosinase-related proteins (TRP) 1 and 2, and several minor proteins. Antibodies to a melanocyte-specific 85 kDa protein have also been described in dogs, cats, and horses. These antibodies damage melanocytes in vitro either through complement-mediated lysis or by ADCC. Cytotoxic T cells are directed against a melanocyte cell-surface 22 kDa antigen called Melan A, suggesting that this too may be a key target in the cytotoxic process.

Vitiligo-like depigmentation occurs in about 26%–67% of gray horses compared to a prevalence of 0.8%–3.5% of horses with other coat colors. Genotyping of gray horses affected by vitiligo has identified seven candidate genes on four chromosomes. Four of these genes are associated with innate immunity, while the others play a role in tumor suppression. Some of these genes may also be implicated in the development of melanomas in these breeds (Chapter 21) (Druml et al., 2021).

Histopathology shows a loss of melanocytes in the epidermis and/or hair follicles, although the epithelial architecture remains normal. There may be pigmentary incontinence with the escape of melanin granules into the intercellular spaces. In active cases, there may also be local infiltration with mononuclear cells.

Alopecia areata

Alopecia areata (AA) is a very rare T cell-mediated disease of horses characterized by non-inflammatory, non-pruritic hair loss. It mainly affects Appaloosas and Quarter horses. It may also have a seasonal pattern, worsening in spring and summer (Hoolahan et al., 2013). This mainly affects the mane, tail, and face, but can occur anywhere on the horse's body. It may also involve hoof dystrophy. The hair loss is usually patchy and localized. Skin histology shows a T cell infiltration of hair follicles (Rosychuk, 2013) Fig. 22.5.

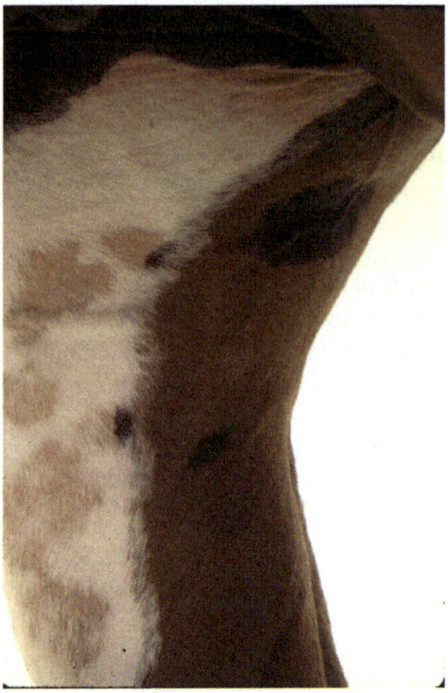

FIGURE 22.5 Alopecia areata in a Paint horse.

- With permission Rosychuk (2013).

Anagen hair follicles normally express immunological tolerance in the region located between the bulge and the bulb. Active suppressive mechanisms limit local MHC class Ia expression as well as NK cell and macrophage activity in this region. Hair follicles are home to much of the skin microbiota. It is possible that this local tolerance within hair follicles may be initiated in part by the immunosuppressive effects of these commensals.

Immunological tolerance is, however, relative and can collapse. Once tolerance collapses, the hair follicles are rapidly invaded by cytotoxic T cells that proceed to destroy the bulb and hence stop hair growth. These diseases may be self-limiting, and it is possible that the eventual restoration of hair growth may be due to a gradual recovery of tolerance.

Alopecia areata is a chronic, non-scarring skin disease that affects anagen (actively growing) hair follicles. Hair growth normally cycles through different stages, while alopecia areata interferes with these cycles. While clinically non-inflammatory, affected hair follicles are infiltrated with cytotoxic $CD8^+$ T cells as well as Langerhans cells. There are few eosinophils and fewer neutrophils in the lesions. Animals also produce IgG directed against antigens in the lower hair follicles. C3 and IgM may accumulate in this region. The autoimmune attack is primarily directed against a protein called trichohyalin located in the inner root sheath of the follicles. Keratins and root matrix proteins may also be targets. The T cells and some plasma cells form an infiltrate that surrounds the hair bulb and the follicular isthmus. Some $CD8^+$ T cells may also enter the hair bulbs. As a result, hair shafts become dysplastic and unpigmented. Pigmentary incontinence occurs. There may also be peri- and intra-bulbar infiltration, peribulbar fibrosis, and degenerated matrix cells with clumped melanosomes.

Equine systemic lupus erythematosus

In some autoimmune diseases, control is lost over most of the immune system. As a result, these animals suffer a generalized breakdown of peripheral tolerance. These diseases or syndromes are interrelated and have many overlapping clinical features. One common feature is extensive and uncontrolled inflammation in multiple tissues or organs. Thus, the dysfunction encompasses both the innate and adaptive immune systems. These diseases may be considered to be located in the middle of the spectrum between purely autoimmune and purely autoinflammatory diseases.

Examples of these systemic, immune-mediated diseases include systemic lupus erythematosus (SLE), and rheumatoid arthritis, as well as systemic arthritis, and vasculitis. Although each of these diseases is associated with some degree of autoimmunity, they do not simply result from tissue damage caused directly by antibodies and T cells. Many of their lesions are associated with the presence of immune complexes and activated complement components in tissues. Many result from uncontrolled inflammatory cytokine production or from defects in the regulation of the complement system. Their initiating factors are largely unknown, although they all exhibit a significant genetic predisposition, commonly with linkage to the MHC. As with other autoimmune diseases, microbial dysbiosis is also consistently associated with their development. As a result, affected animals develop multiple autoantibodies, T cell dysfunction, impaired apoptosis, and multi-organ inflammation. The most significant and complex of these diseases is systemic lupus erythematosus (SLE) Fig. 22.6.

SLE is a complex disease resulting from the interaction of multiple factors, both genetic and environmental, as well as diverse pathogenic processes such as a loss of Treg cells and excessive B cell functionality. Affected animals produce multiple different autoantibodies directed against nuclear, cytoplasmic, and cell membrane antigens (Gershwin, 2005). The most important of these are linked to defects in the way by which dead and dying cells are handled by the immune system.

SLE is a very rare disease of horses. Its severity is highly variable. It usually presents as a generalized skin disease (Geor et al., 2005). Affected horses develop an exfoliative dermatitis with bilaterally symmetrical alopecia, seborrheic dermatitis, mucocutaneous ulceration, scaling, and crusting. Some affected horses may be almost totally hairless. Leukoderma develops on the face and trunk. Systemic manifestations include intermittent fever, tachypnea, progressive anorexia, and weight loss. Affected horses may also drevelop uveitis, and a generalized lymphadenopathy with lymphedema in the lower limbs. An antiglobulin-positive hemolytic anemia and thrombocytopenia with purpura may develop. Affected horses are anti-nuclear

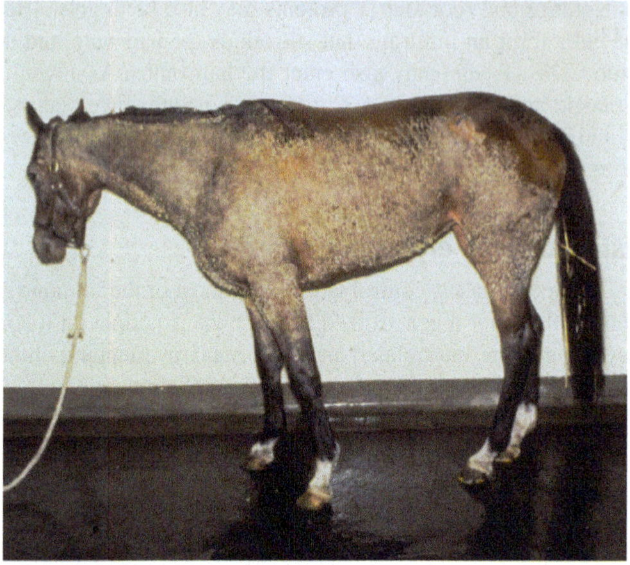

FIGURE 22.6 A filly with systemic lupus erythematosus.

Note the generalized alopecia and crusting.

- *From Geor, R. J., Clark, E. G., Haines, D. M., Napier, P. G. (1990). Systemic lupus erythematosus in a filly.* Journal of the American Veterinary Medical Association, 197, *1489. With Permission.*

antibody (ANA)-positive, although lupus erythematosus (LE) cell tests are equivocal in this species. Skin biopsies show an interface dermatitis containing lymphocytes, plasma cells, and histiocytes with basal cell degeneration, and a thickening of the dermal basement membrane. There is IgG deposition on the skin basement membrane (this forms a "lupus band"). Affected horses also develop a glomerulonephritis and a synovitis, as a result of the deposition of the excessive immune complexes in their kidneys and joints. In some equine SLE cases, the animal may also develop a severe polyarthritis.

If SLE is suspected, a lupus erythematosus (LE) test and an anti-nuclear antibody (ANA) assay should be conducted, and at least two other autoimmune conditions identified. These may include hemolytic anemia, thrombocytopenia, or glomerulonephritis in addition to the skin lesions. Treatment requires immunosuppressive doses of glucocorticoids, perhaps supplemented with other immunosuppressants such as azathioprine or cyclosporine. However, treatment of the reported equine cases has been unsuccessful (Geor et al., 2005) Box 22.1.

Cutaneous (discoid) lupus erythematosus

Despite its name, equine cutaneous lupus erythematosus (CLE) is a skin disease that is distinctly different from systemic lupus erythematosus. It can present clinically in many diverse ways.

Box 22.1 Lupus and herpesviruses

In seeking a cause of systemic lupus, researchers have begun to focus on the role of herpesviruses. Thus, in humans, Epstein–Barr virus (EBV), a herpesvirus, has been linked epidemiologically to systemic lupus. Patients with SLE have consistently high antibody levels against the virus. Recently, it has also been demonstrated that EBV infects B cells and reprograms them. The virus upregulates the genes encoding proteins involved in antigen processing. As a result, these infected B cells are driven to present nuclear antigens to helper T cells. The helper T cells, in turn, expand these B cell clones. The production of antinuclear antibodies is a key feature of SLE. It is tempting to speculate that equine herpesviruses may trigger lupus in susceptible horses (Younis et al., 2025).

The initial steps in the development of CLE are probably triggered by skin damage due to ultraviolet radiation. The UV radiation causes damaged keratinocytes to produce cytokines and other proinflammatory molecules. The cytokines activate local innate immune responses. DNA released from apoptotic cells and neutrophil extracellular traps activates some TLRs. Type 1 interferons are generated and activate adaptive immune responses—first DCs and then Th1 responses and cytotoxic T cells. Nearby NK cells are also activated. These, in turn, activate local Th17 responses, and this results in yet more inflammation. The mixture of T cells, NK cells, and cytokines contributes to the local tissue damage by attacking and killing keratinocytes. The release of cell debris, especially nuclear antigens, reactivates the innate immune pathways, causes the pDCs to produce yet more interferons, and thus generates a self-amplifying inflammatory cycle. Nucleoprotein autoantigens are also induced by the interferons and promote further ANA production. Local accumulation of immune complexes may also contribute to the inflammatory process (Zhou et al., 2020).

Clinical disease

CLE lesions are restricted to the skin. It tends to target the animal's face, ears, and neck. ANA and LE tests are negative or weakly positive. Nasal lesions predominate with patchy erythema, erosions, scaling, crusting ulcers. Scaling and loss of pigment involve the nasal planum and the bridge of the nose. The lesions may spread to the lips, periocular skin, and genitals. CLE may also affect the coronary band in some animals, resulting in erosive lesions, pain, and lameness. CLE has also been described in a donkey. The 5-year-old male, neutered donkey, developed a generalized dermatitis. There were symmetrical areas of alopecia, erythema, crusting, and scaling. Skin biopsy showed the presence of an interface dermatitis infiltrated with $CD8^+$ T cells. The disease was successfully treated with glucocorticoids and methotrexate (Mosca et al., 2020).

A skin biopsy is required for the diagnosis of equine CLE. Histopathology of CLE cases shows characteristic lesions at the dermoepidermal junction and basal cell degeneration. There is an interface inflammation, with vacuolar degeneration, apoptosis, loss of basal cells, and basement membrane thickening, accompanied by a lymphoplasmacytic infiltration. The basement membrane thickening may be patchy and multifocal. This is the classical "band-like" pattern of an interface dermatitis. (Also called a "lichenoid infiltrate"). C3, IgA, IgG, or IgM may be detected in the skin basement membrane in a typical lupus band.

Autoimmune arthritis

The innate immune system, in the form of inflammation, serves as an important stimulus for adaptive immune responses. Triggers of inflammation, such as infections, environmental insults, and signals from the body's microbiota, can initiate some autoimmune diseases. Innate immune responses also play a key role in mediating the consequences of autoimmunity. The organ damage resulting from an autoimmune attack is also a result of innate mechanisms. The activation of cells by proinflammatory cytokines, the generation of tissue-degrading enzymes, and the production of potent oxidants that destroy tissues can all result from uncontrolled innate immunity. This progression from innate immunity to adaptive immunity to innate immunity again is well seen in the erosive inflammatory joint diseases typified by rheumatoid arthritis.

Rheumatoid arthritis (RA) is a common, crippling syndrome that affects about 1% of humans. It is characterized by dysfunctional innate immunity, including immune-complex formation and complement dysregulation; by adaptive autoimmune responses against post-translationally modified proteins; by T cell dysregulation; and by macrophage activation in joints, resulting in cartilage and bone destruction.

Clinically, RA commences as a lymphocytic synovitis with neutrophils in the joint fluid. Cytokines such as IL-6 and TNF-α are released in large quantities, and the inflammation develops progressively. The resulting arthritis is highly erosive and destroys both joint cartilage and bone. Because of the involvement of so many different inflammatory and autoimmune pathways, it has been suggested that rheumatoid arthritis should be considered a common syndrome resulting from the generation of joint inflammation by many different routes.

Way back in 1880, Dr Robert Ward, a veterinarian, published a paper reporting on a case of rheumatoid arthritis in a horse (Ward, 1880). The animal he described was crippled by arthritis, and its fetlocks were "round, swollen, hot and tender." At that time, no diagnostic tests were available, and Dr Ward's diagnosis was based only on clinical signs. In fact, his description suggests that this arthritis was of an infectious nature.

However, with our increasing knowledge of rheumatoid arthritis and its pathogenesis, it is possible to apply modern diagnostic techniques to arthritic horses. For example, affected individuals produce rheumatoid factor (RF), an IgM autoantibody directed against their own IgG. They also develop autoantibodies against citrullinated proteins (ACPA). These, together with an acute-phase response, are significant diagnostic criteria. A study of 60 clinically healthy normal horses has revealed that they possess both rheumatoid factor and ACPA. These autoantibody levels increase progressively as horses age (Hoikhman et al., 2018).

In another study investigating rheumatoid markers in horses suffering from joint disease, investigators measured rheumatoid factor, antinuclear antibodies, and antibodies to 65 kDa heat shock protein. (The 65 kDa heat shock protein is produced by damaged chondrocytes. Human rheumatoid arthritis patients make autoantibodies to it.) These factors showed only modest increases that were not statistically significant and were not correlated with disease severity (Carter et al., 1995). Autoimmunity does not significantly influence equine arthritis, and rheumatoid arthritis does not appear to affect horses.

One common feature of chronic degenerative arthritis in many species is the production of autoantibodies to collagens, the major proteins in articular cartilage. Experimentally an arthritis can be induced in laboratory rats by immunizing them with type II collagen. Likewise, anti-collagen antibodies are present in arthritic humans and dogs. A study on horses with naturally occurring osteoarthritis demonstrated that the synovial fluid from 26% of these animals possessed significant amounts of autoantibodies directed against type II collagen, the major component of articular cartilage (Osborne et al., 1995). In horses suffering from traumatic arthritis, 68% had these antibodies in their synovial fluid. There were also significant quantities of immune complexes in these fluids. These anti-collagen antibodies could not be detected in the horse serum. It remains unclear whether these autoantibodies contributed to the development of the osteoarthritis or, more probably, whether they were secondary to the severe joint damage.

Equine polyarthritis/polysynovitis

Non-erosive, non-infectious arthritis can develop in foals following recovery from an infectious disease. It is believed that this condition is immune-mediated. Polyarthritis has also been reported in foals in association with a lupus-like syndrome (Vrins & Feldman, 1983). Affected foals (up to 3 months of age) develop multiple swollen joints involving all four limbs and a persistent fever. In some cases, synovial sheaths, including tendon sheaths and bursae, are also affected. The synovial effusions are sterile, but synovial biopsies show lymphocyte and plasma cell infiltration with some immunoglobulin deposits. The cells in the joint fluid are mainly neutrophils. These animals are negative for RF, ANA, and LE cells. Many of these foals have a lesion within the thorax, especially *Rhodococcus equi* pneumonia. It is possible that immune complexes originating in the lung lesions may lodge in the synovial vessels and trigger the synovitis. The polyarthritis usually resolves once the primary lesion heals.

A primary idiopathic immune-mediated polyarthritis has also been recorded in adult horses. In these cases, animals lose weight, develop an intermittent fever, and have effusions in multiple joints, leading to severe stiffness. They have systemic signs of inflammation, including anemia, leukocytosis, hyperfibrinogenemia, and hyperglobulinemia. Their synovial fluid is sterile, and immunoglobulins are present in the synovial membrane. The condition usually resolves with steroid and immunosuppressive therapy (Pusterla et al., 2006).

Autoimmune blood diseases

In other domestic species, autoimmune diseases directed against blood erythrocytes, leukocytes, and platelets are not uncommon. Connversely, immune-mediated hemolytic anemia (IMHA) and thrombocytopenia (IMTP) are rare autoimmune diseases in horses. They usually develop secondary to infections or neoplasia. They may occur independently or concurrently.

Immune mediated hemolytic anemia

Both primary and secondary IMHAs have been described in horses. Secondary IMHAs are much more common (Easton-Jones, 2024). For example, secondary anemias develop in horses with lymphosarcomas and melanomas as well as with infections such as *Clostridium perfringens*, Streptococci, and *R. equi*, and of course, equine infectious anemia virus (Weiss & Moritz, 2003). Equine IMHA may also be triggered by drugs such as penicillin, sulfonamides, and organophosphates Fig. 22.7.

Primary hemolytic anemia develops as a result of the spontaneous generation of autoantibodies. Horses with primary disease are usually depressed and febrile. They exhibit weight loss, splenomegaly, jaundice, and hemoglobinuria. They have pale mucus membranes and heart murmurs. They may be weak with significant tachycardia and tachypnea. This all depends upon the severity of the disease. Their serum autoantibodies are usually of the IgG class, but sometimes may be IgM (Wilkerson et al., 2000). Some cases develop spontaneous red cell autoagglutination, and both warm and cold agglutinins have been reported in horses. In these cases, red cell

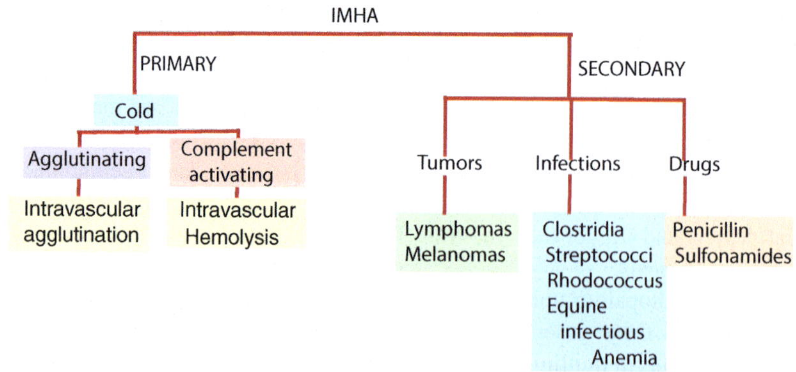

FIGURE 22.7 The different forms of immune-mediated hemolytic anemia that may develop in the horse.

autoagglutination may occur when a drop of blood is diluted with saline on a slide. Icterus is common, especially in chronic cases. These horses have IgG-coated red cells, so the direct Coombs test can be used for diagnosis. Treatment involves the removal of the causes of secondary disease and immunosuppression of the primary disease. Glucocorticoids such as dexamethasone can induce remission, especially in primary disease. This may be supplemented with cyclosporine and/or azathioprine if necessary. Treatment should last for at least for a minimum of 2 weeks. The prognosis depends upon the underlying cause (Easton-Jones, 2024).

Immune-mediated thrombocytopenic purpura

Primary IMTP in horses is characterized by spontaneous epistaxis, petechia, and ecchymoses on the mucus membranes and the conjunctiva. Horses may develop swollen joints, hematomas, and gastrointestinal bleeding (Kimberly et al., 2004). Neurological signs may result from bleeding into the brain. Affected horses have low platelet counts, in the range of 20–30,000/mL. Diagnosis is based on the exclusion of other causes. Secondary thrombocytopenia in horses may be due to infections, drugs, or neoplasia. There is a lack of satisfactory diagnostic tests in this species. Flow cytometry, if available, may be useful in identifying the presence of platelets with increased surface-bound IgG (Nunez et al., 2001). Platelets from affected horses show much greater size diversity than normal horses. Likewise, in one study, about 5% of platelets had IgG on their surface as compared to 0.15% of the platelets from healthy horses. Horses have been treated successfully with dexamethasone supplemented with azathioprine. Administration of platelet-rich plasma may be helpful in a bleeding emergency.

Autoimmune muscle diseases

There are multiple causes of inflammatory myopathies in the horse. One major cause is myosin heavy chain myopathy (MYHM). This is predominantly inherited in Quarter horses and related breeds such as Paints and Appaloosas. It occurs in three distinct phenotypes: non-exertional rhabdomyelitis, immune-mediated myositis, and systemic calcification (calciphylaxis).

Given its predisposition in Quarter horses, it is clear that MYHM has a major genetic component (Durward-Akhurst & Valberg, 2018). Certain stallions are overrepresented in the bloodlines of affected Quarter horses. Genome-wide association studies (GWAS) on Quarter horses and related breeds indicate an autosomal mode of inheritance. GWAS have identified a close association between MYHM and a 6.3 Mb region of chromosome ECA 11. Subsequent analysis identified a mutation located in the myosin heavy chain 1 (MYH1) globular head where a glutamic acid has been exchanged for a normal glycine at position 321. This gene variant is called E321G *MYH1*. It encodes the heavy chain of myosin 2X. It is variably penetrant, thus explaining variations in disease susceptibility. It occurs with a high frequency in some susceptible lines of Quarter horses but not in non-susceptible lines nor in Arabians.

Immune-mediated myositis

The immune-mediated form of myositis (IMM) is characterized by rapid-onset muscle wasting. Affected horses suffer from muscle pain, resulting in stiffness and reluctance to move (Aleman, 2024). The disease usually targets the gluteal and epaxial muscles, leaving other muscle groups such as the semimembranosus and semitendinosus relatively unaffected. Some horses may lose 40% of their muscle mass within 48 h (Durward-Akhurst & Valberg, 2025). Many horses develop a fever during this process. The reason for this localized atrophy is unclear since the affected muscles are not known to express any unique antigens. There is no evidence of IgG binding specifically to gluteal muscle fibers. Normal healthy muscle cells do not normally express MHC molecules. However, in IMM affected horses, some muscle fibers begin to express both MHC class I and class II and therefore acquire the ability to act as antigen-presenting cells and serve as targets for cytotoxic T cells Fig. 22.8.

Affected muscles are infiltrated with lymphocytes and undergo necrosis. In about half of these cases, the predominant infiltrating lymphocytes are $CD4^+$ T cells. However, in about a quarter, $CD8^+$ T cells predominate. B cells, macrophages, and multinucleated giant cells may also be present in the infiltrate. These cells are found within or surrounding myofibers, especially around those myofibers that contain the myosin 2X heavy chain. (2X fibers account for about 40%–80% of muscle fibers, while 2A fibers account for about 30%–40%). There is no evidence of specific binding of immunoglobulins to affected myofibers, confirming the suspicion that this is a T-cell-mediated disease.

While the causes of equine MYHM are largely genetic, it is probable that, as usual, environmental triggers also play an important role. Environmental factors likely include an infectious trigger. Thus, as many as 40% of affected horses may have a history of recent infection. For example, IMM may be triggered by bacteria such as *Streptococcus equi* ssp *equi* or *Corynebacterium pseudotuberculosis*, or by prior vaccination against a respiratory virus such as equine herpesvirus-1 or influenza.

A B
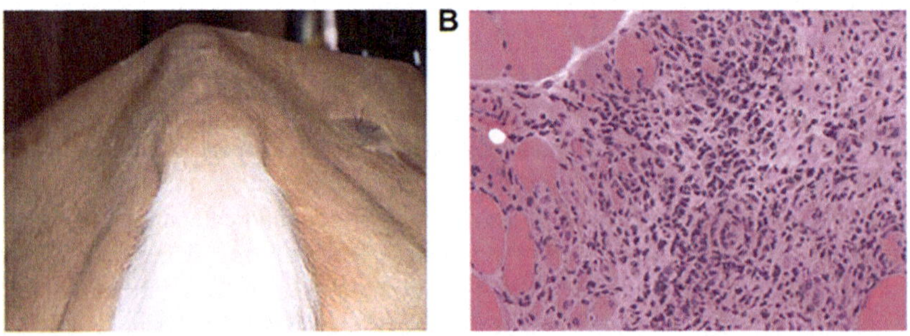

FIGURE 22.8 Equine immune-mediated myositis.

A muscle biopsy showing a marked lymphocyte infiltration of the gluteal muscle.

- With permission Aleman (2008).

Interestingly, the M protein of *Strep. equi* shows considerable homology to myosin heavy chain 2X and thus, molecular mimicry likely plays a role in the induction of IMM. It has been suggested that in the presence of certain environmental triggers, the mutated MYH1 gene can initiate the development of IMM. For example, an innate immune response could be triggered in IMM by the release of myosin 2X from muscle fibers by microtrauma such as that caused by vaccination or severe exercise. Similar mutations in mice predispose them to develop myocarditis.

IMM has a bimodal distribution. Affected Quarter horses tend to be under 4 years of age, whereas affected other breeds tend to be older, with an average onset around 17 years. There is no gender predisposition. The disease presents as rapidly progressive localized symmetrical muscle atrophy affecting predominantly the epaxial and gluteal muscles. The cervical muscles may atrophy as well. The onset of atrophy is rapid and may persist for several months. Affected animals show stiffness, weakness, and malaise, while many are febrile (Hunyadi et al., 2017).

Hematology may be normal or show a leukocytosis. Serum chemistry may show marked increases in serum creatine kinase and aspartate aminotransferase, especially in the acute phase of the disease. The most useful diagnostic procedure is a transcutaneous biopsy. These show a lymphocytic infiltration into the myocytes and perivascular cuffing. Myocytes show evidence of atrophy and myonecrosis, and there may also be signs of myofiber regeneration. Biopsies taken later in the disease process may show fewer lymphocytes.

The prognosis for IMM is good, although horses with a fever or concurrent infections tend to have a somewhat poorer outcome. Anti-inflammatory doses of glucocorticoids administered for about a month are usually effective. The muscle mass will eventually recover, but this may take 2–3 months, and there may be some residual muscle atrophy. About half of apparently recovered horses may undergo recurrent episodes.

Autoimmune kidney disease

As described in Chapter 20, a glomerulonephritis can develop in horse kidneys a result of immune complex deposition. However, some horses may develop autoantibodies to their renal glomerular basement membranes, that also results in the development of glomerulonephritis and renal failure. The two forms of the disease can be differentiated by immunofluorescence examination. Immune complex deposits are "lumpy-bumpy" while autoantibody deposits are smooth. In one study, glomerulonephritis was detected in 3 of 83 horses examined. Immunofluorescence studies in these three horses showed deposits of IgG and complement (C3) on their glomerular basement membranes. Their basement membrane was coated with a smooth, linear deposit of immunoglobulins. These anti-GBM autoantibodies provoked proliferation of the glomerular epithelial cells and resulted in the formation of epithelial crescents containing fibrin, neutrophils, and macrophages. It proved possible to elute the antibodies from the kidney of one affected horse, a 6-year-old Thoroughbred mare.

This horse had a nasal hemangiosarcoma. The immunoglobulins were extracted from its kidney by acid elution and were shown to be directed specifically against the glomerular basement membrane. They did not bind to basement membranes in other body organs (Banks, 1979). A case of a severe protein-losing nephropathy due to an IgM-specific glomerulopathy has also been reported in a Quarter horse (McSloy et al., 2007).

References

Aleman, M. (2024). Inflammatory and immune-mediated myopathies: What do we know? *Veterinary Clinics of North America: Equine Practice, 40*, 207–218.

Aleman, M., Katzman, S. A., Vaughan, B., Hodges, J., et al. (2009). Antemortem diagnosis of polyneuritis equi. *Journal of Veterinary Internal Medicine, 23*, 665–668.

Banks, K. L. (1979). Animal model: Antiglomerular basement membrane antibody in horses. *American Journal of Pathology, 94*(2), 443–446.

Braus, B. K., Miller, I., Kummer, S., Kleinwort, K. J. H., et al. (2017). Investigation of corneal autoantibodies in horses with immune mediated keratitis (IMMK). *Veterinary Immunology and Immunopathology, 187*, 48–54.

Carter, S. D., Osborne, A. C., May, S. A., & Bennett, D. (1995). Rheumatoid factor, anti-heat shock protein (65 kDa) antibodies and antinuclear antibodies in equine joint diseases. *Equine Veterinary Journal, 27*(4), 288–295.

Deeg, C. A., Kaspers, B., Gerhards, H., Thurau, S. R., et al. (2001). Immune responses to retinal autoantigens and peptides in equine recurrent uveitis. *Investigative Ophthalmology & Visual Science, 42*, 393–398.

Degroote, R. L., Hauck, S. M., Amann, B., Hirmer, S., et al. (2014). Unraveling the equine lymphocyte proteome: Differential septin 7 expression associates with immune cells in equine recurrent uveitis. *PLoS One*. https://doi.org/10.1371/journal.pone.0091684

Druml, T., Brem, G., Velie, B., Lindgren, G., et al. (2021). Equine vitiligo-like depigmentation in grey horses is related to genes involved in immune response and tumor metastasis. *BMC Veterinary Research*. https://doi.org/10.1186/s12917-021-03046-x

Durward-Akhurst, S. A., & Valberg, S. J. (2018). Immune-mediated muscle disease in the horse. *Veterinary Pathology Online, 55*, 68–75.

Durward-Akhurst, S. A., & Valberg, S. J. (2025). Myosin heavy chain myopathy and immune-mediated muscle disorders. *Veterinary Clinics of North America: Equine Practice, 41*, 61–75.

Dwyer, A. E., Crockett, R. S., & Kalsow, C. M. (1995). Association of Leptospiral seroreactivity and breed with uveitis and blindness in horses: 372 cases (1986–1993). *Journal of the American Veterinary Medical Association, 207*, 1327–1331.

Easton-Jones, C. A. (2024). Clinical approach to immune-mediated hemolytic anemia and thrombocytopenia. *Veterinary Clinics of North America: Equine Practice, 40*, 263–273.

Edington, N., Wright, J. A., Patel, J. R., et al. (1984). Equine adenovirus 1 isolated from cauda equina neuritis. *Research in Veterinary Science, 37*, 252–254.

Ellison, S. P., Kennedy, T., Li, A., & Schweiss, L. (2015). Serum antibodies against a reactive site of equine myelin protein 2 linked to polyneuritis equi found in horses diagnosed with EPM. *International Journal of Applied Research in Veterinary Medicine, 13*(3), 164–181.

Fadok, V. A. (1995). An overview of equine dermatoses characterized by scaling and crusting. *Veterinary Clinics of North America: Equine Practice, 11*, 43–51.

Fingerhut, L., Yucel, L., Strutzberg-Minder, K., Kockritz-Blickwede, M., et al. (2022). Ex vivo and in vitro analysis identify a detrimental impact of neutrophil extracellular traps on eye structure in equine recurrent uveitis. *Frontiers in Immunology*. https://doi.org/10.3389/fimmu.2022.830871

Fritz, K. L., Kaese, H. J., Valberg, S. J., Hendrickson, J. A., et al. (2014). Genetic risk factors for insidious equine recurrent uveitis in Appaloosa horses. *Animal Genetics*. https://doi.org/10.1111/age.12129

Geor, R. J., Clark, E. G., Haines, D. M., & Napier, P. G. (2005). Systemic lupus erythematosus in a filly. *Journal of the American Veterinary Medical Association, 197*, 1489–1492.

Gerding, J. C., & Gilger, B. C. (2016). Prognosis and impact of equine recurrent uveitis. *Equine Veterinary Journal*. https://doi.org/10.1111/evj.12451

Gershwin, L. J. (2005). Antinuclear antibodies in domestic animals. *Annals of the New York Academy of Sciences, 1050*, 364–370.

Grau-Roma, L., Peckham, R., Paton, J., Stahel, A., et al. (2016). Occurrence of primary lymphocytic hypophysitis in two horses and the presence of scattered T lymphocytes in the normal equine pituitary gland. *Journal of Veterinary Diagnostic Investigation, 29*(1), 115–121.

Hack, Y., Henriksen, M. L., Pihl, T. H., Nielsen, R. K., et al. (2022). Genetic investigation of equine recurrent uveitis in the Icelandic horse breed. *Animal Genetics, 53*, 436–440.

Hahn, C. N. (2008). Polyneuritis equi: The role of T-lymphocytes and importance of differential clinical signs. *Equine Veterinary Journal, 40*, 100.

Hoikhman, R., Kudlackova, H., Babak, V., Faldyna, M., & Jahn, P. (2018). Detection of IgM-rheumatoid factor and anti-citrullinated protein antibodies in healthy horses and their comparison. *Veterinary Immunology and Immunopathology, 202*, 141–146.

Hoolahan, D. E., White, S. D., Outerbridge, C. A., Shearer, P. L., & Affolter, V. K. (2013). Equine alopecia areata: A retrospective clinical descriptive study at the University of California, Davis. (1980–2011). *Veterinary Dermatology, 24*, Article 282-e64.

Horohov, D. W. (2000). Equine T cell cytokines: Protection and pathology. *Veterinary Clinics of North America: Equine Practice, 16*(1), 1–14.

Hunyadi, L., Sundman, E. A., Kass, P. H., Williams, D. C., & Aleman, M. (2017). Clinical implications and hospital outcomes of immune-mediated myositis in horses. *Journal of Veterinary Internal Medicine, 31*, 170–175.

Kimberly, M., McGurrin, J., Arroyo, L. G., & Bienzle, D. (2004). Flow cytometric detection of platelet-bound antibody in three horses with immune-mediated thrombocytopenia. *Journal of the American Veterinary Medical Association, 224*, 83–87.

Kingsley, N. B., Sandmeyer, L., & Bellone, R. R. (2023). A review of investigated risk factors for developing equine recurrent uveitis. *Veterinary Ophthalmology, 26*, 86–100.

Knickelbein, K. E., & Lassaline, M. E. (2024). Approach to immune-mediated ocular diseases. *Clinics: Equine Practice, 40*, 275–286.

Malalana, F., Stylianides, A., & McGowan, C. (2015). Equine recurrent uveitis: Human and equine perspectives. *Veterinary Journal, 206*, 22–29.

Marsella, R. (2024). Autoimmune dermatopathies of horses. *Clinics: Equine Practice, 40*, 237–251.

Matthews, A., & Gilger, B. C. (2009). Equine immune-mediated keratopathies. *Veterinary Opthalmology, 12*(Suppl. 1), 10–16.

McSloy, A., Poulsen, K., Fisher, P. J., Armien, A., et al. (2007). Diagnosis and treatment of a selective immunoglobulin M glomerulopathy in a Quarter Horse gelding. *Journal of Veterinary Internal Medicine, 21*, 874–877.

Michutta, J.-I., Reichelt, U., Crubel, A. D., & Gehlen, H. (2011). Bullous pemphigoid in the horse: Pathogenesis, diagnostic procedures and therapy. *Pferde Equine Medicine, 27*(6), 631–635.

Mosca, M., Randleff-Rasmussen, P., Milhau, N., Panzuti, P., et al. (2020). Long-term successful treatment of a donkey with cutaneous lupus erythematosus with methotrexate. *Veterinary Dermatology, 31*, Article 313-e78.

Mosos, E., Novales, M., & Sierra, M. A. (1991). Focal hypopigmentation in horses resembling Arabian Fading Syndrome. *Equine Veterinary Education, 3*(3), 122–125.

Nunez, R., Gomes-Keller, M. A., Schwartzwald, C., & Feige, K. (2001). Assessment of equine autoimmune thrombocytopenia (EAT) by flow cytometry. *BMC Blood Disorders, 1*, 1. https://doi.org/10.3389/1471-2326-/1/1

Olivry, T., Borrillo, A. K. G., Xu, L., Dunston, S. M., et al. (2000). Equine bullous pemphoid IgG autoantibodies target linear epitopes in the NC16A ectodomain of collagen XVII (BP180, BPAG2). *Veterinary Immunology and Immunopathology, 73*, 45–52.

Osborne, A. C., Carter, S. D., May, S. A., & Bennett, D. (1995). Anti-collagen antibodies and immune complexes in equine joint diseases. *Veterinary Immunology and Immunopathology, 45*, 19–30.

Pate, D. O., Clode, A. B., Olivry, T., Cullen, J. M., et al. (2012). Immunohistochemical and immunohistologic characterization of superficial stromal immune-mediated keratitis in horses. *American Journal of Veterinary Research, 73*, 1067–1073.

Preston, J. F., Mustikka, M. P., Priestnall, S. L., Dunkel, B., & Fischer, M.-C. (2023). Clinical features and outcomes of horses presenting with presumed equine immune-mediated keratitis to two veterinary hospitals in the United Kingdom and Finland: 94 cases (2009–2023). *Equine Veterinary Journal*. https://doi.org/10.1111/evj.14213

Pusterla, N., Pratt, S. M., Magdesian, K. G., et al. (2006). Idiopathic immune-mediated polysynovitis in three horses. *The Veterinary Record, 159*, 13–15.

Reilly, L., & Beech, J. (1994). Bilateral keratoconjunctivitis sicca in a horse. *Equine Veterinary Journal, 26*(2), 171–172.

Rockwell, H., Mack, M., Famula, T., Sandmeyer, L., et al. (2019). Genetic investigation of equine recurrent uveitis in Appaloosa horses. *Animal Genetics, 51*, 111–116.

Rosenkrantz, W. (2013). Immune-mediated dermatoses. *Clinics: Equine Practice, 29*, 607–613.

Rosychuk, R. A. W. (2013). Noninflammatory, nonpruritic alopecia of horses. *Clinics: Equine Practice, 29*, 629–641.

Saldinger, L. K., Nelson, S. G., Bellone, R. R., Lassaline, M., et al. (2020). Horses with equine recurrent uveitis have an activated CD4+ T-cell phenotype that can be modulated by mesenchymal stem cells in vitro. *Veterinary Opthalmology, 23*, 160–170.

Tham, H. L., Linder, K. E., & Olivrey, T. (2019). Autoimmune diseases affecting skin melanocytes in dogs, cats, and horses: Vitiligo and uveodermatological syndrome: A comprehensive review. *BMC Veterinary Research*. https://doi.org/10.1186/s12917-019-2003-9

Tham, H. L., Linder, K. E., & Olivrey, T. (2020). Deep pemphigus (Pemphigus vulgarism, pemohigus vegetans and paraneoplastic pemphigus) in dogs, cats, and horses: A comprehensive review. *BMC Veterinary Research*. https://doi.org/10.1186/s12917-020-02677-w

van Galen, G., Cassart, D., Sandersen, C., et al. (2008). The composition of the inflammatory infiltrate in three cases of polyneuritis equi. *Equine Veterinary Journal, 40*, 185–188.

Vandenabeele, S. I., White, S. D., Affolter, V. K., et al. (2004). Pemphigus foliaceus in the horse: A retrospective study of 20 cases. *Veterinary Dermatology, 15*, 381–388.

Vrins, A., & Feldman, B. F. (1983). Lupus erythematosus-like syndrome in a horse. *Equine Practice, 3*, 8–25.

Ward, R. (1880). Rheumatoid arthritis in the horse. *Veterinary Journal and Annals of Comparative Pathology, 10*(4), 245–2487.

Weigand, M., Hauck, S. M., Deeg, C. A., & Degroote, R. L. (2021). Deviant proteome profile of equine granulocytes associates to latent activation status in organ-specific autoimmune disease. *Journal of Proteomics*. https://doi.org/10.1016/j.jprot.2020.103989

Weiss, D. J., & Moritz, A. (2003). Equine immune-mediated hemolytic anemia associated with *Clostridium perfringens* infection. *Veterinary Clinical Pathology, 32*, 22–26.

Wiedemann, C., Amann, C., Degroote, R. L., Witte, T., & Deeg, C. A. (2020). Aberrant migratory behavior of immune cells in recurrent autoimmune uveitis in horses. *Frontiers in Cell and Developmental Biology*. https://doi.org/10.3389/fcell.2020.00101

Wilkerson, M. J., Davis, E., Shuman, W., Harkin, K., Cox, J., & Rush, B. (2000). Isotype-specific antibodies in horses and dogs with immune-mediated hemolytic anemia. *Journal of Veterinary Internal Medicine, 14*, 190–196.

Williams, M. A., Dowling, P. M., Angarano, D. W., et al. (1995). Paraneoplastic bullous stomatitis in a horse. *Journal of the American Veterinary Medical Association, 207*, 331–334.

Winfield, L. D., White, S. D., Affolter, V. K., Renier, A. C., et al. (2013). Pemphigus vulgaris in a Welsh pony stallion. Case report and demonstration of antidesmoglein autoantibodies. *Veterinary Dermatology, 24*, Article 269-e60.

Wright, J. A., Fordyce, P., & Edington, N. (1987). Neuritis of the cauda equina in the horse. *Journal of Comparative Pathology, 97*, 667–675.

Younis, S., Moutusy, S. I., Rasouli, S., Jahanbani, S., et al. (2025). Epstein-Barr virus reprograms autoreactive B cells as antigen-presenting cells in systemic lupus erythematosus. *Science Translational Medicine, 17*, Article ady0210.

Yvorchuk-St Jean, K. (1987). Neuritis of the cauda equina. *Veterinary Clinics of North America: Equine Practice, 3*, 421–427.

Zabel, S., Mueller, R. S., Fieseler, K. V., et al. (2005). Review of 15 cases of pemphigus foliaceus in horses and a survey of the literature. *The Veterinary Record, 157*, 505–509.

Zhou, X., Yan, J., Lu, Q., Zhou, H., & Fan, L. (2020). The pathogenesis of cutaneous lupus erythematosus: The aberrant distribution and function of different cell types in skin lesions. *Scandinavian Journal of Immunology*. https://doi.org/10.1111/sji.12933

CHAPTER

Equine immunodeficiency diseases 23

The immune systems do not always work properly. Problems, defects, and diseases may arise and result in immune deficiencies. This loss of a properly functioning immune system is usually reflected in an increased susceptibility to infections, especially those caused by opportunistic pathogens. Defects may also develop in the innate immune system. One equine example is Pelger-Huet anomaly that affects neutrophil functions in Arabian horses. More significantly, defects can develop in the adaptive immune system. These may result from inherited genetic mutations and are classified as primary immunodeficiencies. Others may be the consequences of factors not directly involved in the immune system. These include a failure of passive transfer through the mare's colostrum, vitamin deficiencies, transportation stresses, and pituitary pars intermedia dysfunction. These are considered secondary immunodeficiencies.

Primary immunodeficiencies

Immunodeficiencies resulting from genetic defects classically present themselves in young foals once the protection afforded by maternal immunity has waned. Horses are among the few domestic animals whose economic worth has permitted a thorough analysis of neonatal foal mortality. As a result, a significant number of primary immunodeficiency syndromes have been identified in this species (Crisman & Scarratt, 2008; Perryman, 2000).

Pelger-Huët anomaly

As described in Chapter 4, Pelger-Huët anomaly is an autosomal dominant disorder characterized by a failure of granulocyte nuclei to segment into lobes. Pelger-Huët anomaly has been reported to occur in Arabian horses (Gill et al., 2008; Grondin et al., 2007). The hyposegmentation also affects the nuclei of their eosinophils and basophils. It reportedly has a minimal effect on the health of horses. However, these neutrophils are less able to emigrate from blood vessels in vivo (Latimer et al., 2000).

The Immunology of Horses and Donkeys. https://doi.org/10.1016/B978-0-443-44863-8.00003-X

Severe combined immunodeficiency

Severe combined immunodeficiency (SCID) is an autosomal recessive disease that affects some Arabian foals. Affected foals fail to produce functional T or B cells and therefore have very few circulating lymphocytes. If they suckle successfully, they acquire maternal immunoglobulins. Once these have declined, however, these foals cannot produce their own antibodies and eventually become agammaglobulinemic. Affected foals are therefore born healthy but begin to sicken by 2 months of age. The precise time of disease onset depends on the quantity of colostral antibodies absorbed. All affected foals die by 4–6 months as a result of overwhelming gastrointestinal or respiratory infections. Severe bronchopneumonia is the predominant presenting sign. Organisms that have been implicated in this bronchopneumonia include equine adenovirus, *Rhodococcus equi,* and *Pneumocystis carinii* (an opportunistic fungal pathogen). The disease is manifested by a nasal discharge, coughing, dyspnea, weight loss, and fevers. Affected foals may also develop enteritis, omphalophlebitis, and many other infections. The protozoan *Cryptosporidium parvum* and many different bacteria have been implicated in the enteritis.

Affected foals develop a severe, persistent lymphopenia. They make no IgM, and the only IgG in their serum is from their mare's colostrum. On necropsy, their spleens lack germinal centers and periarteriolar lymphoid sheaths. Their lymph nodes lack lymphoid follicles and germinal centers, and there are few cells in the node paracortex. These may contain small clumps of lymphoid cells that resemble plasma cells. Their thymus is severely hypoplastic and may be difficult to find. However, their basic thymic structure is unchanged, despite the absence of thymocytes (McGuire, Banks, & Davis, 1976). Their neutrophil, monocyte, and NK cell numbers and functions appear normal.

SCID is an autosomal recessive disease, and its occurrence therefore indicates that both parents carry the mutation. Accurate diagnosis is of great importance since the presence of the mutation significantly reduces the value of the parent animals. Thus, all suspected cases must be confirmed by postmortem examination. The clinical diagnosis of SCID requires that at least two of the following three criteria be established: (1) very low (consistently below $1000/mm^3$) circulating lymphocytes; (2) histology typical of SCID; that is, gross hypoplasia of the primary and secondary lymphoid organs; and (3) an absence of IgM from presuckle serum. (The normal equine fetus synthesizes small amounts of IgM. As a result, IgM in normal newborn foals is about 160 μg/mL. If the foal successfully suckles, it will obtain immunoglobulins of all isotypes from the mare's colostrum. However, the half-life of equine IgM is only about 6 days, so maternal IgM will disappear within a few days of birth. Thus, a normal foal will always have some IgM in its serum, but an SCID foal will have none.)

Pathogenesis

When B and T cell antigen receptors are generated, large segments of DNA are excised so that the *V, D,* and *J* genes can be rejoined (Chapters 11 and 12). Several enzymes are involved in this recombination process. Some cut the DNA strands, and others join them. Studies on SCID foals show that there is a defect in the large multi-component enzyme that rejoins the cut ends. The specific defect lies in the gene coding for the catalytic subunit of an enzyme called DNA-dependent protein kinase *($DNA\text{-}PK_{cs}$)* (Shin et al., 1997). In the mutant $DNA\text{-}PK_{cs}$ gene, a loss of five nucleotides results in a frameshift, premature termination of the peptide chain with a loss of 967 amino acids from the C-terminus of the molecule, including its entire kinase domain. As a result, functional $DNA\text{-}PK_{cs}$ is totally absent from affected foals. Because of this deficiency, broken DNA strands cannot be rejoined, and neither T cells nor B cells can form functional V regions in their antigen receptors. In the absence of TCRs and BCRs, affected foals cannot respond to any antigens (Perryman, 2004). Since $DNA\text{-}PK_{cs}$ is needed to rejoin broken strands of DNA, it also plays a key role in other DNA repair processes. For example, the cells from SCID foals are unable to repair DNA damaged by radiation Figs. 23.1 and 23.2.

The presence of a mutant *SCID* gene in horses can be detected by means of a PCR test. A sample of DNA is obtained from horse skin cells. A primer set designed to amplify only DNA containing the 5-base pair deletion and another set designed to amplify only the normal gene sequence are used to determine whether the mutant gene is present. This test has demonstrated that the prevalence of the *SCID* gene in Arabian horses is 8.4%. Based on this, it would be expected that 0.18% of Arabian foals would be homozygous for the trait and hence clinically affected. Pedigree

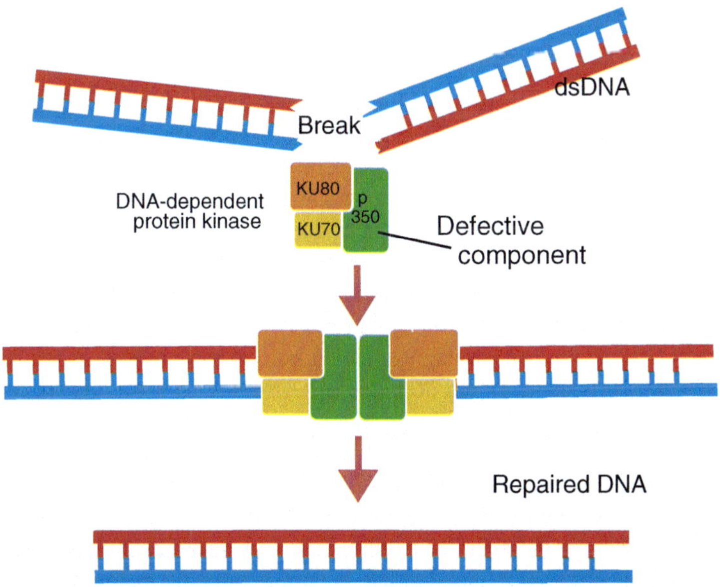

FIGURE 23.1

The defect in DNA-dependent protein kinase (DNA-PK) that prevents DNA repair in SCID foals.

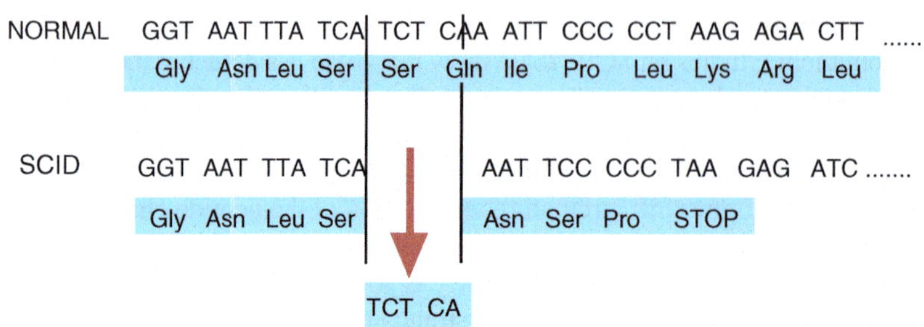

FIGURE 23.2

The deletion of five nucleotides, (TCTCA) in the equine *DNA-PK* gene results in premature termination of the molecule and hence its inactivation.

analysis suggests that the SCID trait was introduced to the United States by a single stallion in the 1920s (Bernoco & Bailey, 1998).

While heterozygous horses are apparently healthy, since they carry one copy of the intact gene, it has been reported that they suffer from an increased prevalence of sarcoid tumors (Ding et al., 2002). Thus, in a survey of sarcoids in Arabians, 19/102 (18.6%) carried the mutant PK gene allele. This is much greater than the 8.4% prevalence in healthy horses (Chapter 21).

Immunoglobulin deficiencies

Primary agammaglobulinemia

Primary agammaglobulinemia is a rare disease of foals. Affected animals totally lack identifiable B cells (cells with surface immunoglobulins) and, once maternal antibodies wane, serum immunoglobulin levels become undetectable (Banks et al., 1976). Affected foals do not mount an antibody response to vaccines. On necropsy, it appears that their lymphoid tissues contain no primary follicles, germinal centers, or plasma cells. Affected foals experience recurrent bacterial infections but may survive for up to 18 months with intensive antibiotic treatment. The disease should be suspected in a foal having a normal lymphocyte count but lacking both IgM and IgG. It may be confirmed by showing normal responses to T cell mitogens and an absence of B cells (Deem et al., 1979). The precise molecular basis of this disease is unknown, but it is similar in many respects to human agammaglobulinemia caused by a mutation in the gene that encodes Bruton tyrosine kinase. In the absence of this kinase, foals are born with a stem cell defect that results in a failure to produce any functional B cells. There may be a persistent low level of immunoglobulin production, suggesting that a few B cells may develop. One report describes five cases of agammaglobulinemia that occurred only in male Thoroughbreds, Quarter Horses, and Standardbreds, so it appears to be an X-linked disorder. The parents of affected foals may be considered to carry the relevant mutations, so they should be excluded from breeding programs (Perryman et al., 1983).

These agammaglobulinemic foals appear to have normal T cell functions. Thus, their blood lymphocyte numbers are normal. Their blood lymphocytes (primarily T cells) can respond to mitogens such as phytohemagglutinin. Likewise, intradermal inoculation of phytohemagglutinin induces a typical type IV delayed hypersensitivity reaction (McGuire, Banks, Evans, & Poppie, 1976).

As in other primary immunodeficiencies, clinical disease presents itself at 2–6 months of age once maternal immunity has waned. Recurrent opportunistic bacterial infections, especially arthritis, laminitis, or respiratory disease develop. Bacterial dermatitis and enteritis have also been reported. Affected foals may become extremely anemic. Complications of sepsis include disseminated intravascular coagulation, acute renal failure, pulmonary thromboembolism, acute respiratory distress syndrome, and intractable hypotension and cardiac arrest.

This disease is uniformly fatal, but affected foals may survive for as long as 1–2 years. Given that these recurrent infections are usually bacterial in origin and may be controlled for a time by aggressive antibiotic therapy, prolonging their lives may be achievable, but may not be the most appropriate course. Supportive care to control opportunistic infections is entirely appropriate until it is determined whether the agammaglobulinemia is persistent rather than transient (Riggs, 1987).

Selective IgM deficiency

An inherited immunodeficiency syndrome characterized by low or absent serum IgM with normal or elevated levels of other immunoglobulin classes has also been reported to occur in foals. Serum IgM levels in these animals are at least two standard deviations below normal (less than 15–25 mg/dL), but IgG and IgA levels and B cell numbers are within normal limits (Weldon et al., 1992). SCID occurs in 2%–3% of Arab foals and is 10 times more common than selective IgM deficiency. Selective IgM deficiency is, in turn, 10 times more common than agammaglobulinemia Fig. 23.3.

The absence of IgM may result from decreased production or increased catabolism, or because of excessive regulatory T-cell activity. Lymphocyte counts are usually within normal ranges, so there is no gross B- or T-cell deficit.Multiple IgM assays must be performed to confirm that the levels are persistently depressed. On necropsy, the lymphoid tissues of affected animals are apparently normal.

Clinical signs first develop around 2–3 months of age as maternal immunity wanes. In most cases, foals develop septicemia or recurrent respiratory tract infections, often involving *Klebsiella pneumoniae* or *R. equi*. Recurrent severe infections, especially diarrhea, arthritis, or respiratory disease leading to death, occur before the age of 10 months. Foals have a history of repeated infections that usually respond to aggressive antibiotic treatment. Unfortunately, infections recur after treatment has stopped. Some affected foals live longer and respond to therapy but fail to grow, have recurrent respiratory infections, and usually die by 24 months. The deficiency has been most often reported in Arabians and Quarter Horses, but other breeds are also affected, suggesting that the disease has a genetic basis.

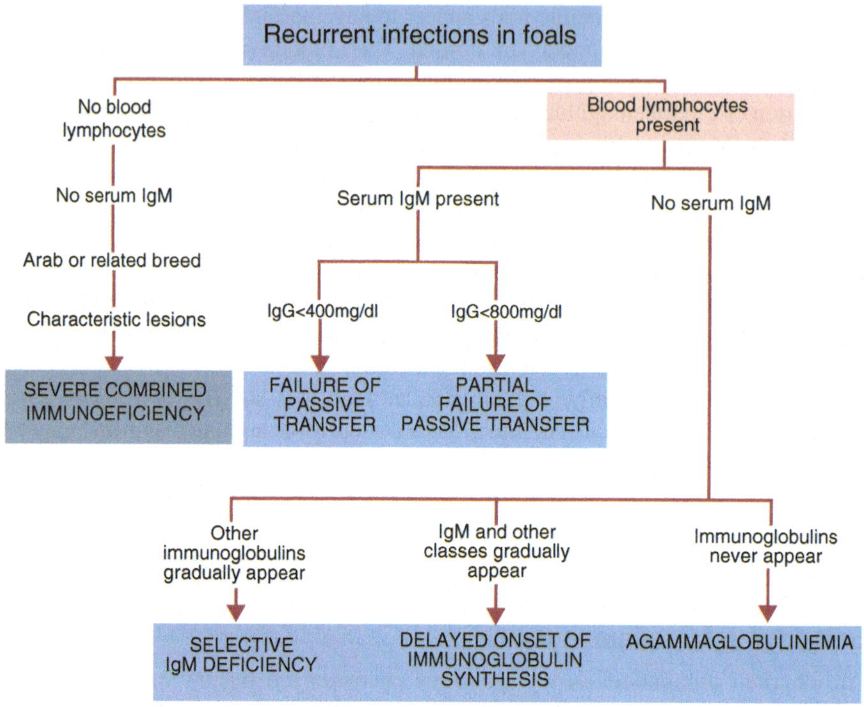

FIGURE 23.3

The differential diagnosis of equine primary immunodeficiencies.

If the foal is identified as lacking IgM before the development of sepsis or pneumonia, then prompt treatment should be instituted to address the deficit. If, however, the foal presents with severe infections, then these must be promptly controlled. Complications of sepsis include disseminated intravascular coagulation, acute renal failure, pulmonary thromboembolism, acute respiratory distress syndrome, intractable hypotension, and cardiac arrest. A transient form of IgM deficiency has been described in foals with chronic infections such as those caused by *R. equi* (Freestone et al., 1989). The IgM levels eventually recover as the animal's immune system responds to the infection (Magdesian, 2024). Another form of IgM deficiency with serum levels under 60 mg/dL has also been described as occurring in adult horses over 2 years of age. In many cases, such horses also have a lymphoid neoplasm (Perkins et al., 2003; Perryman, 1984).

Other selective immunoglobulin deficiencies

A single case of a selective IgG deficiency has been described in a 3-month-old foal with salmonellosis. The animal had normal IgA and IgM but no germinal centers, lymphoid follicles, splenic follicles, or periarteriolar lymphoid sheaths. Serum

IgG was extremely low. In another single case, a 10-month-old Arabian foal had no detectable IgM, IgA, or IgG3/5. but a normal concentration of the remaining IgG subclasses. Its lymphocytes responded normally to T cell mitogens but not to B cell mitogens. There was lymphocyte depletion in its thymus and spleen. Necropsy showed the presence of inflammatory cells throughout all its major organs (Boy et al., 1992).

Foal immunodeficiency syndrome

Fell ponies are a small, hardy breed of mountain pony that originated in northwest England. Dales ponies are a related mountain breed from further south. They are both breeds with very small numbers and employ a limited diversity of favored stallions. As a result, they are seriously inbred. The development of a genetic disease is thus not unexpected. An autosomal recessive syndrome consisting of severe anemia, peripheral ganglionopathy, and immunodeficiency has been reported in their foals. This primary immunodeficiency syndrome was first described in the Fell and Dales pony breeds but can occur in any horse breed (Butler et al., 2006). It occurs in animals of both sexes and is believed to be autosomal in nature. It presents as a B-cell immunodeficiency accompanied by a profound anemia (Scholes et al., 1998). Affected foals appear normal at birth but fail to thrive. Their hematocrit declines over 4–12 weeks until clinical disease, develops (Thomas et al., 2003). Affected animals lack germinal centers and plasma cells. Their B cell numbers decline to less than 10% of normal, and serum immunoglobulin levels drop rapidly once maternal antibodies are catabolized (Thomas et al., 2005). The loss of these immunoglobulins coincides with the development of clinical disease. T cell numbers remain within the normal range (Bell et al., 2001).

Infections develop at 2–32 weeks of age as maternal immunity wanes. The foals become extremely anemic. Some develop a necrotizing enterocolitis with severe diarrhea (Jelinek et al., 2006). Foals may develop severe bronchopneumonia caused by opportunistic pathogens such as adenoviruses, and from diarrhea caused by Cryptosporidium. At the same time, they develop a profound progressive, nonregenerative anemia that alone may be sufficient to cause death. Many develop neurologic disease prior to death. Foals inevitably die or are euthanized by 1–3 months of age (Fox-Clipsham et al., 2009; Gardner et al., 2006).

Affected foals develop severe normochromic to macrocytic anemia as a result of a failure to develop bone marrow erythroid stem cells. Their thymus is hypoplastic, and their secondary lymphoid organs are poorly developed. Affected foals have a marked lymphopenia, and their lymphoid organs lack germinal centers and plasma cells, confirming a B-cell deficiency. Immunoglobulin levels appear to be relatively normal, but any immunoglobulin deficiency may be masked by maternal antibodies. The neurologic signs are a result of a peripheral ganglionopathy that involves the trigeminal, craniomesenteric, and dorsal root ganglia. These result in gastrointestinal dysfunction and muscle weakness (Tallmadge et al., 2020).

Neutrophil counts are normal. Flow cytometry shows that T-cell numbers are within the normal range but B cells are undetectable. $CD4^+$ and $CD8^+$ T-cells show reduced MHC Class II expression. Mitogenic responses to phytohemagglutinin and concanavalin A are normal. Mitogenic responses to bacterial lipopolysaccharide, a B-cell mitogen, are severely depressed. Complications of sepsis include disseminated intravascular coagulation, multiorgan dysfunction syndrome, acute renal failure, pulmonary thromboembolism, acute respiratory distress syndrome, intractable hypotension, and cardiac arrest. This disease is uniformly fatal. The foals usually die or are euthanized by 3 months of age as a result of infections with *Cryptosporidium* spp. or adenoviruses.

Foal immunodeficiency syndrome is inherited as an autosomal recessive disease. It results from a mutation in the gene coding for the sodium/myoinositol cotransporter (*SLC5A3*) located on chromosome ECA26. (The mutation switches a single amino acid from proline to leucine and is homozygous in affected foals.). This protein controls cellular osmotic regulation and is required for lymphoid cell survival and erythropoiesis. A PCR-based test is available that can be used to determine whether a foal carries the mutant gene. Carrier rates are about 40% for Fell ponies and 20% for Dales ponies.) (Tallmadge, Stokol, et al., 2012) The disease prevalence has been markedly reduced as carrier breeding has been avoided, although the carrier rate remains relatively high, as might be expected within such a small breeding population (Carter et al., 2013).

Delayed immunoglobulin synthesis

A syndrome characterized by the delayed onset of immunoglobulin synthesis in newborn foals has been described in Thoroughbreds and Arabians but has not been proven to be genetic in origin. At birth, foals are protected by maternal antibodies acquired through colostrum and are clinically normal. These antibodies provide effective protection for 1–3 months, although their levels decline gradually. As maternal antibodies decline, the foal begins to make its own immunoglobulins. Under normal circumstances, the decline of maternal antibodies occurs at the same time as autologous antibody production begins, so there is no gap in protection and the foal is never without detectable serum antibodies Fig. 23.4.

However, between 2 and 4 months of age, some foals experience hypogammaglobulinemia as a result of a delayed onset of immunoglobulin synthesis. Their IgG, IgM, and IgA concentrations are abnormally low, but not absent. Affected foals have normal blood lymphocytes, and T-cell function assays are normal. Recurrent opportunistic infections, especially diarrhea, arthritis, or respiratory disease, may develop during this period. The prognosis is good, provided bacterial and viral infections are well controlled.

Most of these foals eventually recover and develop normal immunoglobulin levels by 6 months (McGuire et al., 1975). Repeated serum immunoglobulin quantitation is required to document this condition and monitor the onset of

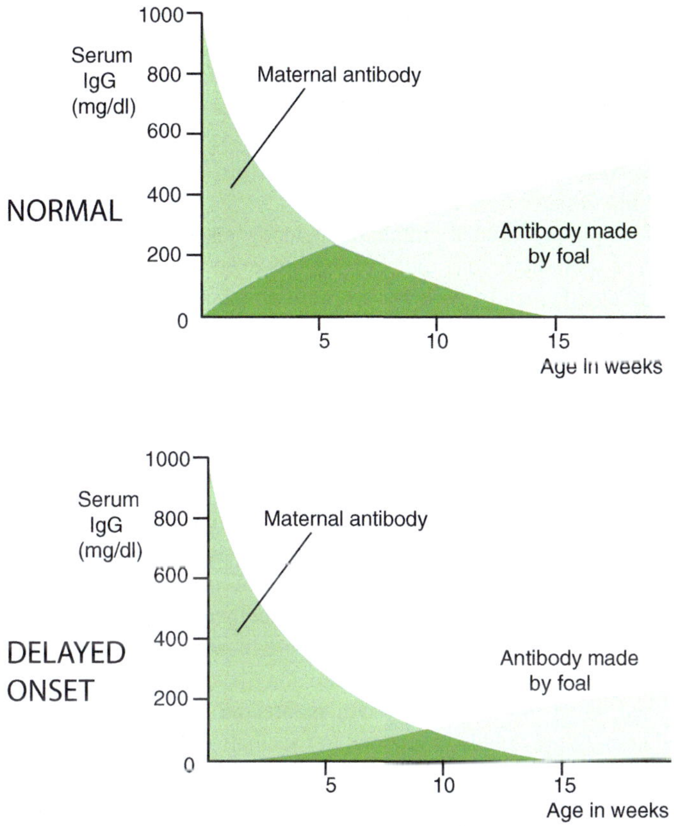

FIGURE 23.4 The effects of delayed onset of immunoglobulin synthesis in the fial.

If a foal delays production of its own antibodies, it will suffer a period of transient hypogammaglobulinemia as maternal antibodies persistently decline.

immunoglobulin synthesis. The true prevalence of this disease is unclear. It may well be much more common than reported, and its severity and duration are highly variable. Because this disease is likely heritable, it is appropriate to discourage future breeding of the parent animals.

Common variable immunodeficiency

Common variable immunodeficiency (CVID) is the second most common primary immunodeficiency syndrome in humans (after selective IgA deficiency). In humans, it is a heterogeneous group of sporadic diseases all characterized by a late-onset B-cell lymphopenia. It is often accompanied by microbial dysbiosis, autoimmunity, or lymphoid malignancies (Flaminio et al., 2009).

In the horse, CVID presents as a B cell deficiency in adult horses that results in a persistent hypogammaglobulinemia with a serum IgG level below 1000 mg/dL (Felippe, 2023). It has been reported to affect multiple breeds, including Thoroughbreds, Quarter Horses, and Arabians, as well as Paints and ponies (Tallmadge et al., 2020). B cells in affected horses account for less than 2% of their total circulating lymphocytes. As a result, affected horses suffer from recurrent bacterial infections (Flaminio et al., 2002).

Cases of common variable immunodeficiency resemble primary immunodeficiencies in their sporadic nature and severity; however, they usually occur in animals over 3 years of age. Typically, these horses present with recurrent infections and fevers that are not responsive to treatment. Chronic respiratory infections are the most common manifestation. Bacterial meningitis may also be a consistent feature (Pelligrini-Masini et al., 2005). Other presentations include cholangiohepatitis, colitis, dermatitis, and severe gastrointestinal parasitism (Felippe, 2023). Their serum contains only trace levels of IgG and IgM, no detectable IgG3, and very low IgA levels (Tallmadge, Such, et al., 2012). Sometimes individual IgG subclasses are deficient, whereas IgA levels are normal. T cell numbers are normal, but B cells may be undetectable, and there is no mitogenic B cell response to bacterial lipopolysaccharide. On necropsy, examination of the lymphoid organs shows the presence of many T cells, but germinal centers are absent, and there are very few scattered B cells in the lymphoid organs, blood, or bone marrow. Some horses may develop severe liver disease, a feature also seen in humans. It is suspected that these individuals may have an underlying defect that is only expressed when the immune system is stressed by infection. In many cases, the affected animals are unable to respond to vaccination. Many develop a concurrent lymphosarcoma, and they may have excessive regulatory T cell function.

Because of the great variability in severity of this syndrome, treatment success and prognosis are unpredictable. Some animals may require minimal support. Others may require euthanasia. As with all immunodeficiency diseases, the prognosis is guarded. However, CVID, as its name suggests, is of variable severity. Some horses succumb rapidly. Some with mild disease may well survive in apparent health, especially if recurrent infections are promptly and aggressively treated (Mullen & Felippe, 2024).

In humans with CVID, four genes, *E2A, PAX5, CD19,* and *IGD,* have significantly reduced expression (Flaminio et al., 2002). Immunohistochemistry has confirmed the absence of PAX5 in the bone marrow of affected horses. PAX5 and the other molecules are known to be transcription factors that regulate the early differentiation of B cells. Their B-cell development seems to be blocked at the transition to pro-B cells (Tallmadge et al., 2015). It is suggested that the late onset of this disease is a result of aberrant epigenetic regulation of the gene that results in PAX5 gene silencing. Thus, studies have confirmed that the PAX5 enhancer region is heavily methylated, a feature that will suppress gene expression and B cell differentiation. Mutations in genes coding for tumor necrosis factor (TNF-α) receptors and other co-stimulatory molecules may also result in loss of helper T cell function (Lobito et al., 2011).

Secondary immunodeficiencies

Equine secondary immunodeficiencies develop as a result of the effects of external factors on the immune system. They are not inherited and may be cured once the inciting cause is identified and eliminated.

Failure of passive transfer

The most common immunodeficiency occurring in foals is not inherited but results from a failure to absorb sufficient colostral antibodies from the mare. This failure of passive transfer may affect up to 20% of all foals. Of these 18% had partial failure while 2% had total failure (Gallacher et al., 2025). Failure is considered partial if IgG concentrations are in the range of 400–800 mg/dL (The average normal serum IgG level is approximately 2000 mg/dL) If their serum levels are below 400 mg/dL (<4 g/L), they are considered to be suffering from a total failure of passive transfer (McGuire et al., 1975). Risk factors for failure include the age of the mare, the month of birth, and the foal's birthweight.

The absorption of IgG from colostrum is required for the protection of a newborn foal against septicemic disease. The continuous intake of IgA or IgG1 from milk is required for protection against enteric disease. Failure of these processes leaves the newborn essentially defenseless. There are three major reasons for the failure of passive transfer through colostrum. First, the mare may produce insufficient or poor-quality colostrum (production failure). Second, there may be sufficient colostrum produced, but inadequate intake by the newborn foal (ingestion failure). Third, there may be a failure of immunoglobulin absorption from the intestine despite an adequate intake of colostrum (absorption failure).

Production failure

Since colostrum represents the accumulated secretions of the mammary glands in late pregnancy, premature births may mean that insufficient colostrum has accumulated. Valuable colostrum may also be lost as a result of premature lactation or excessive dripping. Colostral IgG levels also vary among individuals, with up to 28% of mares producing low-quality colostrum. It is not possible to assess colostral quality simply by looking at it. Its IgG content should be assessed using a colostrometer (a modified hydrometer) to measure its specific gravity. In mares, this is normally in the range of 1.060–1.085, equivalent to an IgG concentration of 3000–8500 mg/dL. Colostrum with an IgG level of less than 3000 mg/dL may be insufficient to protect a foal, and feeding supplemental, high-quality colostrum may become necessary.

Ingestion failure

In some foals, an inadequate intake may be due to poor mothering, an important problem among young, inexperienced mares. It may also be due to weakness in the newborn foal, to a poor suckling drive, or physical problems such as damaged teats or jaw defects.

Absorption failure

Failure of intestinal absorption is especially important in horses not only because of the value of many foals but also because even with good husbandry, about 25% of newborn foals fail to absorb sufficient quantities of immunoglobulins. Foals require serum IgG concentrations of at least 800 mg/dL by 18–24 hours after receiving colostrum to ensure satisfactory protection.

Diagnosis of failure of passive transfer

The success of passive transfer cannot be evaluated in a foal until 18–24 hours after birth, when antibody absorption is essentially complete. Several assays for serum immunoglobulins are available. The most rapid and economic procedure is the zinc sulfate turbidity test, which involves mixing a zinc sulfate solution with foal serum. Zinc sulfate precipitates globulins, and the amount of precipitate is proportional to the immunoglobulin concentration. In total failure of transfer, the reaction mixture remains clear. In sera with an IgG level of more than 400 mg/dL, the mixture becomes cloudy. As an alternative to visual inspection, the optical density of the mixtures can be read in a spectrophotometer, and the IgG concentration read off a standard curve. The relative amount of precipitate can also be read in a hematocrit capillary (immunocrit). Similar techniques include precipitation by ammonium sulfate, glutaraldehyde, or sodium sulfite (Clabough et al., 1989). Single radial immunodiffusion is a more accurate method in that it is both quantitative and specific for IgG. Known standards are compared with the test serum by measuring the diameter of precipitation produced in agar gel containing an antiserum to equine IgG. Unfortunately, radial immunodiffusion takes 18–24 hours to obtain a result and is thus impractical when a rapid diagnosis is needed (Davis et al., 2005).

A third method of measuring IgG levels is by use of a latex agglutination test. The latex particles are coated with anti-equine IgG. In the presence of IgG, they agglutinate. This test can be performed in about 10 minutes using either whole foal blood or serum. It appears to be reliable and rapid but somewhat insensitive.

It is also possible to use a semi-quantitative membrane-filter enzyme-linked immunosorbent assay (ELISA) test to measure IgG in a foal's serum. The color intensity of the reaction on the test filter is compared with color calibration spots. A variant technique uses a dipstick ELISA. Less satisfactory techniques include serum protein electrophoresis and refractometry. Point-of-care portable analyzers also provide acceptable results in a timely manner.

Management of failure of passive transfer

Colostrum may be obtained from mares that have more than is needed for their own young. It can be stored frozen at −15 to −20°C for up to 1 year (Nath et al., 2010). If stored colostrum is not available, fresh colostrum from primiparous mares can be used. If no colostrum is available, serum or plasma may be administered orally (Baldwin et al., 1991).

In foals that are over 15 hours old, oral absorption ceases, and intravenous plasma infusion must be given. Ideally, the dose used can be calculated to attain an IgG level of greater than 400 mg/dL. Frozen horse plasma is available commercially, although this may not contain antibodies against local pathogens. Alternatively, the plasma may be obtained from local donors. Blood should be collected aseptically with heparin or sodium citrate. The plasma is collected after the erythrocytes settle and is stored frozen until used. The plasma must be pre-checked for anti-erythrocyte antibodies and must be free of bacterial contamination. The transfusion should be given slowly while the foal is monitored for any adverse reactions. All foals receiving supplemental colostrum or plasma should have their serum IgG levels rechecked 12–24 hours later (Vivrette, 2001).

Vitamin deficiencies

Mammals depend on certain key dietary vitamins to maintain proper immune functions. Horses and donkeys are no exception. Vitamins E and D are considered the vitamins that are most essential for the proper functioning of their immune systems.

Vitamin E encompasses powerful antioxidants belonging to the tocopherol family. They are required for the effective functioning of cellular bactericidal activity and, most importantly, for the synthesis of IgG. Aged horses on a diet supplemented with vitamin E had increased bactericidal activity in their monocytes and neutrophils as well as higher IgG1 levels in serum (Petersson et al., 2010). More importantly, a vitamin E deficiency resulted in decreased serum immunoglobulin levels to approximately half normal levels in a herd of donkeys (Verdonck et al., 2007).

A second vitamin considered critical to normal immune function is vitamin D. Calcitriol (25(OH)D_3) is a bioactive form of vitamin D_3 and a potent immunomodulator. It is derived from the photoconversion of 7-dihydrocholesterol to vitamin D_3 (cholecalciferol) in the skin by UV sunlight exposure. Vitamin D is then hydroxylated to form calcitriol. Calcitriol plays a critical role in macrophage activation and thus defense against intracellular bacteria. It plays a key role in the modulation of cytokine production and promotes the production of β-defensins. For example, it acts on T cells, regulating their IFN-γ production (White, 2008). The effects of vitamin D are determined not only by its concentration in equine blood but also by the availability of its receptor. For example, the expression of this receptor is significantly higher on alveolar macrophages from 8-week foals than from 2-week foals and adult horses, while serum vitamin D levels remain unchanged. It has been suggested, therefore, that these changes in vitamin D receptor expression have an effect on the production of TNF-α, and IFN-γ, and hence affect the resistance and susceptibility of foals to *R. equi* infection (Berghaus et al., 2024).

Stress and immunity

As described in Chapter 5, the equine immune system acts on key components of the brain to generate the response that we call sickness. However, the signals pass both ways! Stress signals acting on the brain also affect an animal's immune response. In fact, there are close interconnections between the nervous and immune systems. For example, the adrenal cortex is stimulated by adrenocorticotropic hormone (ACTH) from the pituitary under the influence of corticotropin-releasing hormone from the hypothalamus. The sympathetic-adrenergic system is also activated by neurotransmitters such as epinephrine, norepinephrine, and dopamine.

During transportation, for example, these hormonal changes are generated as the horse adjusts to the changing environment. The blood levels of these neurotransmitters rise as early as 10 minutes after the beginning of a journey. These, in turn, induce anxiety and its associated behaviors (Medica et al., 2019). As a result, in stressed animals, glucocorticoids are secreted and suppress T cell function by blocking the NF-κB pathway. IL-1β and IL-6 act on both the hypothalamus and the pituitary to increase ACTH production and subsequent cortisol release. Stress can therefore be profoundly immunosuppressive Fig. 23.5.

Transportation, especially by road, is a key feature of horse management. They are transported more frequently than other livestock species. Transportation stress is well recognized as predisposing to the development of respiratory disease in horses (Arfuso et al., 2023). Even in horses well used to being transported, the physical and mental stimuli collectively stimulate the horse's inflammatory system. Activation of the hypothalamic-pituitary axis is associated with the generation of an acute-phase response and thus influences the immune status of the horse. The stress influences the hypothalamic-pituitary-adrenal axis, as well as activating the sympathetic nervous system. This results in the release of glucocorticosteroids and catecholamines. The glucocorticoids inhibit T cell proliferation and reduce their cytokine synthesis, resulting in immunosuppression. This, in turn, makes the horse more susceptible to transport-related infections, especially after prolonged journeys. In addition to physical injuries, transportation is also associated with the development of respiratory disease, colic, laminitis, and rhabdomyelitis. The most serious of these is equine pleuropneumonia, aka. shipping fever (Padalino et al., 2015).

Donkeys also suffer from stress during transportation and as a result may suffer fom a hyperlipidemia (Mendoza et al., 2018).

One major reason for the impairment of respiratory defenses in transported horses is prolonged head elevation. With the head held high, mucociliary clearance is significantly reduced. Over time, this elevation permits the accumulation of bacteria, particulates, and inflammatory exudates in the trachea. After 24 hours of head elevation, significant pulmonary inflammation develops. It takes about 12 hours of free head movement for this inflammation to decline to normal levels.

When horses are hospitalized, they may also become severely stressed. As a result, they may develop gastrointestinal problems. An analysis of fecal IgA levels in hospitalized horses suggested that they remained relatively constant except

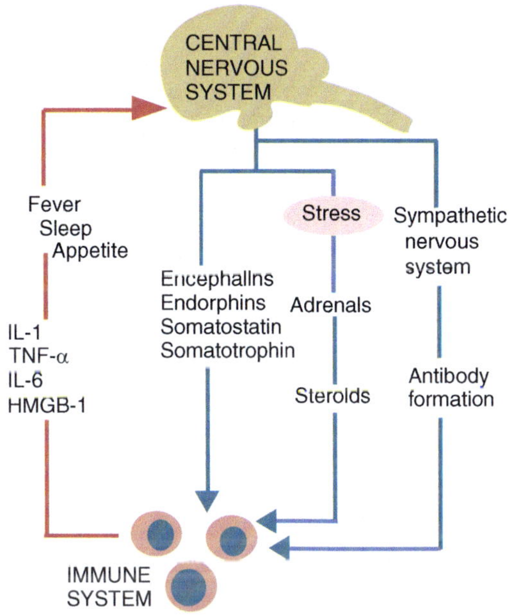

FIGURE 23.5 Some of the ways in which the central nervous system and the immune system interact.

As a result, psychological and physical stress can be profoundly immunosuppressive in horses.

following procedures. For example, after the horses had been subjected to general anesthesia, IgA levels decreased significantly. This was independent of the nature and duration of the surgery. A high plasma cortisol level was weakly correlated with low fecal IgA on the day after surgery. Thus, hospitalization stress has a significant suppressive effect on the local immune response in the gastrointestinal tract (May et al., 2024).

Pituitary pars intermedia dysfunction

As horses and donkeys grow older, the pars intermedia of the pituitary gland fails to function normally—it undergoes hyperplasia (Gehlen et al., 2020). Pituitary pars intermedia dysfunction (PPID) disease may reach a prevalence of 15%–30% in aged equids. Using an ACTH and α-MSH assay as a diagnostic test, 20% of aged horses tested positive for pituitary pars intermedia dysfunction (PPID) (McFarlane, 2011). As a result, affected horses become severely immunosuppressed Fig. 23.6.

The pituitary is located beneath the brain, where it is attached to the hypothalamus. It is divided into two components, an anterior part called the adenohypophysis

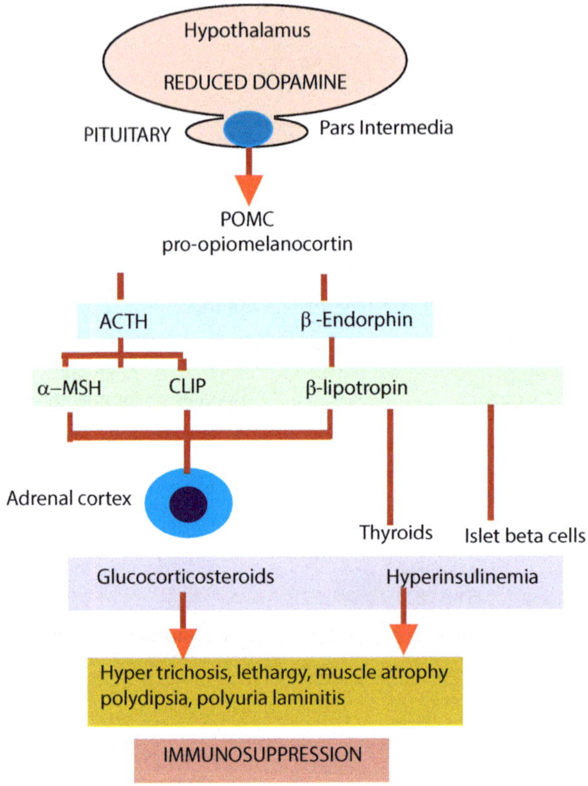

FIGURE 23.6

A simplified diagram showing the pathogenesis of pituitary pars intermedia dysfunction (PPID) and its clinical consequences.

and a posterior part, the neurohypophysis. The pars intermedia is located between the anterior and posterior parts and surrounds the posterior pituitary.

As horses age, there is a progressive loss of dopaminergic control within the pars intermedia. Dopamine levels drop to about 10% of their earlier level. The melanotrophs in the pars intermedia secrete pro-melanocortin peptides As the dopaminergic inhibition is lost, these pars intermedia cells produce increased amounts of their normal product, pro-opiomelanocortin (POMC). This is first cleaved into ACTH and corticotropin-like intermediate peptide (CLIP). ACTH is then cleaved into α-MSH and β-endorphin. These two hormones, as well as ACTH, act on the horse's adrenal cortex, causing it to secrete increased amounts of corticosteroids. PPID is a slowly progressive condition (In humans, it is called Cushing's disease). Affected horses and ponies develop long curly hair, polyuria, and polydipsia as well as excessive sweating. They become progressively debilitated and develop recurrent infections (McCue, 2002). The endocrinopathy also plays an important role in triggering laminitis. Its mechanism is unclear, but the laminitis appears to be a result of elevated insulin levels (McFarlane, 2011). Thus, out of 325 horses with PPID, 32% had hyperinsulinemia, and of these, 66% had laminitis (Kirkwood et al., 2022).

Opportunistic infections occur in about 35% of horses with PPID compared to 11% of healthy aged horses (McFarlane, 2011). These include dermatophilosis, sinus infections, pneumonia, and abscesses. They probably also suffer from occult infections. For example, many are found to have chronic pneumonia at necropsy. They also appear to be more susceptible to parasites, as reflected by higher fecal strongyle egg counts.

Horses suffering from PPID also exhibit defects in their innate immune responses. For example, they have reduced neutrophil functions as reflected by decreased oxidative burst activity and cell adhesion. Chemotaxis is greater in healthy aged horses than in aged horses with PPID. The plasma insulin:α-MSH ratio is correlated with the oxidative burst activity (McFarlane et al., 2015). PPID has a moderate effect on the equine acute-phase response, with SAA levels being correlated with blood insulin levels (Zak et al., 2020).

Given that PPID horses are loaded with excessive ACTH, it is unsurprising that their adaptive immune system also shows significant aberrations. In effect, they suffer from corticosterioid toxicity. Thus, PPID horses have lower absolute lymphocyte counts than healthy horses, although all the other leukocyte counts are normal. PPID horses have increased serum CXCL8 (IL-8) levels. In addition, following stimulation of their lymphocytes with *R. equi* and *E. coli,* the PPID horses have consistently significant decreased IFN-γ production and increased TGF-β expression. Thus, these horses are unable to mount a protective Th1 response to bacterial antigens (Miller et al., 2012). In addition, their responses to some vaccines, such as Rhinopneumonitis or West Nile virus, are suppressed. These horses are at greatly increased risk of opportunistic infections.

ACTH levels in healthy donkeys are significantly higher than in healthy horses. Likewise ACTH levels in donkeys sudffering from PPID are higher than in PPID-affected horses. There is a risk therefore of diagnosing PPID in healthy donkeys bases solely on ACTH levels (Mendoza et al., 2018).

References

Arfuso, F., Rizzo, M., Giannetto, C., Giudice, E., et al. (2023). Inflammatory-like status and acute stress response in horses after road transport. *Scientific Reports*. https://doi.org/10.1038/s41598-023-37069-1

Baldwin, J. L., Cooper, W. L., Vanderwall, D. K., & Erb, H. N. (1991). Prevalence (treatment days) and severity of illness in hypogammaglobulinemic and normogammaglobulinemic foals. *Journal of the American Veterinary Medical Association, 198*, 423–428.

Banks, K. L., McGuire, T. C., & Jerrells, T. R. (1976). Absence of B lymphocytes in a horse with primary agammaglobulinemia. *Clinical Immunology and Immunopathology, 5*, 282–290.

Bell, S. C., Savidge, C., Taylor, P., et al. (2001). An immunodeficiency in Fell ponies: A preliminary study into cellular responses. *Equine Veterinary Journal, 33*, 687–692.

Berghaus, L. J., Cathcart, J., Berghaus, R. D., Ryan, C., et al. (2024). Impact of age on vitamin D receptor expression, vitamin D metabolism and cytokine production in ex vivo *Rhodococcus equi* infection of equine alveolar macrophages. *Veterinary Immunology and Immunopathology*. https://doi.org/10.1016/j.vetimm.2024.110707

Bernoco, D., & Bailey, E. (1998). Frequency of the SCID gene among Arabian horses in the USA. *Animal Genetics, 29*, 41–42.

Boy, M. G., Zhang, C., Antczak, D. F., Hamir, A. N., & Whitlock, R. H. (1992). Unusual selective immunoglobulin deficiency in an Arabian foal. *Journal of Veterinary Internal Medicine, 6*, 201–205.

Butler, C. M., Westermann, C. M., Koeman, J. P., et al. (2006). The Fell pony immunodeficiency syndrome also occurs in the Netherlands: A review and six cases. *Tijdschrift voor Diergeneeskunde, 131*, 114–118.

Carter, S. D., Fox-Clipsham, L. Y., Christley, R., & Swinburne, J. (2013). Foal immunodeficiency syndrome: Carrier testing has markedly reduced disease incidence. *The Veterinary Record, 172*(15), 398.

Clabough, D. L., Clabough, D. L., Conboy, H. S., & Roberts, M. C. (1989). Comparison of four screening techniques for the diagnosis of equine neonatal hypogammaglobulinemia. *Journal of the American Veterinary Medical Association, 194*, 1717–1720.

Crisman, M. V., & Scarratt, W. K. (2008). Immunodeficiency disorders in horses. *Veterinary Clinics of North America: Equine Practice, 24*, 299–310.

Davis, D. G., Schaefer, D. M., Hinchcliff, K. W., et al. (2005). Measurement of serum IgG in foals by radial immunodiffusion and automated turbidimetric immunoassay. *Journal of Veterinary Internal Medicine, 19*, 93–96.

Deem, D. A., Traver, D. S., Thacker, H. L., & Perryman, L. E. (1979). Agammaglobulinemia in a horse. *Journal of the American Veterinary Medical Association, 175*, 469–472.

Ding, Q., Bramble, L., Yuzbasiyan-Gurkan, V., et al. (2002). DNA-PKcs mutations in dogs and horses: Allele frequency and association with neoplasia. *Gene, 283*, 263–269.

Felippe, M. J. B. (2023). Equine common variable immunodeficiency: Lessons from 100 clinical cases. *Equine Veterinary Education*. https://doi.org/10.1111/eve.13948

Flaminio, M. J., LaCombe, V., Kohn, C. W., & Antczak, D. F. (2002). Common variable immunodeficiency in a horse. *Journal of the American Veterinary Medical Association, 221*, 1296–1302.

Flaminio, M. J., Tallmadge, R. L., Salles-Gomes, C. O., & Matychak, M. B. (2009). Common variable immunodeficiency in horses is characterized by B cell depletion in primary and secondary lymphoid tissues. *Journal of Clinical Immunology, 29*(1), 107–116.

Fox-Clipsham, L., Swinburne, J. E., Papoula-Pereira, R. I., et al. (2009). Immunodeficiency/anemia syndrome in a Dales pony. *The Veterinary Record, 165*, 289–290.

Freestone, J. F., Shoemaker, S., & McClure, J. J. (1989). Pulmonary abscessation, hepatoencephalopathy and IgM deficiency associated with *Rhodococcus equi* in a foal. *Australian Veterinary Journal, 66*, 343–344.

Gallacher, K., Champion, K., & Denholm, K. S. (2025). Mare colostrum quality and relationship with foal serum immunoglobulin G concentrations and average daily weight gains. *Equine Veterinary Journal, 57*, 904–914.

Gardner, R. B., Hart, K. A., Stokol, T., et al. (2006). Fell pony syndrome in a pony in North America. *Journal of Veterinary Internal Medicine, 20*, 198–203.

Gehlen, H., Schwarz, B., Bartmann, C., Gernhardt, J., & Stockle, S. D. (2020). Pituitary par intermedia dysfunction and metabolic syndrome in donkeys. *Animals*. https://doi.org/10.3390/ani10122335

Gill, A. F., Gaunt, S., & Sirninger, J. (2008). Congenital Pelger-Huet anomaly in a horse. *Veterinary Clinical Pathology*. https://doi.org/10.1111/j.1939-165x.2006.tb00165.x

Grondin, T. M., DeWitt, S. F., & Keeton, K. S. (2007). Pelger-Huët anomaly in an Arabian horse. *Veterinary Clinical Pathology, 36*, 306–310.

Jelinek, F., Faldyna, M., & Jasurkova-Mikutova, G. (2006). Severe combined immunodeficiency in a Fell pony foal. *Journal of Veterinary Medicine A, 53*, 69–73.

Kirkwood, N. C., Hughes, K. J., & Stewart, A. J. (2022). Pituitary pars intermedia dysfunction (PPID) in horses. *Veterinary Sciences*. https://doi.org/10.3390/vetsci9100556

Latimer, K. S., Campagnoli, R. P., & Danilenko, D. M. (2000). Pelger-Huet anomaly in Australian shepherds: 87 cases (1991–1997). *Comparative Haematology International, 10*, 9–13.

Lobito, A. A., Gabriel, T. L., Medema, J. P., & Kimberley, F. C. (2011). Disease causing mutations in the TNF and TNFR superfamilies: Focus on molecular mechanisms driving disease. *Trends in Molecular Medicine, 17*(9), 494–505.

Magdesian, K. G. (2024). Immunodeficiencies in foals. *Veterinary Clinics: Equine Practice, 40*, e1–e49.

May, A., Gerhards, H., & Wollanke, B. (2024). Effect of hospitalization on equine local intestinal immunoglobulin A (IgA) concentration measured in feces. *Journal of Equine Veterinary Science*. https://doi.org/10.1016/j.jevs.2024.105078

McCue, P. M. (2002). Equine Cushing's disease. *Veterinary Clinics of North America: Equine Practice, 18*, 533–543.

McFarlane, D. (2011). Equine pituitary pars intermedia dysfunction. *Veterinary Clinics: Equine Practice, 27*, 93–113.

McFarlane, D., Hill, K., & Anton, J. (2015). Neutrophil function in healthy aged horses and horses with pituitary dysfunction. *Veterinary Immunology and Immunopathology, 165*, 99–106.

McGuire, T. C., Banks, K. L., & Davis, W. C. (1976a). Alterations in the thymus and other lymphoid tissues in young horses with combined immunodeficiency. *American Journal of Pathology, 84*, 39–54.

McGuire, T. C., Banks, K. L., Evans, D. R., & Poppie, M. J. (1976b). Agammaglobulinemia in a horse with evidence of functional T lymphocytes. *American Journal of Veterinary Research, 37*(1), 41–46.

McGuire, T. C., Poppie, M. J., & Banks, K. L. (1975). Hypogammaglobulinemia predisposing to infection in foals. *Journal of the American Veterinary Medical Association, 166*, 71–75.

Medica, P., Bruschetta, G., Cravana, C., Ferlazzo, A., & Fazio, E. (2019). Effect of transportation on the sympatho-adrenal system responses in horses. *Research in Veterinary Science, 125*, 401–404.

Mendoza, F. J., Toribio, R. E., & Perez-Ecija, A. (2018). Donkey internal medicine—Part I. Metabolic, endocrine, and alimentary tract disturbances. *Journal of Equine Veterinary Science, 65*, 66–74.

Miller, A. B., Loynachan, A. T., Bush, H. M., Hart, R. A., et al. (2012). Effects of pituitary pars intermedia dysfunction and Prascend (pergolide tablets) treatment on endocrine and immune function in horses. *Domestic Animal Endocrinology*. https://doi.org/10.1016/j.bpmanieend.2020.106531

Mullen, K. R., & Felippe, M. J. B. (2024). The horse with recurrent fevers and infections: Approach to common variable immunodeficiency. *Veterinary Clinics of North America: Equine Practice, 40*, 179–188.

Nath, L. C., Anderson, G. A., Savage, C. J., & McKinnon, A. O. (2010). Use of stored equine colostrum for the treatment of foals perceived to be at risk for failure of transfer of passive immunity. *Journal of the American Veterinary Medical Association, 236*, 1085–1090.

Padalino, B., Hall, E., Raidal, S., Celi, P., et al. (2015). Health problems and risk factors associated with long haul transport of horses in Australia. *Animals*. https://doi.org/10.3390/ani5040412

Pelligrini-Masini, A., Bentz, A. I., Johns, I. C., et al. (2005). Common variable immunodeficiency in three horses with presumptive bacterial meningitis. *Journal of the American Veterinary Medical Association, 227*, 114–122.

Perkins, G. A., Nydam, D. V., Flaminio, M. J., & Ainsworth, D. M. (2003). Serum IgM concentrations in normal fit horses and horses with a lymphoma or other medical conditions. *Journal of Veterinary Internal Medicine, 17*, 337–342.

Perryman, L. E. (1984). Biochemical and functional characterization of lymphocytes from a horse with lymphosarcoma and IgM deficiency. *Comparative Immunology, Microbiology and Infectious Diseases, 7*, 53–62.

Perryman, L. E. (2000). Primary immunodeficiencies of horses. *Veterinary Clinics of North America: Equine Practice, 16*, 105–116.

Perryman, L. E. (2004). Molecular pathology of severe combined immunodeficiency in mice, horses, and pigs. *Veterinary Pathology Online, 41*, 95–100.

Perryman, L. E., McGuire, T. C., & Banks, K. L. (1983). Animal model of human disease. Infantile X-linked agammaglobulinemia. Agammaglobulinemia in horses. *American Journal of Pathology, 111*, 125–127.

Petersson, K. H., Burr, D. B., Gomez-Chiarri, M., & Petersson-Wolfe, C. S. (2010). The influence of vitamin E on immune function and response to vaccination in older horses. *Journal of Animal Science, 88*, 2950–2958.

Riggs, M. W. (1987). Evaluation of foals for immune deficiency disorders. *Veterinary Clinics of North America: Equine Practice, 3*, 515–528.

Scholes, S. F., Holliman, A., May, P. D., & Holmes, M. A. (1998). A syndrome of anemia, immunodeficiency and peripheral ganglionopathy in Fell pony foals. *The Veterinary Record, 142*, 128–134.

Shin, E. K., Perryman, L. E., & Meek, K. (1997). A kinase-negative mutation of DNA-PKcs in equine SCID results in defective coding and signal joint formation. *Jounal of Immunology, 158*, 3565–3569.

Tallmadge, R. L., Antczak, D. F., & Felippe, M. J. (2020). Genetics of immune disease in the horse. *Veterinary Clinics: Equine Practice, 36*, 273–288.

Tallmadge, R. L., Shen, L., Tseng, C. T., Miller, S. C., et al. (2015). Bone marrow transcriptome and epigenome profiles of equine common variable immunodeficiency patients unveil block of B lymphocyte differentiation. *Clinical Immunology, 160*(2), 261–276.

Tallmadge, R. L., Stokol, T., Gould-Earley, M. J., Earley, et al. (2012). Fell Pony syndrome: Characterization of developmental hematopoiesis failure and associated gene expression profiles. *Clinical and Vaccine Immunology, 19*, 1054–1064.

Tallmadge, R. L., Such, K. A., Miller Kc, K., Bu, M., et al. (2012). Expression of essential B cell development genes in horses with common variable immunodeficiency. *Molecular Immunology, 51*, 169–176.

Thomas, G. W., Bell, S. C., & Carter, S. D. (2005). Immunoglobulin and peripheral B-lymphocyte concentrations in Fell pony foal syndrome. *Equine Veterinary Journal, 37*, 48–52.

Thomas, G. W., Bell, S. C., Phythian, C., et al. (2003). Aid to the antemortem diagnosis of Fell pony foal syndrome by the analysis of B lymphocytes. *The Veterinary Record, 152*, 618–621.

Verdonck, F., Merlevede, I., Godderis, B. M., DePrez, P., & Cox, E. (2007). Vitamin E deficiency and decreased serum immunoglobulin concentrations in a population of donkeys. *Veterinary Record, 160*, 232–233.

Vivrette, S. (2001). Colostrum and oral immunoglobulin therapy in newborn foals. *Compendium on Continuing Education for The Practicing Veterinarian, 23*, 286–291.

Weldon, A. D., Zhang, C., Antczak, D. F., & Rebhun, W. C. (1992). Selective IgM deficiency and abnormal B-cell response in a foal. *Journal of the American Veterinary Medical Association, 201*, 1396–1398.

White, J. H. (2008). Vitamin D signaling, infectious diseases, and regulation of innate immunity. *Infection and Immunity, 76*(9), 3837–3843.

Zak, A., Siwinska, N., Elzinga, S., Barker, V. D., et al. (2020). Effects of advanced age and pituitary pars intermedia dysfunction on components of the acute phase reaction in horses. *Domestic Animal Endocrinology*. https://doi.org/10.1016/j.domaniend.2020.106476

CHAPTER

Racing, exercise, and the equine immune system 24

The wild ancestors of the modern horse evolved an anatomy and physiology that enabled them to effectively escape predators. In general, they chose to flee rather than stay and fight, although they could fight with their hooves if foals had to be protected. As a result, horses are unrivaled in their alertness, agility, speed, and endurance. Once the horse was domesticated, humans exploited these properties in warfare, in load carrying, and subsequently, in competitive racing. One of their attractions to early humans was their ability to vastly increase the speed and duration of human mobility.

Unlike livestock raised for their meat, horses, mules, and donkeys are expected to work. This work can involve carrying or pulling heavy loads, such as carts and plows, over very long distances. It can also involve strenuous sports ranging from long-distance endurance races to short, intensive horse racing. All these efforts require that the animals be physically fit. Especially in the case of racing, Thoroughbred horses are required to undergo strenuous training. Both racing and load carrying/pulling can be highly stressful, especially if the burden is excessive, and, as a result, can have significant effects on the equine muscular, skeletal and immune systems. It is often difficult to separate psychological stress and physical stress. It is also difficult to separate the effects of the exercise from its accompanying stress. Additional significant stress may be added if animals are beaten to force them to work harder or gallop faster.

In general, increased exercise improves bodily fitness, including the functioning of the immune system. However, beyond a certain level, this exercise can become damaging and suppress multiple immune functions. Thus, horse racing can have profound effects on both innate and adaptive immunity. Additional complexity is added to the process by the great variations in this exercise. Thus, the exercise may be "acute" in short fast races, or "chronic" in long-duration endurance rides. Both types are stressful and profoundly influence equine immune capabilities. It is also important to point out the effects. of extreme exercise have been intensively studied in human athletes. In general, extreme exercise has a similar effect on humans and horses (Fitzgerald, 1988). Given the athleticism of horses and their important roles in racing, it is clear that the horse is an excellent model to study the effects of exercise stress on human immune functions.

The Immunology of Horses and Donkeys. https://doi.org/10.1016/B978-0-443-44863-8.00021-1

Neural regulation of immunity

Stress response

Hypothalamic-pituitary-adrenal cortical axis

Physical or mental stress can be profoundly immunosuppressive. When confronted by a predator or other threat, a threatened horse triggers a response in the hypothalamus that leads to activation of the pituitary and the production of adrenocorticotropic hormone (ACTH). This, in turn, triggers the adrenal gland to release both epinephrine and norepinephrine, as well as the production of cortisol. The epinephrine and norepinephrine prepare the horse's vascular system for physical activity, but the cortisol is immunosuppressive and antiinflammatory.

As a result, in stressed animals, glucocorticoids are secreted and suppress T cell function by interfering with the NF-κB pathway. The inflammatory cytokines, IL-1β and IL-6 act on both the hypothalamus and the pituitary to increase ACTH production and subsequent cortisol release.

Corticosteroids such as cortisol are lipid soluble and are absorbed directly into cells, where they bind to receptors in the cytosol. The corticosteroid-receptor complexes are then translocated to the nucleus, where they bind to DNA sequences called glucocorticoid response elements and regulate gene transcription. For example, they stimulate the synthesis of IκBα, an inhibitor of the key regulator of gene transcription, NF-κB. In a resting cell, NF-κB remains inactive since its nuclear binding site is masked by IκBα. When a lymphocyte is stimulated by antigens or cytokines, the two molecules dissociate, the IκBα is degraded, and the released NF-κB can then move into the nucleus, where it activates the genes involved in inflammation and immunity. Because corticosteroids, however, stimulate the production of IκBα, it persists and continues to block NF-κB-mediated processes, including cytokine synthesis and T cell responses in activated cells. Corticosteroids are therefore able to suppress both innate and adaptive immune responses (De Bosscher et al., 2000).

Corticosteroids thus influence three aspects of the immune system: they affect leukocyte production and circulation and so reduce innate immunity; they influence the effector mechanisms of lymphocytes and so suppress adaptive immunity; and they modulate the activities of inflammatory mediators.

Effects on lymphocytes

Corticosteroids inhibit the ability of T cells to produce IL-1β, IL-6, IL-8, IL-12, IFN-γ and TNF-α (Banuelos, 2016). These are the major cytokines that promote type 1 immune responses and inflammation. However paradoxically, glucocorticoids can also upregulate the production of IL-4, IL-10 and IL-13 by Th2 cells! As a result, they cause a change in the Th1/Th2 balance rather than a nonspecific immunosuppression (Elenkov, 2004). Corticosteroids also upregulate the expression of the IL-1β receptor, CD121b. This is a decoy receptor that can bind active IL-1β but does not generate a signal, thus blocking IL-1β functions. In addition to suppressing Th1 responses, glucocorticoids increase Treg numbers and stimulate Treg activity. They do this in part by upregulating the expression of the transcription factor, FoxP3, as well as by modulating the cytokine mixture within the T cell environment.

The effects of corticosteroids on antibody responses are variable and depend on timing and dose. In general, B cells tend to be corticosteroid resistant, and large doses are usually required to suppress antibody synthesis (Cupps et al., 1985).

Effects on leukocytes

In horses the number of circulating eosinophils, basophils, and lymphocytes declines within a few hours following corticosteroid administration as a result of sequestration in the bone marrow. The number of neutrophils, on the other hand, increases as a result of decreased adherence to vascular endothelium and reduced emigration into inflamed tissues. Neutrophil, monocyte, and eosinophil chemotaxis are suppressed by corticosteroids. However, they have no apparent effect on neutrophil phagocytosis in horses. The production of antimicrobial proteins, such as the defensins is also regulated by the autonomic nervous system, and stress reduces cutaneous epithelial antimicrobial activity. This appears to be a result of increased glucocorticoid and acetylcholine production (Targowski, 1975).

Other nervous system—Immune links

The nervous and immune systems also communicate through parasympathetic and sympathetic nerves as well as through soluble neurotransmitters. Neuroendocrine hormones such as corticotropin-releasing factor and α-melanocyte-stimulating hormone, as well as some neurotransmitters, act on the cells of the immune system to regulate cytokine production (Borghetti et al., 2009).

Autonomic nervous system

Almost all primary and secondary lymphoid organs are supplied by nerves through the autonomic nervous system. Additionally, many cells of the immune system express receptors for the neurotransmitters released by both arms of the autonomic nervous system. This may occur either through adrenergic signals from the sympathetic nervous system or cholinergic signals from the parasympathetic nervous system (Kenney & Ganta, 2014).

Parasympathetic

Stimulation of the vagus nerve inhibits cytokine release from the spleen and reduces inflammation-mediated injury in endotoxemia and sepsis. This is called the "inflammatory reflex" and requires acetylcholine production. The acetylcholine inhibits inflammasome activity and thus reduces cytokine production. Both TNF-α and IL-1β in turn affect vagus nerve activity (Zanos et al., 2018). Immune cells also have a complete set of cholinergic receptors. Efferent activity in the vagus nerve activates a cholinergic anti-inflammatory pathway. Vagal stimulation suppresses the systemic response to endotoxin by downregulating hepatic TNF-α synthesis. Activation of acetylcholine receptors on macrophages inhibits their production of IL-1β and TNF-α.

Sympathetic

The sympathetic nerves act through the neurotransmitter norepinephrine. They innervate the thymus, the splenic white pulp, and the lymph nodes. They influence blood flow, vascular permeability, and lymphocyte migration and differentiation. Surgical or chemical sympathectomy of the spleen enhances antibody production and can induce changes in the distribution of lymphocyte subpopulations. NK cell activity appears to be modulated directly by the hypothalamus through the splenic nerve. Autonomic nerves also innervate Langerhans cells in the skin. By releasing neuropeptides, these nerves can depress their antigen-presenting ability. This might explain why some skin lesions in horses worsen with anxiety. Denervated skin shows reduced inflammation after tissue damage and heals more slowly. Most importantly, sympathetic nerves innervate the adrenal medulla (Downing & Miyan, 2000).

Both adrenergic and cholinergic stimulation increase noradrenaline signaling, leading to NF-κB activation of mononuclear cells. The sympathetic nervous system can alter the Th1/Th2 balance through the β-adrenergic receptors. Stimulation of sympathetic nerves enhances the production of Th2 cytokines while inhibiting the production of Th1 cytokines. Norepinephrine suppresses the production of IL-6 and TNF-α.

Neuropeptides and lymphocytes

Lymphocytes have receptors for neuropeptides such as the enkephalins and endorphins that can thus influence lymphocyte activity. The generation of cytotoxic T cells is enhanced by metenkephalin and β-endorphin, whereas α-endorphin suppresses antibody formation and β-endorphin reverses this suppressive effect. Other neuropeptides that influence the immune system include ACTH, oxytocin, vasoactive intestinal peptide, somatostatin, prolactin, and substance P (Brogden et al., 2005).

Many neuropeptides, such as vasoactive intestinal peptide and substance P, also have antimicrobial properties and may therefore be involved in host defense. For example, substance P not only mediates pain and inflammation but also kills bacteria. Other neuropeptides have similar effects. As a result, appropriate nervous stimulation can promote neuropeptide release and enhance local antibacterial activity. The pain associated with acute inflammation may well reflect this local resistance to infection. Some neuropeptides can also promote Th17 activity by triggering monocyte production of IL-23.

Immune responses are also modulated by environmental factors. Changes in day length (photoperiod) influence immunity. These effects can be complex, but in general, reduced day length appears to promote immune reactivity. The effect appears to be mediated through the hormone melatonin. Circadian rhythms also regulate some immune functions, such as the activities of hematopoietic stem cells and lymphocyte recruitment from the blood. These appear to be a result of oscillations in chemokine levels and the expression of adhesion molecules on vascular endothelial cells (Scheiermann et al., 2013).

Conversely, the innate immune system can influence nervous system function. For example, cytokines such as IL-1β, IL-6, and TNF-α, as well as other inflammatory mediators, induce "sickness behavior," including fever, fatigue, and impaired performance. Cytokines and chemokines modulate nervous system activities such as appetite and mood. In addition, exercise-induced inflammation can lead to activation of sensory nerves (and cause pain) that then relay messages to the brain. Many cytokines are produced by the brain and meningeal macrophages—microglia. For example, IL-1β is produced in the brain in response to endotoxin. All these are closely associated with the systemic response to infectious agents and chronic inflammation.

Exercise stress

Physical exercise, depending upon its duration and severity, affects the immune systems of both humans and equids in many different ways (Witkowska-Pilaszewicz et al., 2024). The degree of physical stress caused by exercise in the horse depends in large part on the animal's physical fitness, in addition to the exercise intensity and duration. High intensity exercise, prolonged exhaustive exercise, and overtraining are highly stressful and, as a result, tend to be significantly immunosuppressive. Conversely, moderate training and increased fitness may enhance host defenses (Trogdon Hines et al., 1996).

A single intense bout of exercise can cause a transient immunosuppression as reflected in a suppressed lymphocyte response to mitogens, a decreased CD4:CD8 ratio, and reduced levels of salivary IgA and IgM. NK cell numbers and functions may also be suppressed. Moderate exercise in a fit horse may actually enhance some immune responses (Fitzgerald, 1988). However, progressive intensification of training can result in long-term immunosuppression. Exercise-induced stress also affects the margination and distribution of blood leukocytes and influences the levels of circulating Th2 cells, and as a result, increases the levels of regulatory cytokines (Shaw et al., 2018). Consequently, equine athletes may show increased susceptibility to influenza virus infection (Folsom et al., 2001), in addition to other respiratory infections (Raidal et al., 1997).

Exercised-induced pulmonary hemorrhage

It is relevant to point out here that exercise-induced pulmonary hemorrhage is not uncommon in horses immediately after racing. In some animals the condition may be fatal. The pathogenesis of this syndrome remains unclear. It appears that a rise in pulmonary intravascular pressure resulting from increased cardiac output and rapid acceleration may be greater than the pulmonary blood vessels can withstand. This results in stress failure and vascular rupture (Moore, 1996). However, it also appears that the bronchiolar damage associated with inflammatory airway disease (IAD) may play a key role in predisposing some horses to this condition. Repeated episodes of bronchiolitis result in neovascularization The newly formed blood vessels in IAD-affected horses may be especially fragile (Derksen et al., 1992). It is also possible that the hemorrhage may predispose horses to IAD by triggering local inflammation. Hemosiderin is commonly found in equine alveolar macrophages.

Exertional hyperthermia

During intense physical activity such as racing, Thoroughbred horses generate large amounts of heat which they may be unable to dissipate by evaporative sweating and panting. As a result, their body temperatures may reach as high as 42°C (Brownlow & Mizzi, 2023). This may be sufficient to cause cardiovascular failure, collapse, and death. In less severe cases, it may affect the horse's immune functions. The effects of a fever on immune functions are described in Chapter 5. Fevers usually present as a prolonged elevation in body temperature, whereas exercise-induced hyperthermia is generally of short duration. Nevertheless, very high body temperatures may be sufficient to temporarily enhance antigen presentation, dendritic cell activity, and effectively boost innate immunity. Some examples of this boosting are described later in this chapter (Baronzio et al., 2006).

Duration

There is a significant difference in the intensity and duration of stress between horses participating in short-distance racing and those engaged in endurance races. Thus, horses participating in prolonged races appear to be more susceptible to bacterial and viral respiratory diseases. For example, immediately following a race that lasted about 5 h over 80 km, mean serum cortisol, blood monocyte and neutrophil counts in horses were higher, whereas blood lymphocyte numbers and glucose levels were lower than before the race. Both neutrophil and monocyte oxidative burst activity decreased following the race and only returned to pre-race values 3 days later (Robson et al., 2003). In contrast, cortisol levels had returned to normal by the next day.

Studies using gene transcription on horses that just completed a 160 km endurance ride demonstrated significant upregulation of TLR4, CXCL8, and CCL5 gene transcription. There were gender differences noted in this study as well. Thus, mares showed upregulation of ribosomal protein genes, suggesting enhanced protein synthesis and recovery. In contrast, geldings showed upregulation of inflammatory and stress-related genes, perhaps reflecting a lower level of fitness (Akcay et al., 2025).

Another study investigated the effects of repeated bouts of exercise on neutrophil functions in trained Standardbred trotters. These horses were exercised on two days with a 3-day interval between. On each day, they underwent three exercise bouts with increasing intensity at 60-minute intervals (Korhonen et al., 2000). Following these exercises, the horses exhibited a leukocytosis with an increase in the neutrophil: lymphocyte ratio. They also increased their ability to mount a respiratory burst, as evidenced by an increase in whole blood chemiluminescence. The neutrophilia lasted for about 6 h. However, cortisol levels did not change significantly after these exercises. These trained horses were clearly not highly stressed.

Training

As described above, intense exercise clearly promotes a transient inflammatory response. However, homeostasis also functions in these horses, and they mount a corresponding anti-inflammatory response mediated by cytokines. Studies have been conducted on the levels of the anti-inflammatory cytokine antagonist IL-1RA, as well as IL-10 and IL-13 produced during endurance (aerobic) and race (anaerobic) exercises in horses of different fitness levels (Fig. 24.1).

Blood samples were analyzed before and after the exercise. In endurance horses, there was an increase in IL-13 after a 100 km ride and in IL-1RA after a 120 km ride. The changes in IL-10 were not statistically significant. In the racehorses, there was a higher IL-13 basal serum concentration in the untrained than in the trained animals, and this decreased after exercise. In the trained racehorses, there was an increase in both IL-1RA and IL-13 after exercise. This implies that training affects the production of these cytokines (Plisak et al., 2023). In a study comparing the peripheral blood mononuclear cells of trained and sedentary mares, transcripts of both IL-6 and IL-6R were upregulated in the trained horses (Capomaccio et al., 2011) (Fig. 24.2).

Overtraining syndrome causes a decline in a horse's performance due to excess exercise activity, a lack of proper recovery time, resulting in chronic energy shortage, and failure to repair damaged tissues. Analysis of gene transcription in American Quarter horses, either after resting for 3 days or immediately after intense exercise for 1.8 miles, was investigated. Five genes were differentially expressed. The upregulated genes were IL-13 (male only, CCR4 (female only), TLR6, and TLR9 (female only). The downregulated genes were CD4 (male only) and MyD88. Thus, the affected pathways included those involving both Th1 and Th2 activation as well as the NF-κB and chemokine signaling pathways. Overtraining appeared to activate inflammatory pathways as a result of the ongoing stress (Wilson et al., 2023).

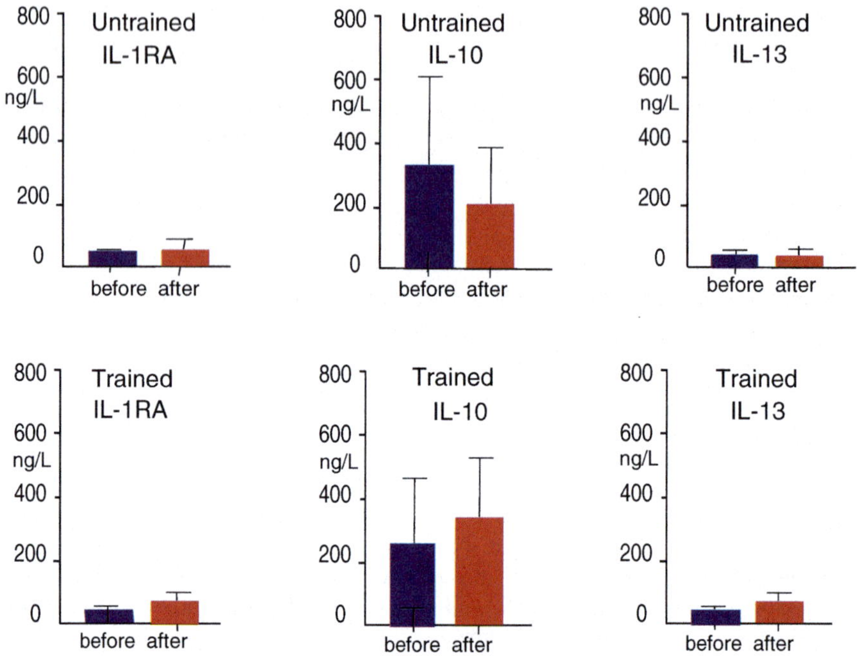

FIGURE 24.1

Comparison of IL-1RA, IL-10 and IL-1 serum concentrations before and after exercise in trained and untrained race horses.

- With permission Plisak et al. (2023).

Exercise and innate immunity

Physical exercise places great stress on the physiology of a horse. After all, in racing, the goal is to reach the upper limits of the animal's abilities. These limits include vascular and respiratory efficiency, muscle strength, and joint stability. When these limits are reached or exceeded, the tissues are damaged so that pulmonary hemorrhage and inflammation result.

It is also well recognized that 70%–80% of young racehorses beginning training commonly develop airway inflammation. This appears to result, in part, from an induced immunodeficiency. It appears that exercise induces a reduction in the phagocytic ability of equine alveolar macrophages as well as a reduced response to TLR ligands. Analysis of bronchoalveolar cells also shows alterations in their expression of the genes associated with airway immunity (Karagianni et al., 2022). However, it is important to point out that three key factors influence the severity of exercise-induced stress in horses: the intensity and duration of the stress,

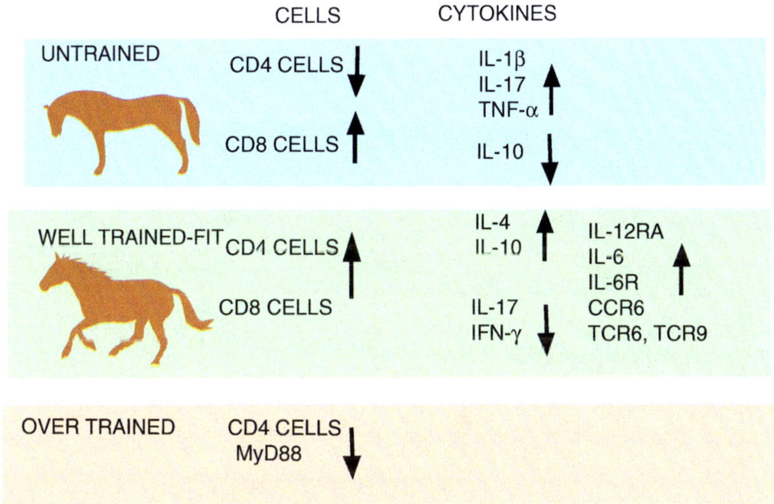

FIGURE 24.2 A summary of some of the effects of training on equine immune responsess.

Note that overtraining is both stressful and immunosuppressive.

the increase in body temperature, and the fitness of the horses. These, in turn, determine the amount of cortisol generated and the degree of immunosuppression induced. Thus, that short-duration, high-intensity exercise is sufficiently stressful to provoke a decline in leukocyte effectiveness and thus permits the development of respiratory disease. It has also been suggested, however, that the immunosuppression that develops post-exercise may have a beneficial effect since it may permit a degree of tolerance to antigens released as a result of muscle damage and may prevent the development of immune-mediated muscle lesions (McKeever et al., 2014) (Fig. 24.3).

Neutrophilic airway inflammation is very common in racehorses during training. In effect, they develop mild to moderate equine asthma. Studies have been conducted on the effects of training on the respiratory immune system by defining gene and protein expression patterns in transtracheal washes before and after training. It was found that there were 2138 differentially expressed genes and 260 proteins expressed during the training period. These genes and proteins are enriched for processes including the acute phase response, oxidative stress, and hematopoiesis, in addition to immune responses and inflammation (Karagianni et al., 2022). Many components of the interferon signaling pathways were also upregulated, whereas many other pathways involved in immune and inflammatory responses were downregulated.

In horses, one feature of the exercise-induced response is an increase in the acute-phase protein serum amyloid A. For example, a tenfold increase in SAA was detected in horses completing long-distance endurance rides. CRP and haptoglobin levels were unchanged (Cywinska et al., 2013). This acute-phase response

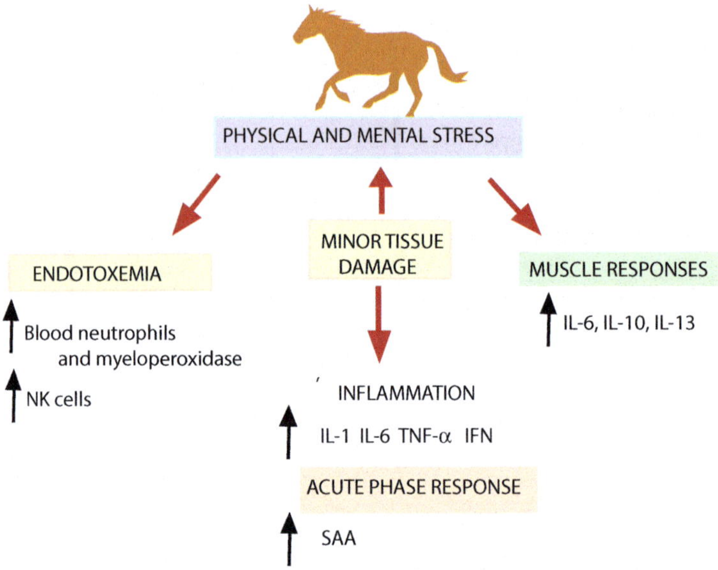

FIGURE 24.3

The effect of strenuous exercise on innate immunity in the horse.

is almost certainly due to the activities of IL-6 produced by muscle activity and acting on the liver. Other studies have suggested that this increase in SAA occurs only in unfit/inexperienced horses (Grzedzicka et al., 2023). Interestingly, this rise in SAA is not observed in racehorses after acute exercise (Witkowska-Pilaszewicz et al., 2024). Standardbred trotting horses also demonstrate a decline of up to 40% in their serum haptoglobin levels after a 2500 m race (Kristensen et al., 2014). In general, therefore, an acute phase response only develops in horses subjected to prolonged strenuous exertion. When it does occur, only SAA concentrations are significantly increased (Cywinska et al., 2012).

Neutrophil functions

When horses exercise, blood flow through many vessels, especially those in the muscles increases. The increased shearing force of this blood displaces some of the marginal neutrophils within these vessels. As a result, a transient neutrophilia develops. Lymphocyte numbers also increase immediately during exercise but then drop rapidly, so that a lymphopenia occurs during the post-exercise recovery period. Brief periods of intensive exercise result in a decrease in arterial blood pH and the development of lactic acidosis. They also induce changes in neutrophil function that may persist for at least 72 h. In a study that examined neutrophil functions in horses exercised to exhaustion, it was demonstrated that their response to bacterial lipopolysaccharide, as measured by the production of reactive oxygen species, was increased and remained elevated for up to 6 h after the exercise. A neutrophilia also developed during these first 6 hours. Leukocytosis was apparent for 24 h after the exercise. In general, the magnitude of the leukocytosis tended to increase with the duration and intensity of the exercise. There was also a significant increase in neutrophil apoptosis when the horses were exhausted, but this declined rapidly once the exercise ceased (Donovan et al., 2007).

Despite the size and complexity of the equine intestinal microbiota, bacterial endotoxins are normally confined to the gut. However, a transient endotoxemia can be detected in horses immediately following a race (Baker et al., 1988). These endotoxin levels are significantly higher in fit, trained horses than in unfit animals. It is possible that training promotes this "leakage" of endotoxin into the systemic circulation. Its clinical significance is unclear. A similar efflux of endotoxin also occurs after long-distance endurance competitions. It is correlated with plasma lactate levels (Barton et al., 2003).

In a related study, the level of neutrophil elastase activity was measured after intense exercise. Its level was significantly increased, and this correlated with the increase in myeloperoxidase. There was, however, great individual variation in this study, demonstrating that not all horses develop the same level of systemic inflammatory response (Lejeune et al., 2010).

Studies conducted on Thoroughbred racehorses immediately after races as well as after training, have also shown changes in neutrophil phagocytic ability. There was a decrease in the amount and intensity (number of particles phagocytosed) of phagocytosis immediately after each race. There was also a decline in the mean level of the oxidative burst (Meleiro et al., 2022). However, there were no significant differences in the numbers of apoptotic cells or lymphoproliferation assays. Mean serum cortisol levels were increased immediately following each race. There was also a neutrophilia immediately after each race.

Exercise and adaptive immunity

Regular moderate exercise boosts adaptive immune function. For example, increased antibody responses are mounted by mice that get moderate exercise, when compared to unexercised control mice. Moderate exercise also increases blood neutrophil counts, enhances NK cell activity, promotes lymphocyte responses to mitogens, and increases blood levels of IL-1β, IL-6, and TNF-α (Rogers et al., 2008). A similar situation occurs in horses (Fig. 24.4).

IgA levels in the bloodstream are significantly lower in horses housed in stables with limited exercise opportunities compared to free-ranging horses (Souza et al., 2010). Although mild exercise is good for immune function, high-intensity exercise, prolonged exhaustive exercise, or overtraining may induce a functional immunodeficiency. In horses, blood lymphocytes show a decreased proliferative response to mitogens for up to 16 h after a race. Acute exercise in the unfit animal can be especially stressful. Unfit horses subjected to strenuous exercise showed significantly

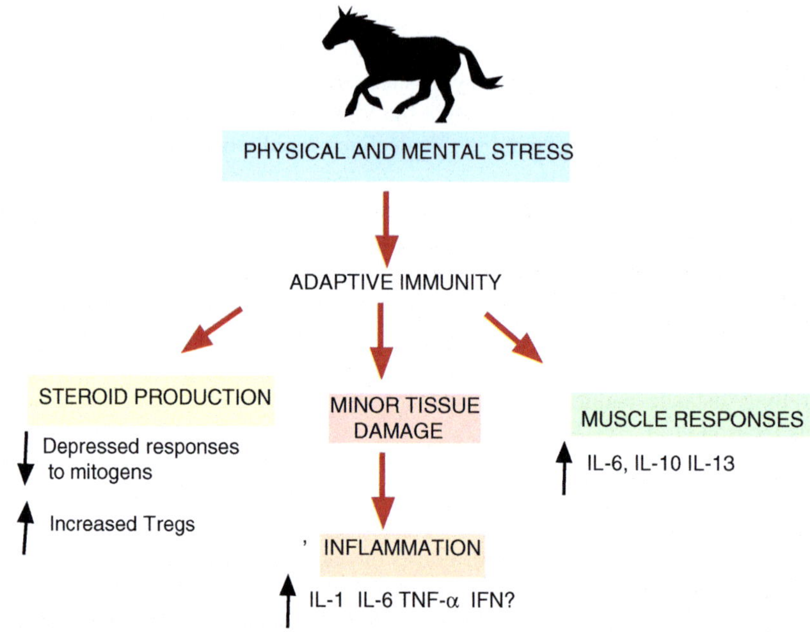

FIGURE 24.4

The effects of exercise on adaptive immunity.

raised steroid levels, resulting in reduced lymphocyte responses to mitogens or influenza virus antigens and reduced neutrophil chemotactic responsiveness and chemoluminescence (a measure of respiratory burst activity). These animals show a decline in their CD4:CD8 ratio as well as in both the number and activity of their NK cells. The age of an animal may also influence the effect of exercise on immune responses. For example, strenuous exercise significantly reduces lymphocyte proliferative responses in young horses, yet has much less effect on older animals. This resistance of older horses to exercise-induced immunosuppression may be due to their reduced steroid production.

Mononuclear cell functions

In a study of acute, short-term physical stress, horses were subjected to a short treadmill-based exercise challenge. Peripheral blood mononuclear cells were used to determine their responses to plant mitogens such as pokeweed mitogen, antigen (influenza-specific proliferation) and lymphokine activated killer cell (LAK) activity reflecting T cell function Thus in unfit horses galloping on an incline reaching a heart rate of 200 bpm and plasma cortisol levels were 76% higher than in unstressed animals. The response of their peripheral blood mononuclear cells to pokeweed mitogen and influenza virus was significantly suppressed, whereas their T cell cytotoxic (LAK) functionality was enhanced (Keadle et al., 1993). Experienced racehorses showed an increase in $CD14^-$ MHCII + cells after exercise, while $CD14^+$ $MHCII^-$ cells were unaffected. Conversely, untrained horses demonstrated an opposite effect. Their $CD14^+MHCII^-$ cells increased while their $CD14^-$ $MHCII^+$ cells declined (Witkowska-Pilaszewicz et al., 2020).

B cell functions

Vigorous exercise appears to have minimal effects on B-cell functions. Following a single strenuous exercise, equine immunoglobulin levels remain unchanged (Wong et al., 1992). This is entirely consistent with the limited responses of the B cell system to stress-induced corticosteroids. Following 3-day endurance racing events both serum IgA levels were relatively unchanged. However serum IgM levels had dropped by days two and three. IgG3/5 and IgG1 levels were unchanged. However, serum IgG4/7 levels were significantly lower in untrained control horses compared to trained endurance horses by day two (McKenzie et al., 2014).

T cell functions

Trained racehorses appear to have a significant increase in their number of $FoxP3^+$ $CD4^+$ and $CD8^+$ cells in their bloodstream when compared to untrained horses (Witkowska-Pilaszewicz et al., 2020). Single bouts of exercise are associated with an increase in NK or LAK cell activities in horses (Horohov, 2008, pp. 410–422).

Antiviral immunity

As described above, strenuous exercise such as racin not only affects innate immunity but also adaptive immune responses as well. For example, subjecting vaccinated ponies to a 5-day strenuous exercise program on a treadmill resulted in a significant suppression of their T cell-mediated responses to equine influenza vaccine compared to both the control animals and their pre-exercise results. Their blood lymphocytes showed a decreased antigen-specific lymphoproliferative response as well as reduced gamma interferon production. The addition of IL-2 failed to restore their proliferative response. Their IFN-γ mRNA levels were significantly reduced after 5 days of exercise compared to pre-exercise levels. Three of the four ponies in the exercised group also demonstrated increased susceptibility to experimental influenza challenge by developing clinical disease. Conversely, rested ponies that had received the same vaccine remained resistant to influenza (Folsom et al., 2001). The exercised ponies had lower (but not significant) anti-influenza antibody titers. In conclusion, limited exercise is good for humans and horses, but if excessive, it can be immunosuppressive.

Muscles and the immune system

As is clear throughout this book, the immune system does not act in isolation. It interacts with other body systems, including the muscular system. The two systems interact by way of their cytokines. In effect, cytokines from the immune system affect muscles, while cytokines (or myokines) from muscles influence immunity. Extreme exercise, as described above, is an example of this two-way conversation.

Muscle functions

Immune cells are not the only source of the cytokines that contribute to muscle repair. Myokines themselves also promote stem cell differentiation in an autocrine manner. These include growth factors such as TGF-β, and a related protein, myostatin as well as the growth factors, FGF and PDGF (Waldemer-Streyer et al., 2022). Skeletal muscle is increasingly recognized as a secretory organ that produces cytokines in response to repeated contraction. These cytokines include IL-6, IL-7, and myostatin. Thus, the activation of inflammatory pathways during the course of intense exercise results in the release of cytokines that modulate or mitigate exercise-induced inflammation as well as the health of skeletal muscles (Docherty et al., 2022).

Muscles are the source of many of the different myokines released during exercise For example, the proinflammatory cytokine, IL-6 is produced mainly by muscle cells (Liburt et al., 2010). The IL-6 appears to serve an anti-inflammatory role by inhibiting the actions of TNF-α. It is produced in large quantities by skeletal muscle cells. and plays a role in suppressing inflammation and promoting healing (Rogeri et al., 2020). As described in Chapter 6, IL-6 is a major stimulant of the acute phase response. Its level is upregulated in direct correlation with the intensity of the exercise. It may rise up to 100-fold during exercise, especially if the exercise is prolonged (Lee et al., 2019.). Thus, IL-6 levels are significantly increased in endurance horses. The inflammatory cytokine IL-1β may also be significantly upregulated immediately after exercise. Liburt et al. have also demonstrated a significant increase in other cytokines such as IFN-γ (Liburt et al., 2010). It has also been demonstrated that IL-10 levels increase in conjunction with IL-6 levels. Both peak at the same time, suggesting that the IL-10 may play a regulatory role (Cywinska et al., 2014; Page et al., 2019). Another cytokine that is elevated following intensive exercise in horses is IL-13. It is a cytokine that can promote myogenesis. It may play a significant role in the adaptation of muscles to training (Witkowska-Pilaszewicz et al., 2020) It appears to play a role in the post-exercise recovery process (Plisak et al., 2023; Wilson et al., 2023). In a study of Thoroughbreds participating in a 1300-meter race found that after racing, the horses had higher levels of cortisol, IL-1 receptor antagonist (IL-1RA), leukocytes, and erythrocytes. This elevated IL-1RA level is unsurprising since its production is stimulated by IL-6 produced by contracting muscles (Arfuso et al., 2022).

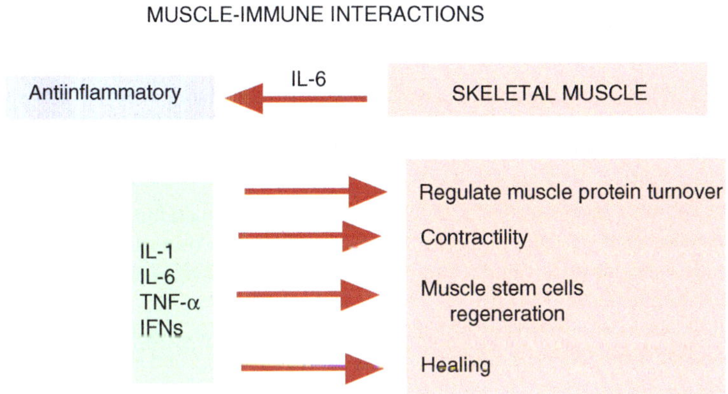

FIGURE 24.5 Muscle-immune cell interactions. Skeletal muscle cells produce IL-6 which in this situation has an anti-inflammatory effeci.

Conversely, the inflammatory cytokines have multiple effects on skeletal muscle.

In considering the role of myokines in response to intensive muscle usage, it should also be remembered that myokine gene expression appears to be specific to each muscle type and as described above, changes with time and training (Hammack et al., 2025) (Fig. 24.5).

The major inflammatory cytokines TNF-α, IL-1β, as well as the interferons, all have direct effects on muscle cell functions. For example, they regulate protein metabolism (Zoico & Roubenoff, 2002). They also stimulate muscle growth and regeneration. Thus, if muscles are traumatized, then local inflammation will result, and this has multiple significant results. The inflammatory cytokines promote the growth and proliferation of muscle stem cells. The initial inflammatory response, which involves the development of M1 macrophages, transitions to promoting an M2 phenotype that promotes muscle damage repair and regeneration. The four proinflammatory cytokines IL-1β, IL-13, TNF-α, and IFN-γ all stimulate muscle stem cell proliferation. These stem cells are essential for the repair of muscle injuries (Fu et al., 2015).

References

Akcay, S., Gurkok-Tan, T., & Ekici, S. (2025). Identification of key genes in immune response post endurance run in horses. *Journal of Equine Veterinary Science*. https://doi.org/10.1016/j.jevs.2025.105418

Arfuso, F., Giudice, E., Panzera, M., Rizzo, M., et al. (2022). Interleukin-1Ra (IL-1Ra) and serum cortisol level relationship in horse as dynamic adaptive response during physical exercise. *Veterinary Immunology and Immunopathology, 243*. https://doi.org/10.1016/j.vetimm.2021.110368

Baker, B., Gaffin, S. L., Wells, M., Wessels, B. C., & Brock-Utne. (1988). Endotoxaemia in racehorses following exertion. *Journal of the South African Veterinary Association, 59*, 63–66.

Banuelos, J. (2016). A gradient of glucocorticoid sensitivity among helper T cell cytokines. *Cytokine & Growth Factor Reviews, 31*, 27–35.

Baronzio, G., Gramaglia, A., & Fiorentini, G. (2006). Hyperthermia and immunity. A brief overview. *In Vivo, 20*, 689–696.

Barton, M. H., Williamson, L., Jacks, D., et al. (2003). Effects on plasma endotoxin and eicosanoid concentrations and serum cytokine activities in horses competing in 48-, 83-, or 159 km endurance ride under similar terrain and weather conditions. *American Journal of Veterinary Research, 64*, 754–761.

Borghetti, P., Saleri, R., Mocchegiani, E., Corradi, A., & Martelli, P. (2009). Infection, immunity and the neuroendocrine response. *Veterinary Immunology and Immunopathology, 130* (3-4), 141–162.

Brogden, K. A., Guthmiller, J. M., Salzet, M., & Zasloff, M. (2005). The nervous system and innate immunity: The neuropeptide connection. *Nature Immunology, 6*, 558–564.

Brownlow, M., & Mizzi, J. X. (2023). An overview of exertional heat illness in thoroughbred racehorses. Pathophysiology, diagnosis, and treatment rationale. *Animals*. https://doi.org/10.3390/ani13040610

Capomaccio, S., Cappelli, K., Spinsanti, G., Mencarelli, M., et al. (2011). Athletic humans and horses: Comparative analysis of interleukin-6 (IL-6) and IL-6 receptor (IL-6R) expression in peripheral blood mononuclear cells in trained and untrained subjects at rest. *BMC Physiology, 11*, 3.

Cupps, T. R., Gerrard, T. L., Falkoff, R. J., Whalen, G., & Fauci, A. S. (1985). Effect of in vitro corticosteroids on B cell activation, proliferation, and differentiation. *Journal of Clinical Investigation, 75*(2), 754–761.

Cywinska, A., Szarska, E., Gorecka, R., Witkowski, L., et al. (2012). Acute phase protein concentrations after limited distance and long distance endurance rides in horses. *Research in Veterinary Science, 93*, 1402–1406.

Cywinska, A., Turlo, A., Witkowski, L., Szarska, E., & Winnicka, A. (2014). Changes in blood cytokine concentrations in horses after long-distance endurance rides. *Medycyna Weterynaryjna, 70*, 568–571.

Cywinska, A., Witkowski, L., Szarska, E., Schollenberger, A., & Winnicka, A. (2013). Serum amyloid A (SAA) concentration after training sessions in Arabian race and endurance horses. *BMC Veterinary Research, 9*, 91.

De Bosscher, K., Vnden Berghe, W., Vermuelen, L., & Haegeman, G. (2000). Glucocorticoids repress NF-κB-driven genes by disturbing the interaction pf p65 with the basal transcription machinery irrespective of coactivator levels in the cell. *Proceedings of the National Academy of Sciences, 97*(8), 3919–3924.

Derksen, F. J., Slocombe, R. F., Gray, P. R., & Robinson, N. E. (1992). Exercise-induced pulmonary hemorrhage in horses with experimentally induced allergic lung disease. *American Journal of Veterinary Research, 53*(1), 15–21.

Docherty, S., Harley, R., McAuley, J. J., Crowe, L. A. N., et al. (2022). The effect of exercise on cytokines: Implications for musculoskeletal health: A narrative review. *BMC Sports Science, Medicine and Rehabilitation*. https://doi.org/10.1186/s13102-022-00397-2

Donovan, D. C., Jackson, C. A., Colahan, P. T., Norton, N. N., et al. (2007). Assessment of exercise induced alterations in neutrophil function in horses. *American Journal of Veterinary Research, 68*, 1198–1204.

Downing, J. E. G., & Miyan, J. A. (2000). Neural immunoregulation: Emerging roles for nerves in immune homeostasis and disease. *Immunology Today, 21*, 281–289.

Elenkov, E. J. (2004). Glucocorticoids and the Th1/Th2 balance. *Annals of the New York Academy of Sciences, 1024*, 138–146.

Fitzgerald, L. (1988). Exercise and the immune system. *Immunology Today, 9*, 337–339.

Folsom, R. W., Littlefield-Chabaud, M. A., French, D. D., Pourciau, S. S., et al. (2001). Exercise alters the immune response to equine influenza virus and increases susceptibility to infection. *Equine Veterinary Journal, 33*(7), 664–669.

Fu, X., Xiao, J., Wei, Y., Li, S., et al. (2015). Combination of inflammation-related cytokines promotes long-term muscle stem cell expansion. *Cell Research, 25*, 655–673.

Grzedzicka, J., Dabrowska, I., Malin, K., & Witkowska-Pilaszewicz, O. (2023). Exercise-related changes in the anabolic index (testosterone to cortisol ratio) and serum amyloid A concentration in endurance and racehorses at different fitness levels. *Frontiers in Veterinary Science, 10*, Article 1148990.

Hammack, S. M., Moshage, S. G., Kersh, M. E., & McCoy, A. M. (2025). Exercise-induced changes in foal myokine gene expression are specific to muscle type. *Journal of Equine Veterinary Science*. https://doi.org/10.1016/j.jevs.2025.105487

Horohov, D. W. (2008). *Immunological Responses to Exercise and Training. Equine Exercise Physiology* (pp. 410–422). Elsevier.

Karagianni, A. E., Kurian, D., Cillán-Garcia, E., Eaton, S. L., et al. (2022). Training associated alterations in equine respiratory immunity using a multiomics comparative approach. *Scientific Reports, 12*, 427. https://doi.org/10.1038/s41598-021-04137-3

Keadle, T. L., Pourciau, S. S., Melrose, P. A., Kammerling, S. G., & Horohov, D. W. (1993). Acute exercise stress modulates immune function in unfit horses. *Journal of Equine Veterinary Science, 13*(4), 226–231.

Kenney, M. J., & Ganta, C. K. (2014). Autonomic nervous system and immune system interactions. *Comparative Physiology, 4*, 1177–1200.

Korhonen, P. A. S., Lilius, E.-M., Hyyppa, S., Rasanen, L. A., & Posp, A. R. (2000). Production of reactive oxygen species in neutrophils after repeated bouts of exercise in standardbred trotters. *Journal of Veterinary Medicine A, 47*, 565–573.

Kristensen, L., Buhl, R., Nostell, K., Bak, L., et al. (2014). Acute exercise does not induce an acute phase response (APR) in standardbred trotters. *Canadian Journal of Veterinary Research, 78*, 97–102.

Lee, H. G., Choi, J.-Y., Park, J.-W., Song, K. D., et al. (2019). Effects of exercise on myokine gene expression in horse skeletal muscles. *Journal of Animal Science, 32*, 350–356.

Lejeune, J. P., Sandersen, C., Votion, D., Caudron, I., et al. (2010). Effect of intensive exercise on plasmatic neutrophil elastase level in eventing and endurance horses. *Equine Veterinary Journal, 42*, 12–16.

Liburt, N. R., Adams, A. A., Betancourt, A., Horohov, D. W., & McKeever, K. H. (2010). Exercise -induced increases in inflammatory cytokines in muscle and blood of horses. *Equine Veterinary Journal, 42*, 280–288.

McKeever, K. H., Arent, S. M., & Davitt, P. (2014). Endocrine and immune responses to exercise and training. In *The athletic horse* (pp. 88–107). Amsterdam, The Netherlands: Elsevier.

McKenzie, E., Esser, M., & Payton, E. (2014). Serum immunoglobulin concentrations in racing endurance horses. *Equine Veterinary Journal*. https://doi.org/10.1111/evj.12267-54

Meleiro, M. C. Z., Costa de Carvalho, H. J., Ribeiro, R., Duarte da Silva, M., et al. (2022). Immune functions alterations due to racing stress in thoroughbred horses. *Animals*. https://doi.org/10.3390/ani12091203

Moore, B. R. (1996). Lower respiratory tract disease. *Veterinary Clinics NA. Equine Practices, 12*(3), 457–472.

Page, A. E., Stewart, J. C., Fielding, C. L., & Horohov, D. W. (2019). The effect of a 160-kilometer competitive endurance ride on inflammatory marker MRNA expression in horses. *Equine Veterinary Journal, 79*, 45–49.

Plisak, U., Szczepaniak, J., Znigrodzka, M., Giercuszkiewicz-Hecold, B., & Witkowska-Pilaszewicz, O. (2023). Changes in novel antiinflammatory cytokine concentration in the blood of endurance and race horses at different levels of training. *Computational and Structural Biotechnology Journal, 21*, 418–424.

Raidal, S., Love, D., & Bailey, G. (1997). Effect of a single bout of high intensity exercise on lower respiratory tract contamination in the horse. *Australian Veterinary Journal, 75*, 293–295.

Robson, R. J., Alston, T. D., & Myburgh, K. H. (2003). Prolonged suppression of the innate immune system in the horse following an 80 km endurance race. *Equine Veterinary Journal, 35*(2), 133–137.

Rogeri, P. S., Gasparini, S. O., Martins, G. L., Costa, L. K. F., et al. (2020). Crosstalk between skeletal muscle and immune system: Which roles do IL-6 and glutamine play? *Frontiers in Physiology*. https://doi.org/10.3389/fphys.2020.582258

Rogers, C. J., Zaharoff, D. A., Hance, K. W., et al. (2008). Exercise enhances vaccine-induced antigen-specific T cell responses. *Vaccine, 26*, 5407–5415.

Scheiermann, C., Kunisaki, Y., & Frenette, P. S. (2013). Circadian control of the immune system. *Nature Reviews Immunology, 13*, 190–198.

Shaw, D. M., Merien, F., Braakhuis, A., & Dulson, D. (2018). T cells and their cytokine production. The anti-inflammatory and immunosuppressive effects of strenuous exercise. *Cytokine, 104*, 136–142.

Souza, C. M., Miotto, B. A., Bonin, C. P., & Camargo, M. M. (2010). Lower serum IgA levels in horses kept under extensive sanitary management and physical training. *Animal, 4*(12), 2080–2083.

Targowski, S. P. (1975). Effect of prednisolone on the leukocyte counts of ponies and on the reactivity of lymphocytes in vitro and in vivo. *Infection and Immunity, 11*(2), 252–256.

Trogdon Hines, M., Schott, H. C., Bayly, W. M., & Leroux, A. J. (1996). Exercise and immunity: A review with emphasis on the horse. *Journal of Veterinary Internal Medicine, 10*(5), 280–289.

Waldemer-Streyer, R. J., Kim, D., & Chen, J. (2022). Muscle cell-derived cytokines in skeletal muscle regeneration. *FEBS Journal*. https://doi.org/10.1111/febs.16372

Wilson, J., De Donato, M., Appelbaum, B., Garcia, C. T., & Peters, S. (2023). Differential expression of innate and adaptive immune genes during acute physical exercise in American quarter horses. *Animals*. https://doi.org/10.3390/ani13020308

Witkowska-Pilaszewicz, O., Pingwara, R., & Winnicka, A. (2020). The effect of physical training on peripheral blood mononuclear cell ex vivo proliferation, differentiation, activity, and reactive oxygen species in racehorses. *Antioxidants*. https://doi.org/10.3390/antiox9111155

Witkowska-Pilaszewicz, O., Malin, K., Dabrowska, I., Grzedzicka, J., et al. (2024). Immunology of physical exercise: Is *Equus caballus* an appropriate animal model for human athletes? *International Journal of Molecular Sciences.* https://doi.org/10.3390/ijms25105210

Wong, C. W., Smith, S. E., Thong, Y. H., Opdebeeck, J. P., & Thornton, J. R. (1992). Effects of exercise stress on various immune functions in horses. *American Journal of Veterinary Research, 53*(8), 1414–1417.

Zanos, T. P., Sikverman, H. A., Levy, T., Tsaava, T., et al. (2018). Identification of cytokine-specific sensory neural signals by decoding murine vagus nerve activity. *Proceedings of the National Academy of Sciences, 115.* https://doi.org/10.1073/pnas.1719083115

Zoico, E., & Roubenoff, R. (2002). The role of cytokines in regulating protein metabolism and muscle function. *Nutrition Reviews, 60*(2), 39–51.

CHAPTER

Obesity, old age, and immunosenescence

25

The horse is the longest-lived of the domestic mammals. In 2011, it was estimated that about 7.6% of the US and 13% of the UK equine population were over 20 years of age (Ireland et al., 2011). Over the past several years, the number of horses over 15 years of age has grown to 22%–34% (National Animal Health Monitoring System, 2015). Many remain active in competitions, some are still being bred, and many are simply companions. Just as in humans, old age in horses is associated with a reduction in muscle mass, increased obesity, and poorer body condition. Like older humans, elderly horses gradually develop age-related diseases such as osteoarthritis and lameness, as well as pituitary dysfunction (PPID), and cancers (Herbst et al., 2025). In addition, like other mammals, changes also occur in their immune systems. In general, aging is associated with a decline in the functioning of the adaptive immune system. The animal's ability to protect itself against infection declines, and their responses to vaccines diminishes. There is a progressive loss of T-cell-mediated immunity and an increase in certain aspects of innate immunity, especially chronic inflammation. Thus, as the immune system ages and declines functionally, a phenomenon called immunosenescence develops (McFarlane, 2013).

For obvious reasons, immunosenescence has been largely studied in humans. It does, however, also occur in horses but with some significant and interesting differences (DeNotta & McFarlane, 2023). Thus, as in humans, aged horses undergo a decline in lymphocyte activities, antibody production, and responses to vaccination. This does not appear to result in a significantly increased susceptibility to infectious diseases. Likewise, horses appear to be less susceptible to the chronic afflictions of older humans such as cancer and heart disease although this likely reflects their shorter life-span.

Telomeres are structures located at the ends of chromosomes that serve to maintain their stability and integrity. The length of these telomeres progressively shortens each time a cell undergoes mitosis. This, in effect, acts as a molecular aging clock, and telomere length correlates closely with an animal's age. This relative length also correlates closely with their lymphocyte proliferative ability as measured by tritiated thymidine incorporation, as well as with total IgG levels. Thus, there is a positive correlation between peripheral blood mononuclear cell activities and equine telomere length (Katepalli et al., 2008). The telomere shortening is not only related to their numbers but also to their production of proinflammatory cytokines. Thus, there is a negative correlation between the relative telomere length and pro-inflammatory cytokine (IFN-γ and TNF-α) expression. Shorter telomeres mean more inflammation (Fig. 25.1).

The Immunology of Horses and Donkeys. https://doi.org/10.1016/B978-0-443-44863-8.00022-3

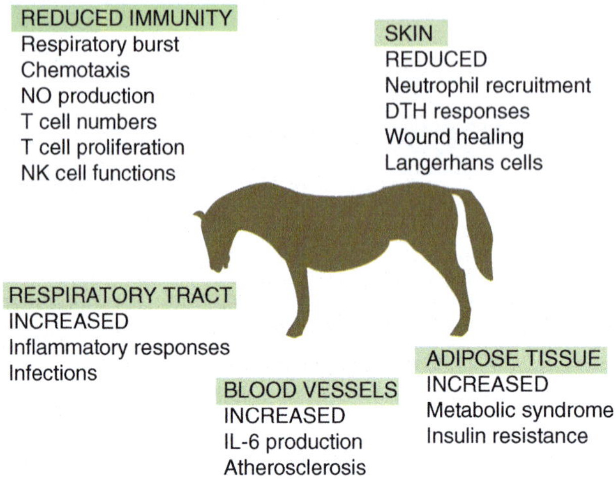

FIGURE 25.1

The major features of aging in the horse.

Obesity

Mammals posses two forms of adipose tissue, white and brown. Brown adipose tissue has not been identified in adult horses. The amount of white adipose tissue varies greatly between individual horses and is influenced by age, breed, and gender, in addition to diet (McCullagh et al., 2024). White adipose tissue was long considered a resting tissue where fat reserves were stored until needed. We now know, however, that adipose tissue plays an active role in both innate and adaptive immunity. It is an important (and large) endocrine organ. The major cell types found in adipose tissue are adipocytes and macrophages. The macrophages produce multiple proinflammatory cytokines including IL-1β, IL-6, MCP-1, and TNF-α. The adipocytes produce three cytokines (also called adipokines), leptin, adiponectin, and resistin. All three of these molecules, influence the functioning of the equine the immune system (Park & Ahima., 2015) (Fig. 25.2).

Leptin

Leptin levels increase in obese animals, and this suppresses appetite. For example, equine leptin levels are greater in horses with a higher body condition score than in slim, fit horses (Buff et al., 2002). Equine leptin is a protein of 145 amino acids (15 kDa) produced by adipocytes. While first described as an anti-obesity hormone, it also influences both innate and adaptive immunity and promotes inflammatory responses. It binds to receptors in the hypothalamus and suppresses the appetite. The amount of leptin in the blood is proportional to the amount of fat in the body. The fatter an animal, therefore, the more leptin is produced, and appetite is

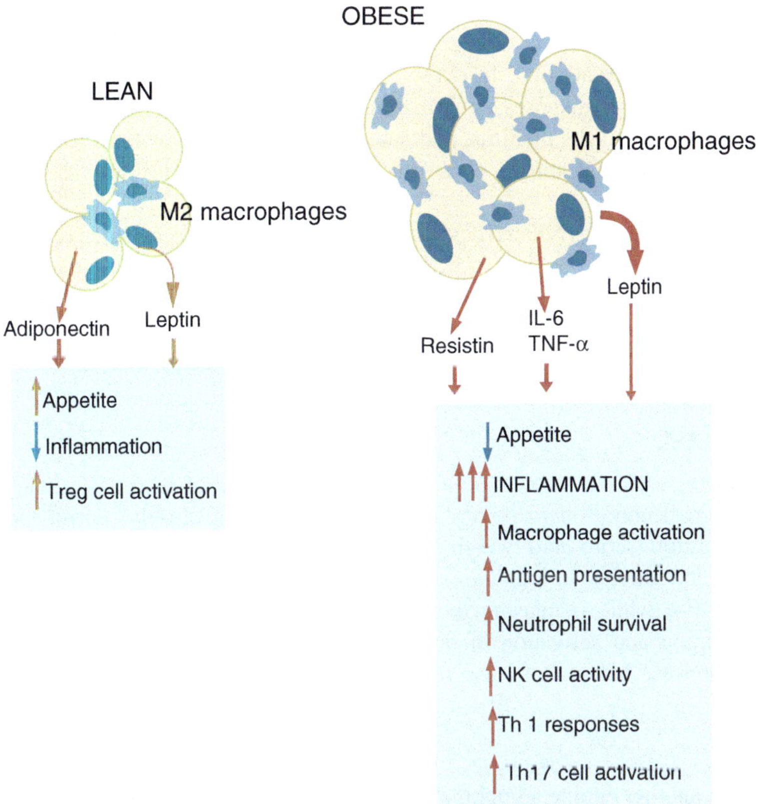

FIGURE 25.2 The interactions between adipocytes, macrophages, and the immune system.
These effects are especially important in old, obese horses.

correspondingly suppressed. Conversely, caloric restriction and weight loss lead to a loss of adipocytes, a drop in leptin levels, and an increase in appetite. In mares, leptin levels in colostrum are two to three times higher than those in blood, and it has been suggested that this leptin may be required for intestinal development in foals. It may also stimulate suckling by the foal (Naylor & Petri, 2016). The levels of leptin in equine serum are also affected by exercise. Thus, intensive exercise in young, or untrained horses raises blood leptin levels. In well-trained horses, plasma leptin levels do not change. Training effectively reduces leptin levels (Kedzierski, 2016).

Donkeys are often obliged to survive on low quality forages. If however they are fed high quality, calorie rich foods they are prone to obesity and its associated diseases. Serum leptin concentrations in donkeys are similar to those in horses (Mendoza et al., 2018).

White adipose tissue may contain up to 50% macrophages. These adipose tissue macrophages are M1 cells activated by leptin. Leptin increases their TNF-α, IL-6, and IL-1β production and upregulates their MHC class II expression. This increased

IL-6 production also promotes Th17-mediated inflammatory responses. Leptin also enhances Th17 responses by upregulating the transcription factor ROR-γt and suppressing Treg differentiation. In obese animals, therefore, this widespread macrophage activation predisposes to inflammatory diseases such as atherosclerosis, arthritis, type 2 diabetes mellitus, and autoimmunity, as well as to cancer (German et al., 2010). There is thus a clear link between obesity and chronic low-grade inflammation.

Leptin also enhances NK cell development and activation (de Andrade et al., 2025). It promotes Th1 cell production of IFN-γ, tumor necrosis factor-α (TNF-α), and leptin itself, thus generating an autocrine feedback loop. In lean animals where leptin levels are low, macrophage activation is suppressed, inflammatory responses are reduced, and there is a shift from Th1 to Th2 responses while increasing Treg cells.

Adiponectin

Adiponectin, a 28 kDa protein, counteracts the activities of leptin (German et al., 2010). Its concentration in ponies is positively (but not closely) correlated with body condition score and weight (Barnabe et al., 2024). It has strong anti-inflammatory activity. In lean animals, it decreases production of IL-8, IFN-γ, IL-6, and TNF-α while increasing the production of IL-1RA and IL-10. It induces the maturation and activation of dendritic cells. As a result, it reduces Th1 and Th17 responses. Adiponectin also regulates glucose and fatty acid metabolism.

Resistin

Resistin is another equine adipokine that mediates interactions between adipose tissue and immunity/inflammation. In the horse it is a protein of 214 amino acids and 22.5 kDa encoded by a gene on chromosome ECA 7. It is primarily produced by immune cells. In obesity, adiponectin production drops, and adipose tissue macrophages then produce resistin that increases insulin resistance, leading to diabetes (Nguyen, 2020). However, in a study that examined resistin levels in healthy horses and horses suffering from inflammatory diseases of different severity, it was found that their levels were also significantly correlated with the severity of the inflammation. Thus, horses with severe inflammation have elevated resistin levels, whereas these levels are very low in healthy horses. It was not correlated with insulin levels. However resistin levels are closely correlated with serum amyloid A levels (Fuentes-Romero et al., 2022).

Immunosenescence

Aging is a complex, multifactorial process that involves many body systems. Much depends upon the progressive accumulation of epigenetic changes such as DNA methylation. This tends to be a linear process in humans, as well as in horses.

Progressive aging results in a reduction in skeletal muscle mass, a general loss of bone mass, cartilage degradation in joints, and brain atrophy. White adipose tissue may increase as lean body mass declines. Genetic damage accumulates, telomeres shorten, epigenetic changes persist, nutrient signaling is altered, mitochondria begin to dysfunction, stem cells decline, and inflammation increases (McKenzie, 2022).

As animals age, their immune system changes. These changes affect many immune parameters when compared to the young and healthy. For example, aging of the immune system is associated with a decline in cell-mediated immunity and an increase in innate immunity. Beginning with thymic involution, T cell numbers drop over time while memory cells accumulate. There is also a shift in the helper T cell balance from Th1 to Th2 responses associated with a decline in IL-2 production (Schumacher et al., 2021). These changes contribute to the increased severity of infections in aged animals, as well as a decline in vaccination efficacy. They may also contribute to the increased prevalence and lethality of cancers (Franceschi et al., 2017). Thus, as the immune system ages, a phenomenon called immunosenescence develops. This is defined as the series of age-related changes that adversely affect the immune system. These, in turn, result from chronic stimulation by inflammatory immune responses (Candore et al., 2006).

Obviously, the ability of the immune system to permit an animal to survive in a microbial world until successful reproduction and parenting have occurred is central to species survival. After that critical period, in post-reproductive life, chronic inflammation progressively develops. In this situation, a weak inflammatory response may serve to increase lifespan provided the pathogen burden remains low (Fig. 25.3).

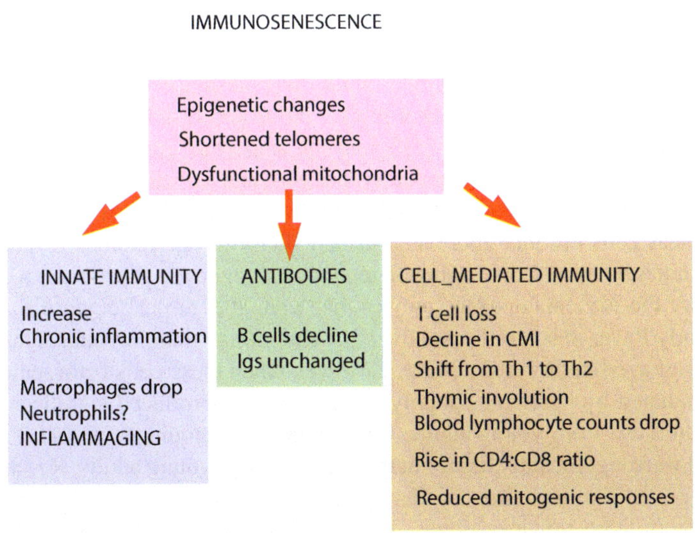

FIGURE 25.3

The key features of immunosenescence.

It is not only changes in the immune system that develop with increasing age. Other organs, including the heart and respiratory system, age as well. For example, the lungs of aged horses show an age-related decline in the transcription of IL-1β and CXCL8 but not in IL-6 or TNF-α. The frequency of IFN-γ-producing lymphocytes in BALF increases with age. The number of alveolar macrophages, however, is unaffected by aging (Hansen et al., 2015).

Most of the intrinsic factors that influence lifespan and thus immunosenescence are under genetic control. They do this because genes control critical housekeeping and cellular maintenance functions such as the elimination of invaders and the repair of tissue damage. In fact, longevity is directly correlated with optimal performance of the immune system (Liu et al., 2023).

Innate immunity

Innate, cell-mediated, and humoral immune responses all change with advancing age. They are characterized by chronic activation, decreased responsiveness to stimulation, and reductions in the efficiency of antigen processing and presentation (Candore et al., 2006). The aging process also differs between individuals. Some animals experience increased inflammation, whereas others show a decrease. In healthy aged horses, neutrophil adherence, the oxidative burst, and phagocytosis are unchanged, but their chemotactic responsiveness is increased (McFarlane & McDaniel, 2010). In those individuals where inflammation appears to decrease with age, macrophage numbers decline, and they express lower levels of TLRs. Aging is associated with impaired TLR signaling. When stimulated with TLR ligands, these aged macrophages secrete reduced amounts of IL-6 and TNF-α. Aged macrophages also mount reduced responses to activators such as IFN-γ and produce less nitric oxide. Aged horses also have decreased monocyte counts and plasma myeloperoxidase (Miller et al., 2021). However, they produce more TNF-α and less IL-17—Perhaps this is a compensatory response. Th17 cells play an important role in the pathogenesis of many immune-mediated inflammatory diseases, and a decline in IL-17 production has an anti-inflammatory effect. It has also been reported that the peripheral blood mononuclear cells produce more TNF-α and IFN-γ in aged horses (Adams et al., 2008). Studies on the effect of aging on monocyte phagocytic functions have demonstrated that the percentage of monocytes that were able to phagocytose *E. coli* was significantly lower in senior horses over 20 years of age than in young adult horses, 4–6 years of age (Herbst et al., 2022). However, when these cells from senior horses were stimulated by bacterial lipopolysaccharide, they produced significantly more IL-1β than those from young adults. Conversely, the amounts of CXCL8 and IL-6 produced were significantly higher in the cells from the young adults. Recent studies have suggested that signaling by IL-4 slows macrophage aging by promoting the production of DNA repair enzymes. Thus, the activities of Th2 cells may maintain macrophage functionality and slow macrophage senescence (Zhou et al., 2024, p. p513).

Inflammaging

Aging is associated with a progressive increase in a chronic low-grade inflammation - a process called inflammaging. This is a result of the gradual accumulation of damaged or dying cells and organelles over time. These dying cells generate senescence-associated DAMPs that act through TLR2 and IL-1β to activate the NF-κB pathway. This, in turn, results in chronic activation of the innate immune system. This chronic activation eventually leads to changes in the phenotype of some cells, such as macrophages. As a result, pro-inflammatory cytokine levels in the bloodstream gradually increase over time (Candore et al., 2006). These, in turn, are responsible for the age-associated increase in chronic diseases. Aged horses show a change in their inflammatory cytokine profile. For example, they show increased gene expression of TNF-α, IL-1β, IL-6, CXCL8, IFN-γ, IL-15, and IL-18 (Adams et al., 2008; McFarlane & Holbrook, 2008). These changes also depend, to a large extent, on the health of the animal and whether it is also suffering from concurrent but inapparent infections. As in humans, horses also increase their production of proinflammatory cytokines as their body weight increases and obesity develops. Old fat horses have more lymphocytes and monocytes producing TNF-α and IFN-λ compared to old thin horses (Adams et al., 2009). Serum levels of TNF-α in horses were significantly reduced when the animals lost weight.

Recent studies in mice have identified a subpopulation of adipose-tissue macrophages that also control the production of inflammaging cyokines. The specific macrophage population is $CD169^+$ $CD11c^-$ and they appear to be closely associated with nerves. However this regulatory population declines with age so permitting inflammaging to increase (Gonzalez-Hurtado et al., 2025).

Senescence-associated secretory phenotype

As cells age, they undergo alterations in structure, chromatin organization, and metabolism. Their organelles such as mitochondria, release damaged or disrupted DNA into their cytoplasm. Mitochondria have evolved from a population of intracellular bacteria. As a result affected cells are triggered to activate their defenses. For example, mitochondrial DNA activates the cGAS-STING pathway, which affects the cell behavior (Bahat et al., 2025). Their growth is arrested, and they begin to generate senescence-associated DAMPs that act through TLR2 and IL-1β to activate the NF-κB pathway. These chronically activated senescent cells eventually develop a state known as the senescence-associated secretory phenotype (SASP). They undergo metabolic reprogramming and, as a result, produce increasing quantities of inflammatory mediators, immune modulators, growth factors, such as TNF-α, IL-1β, IL-6, metalloproteases, enzymes, and chemokines. They also generate exosomes containing not only enzymes but also microRNA, and DNA fragments. As a result, TNF-α, IL-6, IL-8, and C-reactive protein levels in the bloodstream increase gradually over time while these senescent cells progressively accumulate (Behmoaras & Gil, 2020). SASP cells are metabolically active and, while just a relatively small proportion (2%–3%) of tissue cells, are a significant contributor to the diseases of aging (Fig. 25.4).

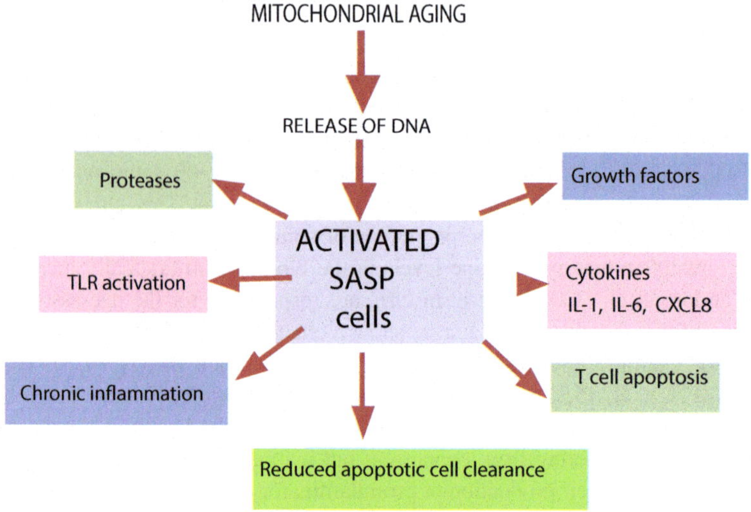

FIGURE 25.4 The production and phenotype of SASP cells.

This phenotype is triggered by mitochondrial aging. Since mitochondria have evolved from intracellular bacteria the cell responds as if infected. It thus activates its intracellular defensive responses.

The generation of SASP macrophages is the main driver of age-related inflammation. At low levels, these cells may be protective, but as the levels of proinflammatory cytokines increase, they eventually provoke the development of many of the chronic diseases of aging, such as heart disease, neurodegeneration, and arthritis. In some respects, therefore, inflammaging can be considered a manifestation of innate autoimmunity (Kale et al., 2020). Eliminating these SASP cells can delay age-related tissue dysfunction and potentially increase a horse's lifespan (Baker et al., 2016). SASP cells can also promote tissue repair and wound healing (Kale et al., 2020). The generation of a SASP phenotype is, however, a detrimental process. Under normal circumstances, macrophages eliminate unwanted dead, dying, and neoplastic cells. Thus, TNF-α secreted by macrophages, can serve to induce apoptosis in senescent dermal fibroblasts. Once this has occurred, the dead cells are phagocytosed by the macrophages. However, SASP cells suppress these clearance functions, and as a result, senescent cells tend to accumulate (Ogata et al., 2020).

Zak et al. (2020) investigated the role of aging on the acute-phase protein levels of horses. They found that the concentrations of serum amyloid A, C-reactive protein, haptoglobin, activin A, a1-antichymotrypsin, and procalcitonin were unaffected by age. There were no significant differences between aged and healthy horses. Absolute numbers of NK cells are lower in aged animals. In addition, their proliferative responses decline with age (DeNotta & McFarlane, 2023).

Adaptive immunity

Both cell-mediated and humoral immune responses decline with advancing age. This is characterized by decreased responsiveness to antigenic stimulation (Candore et al., 2006).

Lymphoid organs

Thymic involution is the most obvious of the age-related changes in lymphoid organs. As a result, the size of the functional T cell pool drops over time while memory cells accumulate. There is also a progressive shift in the helper T cell balance from Th1 to Th2 responses associated with a decline in IL-2 production (Schumacher et al., 2021). Ileal Peyer's patches involute after sexual maturity. Old animals also have a reduced splenic white pulp. Lymph node changes vary depending on their location but include cortical atrophy and medullary fibrosis. The bone marrow appears to be relatively unaffected by old age, and an aged bone marrow can reconstitute the body as well as a young one can.

Blood leukocyte counts

The most obvious change in aged horse hematology is a decline in total leukocyte counts. This is especially obvious in lymphocyte populations that decrease significantly with age (Blount et al., 2005). There is consequently reduced T cell diversity in older horses. Conversely, the number of Th17 cells increases with age, a finding compatible with the concept of inflammaging.

Because of this T cell senescence, the relative percentages of lymphocytes and $CD4^+$ T cells in the bloodstream decrease, whereas the percentage of granulocytes and $CD8^+$ T cells increases with age (Nikolich-Zugich, 2018). In old horses (>20 years), there is a significant decrease in the proportion of $CD8^+$ T cells and a rise in the CD4:CD8 ratio compared with young animals. Horses over 20 years of age have reduced lymphocyte responses to mitogens, and this deficiency cannot be overcome by exposure to additional IL-2 (Horohov et al., 2002). McFarlane et al. (2001) reported a decrease with age of total T cells as well as CD54 and $CD8^+$ cells. Conversely, Adams et al. (2008) reported an increase in total T cell numbers.

There is also an increase in the relative percentage of $CD4^+$ T cells in aged horses. These aged T cells respond poorly to the T cell mitogen, concanavalin A. However, these horses have an increased frequency of $CD8^-$, IFN-γ^+, and TNF-α^+ T cells. They also have elevated serum levels of IL-1β, IL-15, CXCL-8, and TNF-α gene expression in peripheral blood, - evidence of inflammaging (Adams et al., 2008). In ponies, it has been reported that there is also a decrease in monocyte and eosinophil counts (Horohov et al., 2002).

Horohov and his colleagues have demonstrated that old horses (~25 years) had similar T cell lymphokine activated killer cell activity as young horses (<7.5 years) (Horohov et al., 1999).

Adaptive immunity

Aging is associated with a progressive increase in defects in lymphoid cell hematopoiesis, especially T and B cells. It has been theorized that one reason for this is the development of a bias in hematopoietic stem cells (HSCs) toward producing myeloid cells and megakaryocyte precursors. However, it appears that all lineages, lymphoid, myeloid, and megakaryocyte, show a progressive loss of differentiation. HSCs can compensate for these defects in the myeloid cell line and B cell precursors, but not in the T cell precursors. As a result of this stem cell uncoupling, T cell production is selectively impaired (Jang et al., 2023).

Although the thymus involutes with age, the T cell pool has to be maintained. This is accomplished by periodic expansions of the T cell population. However, repeated proliferative episodes erode telomere length and, as a result, T cells continue to age. End-stage T cells with shortened telomeres accumulate. The thymic involution results in the reduced export of cells from the thymus and a decline in the numbers of $CD8^+$ T cells. In addition, the lymphocyte population of the aged animal changes from a naïve population to a memory cell population. T cells from aged animals lose their ability to progress through the cell cycle. As a result, early events in the T cell response to antigens, such as activation of protein kinase C and the rise in intracellular calcium, are impaired. Even after expressing IL-2 receptors and being exposed to IL-2, aged T cells may not respond effectively to antigens. Analysis shows that some aged T cells continue to produce normal amounts of IL-2, but many do not. Horses show an age-dependent decline in lymphocyte proliferation in response to exposure to IL-2 (Horohov et al., 2002).

As a result, aged T cell populations are mixtures of fully functional and impaired cells. It also appears that aged T cells begin to express the enzyme pathways associated with NK cells (Laphanuwat et al., 2023). IL-17 controls the homeostasis of Treg cells and also the maintenance of core body temperature (Papotto & Silva-Santos., 2018). IL-10-producing Tfh cells also accumulate with age and so contribute to age-related immunosuppression (Almanan et al., 2020). Robbin et al. (2011) however, reported that the percentage of equine Treg cells decreases with age.

B cell responses

The bone marrow is relatively unaffected by old age, and an aged bone marrow can reconstitute the body as well as a young one. If aged B cells are mixed with young T cells, the response is relatively normal. If the reverse is attempted (i.e., mixing young B cells with aged T cells), the B cells respond poorly. Somatic hypermutation in immunoglobulin V region genes declines in old animals, so that antibody affinity tends to be lower than in young animals. Nevertheless, immunoglobulin concentrations do not decline in old age. Aged horses show a significant decrease in B cell numbers compared to young animals. However, the serum levels of IgG3/5, IgM, and IgA are not significantly different between age groups (McFarlane et al., 2001).

Vaccine responsiveness

Aged horses have been reported to mount a weaker immune response to influenza vaccination when compared to young, healthy horses (Ralston et al., 1988). This difference may be as much as tenfold (Horohov et al., 2002). In a study that compared the immune responses of young and aged horses to influenza and rabies vaccination. It was found that healthy aged horses mounted an antibody response to the rabies vaccine that was similar to that observed in young adult horses. However, the aged horses had a significantly reduced anamnestic response to the influenza vaccine when compared to the young horses (Muirhead et al., 2010) (Fig. 25.5).

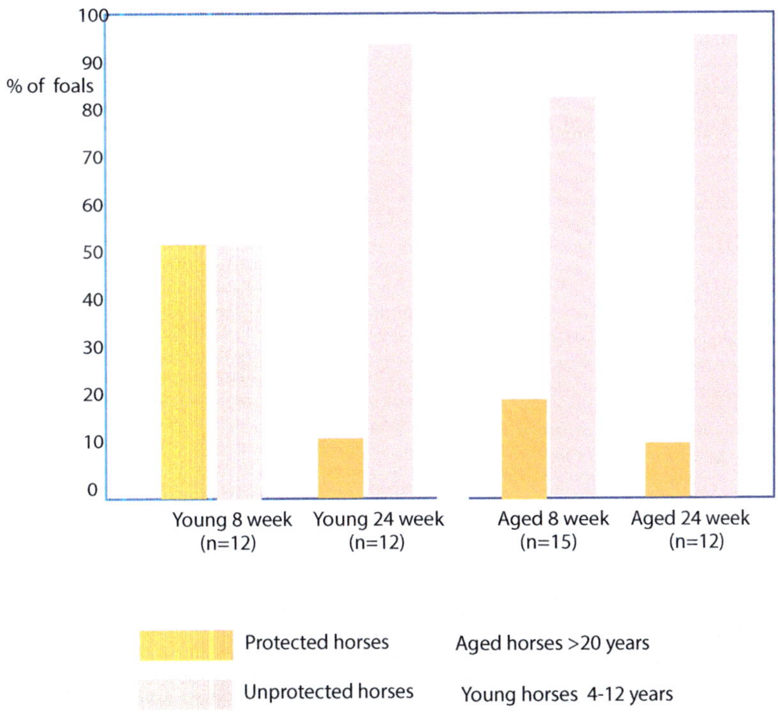

FIGURE 25.5 Immune responses to vaccination in aged horses.

The antibody response of horses vaccinated against rabies depends upon their age. This chart shows the proportion of young ($-10 yrs) and aged (>20 years) horses that have a protective antibody titer eight and 24 weeks following rabies vaccination. Note that the aged horses mounted a weak primary response. In both the young and aged animals the antibody response had declined significantly by 24 weeks.

- With permission Muirhead et al. (2010).

The aged microbiota

Equine intestinal physiology and function also change during the aging process. Given the importance of the gastrointestinal lymphoid tissues and their interactions with the microbiota, it is unsurprising that the intestinal microbiota may have a significant effect on the aging of the adaptive immune system and the intestinal lymphoid tissues.

The most significant of these changes occur in young foals and during the aging process at times when the immune system is most vulnerable. It is also well established that the microbiota also changes with age, and these changes may likely affect the health of the aged horse. For example, in the aged horse, there is a decrease in microbial diversity and a rise in the populations of pathobionts (Nagpal et al., 2018).

Recent studies on aged humans and mice have found that as they age, their intestinal microbiota produces increased quantities of phenylacetic acid and its metabolite phenylacetylglutamine. These two molecules induce vascular endothelial senescence. As a result of enhancing mitochondrial peroxide production, they exacerbate the development of the senescence-associated secretory phenotype and drive cardiovascular aging (Saravi et al., 2025).

References

Adams, A. A., Breathnach, C. C., Katepalli, M. P., et al. (2008). Advanced age in horses affects divisional history of T cells and inflammatory cytokine production. *Mechanism of Ageing and Development, 129*, 656–664.

Adams, A. A., Katepalli, M. P., Kohler, K., et al. (2009). Effect of body condition, body weight and adiposity on inflammatory cytokine responses in old horses. *Veterinary Immunology and Immunopathology, 127*, 286–294.

Almanan, M., Raynor, J., Ogunsulire, I., Malyshkina, A., et al. (2020). IL-10-producing Tfh cells accumulate with age and link inflammation with age-related immunosuppression. *Science Advances, G*, Article eabb0806.

Bahat, A., Milenkovic, D., Cors, E., Barnette, M., et al. (2025). Ribonucleotide incorporation into mitochondrial DNA drives inflammation. *Nature*. https://doi.org/10.1038/s41586-025-09541-7

Baker, D. J., Childs, B. G., Durik, M., Wijers, M. E., et al. (2016). Naturally occurring p16lnk4a-positive cells shorten healthy lifespan. *Nature, 530*, 184–189.

Barnabe, M. A., Elliott, J., Harris, P. A., & Menzies-Gow, N. J. (2024). Relationships between total adiponectin concentrations and obesity in native-breed ponies in England. *Equine Veterinary Journal, 56*, 264–272.

Behmoaras, J., & Gil, J. (2020). Similarities and interplay between senescent cells and macrophages. *The Journal of Cell Biology*. https://doi.org/10.1083/jcb.202010162

Blount, D. G., Pritchard, D. L., & Heaton, P. R. (2005). Age-related alterations in immune parameters in labrador retriever dogs. *Veterinary Immunology and Immunopathology, 108*, 399–407.

Buff, P. R., Dodds, A. C., Morrison, C. D., Whitley, N. C., et al. (2002). Leptin in horses: Tissue localization and relationship between peripheral concentrations of leptin and body condition. *Journal of Animal Science, 80*, 2942–2949.

Candore, G., Colonna-Romano, G., Balistreri, C. R., Di Carlo, D., et al. (2006). Biology of longevity: The role of the innate immune system. *Rejuvenation Research, 1*, 143–148.

de Andrade, A. G., Vanderley, S. E. R., Marques, L. F., Almeida, F. S., et al. (2025). Leptin, NK cells, and the weight of immunity: Insights into obesity. *International Immunopharmacology.* https://doi.org/10.1016/j.intimp.2024.113992

DeNotta, S., & McFarlane, D. (2023). Immunosenescence and inflammaging in the aged horse. *Immunology & Aging.* https://doi.org/10.1186/s12979-022-00325-5

Franceschi, C., Garagnani, P., Vitale, G., Capri, M., & Salviolo, S. (2017). Inflammaging and garb-aging. *Trends in Endocrinology and Metabolism.* https://doi.org/10.1016/j.tem.2016.09.005

Fuentes-Romero, B., Munoz-Prieto, A., Ceron, J. J., Martin-Cuervo, M., et al. (2022). Measurement of plasma resistin concentrations in horses with metabolic and inflammatory disorders. *Animals.* https://doi.org/10.3390/ani2010077

German, A. J., Ryan, V. H., German, A. C., et al. (2010). Obesity, its associated disorders and the role of inflammatory adipokines in companion animals. *The Veterinary Journal, 185*, 4–9.

Gonzalez-Hurtado, E., Leveau, C., Li, K., Mishra, M., et al. (2025). Nerve-associated macrophages control adipose tissue homeostasis across lifespan and restrain age-related inflammation. *Nature.* https://doi.org/10.1038/s43587-025-00952-9

Hansen, S., Baptiste, K. E., Fjeldborg, J., & Horohov, D. W. (2015). A review of equine age-related changes in the immune system: Comparisons between human and equine aging, with focus on lung-specific immune aging. *Aging Research Revs, 20*, 11–23.

Herbst, A. C., Coleman, M. C., Macon, E. L., Harris, P. A., & Adams, A. A. (2025). Owner-reported health and disease in US senior horses. *Equine Veterinary Journal, 57*, 684–702.

Herbst, A. C., Reedy, S. E., Page, A. E., Horohov, D. W., & Adams, A. A. (2022). Effect of aging on monocyte phagocytic and inflammatory functions, and on the ex vivo inflammatory response to lipopolysaccharide in horses. *Veterinary Immunology and Immunopathology.* https://doi.org/10.1016/j.vetimm.2022.110459

Horohov, D. W., Dimmock, A., Guirnalda, P., Folsom, R. W., et al. (1999). Effect of exercise on the immune response of young and old horses. *American Journal of Veterinary Research, 60*, 643–647.

Horohov, D. W., Kydd, J. H., & Hannant, D. (2002). The effect of aging on T cell responses in the horse. *Developmental & Comparative Immunology, 26*, 121–128.

Ireland, J. L., Clegg, P. D., McGowan, C. M., McKane, S. A., & Pinchbeck, G. L. (2011). A cross-sectional study of geriatric horses in the United Kingdom. Part 1: Demographics and management practices. *Equine Veterinary Journal, 43*, 30–36.

Jang, G., Castillo, S. C., Esteva, E., Upadhaya, S., et al. (2023). Stem cell decoupling underlies impaired lymphoid development during aging. *Proceedings of the National Academy of Sciences of the United States of America, 120*(22). https://doi.org/10.1073/pnas.2302019120

Kale, A., Sharma, A., Stolzing, A., Desprez, P.-Y., et al. (2020). Role of immune cells in the removal of deleterious senescent cells. *BMC Immunity and Ageing.* https://doi.org/10.1186/s12979-020-00187-9

Katepalli, M. P., Adams, A. A., Lear, T. L., & Horohov, D. W. (2008). The effect of age and telomere length on immune function in the horse. *Developmental & Comparative Immunology, 32*, 1409–1415.

Kedzierski, W. (2016). The effect of exercise on plasma leptin concentrations in horses. *Journal of Equine Veterinary Science, 47*, 36–41.

Laphanuwat, P., Gomes, D. C. O., & Akbar, A. N. (2023). Senescent T cells; beneficial and detrimental roles. *Immunological Reviews, 316*(1), 160–175.

Liu, Z., Liang, Q., Ren, Y., Guo, C., et al. (2023). Immunosenescence: Molecular mechanisms and diseases. *Signal Transduction and Targeted Therapy*. https://doi.org/10.1038/s41392-023-01451-2

McCullagh, S., Keen, J., Dosi, M., & Morgan, R. (2024). Bringing equine adipose tissue into focus. *Equine Veterinary Education, 36*, 145–151.

McFarlane, D. (2013). Immunosenescence in horses. *AAEP Proceedings, 59*, 1–3.

McFarlane, D., & Holbrook, T. C. (2008). Cytokine dysregulation oin aged horses and horses with pituitary pars intermedia dysfunction. *Journal of Veterinary Internal Medicine, 22*, 436–442.

McFarlane, D., & McDaniel, K. (2010). Neutrophil function in healthy aged horses and horses with pituitary dysfunction. *Journal of Veterinary Internal Medicine, 24*, 688–689.

McFarlane, D., Sellon, D. C., & Gibbs, S. A. (2001). Age-related quantitative alterations in lymphocyte subsets and immunoglobulin isotypes in healthy horses. *American Journal of Veterinary Research, 62*, 1413–1417.

McKenzie, B. A. (2022). Comparative veterinary gerosenescence: Mechanism of molecular, cellular, and tissue aging in humans, laboratory animal models, and companion dogs and cats. *American Journal of Veterinary Research*. https://doi.org/10.2460/ajvr.22.02.0027

Mendoza, F. J., Toribio, R. E., & Perez-Ecija, A. (2018). Donkey internal medicine - Part I: Metabolic, endocrine, and alimentary tract disturbances. *Journal of Equine Veterinary Science, 65*, 66–74.

Miller, A. B., Loynachan, A. T., Barker, V. D., & Adams, A. A. (2021). Investigation of innate immune function in adult and geriatric horses. *Veterinary Immunology and Immunopathology, 235*. https://doi.org/10.1016/j.vetimm.2021.110207

Muirhead, T. L., McClure, J. T., Wichtel, J. J., Stryhn, H., et al. (2010). The effect of age on the immune response of horses to vaccination. *Journal of Comparative Pathology, 1421*, s85–s90.

Nagpal, R., Mainali, R., Ahmadi, S., Wang, S., et al. (2018). Gut microbiome and aging: Physiological and mechanistic insights. *Nutrition and Healthy Aging, 4*, 267–285.

National Animal Health Monitoring System Studies. (2015). *Age-related trends in demographics of equids in the United States*. https://www.aphis.usda.gov/animal_health/hahms/equine/downloads/equine15.equine15_is_Trends Age.pdf.

Naylor, C., & Petri, W. A. (2016). Leptin regulation of immune responses. *Trends in Molecular Medicine, 22*, 88–98.

Nguyen, T. M. D. (2020). Adiponectin: Role in physiology and pathophysiology. *International Journal of Preventive Medicine, 11*, 136–144.

Nikolich-Zugich, J. (2018). The twilight of immunity: Emerging concepts in aging of the immune system. *Nature Immunology, 19*, 10–19.

Ogata, Y., Yamada, T., Hasegawa, S., Sanada, A., et al. (2020). SASP-induced macrophage dysfunction may contribute to accelerated fibroblast accumulation in the dermis. *Experimental Dermatology, 30*(1), 84–91.

Papotto, P. H., & Silva-Santos, B. (2018). Got my γδ17T cells to keep me warm. *Nature Immunology, 19*, 426–434.

Park, H.-K., & Ahima, R. S. (2015). Physiology of leptin: Energy homeostasis, neuroendocrine function and metabolism. *Metabolism, 64*(1), 24–34.

Ralston, S. L., Nockels, C. F., & Squires, E. L. (1988). Differences in diagnostic test results and hematologic data between aged and young horses. *American Journal of Veterinary Research, 49*, 1387–1392.

Robbin, M. G., Wagner, B., Norhona, L. E., Antczak, D. F., & de Mestre, A. M. (2011). Subpopulations of equine blood lymphocytes expressing regulatory T cell markers. *Veterinary Immunology and Immunopathology, 140*, 90–101.

Saravi, S. S. S., Pugin, B., Constancias, F., Shabanian, K., et al. (2025). Gut microbiota-dependent increase in phenylacetic acid induces endothelial senescence during aging. *Nature Aging, 5*, 1–25=1045.

Schumacher, B., Pothof, J., Vijg, J., & Hoeijmakers, J. H. (2021). The central role of DNA damage in the aging process. *Nature, 592*, 695–703.

Zak, A., Siwinska, N., Elzinga, S., Barker, V. D., et al. (2020). Effects of equine metabolic syndrome on inflammation and acute-phase markers in horses. *Domestic Animal Endocrinology, 72*. https://doi.org/10.1016/j.domianiend.2020.10647

Zhou, Z., Yao, J., Wu, D., Li, X., et al. (2024). Type 2 cytokine signaling in macrophages protects from cellular senescence and organismal aging. *Immunity, 57*(3), p513–527.

Abbreviations

ACTH	Adrenocorticotropic hormone
AD	Allergic (or atopic) dermatitis
ADCC	Antibody-dependent cell-mediated cytotoxicity
AGP	Alpha-1-acid glycoprotein
AHS	African horse sickness
AIM2	Absent in melanoma 2
AIRE	Autoimmune regulator
AITP	Autoimmune thrombocytopenia
ANA	Antinuclear antibody
APC	Antigen-presenting cell
APP	Acute phase protein
APRIL	A proliferation-inducing ligand
BAFF	B-cell activating factor
BALF	Bronchoalveolar lavage fluid
BALT	Bronchus-associated lymphoid tissue
BCE	Before the Christian era
BCG	Bacillus Calmette–Guerin (*Mycobacterium bovis*)
BCR	B-cell (antigen) receptor
C	Complement
CAM	Cell adhesion molecule
CBH	Cutaneous basophil hypersensitivity
CCL	A chemokine ligand with paired cysteine (C) residues
CD	Cluster of differentiation
cDC	Classical (or conventional) dendritic cell
CDR	Complementarity-determining region
cGAS	Cyclic GMP–AMP synthase
Con A	Concanavalin A
COX	Cyclooxygenase
CpG DNA	Cytosine–guanosine-rich DNA
CR	Complement receptor
CRP	C-reactive protein
CSF	Colony-stimulating factor (or cerebrospinal fluid)
CTL	C-type lectin
CTLA-4	Cytotoxic T-lymphocyte–associated (protein)-4
CXCL	A chemokine
DAF	Decay accelerating factor
DAMP	Damage-associated molecular pattern
DC	Dendritic cell

DC-SIGN	Dendritic cell-specific ICAM-Grabbing Nonintegrin
DIC	Disseminated intravascular coagulation
dsRNA	Double-stranded RNA
DTH	Delayed-type hypersensitivity
EAS	*Equus asinus*. The designation of donkey chromosomes
EAV	Equine arteritis virus
EBD	Equine beta-defensin
ECA	*Equus caballus*. The designation of horse chromosomes
EHV	Equine herpesvirus
EIA	Equine infectious anemia
ELA	Equine leukocyte antigen
ELISA	Enzyme-linked immunosorbent assay
ERU	Equine recurrent uveitis
EVA	Equine viral arteritis
Fab	Antigen-binding fragment
FACS	Fluorescence-activated cell sorter
Fc	Crystallizable fragment (of immunoglobulin)
FcR	Immunoglobulin (Fc) receptor
FcRn	Neonatal Fc receptor
fDC	Follicular dendritic cell
FGF	Fibroblast growth factor
FH	Factor H
FoxP3	Forkhead box P3—a transcription factor
GALT	Gut-associated lymphoid tissue
GATA	A transcription factor that can bind to the amino acid sequence G
GM-CSF	Granulocyte–macrophage colony-stimulating factor
GPI	Glycosylphosphatidylinositol
GVH	Graft-versus-host (disease)
GWAS	Genome-wide association studies
HDN	Hemolytic disease of the newborn
HEV	High endothelial venule
HMGB1	High-mobility group box protein-1
Hp	Haptoglobin
HSC	Hematopoietic stem cell
HSP	Heat shock protein
IBD	Inflammatory bowel disease
ICAM	Intercellular adhesion molecule
IDDM	Insulin-dependent diabetes mellitus
IDO	Indoleamine 2,3-dioxygenase
IEL	Intraepithelial lymphocyte
IFA	Indirect fluorescence assay
IFN	Interferon
Ig	Immunoglobulin
IL	Interleukin
ILC	Innate lymphoid cell
IMHA	Immune-mediated hemolytic anemia

iNOS	Induced nitric oxide synthase
ISG	interferon-stimulated gene
ITAM	Immunoreceptor tyrosine-based activation motif
J chain	Joining chain
JAK	Janus tyrosine kinase
kb	Kilobases, a measure of gene size
kDa	Kilodalton
KIR	Killer immunoglobulin–like receptor
LAK	Lymphokine-activated killer (cells)
LE	Lupus erythematosus
LFA	Leucocyte function–associated antigen
LGL	Large granular lymphocyte
LILR	Leukocyte immunoglobulin–like receptor
LPS	Lipopolysaccharide
LT	Lymphotoxin (or leukotriene)
M-cell	Microfold cell
M-CSF	Macrophage colony–stimulating factor
MAb	Monoclonal antibody
MAdCAM-1	Mucosal addressin cell adhesion molecule-1
MAIT	Mucosal-associated invariant T (cells)
MAMP	Microbial-associated molecular pattern
MBL	Mannose-binding lectin
MCP	Monocyte chemoattractant protein (or male chauvinist pig)
MEED	Multisystemic eosinophilic epitheliotropic disease
MHC	Major histocompatibility complex
MIP	Macrophage inflammatory protein
MLV	Modified live virus
MODS	Multiple organ dysfunction syndrome
MPGN	Mesangioproliferative glomerulonephritis
MSH	Melanocyte-stimulating hormone
mTEC	Medullary thymic epithelial cell
mya	Million years ago
NAP	Neutrophil antibacterial peptide
NET	Neutrophil extracellular trap
NF-κB	Nuclear factor-kappa B
NI	Neonatal isoerythrolysis
NK	Natural killer (cell)
NKT	Natural killer T (cell)
NLR	NOD domain, leucine-rich repeat (receptor)
NOD	Nucleotide-binding oligomerization domain
NOS	Nitric oxide synthase
NOX	NADPH oxidase
OAD	Inflammatory airway disease
ORF	Open reading frame
PAF	Platelet-activating factor
PAMP	Pathogen-associated molecular pattern

PCR	Polymerase chain reaction
PD-1	Programed death-1
pDC	Plasmacytoid dendritic cell
PDGF	Platelet-derived growth factor
PGE	Prostaglandin E
PHA	Phytohemagglutinin
pIgR	Receptor for polymeric immunoglobulin
PIM	Pulmonary intravascular macrophage
PKC	Protein kinase C
PMA	Phorbol myristate acetate
PP	Peyer's patch
PRM(R)	Pattern-recognition molecule (receptor)
PTX	Pentraxin
PWM	Pokeweed mitogen
RA	Receptor antagonist (or rheumatoid arthritis)
RAGE	Receptor for advanced glycation end products
RAO	Recurrent airway obstruction
RF	Rheumatoid factor
RIG	Retinoic acid–inducible gene
RLR	Retinoic acid–inducible gene-like receptor
ROS	Reactive oxygen species
RT-PCR	Reverse transcriptase–polymerase chain reaction
SAA	Serum amyloid A
SAP	Serum amyloid P
SASP	senility-associated secretory phenotype
SCID	Severe combined immunodeficiency
SIgA	Secretory IgA
SIRS	Systemic inflammatory response syndrome
SLAM	Signaling lymphocyte activation molecule
SLE	Systemic lupus erythematosus
SMAC	Supramolecular activation cluster
SNP	Single-nucleotide polymorphism
SP	Surfactant protein
SRCR	Scavenger -Receptor, Cysteine Rich (protein family)
ssRNA	Single-stranded RNA
STAT	Signal transducers and activators of transcription
STING	Stimulator of interferon genes
TAP	Transporter for antigen processing
TCC	Terminal complement complex
TCR	T-cell (antigen) receptor
TdT	Terminal deoxynucleotidyl transferase
TF	Tissue factor
TGF-β	Transforming growth factor-beta
TK	Thymidine kinase
TLR	Toll-like receptor
TNF	Tumor necrosis factor

TNFR	Tumor necrosis factor receptor
Treg	Regulatory T (cell)
TSLP	Thymic stromal lymphopoietin
VEE	Venezuelan equine encephalitis
VEGF	Vascular endothelial cell growth factor
WC	Workshop cluster
WEE	Western equine encephalitis
WNV	West Nile virus
β_2M	β_2-microglobulin

Glossary

Activated macrophage A macrophage in a state of polarized metabolic and functional activity as a result of cytokine stimulation.

Active Immunity Immunity generated within a horse or donkey as a result of the administration of an antigen, thus triggering an immune response.

Acute-phase proteins Proteins, synthesized by the liver and other tissues, whose level in serum rises rapidly during the response to cytokines produced by acute inflammation and tissue damage.

Adipokines Adipose tissue cells produce cytokines called adipokines: Two important examples are leptin and adiponectin. Both molecules influence the functions of the immune system.

Alarmins Molecules such as IL-33 released by dead or damaged tissues that trigger innate immune responses, especially inflammation. See also: Damage-associated molecular patterns.

Allergic contact dermatitis An inflammatory skin reaction mediated by Th1 cells responding to low-molecular-weight reactive chemicals chemically bound to skin cells.

Allergies Type I hypersensitivity responses that are initiated by IgE-mediated mast cell degranulation.

Alternative complement pathway The complement pathway triggered by the activation of C3 by the presence of an activating microbial surface.

Amyloid An extracellular, amorphous, waxy protein deposited in the tissues of horses suffering from chronic inflammation or a myeloma. It consists of misfolded, insoluble protein fibers.

Anaphylatoxins Complement-derived peptides that trigger mast cell degranulation resulting in inflammation and smooth muscle contraction.

Anaphylaxis A life-threatening, acute, immediate hypersensitivity reaction resulting from the rapid release of inflammatory mediators from large numbers of mast cells. Affected horses develop acute respiratory distress, cardiovascular collapse, and death.

Antibody An immunoglobulin molecule made by an appropriately stimulated B cell following exposure to antigen, which can combine specifically with that antigen.

Antibody Classes The five major forms of immunoglobulin molecules common to all horses and donkeys IgM, IgD, IgG, IgA, and IgE.

Antigen Any foreign substance that can bind to specific lymphocyte receptors and so induce an adaptive immune response.

Antigen-presenting cells Cells that can ingest, process, and present antigen to T cells. These cells express MHC class I or class II molecules on their surface. These form a complex with antigenic peptides that can activate T cell antigen receptors.

Apoptosis The self-destruction of a cell; one form of programmed cell death.

Asthma A hypersensitivity disease characterized by a reduction in airway diameter, leading to difficulty in breathing (dyspnea). There are many possible causes but type I hypersensitivity to aeroallergens is most common.

Atopy A genetic predisposition to become sensitized and produce IgE antibodies in response to common environmental allergens.

Autoimmune diseases Diseases caused by an immune attack against normal antigens expressed in an animal's own tissues. It may affect either a single organ or multiple body organs depending upon the location of the autoantigen.

B cells Lymphocytes that have undergone development within the bone marrow rather than the thymus. When they mature, they differentiate into plasma cells and are responsible for antibody production. They are characterized by using immunoglobulins as antigen receptors.

Bacille Calmette-Guérin (BCG) vaccine An attenuated strain of *Mycobacterium bovis*. This may be used as a non-specific immune stimulator.

Bacterin A killed bacterial vaccine.

Basophils The least common polymorphonuclear leukocyte. They contain large numbers of granules with a high avidity for basic dyes. They participate in type I hypersensitivity reactions such as allergic dermatitis and asthma.

Blood groups Antigens expressedon the surface of red blood cells. Their expression is inherited. They play a critical role in transfusion reactions and hemolytic disease of foals.

Cell-mediated cytotoxicity The killing of antigenic target cells induced by contact with cytotoxic T cells, NK cells, or macrophages.

Cell-mediated immunity A form of immune response mediated by T lymphocytes and macrophages; it can be conferred on an animal by adoptive transfer of these cells. Also called Type 1 Immunity.

Chemokines A family of proinflammatory and chemotactic cytokines with a characteristic sequence of four cysteine residues. They regulate the migration of leukocytes.

Chromosome translocation A mutation in which portions of two chromosomes switch position.

Class switch The change in immunoglobulin class production by B cells that occurs during the course of an immune response as a result of a change in heavy chain gene use.

Classical complement pathway The complement pathway triggered by activation of C1 by antigen-antibody complexes located on a microbial or cell surface.

Cluster of differentiation (CD) The classification of cell surface proteins based upon their identification by monoclonal antibodies. A CD antigen is, by extension, therefore, a defined protein on the surface of a cell. There are about 360 of them.

Collectins A family of carbohydrate-binding lectins that depend on calcium for their adhesion.

Colostrum The secretion that accumulates in the mare's mammary gland in the last weeks of pregnancy. It is very rich in immunoglobulins and so transfers immunity to suckling newborn foals.

Combined immunodeficiency A deficiency in both the T cell– and B cell–mediated components of the immune system.

Complement A family of serum and cell surface proteins activated by factors such as the combination of antigen and antibody. This results in the generation of enzyme cascades that have a variety of biological consequences, including chemotaxis, cell lysis, and opsonization.

Complementarity determining region Those areas within the variable regions of antibodies and T cell antigen receptors that bind to antigen and so determine the molecule's antigen-binding specificity. Synonymous with hypervariable region.

Concanavalin A (Con A) A lectin extracted from the Jack bean that makes T cells divide.

Corticosteroids Steroid hormones released from the adrenal cortex that have profound immunosuppressive effects on the cells of the immune system. Some corticosteroids may be synthetic in origin.

Cutaneous basophil hypersensitivity A form of delayed hypersensitivity reaction in skin associated with an extensive basophil infiltration.

Cytokine storm The pathological effects induced by the uncontrolled activation of T cells, and as a result, the unregulated and excessive production of many different cytokines.

Cytokines Proteins that mediate cellular interactions and regulate cell growth and secretion. They are generated during both innate and adaptive immune responses. As a result, they regulate most aspects of the immune system.

Cytotoxic lymphocytes Lymphocytes that can bind to target cells and trigger their killing by inducing apoptosis.

Damage-associated molecular patterns (DAMPs) Conserved molecular structures derived from damaged cells and diseased tissues that trigger inflammation.

Delayed hypersensitivity reaction A T cell-mediated inflammatory reaction in the skin, so called because it takes 24–48 hours to reach maximum intensity following injection of antigen.

Dendritic cells Specialized antigen-processing cells. They possess long cytoplasmic processes (dendrites), and their primary role is to function as highly effective antigen-trapping and antigen-presenting cells.

Disseminated intravascular coagulation A severe clinical syndrome characterized by dysregulation of the clotting and fibrinolytic cascades.

Domain Discrete structural units from which protein molecules are constructed.

Dysbiosis A disturbance or imbalance in the types and numbers of bacterial species in the normal intestinal, respiratory, or skin microbiota.

Effector cell A cell that is able to "effect" an immune response. These cells include cytotoxic T cells and natural killer cells.

Eicosanoids A family of lipids mainly synthesized from arachidonic acid. They include the prostaglandins and leukotrienes and play a key role in inflammation and allergic diseases.

Endogenous antigen A foreign antigen synthesized within body cells. Examples include newly formed virus proteins.

Endosomes Intracellular vesicles formed by endocytosis.

Endotoxins Lipopolysaccharide components of Gram-negative bacterial cell walls.

Eosinophils A polymorphonuclear leukocyte containing characteristic granules that stain intensely with the acid dye eosin. They play a key role in resistance to parasites.

Eosinophilia Increased numbers of eosinophils in the blood.

Epitope A site on the surface of an antigenic molecule that is recognized by an antigen receptor. As a result, immune responses are directed against specific epitopes. Synonymous with antigenic determinant.

Equidae The family of equids including horses, asses, and zebras

Exogenous antigen A foreign antigen that originates outside the body, for example, invading bacterial antigens.

Exotoxins Soluble protein toxins, usually produced by Gram-positive bacteria, that have a specific toxic effect. Examples include tetanus and botulinum toxin.

Fab fragment The antigen-binding fragment of a partially digested antibody. It consists of the light chains and the N-terminal halves of heavy chains.

Facultative intracellular organism An organism that can, if opportunity presents, grow within cells. A good example is *Rhodococcus equi.*

Fc receptor A cell surface receptor that specifically binds antibody molecules through their Fc region.

Fc region That part of an immunoglobulin molecule consisting of the C-terminal halves of heavy chains. It is responsible for the biological activities of the molecule.

Firmicutes A bacterial phylum consisting mainly of Gram-positive bacteria characterized by having a low G+C ratio. They include important bacteria such as the Clostridia, *Listeria*, and *Bacillus*.

G-proteins Guanosine triphosphate (GTP)-binding proteins that act as signal transducers for many cell surface receptors.

Gel diffusion An immunoprecipitation technique that involves letting antigen and antibody interact and precipitate in a clear gel, such as agar. A relevant example is the Coggins' test for equine infectious anemia.

Gene conversion The exchange of blocks of DNA between different genes.

Gene segment Another term for exon. It tends to be used exclusively to denote the exons that code for immunoglobulin and TCR V, D, and J regions.

Germinal centers Structures found in secondary lymphoid organs, in which rapidly dividing B cells form a pale-staining spherical mass surrounded by a zone of dark-staining cells. This is the site where somatic hypermutation occurs, and memory cells are generated.

Glomerulonephritis Pathological lesions that develop in the glomeruli of the kidney in response to immune-complex deposition within glomerular blood vessels.

Granuloma An inflammatory lesion characterized by chronic inflammation with mononuclear cell infiltration and extensive fibrosis.

Granzymes A family of proteases found in the granules of cytotoxic T cells.

Growth factors Cytokines that promote cell growth.

Haplotype The complete set of linked alleles within a gene complex. They are inherited as a group and determine a specific phenotype. They are especially important in the MHC complex.

Heat-shock proteins Proteins synthesized by cells such as bacteria in response to many different physiological stresses, including increased temperature.

Helminths Worms, many of which are important equine parasites that stimulate protective immune responses.

Helper T cells The subpopulation of T cells that promotes immune responses by providing the required co-stimulation from cytokines and co-stimulatory receptors. There are two types, Th1 and Th2 cells.

Hemolytic disease of the newborn Disease occurring as a result of the destruction of red blood cells by antibodies to blood groups transferred to the foal from its mother through colostrum.

Herd immunity Immunity conferred on a population as a whole as a result of the presence of immune individuals within that population.

High endothelial venule A specialized blood vessel lined with high epithelium, found in the paracortex of lymph nodes and other lymphoid organs.

Hinge region The region located between the first and second constant domains in some immunoglobulin heavy chains that permits them to bend freely.

Hinny The offspring of a male horse and a female donkey.

Histiocytes Tissue macrophages.

Humoral immunity An immune response mediated by antibodies.

Hypersensitivity pneumonitis An immune-complex-mediated hypersensitivity disease affecting the lungs when sensitized horses inhale large quantities of foreign antigens over a long period.

Hypervariable regions Areas within immunoglobulin or TCR variable regions where the greatest variations in amino acid sequence occur, and which therefore bind antigens.

Immediate hypersensitivity The hypersensitivity reaction is mediated by IgE and mast cells. Otherwise known as type I hypersensitivity. It usually occurs within minutes of encountering an allergen.

Immune checkpoint therapy The use of monoclonal antibodies to prevent T cell inhibition by checkpoint molecules. Checkpoint molecules are T cell surface receptors and their ligands that normally regulate immune responses by suppressing T cell proliferation and cytotoxicity.

Immune complex Another term for antigen antibody complexes that form following an antibody response and may trigger hypersensitivity responses.

Immune exclusion The prevention of absorption of antigens into the body through epithelial surfaces by binding to immunoglobulin A.

Immune globulin An antibody preparation containing specific antibodies against a pathogen and used for passive immunization. A relevant example is tetanus immune globulin (antitoxin).

Immune surveillance The concept that lymphocytes, such as T cells and NK cells, survey the body for cancerous or abnormal cells and then eliminate them.

Immune synapse An organized molecular structure that forms when receptors cluster in the area of contact between a T cell and an antigen-presenting cell or a target cell.

Immunodeficiencies A loss of effective immune function. They may be classified as primary if it is a result of a genetic defect. They are secondary if they develop in response to infections, toxins, malnutrition, or extreme stress.

Immunodiffusion Another name for the gel diffusion technique used in the Coggins' test.

Immunoglobulins The protein class to which antibodies belong.

Immunosenescence The series of age-related changes that adversely affect the functioning of the immune system as an animal grows older.

Inactivated vaccine A vaccine containing an infectious agent that has been treated in such a way that it can no longer replicate

Inflammaging A progressive increase in chronic low-grade inflammation that occurs as an animal ages. This is a result of the gradual accumulation of damaged or dying cells and organelles over time.

Inflammasomes Multiprotein complexes that form in sentinel cells in response to the triggering of certain pattern-recognition receptors. Their function is to initiate synthesis of inflammatory cytokines, as well as pyroptosis and necroptosis.

Inflammation The responses of tissues to injury or invasion. It involves both vascular and cellular changes. As a result, defensive molecules and cells accumulate at sites of microbial invasion, enhance tissue defenses, and eventually initiate tissue repair.

Inflammatory airway disease A mild respiratory disease of horses in which breathing appears normal at rest. Affected horses show poor performance, exercise intolerance, and a chronic cough.

Innate immunity Immunity present in all animals that is triggered on exposure to a foreign agent. It is mediated by proteins encoded in the germline.

Innate lymphoid cells (ILC) A type of lymphocyte that does not express antigen-specific receptors. However, they bind MHC molecules and produce multiple cytokines. Some act as helper cells, and some (NK cells) are cytotoxic.

Integrins A family of adhesion proteins found on cell membranes that bind either to ligands on the surface of other cells or to connective tissue proteins such as fibronectin or collagen.

Interferons Three large families of cytokines that interfere with viral replication. Some interferons also play an important role in the regulation of equine immunity.

Interleukins Cytokines that act as growth and differentiation factors for the cells of the immune system.

Intraepithelial lymphocytes Lymphocytes, mainly T cells, located among the epithelial cells lining the intestinal and respiratory tracts.

Isotype Closely related proteins that arise as a result of gene duplication. They are found in all animals of a species. Thus, the subclasses of equine or donkey IgG are actually isotypes.

Isotype switching The change in immunoglobulin class that occurs during the course of the immune response as a result of heavy chain gene switching.

J chain A short peptide that joins units in the polymeric immunoglobulins IgM and IgA.

Joining (J) gene segment A short gene segment that is located 3′ to the *V* gene segments in immunoglobulin and TCR *V* genes and codes for part of the variable region.

Killer cell See Cytotoxic T cell and Natural killer cell.

Kinins Vasoactive peptides produced in injured or inflamed tissue.

Kupffer cells A specialized population of macrophages that line the sinusoids of the liver.

Laminitis A common debilitating disease syndrome in horses and donkeys. Caused by inflammation within the hoof that results in failure of the bonds between the hoof wall and the distal phalanx.

Langerhans cells A population of specialized dendritic cells found in equine skin. They are effective antigen-presenting cells.

Lectin A protein that can bind specifically to a carbohydrate. Some lectins of plant origin can also induce lymphocytes to divide. Lectins may also activate the complement system.

Leukopenia The absence of leukocytes.

Leukotrienes Lipid mediators derived from arachidonic acid by the actions of 5-lipoxygenase, and responsible for potent proinflammatory responses. Released by degranulating mast cells.

Looping out A method of excising a segment of intervening DNA (intron) in order to join two gene segments (exons).

Lymphadenopathy Literally, "disease of lymph nodes." In practice, it is used to describe enlarged lymph nodes.

Lymphocytes Small mononuclear cells with a round nucleus found in equine blood and lymphoid tissues. They recognize foreign antigens through specialized receptors.

Lymphokine-activated killer (LAK) cells Lymphocytes activated by exposure to cytokines such as IL-2 in vitro.

Lymphopenia Abnormally low numbers of lymphocytes in the blood.

Lymphotoxins Cytotoxic cytokines secreted by lymphocytes.

Lysosomal enzymes The complex mixture of enzymes, many of which are proteases, found within the lysosomes of phagocytic cells such as neutrophils and macrophages.

Macrophages Large phagocytic cells containing a single rounded nucleus. They are derived from blood monocytes and are found in many different tissues and organs.

Major histocompatibility complex (MHC) The genomic region that contains the genes for the major histocompatibility molecules, as well as for some complement components and related proteins. It is called ELA in the horse and MHC-Eqas in the donkey.

Maternal antibodies Antibodies that originate in the mother but enter the bloodstream of her offspring by adsorption of ingested colostrum.

Memory cells Populations of long-lived B and T cells that develop in response to an antigen. On subsequent exposure to that antigen, they mount a faster and stronger response.

Mesangial cells Modified smooth muscle cells found within a glomerulus. They may proliferate in response to immune complex deposition.

MHC restriction The requirement that a helper T cell can only recognize an antigen presented in close association with an MHC molecule.

Microbiota The collective term for the microbial populations that colonize normal healthy body surfaces. These include the skin, genital, respiratory, and gastrointestinal tracts.

Microglia Macrophages resident within the brain.

Mitogen Any substance that makes cells divide.

Modified live virus A virus whose virulence has been artificially reduced so that it can replicate in the host but cannot cause disease in normal healthy animals.

Molecular mimicry Molecules from infectious agents whose structure closely resembles molecules found in their host. In this way, the invaders may be able to trigger autoimmunity.

Monoclonal antibody Antibody derived from a single clone of cancerous plasma cells and hence biochemically homogeneous.

Monoclonal gammopathy The appearance in serum of a high level of a monoclonal immunoglobulin. This is commonly associated with the presence of a myeloma.

Monocytes The largest of the blood leukocytes in the horse. They are immature macrophages circulating in the bloodstream and can differentiate into either macrophages or dendritic cells.

Mononuclear cells Leukocytes with a single round nucleus; for example, lymphocytes and macrophages.

Mononuclear-phagocytic system The cells that belong to the macrophage family.

Mule The offspring of a male donkey and a female horse.

Multiple organ dysfunction syndrome (MODS) Altered organ function in a seriously ill horse such that normal functioning cannot be maintained. It is a sequel to severe sepsis or septic shock.

Myeloid system All the granulocytes and their precursors. These precursor cells are found in the bone marrow.

Myelomas Tumors consisting of plasma cells. They are uncommon in horses.

Natural killer cells Large granular cytotoxic lymphocytes that are found in normal, unsensitized animals and that can recognize and kill abnormal cells such as tumor- and virus-infected cells. They can also kill bacteria, fungi and viruses.

Negative selection The killing of immature T cells that have the potential to react to self-antigens. A key mechanism in the prevention of autoimmunity.

Neonatal isoerythrolysis Otherwise called hemolytic disease of the newborn. It results from a foal ingesting antiblood group antibodies in its mare's colostrum.

Neutropenia Low numbers of neutrophils in the blood.

Neutrophilia High numbers of neutrophils in the blood.

Neutrophils Polymorphonuclear neutrophil granulocytes. The predominant blood leukocyte in horses.

Nucleocapsid The key structural component of a virus consisting of the viral nucleic acid enclosed within its protective capsid coat.

Obligate intracellular parasite An organism such as a virus that cannot grow outside cells.

Oncofetal antigens Antigens found on both fetal and tumor cells.

Oncogenic virus A virus that causes cancer.

Ontogeny The progressive embryonic development of a body system.

Opportunistic pathogen An organism that, although unable to cause disease in a healthy individual, may invade and cause disease in an individual whose immunological defenses are impaired.

Opsonin A molecule that facilitates phagocytosis by coating foreign particles.

Orthologous Genes that have a conserved structure and are clearly descended from a common ancestral gene.

Paralogous Genes or gene clusters that, although descended from a single ancestral gene have diverged significantly following the original duplication.

Passive immunization Protection of an individual animal conferred by the administration of immunoglobulins produced in another individual. This can involve either antiserum or colostrum.

Pathobiont A member of the normal microbiota that can become a pathogen should circumstances permit.

Pathogen-associated molecular patterns (PAMPs) Conserved molecular structures widely distributed among pathogenic microbes that, when recognized by sentinel cells, can trigger inflammation.

Pattern-recognition receptors and molecules (PRR and PRMs) Cellular receptors that can recognize conserved microbial structures (PAMPs) as well as products released by damaged cells (DAMPs). PRRs include toll-like receptors, among others.

Perforins A family of proteins made by T cells and NK cells that, when polymerized, can form tubular structures and insert themselves into target cell membranes to cause cell lysis.

Perissodactyla The odd-toed ungulates. Horses, rhinos, and tapirs.

Phagocytes Leukocytes whose prime function is to eat foreign particles, especially bacteria. They include macrophages and related cells, neutrophils, and eosinophils.

Phagolysosome A structure produced within a phagocytic cell by the fusion of a phagosome and lysosomes following phagocytosis. The site where bacteria are destroyed.

Phagosome The cytoplasmic vesicle in a phagocytic cell that encloses an ingested organism.

Phytohemagglutinin (PHA) A lectin derived from the red kidney bean. It acts as a T-cell mitogen.

Pinocytosis The endocytosis of small fluid droplets - drinking by cells.

Plasma cells Fully differentiated B cells that are structurally optimized for synthesizing and secreting large amounts of immunoglobulin.

Positive selection The enhanced proliferation of cells within the thymus that can respond optimally to foreign antigens.

Primary immune response The immune response resulting from an individual's first encounter with an antigen.

Primary lymphoid organ An organ, such as the thymus, that serves as a source of lymphocytes or in which lymphocytes mature.

Primary pathogen An organism that can cause disease without first suppressing an individual's immune defenses.

Proteasomes Tubular multienzyme proteolytic structures found in the cytosol of many cell types. They act on ubiquinated cellular proteins to cleave them into small fragments. A necessary first step in endogenous antigen presentation.

Protein kinase An enzyme that phosphorylates proteins.

Pruritus Another word for itch

Pseudogenes DNA sequences that resemble functional genes but that cannot be transcribed.

Purpura hemorrhagica A response to *Streptococcus equi* infection characterized by urticaria, severe subcutaneous edema, especially involving the limbs, and the development of hemorrhages in the mucosa and subcutaneous tissues.

Respiratory burst The rapid increase in metabolic activity that occurs in phagocytic cells while particles are being ingested. It generates potent oxidants that can kill invading microorganisms.

Rheumatoid factor An autoantibody directed against epitopes on immunoglobulin Fc regions. It is present in the blood of some horses suffering from arthritis.

Secondary immune response An enhanced adaptive response that results from second or subsequent exposure to an antigen.

Secondary immunodeficiencies Immunodeficiency diseases resulting from a known, noninherited cause

Secondary infections Infections by organisms that can invade only a host whose defenses are first weakened or destroyed by other infectious agents or toxins.

Secondary lymphoid organ The lymphoid organs that contain mature lymphocytes whose function is to trap and respond to foreign antigens. Examples include lymph nodes, tonsils, and the spleen.

Secretory component A protein produced by mucosal epithelial cells; it functions as an IgA receptor and, on binding to IgA, protects IgA against proteases in the intestine.

Selectin A family of cell surface adhesion proteins that bind cells to glycoproteins on vascular endothelium.

Self-cure The rapid elimination of parasitic worms caused by a localized type I hypersensitivity reaction in the intestinal tract.

Signal transduction The transmission of a signal through a receptor to a cell by means of a series of linked reactions.

Skin test A diagnostic procedure that induces a local inflammatory response following intradermal inoculation of an antigen or allergen.

Somatic hypermutation Mutations that occur in somatic rather than germline cells. In immunology, this refers to the extensive mutations that occur in the *V* genes of B cells during the course of an immune response.

Subclass Different immunoglobulin isotypes closely related within a specific class.

Symbiosis The relation between species that live together.

Systemic inflammatory response syndrome Uncontrolled inflammation resulting from the massive overproduction of cytokines as a result of serious infection and/or tissue damage

T cells Lymphocytes that have matured within the thymus, and are responsible for mediating cell-mediated immune responses.

T-cell receptor (TCR) The antigen-binding receptors of T lymphocytes. They are heterodimers of the antigen-binding peptide chains α and β or γ and δ. They associate with the CD3 complex.

Terminal complement complex A multimolecular structure formed by polymeric C9 that generates pores in target cell membranes, resulting in their osmotic lysis and cell death.

Tolerance A state of specific immune unresponsiveness to an antigen or foreign tissue. A key example of this is the failure of a mare to reject her fetus despite it being significantly genetically different from her. Another example is a horse's tolerance of dietary allergens.

Toxic shock A disease resulting from exposure to large amounts of staphylococcal toxin, a superantigen.

Toxoid Nontoxic derivatives of chemically treated toxins used as vaccines.

Trained immunity The temporary improvement observed in the functioning of innate immune cells following an inflammatory episode.

Transcription factors Specialized proteins that regulate gene activity by binding to the promoter region of genes. They thus turn gene transcription on or off.

Transporter protein Proteins that bind fragments of endogenous antigen and carry them to newly assembled MHC class I molecules in the endoplasmic reticulum.

Treg cells Regulatory T cells that secrete suppressive cytokines and prevent excessive immune responses

Tuberculin An extract of tubercle bacilli used in a diagnostic skin test for tuberculosis.

Tuft cells A specialized population of chemosensory cells found among the epithelial cell layer of the gastrointestinal tract. They sense and respond to the presence of intestinal parasites.

Tumor necrosis factors Macrophage and lymphocyte-derived cytokines that are key triggers of inflammation. They can also exert a direct toxic effect on neoplastic cells.

Type 1 immune responses Cell-mediated immune responses mediated through the activities of Th1 helper cells, and DC1 cells.

Type 2 immune responses Immune responses mediated by Th2 cells, ILC2 cells, and M2 macrophages. They result in antibody production.

Type 3 immune responses These are primarily antibacterial inflammatory responses mediated by interleukin -17 (IL-17) produced by Th17 cells.

Tyrosine kinase An enzyme that phosphorylates tyrosine residues in proteins. It plays a key role in signal transduction.

Urticaria Inflammatory and edematous skin reactions due to allergic mechanisms. Horses develop well-defined raised bumps with lumps, wheals, or rings of variable sizes in the superficial dermis.

Variable regions That part of the immunoglobulin or TCR peptide chains in which the amino acid sequence shows significant variation among molecules. This forms the antigen-binding site.

Vasculitis Inflammation of blood vessel walls. It may be caused by a hypersensitivity reaction in horses.

Virulence The ability of an organism to cause disease.

Index

'*Note:* Page numbers followed by "f" indicate figures, "t" indicate tables and "b" indicate boxes.'

C

D

G

H

M

N

O

P

Q

R

T

U

V

W

Z